CARDIOTHORACIC SURGICAL NURSING

CARDIOTHORACIC SURGICAL NURSING

Betsy A. Finkelmeier, R.N., M.S.

Manager of Clinical Services
Division of Cardiothoracic Surgery
Northwestern University Medical School

Clinical Appointment
Department of Nursing
Northwestern Memorial Hospital
Chicago, Illinois

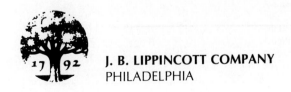

J. B. LIPPINCOTT COMPANY
PHILADELPHIA

Sponsoring Editor: DIANE SCHWEISGUTH
Coordinating Editorial Assistant: SARAH ANDRUS
Project Editor: TOM GIBBONS
Indexer: VICTORIA BOYLE
Design Coordinator: MELISSA OLSON
Interior Designer: MARIA KARKUCINSKI
Cover Designer: JERRY CABLE
Production Manager: HELEN EWAN
Production Coordinator: KATHRYN RULE
Compositor: BI-COMP, INCORPORATED
Printer/Binder: COURIER BOOK COMPANY/WESTFORD

6   5   4   3   2   1

Library of Congress Cataloging-in-Publication Data

Finkelmeier, Betsy A.
    Cardiothoracic surgical nursing / Betsy Finkelmeier.
        p.   cm.
    Includes bibliographical references and index.
    ISBN 0-397-54796-X
    1. Chest—Surgery—Nursing.   2. Heart—Surgery—Nursing.
  I. Title
    [DNLM: 1. Surgical Nursing—methods.   2. Cardiovascular
    Diseases—nursing. 3. Cardiovascular Diseases—surgery.
    4. Thoracic Diseases—nursing. 5. Thoracic Diseases—surgery.
    WY 161 F499c 1995]
RD536.F465   1995
610.73'677—dc20
DNLM/DLC
for Library of Congress   94-13162
                                                                 CIP

Any procedure or practice described in this book should be applied by
the health-care practitioner under appropriate supervision in accordance with professional standards of care used with regard to the
unique circumstances that apply in each practice situation. Care has
been taken to confirm the accuracy of information presented and to
describe generally accepted practices. However, the authors, editors,
and publisher cannot accept any responsibility for errors or omissions
or for any consequences from applications of the information in this
book and make no warranty express or implied, with respect to the
contents of the book.
    Every effort has been made to ensure drug selections and dosages
are in accordance with current recommendations and practice. Because of ongoing research, changes in government regulations and the
constant flow of information on drug therapy, reactions and interactions, the reader is cautioned to check the package insert for each drug
for indications, dosages, warnings, and precautions, particularly if the
drug is new or infrequently used.

*To my mother, Marjorie Thompson Finkelmeier,
and my father, Louis John Finkelmeier, M.D.,
for their steadfast love and guidance.*

REVIEWERS

Robert W. Anderson, M.D.
Professor of Surgery and Chief
Division of Cardiothoracic Surgery
Northwestern University Medical School
Chicago, Illinois

Carl E. Arentzen, M.D.
Assistant Professor of Surgery
Division of Cardiothoracic Surgery
Northwestern University Medical School
Chicago, Illinois

Carl L. Backer, M.D.
Assistant Professor of Surgery
Division of Cardiothoracic Surgery
Northwestern University Medical School
Chicago, Illinois

Susan Bailey Black, R.N., M.H.A.
Augusta, Georgia

Ivan K. Crosby, M.D.
Chief of Cardiac Surgery
Forsyth Memorial Hospital
Winston-Salem, North Carolina

Catherine S. Dunnington, R.N., M.S.
Clinical Nurse Specialist
Clinical Cardiac Electrophysiology Department
Illinois Masonic Hospital
Chicago, Illinois

John E. Fetter, M.D.
Lieutenant Commander, Medical Corps
Cardiothoracic Surgery Division
Navy Medical Center
San Diego, California

James W. Frederikson, M.D.
Associate Professor of Surgery
Division of Cardiothoracic Surgery
Northwestern University Medical School
Chicago, Illinois

Willard Fry, M.D.
Professor of Surgery
Division of Cardiothoracic Surgery
Northwestern University Medical School
Chicago, Illinois

Kathleen L. Grady, R.N., M.S.
Clinical Nurse Specialist
Department of Nursing
Loyola University Medical Center
Maywood, Illinois

I. Martin Grais, M.D.
Assistant Professor of Clinical Medicine
Division of Cardiology
Northwestern University Medical School
Chicago, Illinois

Renee S. Hartz, M.D.
Professor of Surgery and Chief
Division of Cardiothoracic Surgery
University of Illinois at Chicago College of Medicine
Chicago, Illinois

Mary H. Hawthorne, Ph.D., R.N.
Assistant Professor
School of Nursing
Duke University
Durham, North Carolina

Linda F. Hellstedt, M.S., R.N., CCRN
Clinical Nurse Specialist
Department of Nursing
Northwestern Memorial Hospital
Chicago, Illinois

Axel W. Joob, M.D.
Assistant Professor of Surgery
Division of Cardiothoracic Surgery
Northwestern University Medical School
Chicago, Illinois

Irving L. Kron, M.D.
Professor of Surgery and Chief
Division of Cardiothoracic Surgery
University of Virginia Medical School
Charlottesville, Virginia

Carol Lake, M.D.
Professor of Anesthesiology
Department of Anesthesiology
University of Virginia Medical School
Charlottesville, Virginia

Joseph LoCicero III, M.D.
Associate Professor of Surgery
Division of Cardiothoracic Surgery
Harvard University Medical School
Boston, Massachusetts

C. Gregory Lockhart, M.D.
Attending Surgeon
Surgical Associates of Richmond
Richmond, Virginia

Robert G. Matheny, M.D.
Attending Surgeon
Division of Cardiovascular Surgery
St. Vincent's Hospital
Indianapolis, Indiana

Jane S. McMurray, R.N., M.S.N.
Clinical Nurse Specialist
Department of Nursing
Northwestern Memorial Hospital
Chicago, Illinois

David D. McPherson, M.D.
Associate Professor of Medicine
Division of Cardiology
Northwestern University Medical School
Chicago, Illinois

David Mehlman, M.D.
Associate Professor of Medicine
Division of Cardiology
Northwestern University Medical School
Chicago, Illinois

Robert M. Mentzer, Jr., M.D.
Professor of Surgery and Chairman
Division of Cardiothoracic Surgery
University of Wisconsin Medical School
Madison, Wisconsin

Lawrence L. Michaelis, M.D.
Professor of Surgery
Division of Cardiothoracic Surgery
Northwestern University Medical School
Chicago, Illinois

Stanton P. Nolan, M.D.
Professor of Surgery
Division of Cardiothoracic Surgery
University of Virginia Medical School
Charlottesville, Virginia

Arthur S. Palmer, M.D.
Assistant Professor of Surgery
Division of Cardiothoracic Surgery
Northwestern University Medical School
Chicago, Illinois

John R. Pellet, M.D.
Professor of Surgery
Department of Surgery
University of Wisconsin Medical School
Madison, Wisconsin

Pamela B. Pfeifer, M.S., R.N., CCRN
Clinical Nurse Specialist
Cardiac Transplant Program
Edward Hines Jr. VA Hospital
Hines, Illinois

Jane E. Reedy, R.N., B.S.N.
Cardiothoracic Service Clinical Coordinator
Department of Surgery
St. Louis University Medical School
St. Louis, Missouri

Robert J. Robison, M.D.
Attending Surgeon
Division of Cardiovascular Surgery
St. Vincent's Hospital
Indianapolis, Indiana

James E. Rosenthal, M.D.
Associate Professor of Medicine
Division of Cardiology
Northwestern University Medical School
Chicago, Illinois

Michael H. Salinger, M.D.
Associate Professor of Clinical Medicine
Division of Cardiology
Northwestern University Medical School
Chicago, Illinois

John H. Sanders, Jr., M.D.
Professor of Surgery
Division of Cardiothoracic Surgery
Northwestern University Medical School
Chicago, Illinois

Thomas W. Shields, M.D.
Professor Emeritus of Surgery
Department of Surgery
Northwestern University Medical School
Chicago, Illinois

Neil Stone, M.D.
Associate Professor of Medicine
Division of Cardiology
Northwestern University Medical School
Chicago, Illinois

Medhat Takla, M.D.
Chief Resident in Cardiothoracic Surgery
Division of Cardiothoracic Surgery
Northwestern University Medical School
Chicago, Illinois

Robert M. Vanecko, M.D.
Professor of Surgery
Division of Cardiothoracic Surgery
Northwestern University Medical School
Chicago, Illinois

Timothy V. Votapka, M.D.
Assistant Professor of Surgery
Division of Cardiothoracic Surgery
St. Louis University Medical School
St. Louis, Missouri

Leonard D. Wade, M.S.
Assistant Professor of Anesthesia
Department of Anesthesia
Northwestern University Medical School
Chicago, Illinois

Anne P. Weiland, R.N., M.B.A.
Assistant Vice President, Clinical Services
Washington Hospital Center
Washington, D.C.

Gayle R. Whitman, M.S.N., R.N., FAAN
Director, Cardiothoracic Nursing
Cleveland Clinic Foundation
Cleveland, Ohio

Edward Winslow, M.D.
Associate Professor of Clinical Medicine
Division of Cardiology
Northwestern University Medical School
Chicago, Illinois

Terry A. Zheutlin, M.D.
Director, Progressive Coronary Care Unit
Clinical Cardiac Electrophysiology Department
Illinois Masonic Hospital
Chicago, Illinois

PREFACE

Extraordinary progress has been achieved during the past several decades in surgical treatment of cardiac and thoracic diseases. Improvements in cardiopulmonary bypass and myocardial protection and the development of sophisticated perioperative nursing units and monitoring capabilities have greatly expanded the opportunities for surgical therapy. As a result of these advances, cardiothoracic surgical nursing has emerged as an important and challenging area of specialty practice, encompassing the care of patients with a wide variety of acute, chronic, malignant, and life-threatening cardiac and thoracic diseases of the chest.

Cardiothoracic Surgical Nursing is intended to provide a comprehensive reference for nurses specializing in the care of adult patients with cardiac and thoracic surgical diseases. Current information is included about specific diseases, surgical therapy, and all aspects of pre- and postoperative nursing care in both routine and complex patient care situations. Unit I, which addresses cardiac surgery, is divided into five parts: cardiovascular diseases, preoperative evaluation and preparation, intraoperative considerations, cardiovascular operations, and postoperative management. In Unit II, cardiothoracic transplantation and trauma are discussed. Thoracic surgery is discussed in Unit III, including surgical diseases of the chest, preoperative evaluation and preparation, thoracic operations, and postoperative management.

The text has been designed for nurses working with cardiothoracic surgical patients. It is hoped that they will find in the contents a broad foundation of relevant information upon which to base their clinical practice.

ACKNOWLEDGMENTS

Many individuals contributed to the completion of this book. Countless patients and families through the years have taught me much of what is contained in the text. Many nursing and physician colleagues have tolerated endless requests for advice and information and have provided invaluable support in shaping the book. I would particularly like to thank my family and friends, the surgeons and staff in the Northwestern University Division of Cardiothoracic Surgery, my nursing colleagues at Northwestern Memorial Hospital, the reviewers of the text, and my sister, Mary F. Havener, who assisted in preparation of the manuscript.

I would also like to acknowledge the following mentors and colleagues who have contributed greatly to my professional growth. Louis J. Finkelmeier, M.D., who practiced as a general surgeon for nearly fifty years in rural Ohio, profoundly influenced my deep commitment to the care of patients. Stanton P. Nolan, M.D., and Helen Ripple, R.N., M.S., had a major impact on my career development during my years at the University of Virginia. John H. Sanders, Jr., M.D., Lawrence L. Michaelis, M.D., and Robert W. Anderson, M.D., have made it possible for me to continue to achieve professional growth and satisfaction during my tenure at Northwestern Memorial Hospital. These individuals share in common a strong commitment to patients and the ability to promote excellence in the people around them.

CONTENTS

CARDIOTHORACIC SURGICAL NURSING

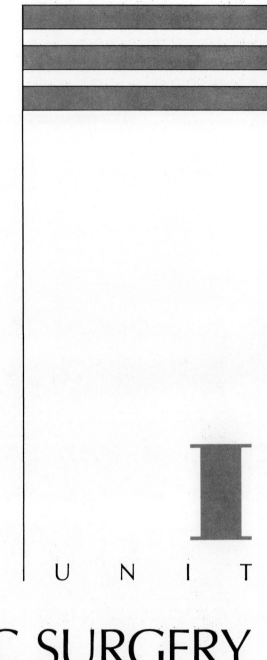

U N I T

I

CARDIAC SURGERY

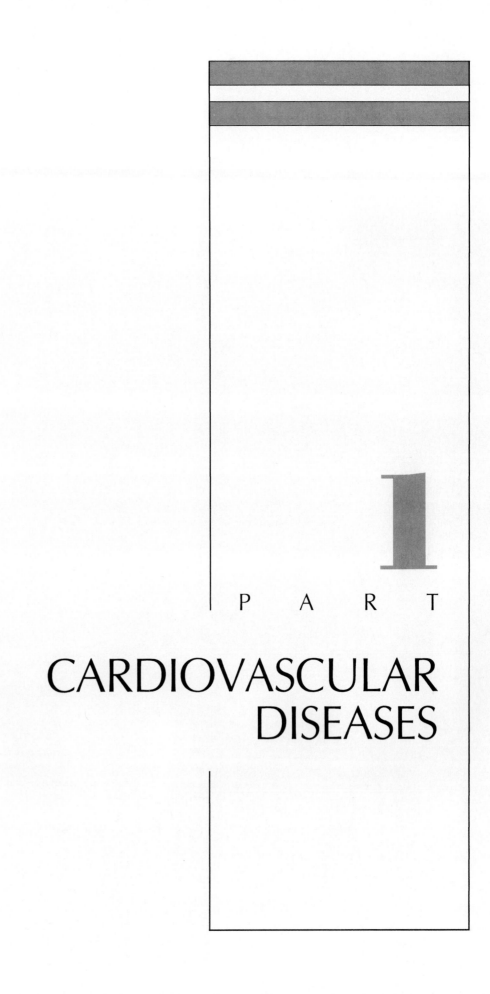

P A R T

1

CARDIOVASCULAR DISEASES

CORONARY ARTERY DISEASE

OVERVIEW
  Etiology
  Clinical Manifestations
  Diagnosis
  Treatment
ACUTE MYOCARDIAL ISCHEMIC SYNDROME
  Definitions
  Diagnosis and Treatment

COMPLICATIONS OF MYOCARDIAL
  INFARCTION
Ventricular Dysfunction
Ventricular Aneurysm
Thromboembolism
Acute Mechanical Defects

OVERVIEW

Coronary artery disease (CAD) is one of the most common diseases affecting the adult population and the leading cause of death in the United States (Wenger, 1990). An estimated 7 million Americans have clinically active CAD (Rutherford & Braunwald, 1992). Each year, approximately 1.5 million people suffer a myocardial infarction (MI), 500,000 of which are fatal (American Heart Association, 1991).

ETIOLOGY

Pathogenesis of Atherosclerosis

The major cause of CAD is *atherosclerosis,* a pathologic process that causes irregularity and thickening of artery walls. Atherosclerotic lesions occur primarily within the intima, or innermost layer of the wall. The process begins early in life with the development of lipid-rich lesions (fatty streaks) composed of macrophages and smooth muscle cells (Ross, 1992). Over time, the smooth muscle cells proliferate and a connective tissue matrix forms, leading to accumulation of more intracellular and extracellular lipid (Ross, 1990).

In susceptible individuals, the lesion develops into an *atheroma* or fibrous plaque (Fig. 1-1). Small blood vessels grow into the plaque and may rupture, result-

ing in areas of subintimal hemorrhage that increase the plaque's size. Thrombus formation and ulceration and calcification of the lesion are common. Fatty streaks are present in almost all individuals after 20 years of age; in those in whom the lesions progress, fibrous plaques appear about the third decade and more complicated lesions and their clinical consequences typically begin to develop in the fourth decade (Fuster et al., 1992).

Atherosclerotic lesions usually produce localized narrowing, often in proximal portions of the major coronary arteries and their branches. As a lesion increasingly occupies an artery lumen, blood supply to the myocardium can be impeded by one of several mechanisms: (1) the lesion creates a fixed obstruction so that blood flow through the artery cannot increase in response to increased demand, (2) the vessel lumen becomes completely occluded with atheromatous material or thrombus, or (3) portions of clot or plaque embolize, occluding the distal portion of the vessel. The growth of obstructive lesions in the coronary arteries causes formation of collateral blood vessels that provide alternative routes of blood flow to the myocardium. However, when one or more of the major arteries becomes significantly obstructed (i.e., the artery lumen is reduced to a small proportion of its normal circumference), myocardial ischemia is likely to occur.

Betsy Finkelmeier: CARDIOTHORACIC SURGICAL NURSING.
© 1995 J.B. Lippincott Company.

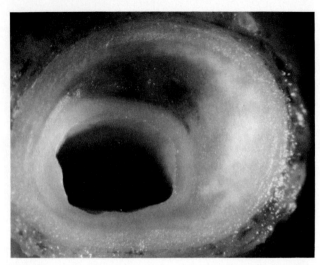

FIGURE 1-1. Cross section of coronary artery demonstrating eccentric fibrofatty atherosclerotic plaque. (Courtesy of Cornelius Davis, M.D., Northwestern University)

Myocardial metabolism is predominantly aerobic, supported by extraction of 70% to 80% of oxygen from the coronary arterial blood even at rest (Chung, 1988). Therefore, to augment supply, blood flow must increase. The presence of obstructive lesions in the coronary circulation limits increased flow. Generally blood flow is not significantly obstructed until the vessel lumen is more than 75% narrowed (Yee, 1986). Even with that degree of narrowing, blood flow is often sufficient to meet baseline myocardial oxygen demands except when precipitating factors produce a demand–supply imbalance.

Risk Factors

Although fatty streaks are present in almost all adults, their evolution into clinically relevant fibrous plaques and more complicated lesions varies in incidence and extent among different geographic and ethnic groups (Fuster et al., 1992). A number of risk factors have been linked with the occurrence and progression of CAD (Table 1-1). Risk factors are those personal traits or life-styles that convey an increased propensity for development of the disease (Stone, 1990).

Perhaps of greatest significance are the three major modifiable risk factors for CAD: hypertension, hypercholesterolemia, and cigarette smoking. Elimination or control of these factors offers the most hope of preventing disease and slowing disease progression. Both systolic and diastolic hypertension independently increase risk for developing CAD as well as other forms of cardiovascular disease. The prevalence of early heart disease increases exponentially when blood pressure exceeds 140/90 mm Hg (Klein, 1991). Additionally, the risk associated with hypertension increases markedly when hyperlipidemia, cigarette

smoking, glucose intolerance, and other factors are present (Wenger, 1990)

A relationship between elevated serum cholesterol levels and CAD is also well established. Risk increases exponentially with higher serum cholesterol levels, particularly levels above 240 mg/dL (Stone, 1990). The predictive value of serum cholesterol is more powerful in younger persons and in those who have other associated risk factors (Stone & Green, 1980). Two lipoproteins (i.e., complex molecules that transport cholesterol in the bloodstream) also have prognostic significance for development and progression of CAD: *high-density lipoprotein (HDL-c)* and *low-density lipoprotein (LDL-c)*.

HDL-c levels are inversely related to risk of cardiovascular disease. In fact, elevated HDL-c appears to slow atherosclerosis. Accordingly, HDL-c levels are considered an important predictor of CAD, independent of serum cholesterol levels. Also, other risk factors for CAD, such as physical inactivity, obesity, and cigarette smoking, are known to decrease HDL-c (Goe, 1989). Conversely, exercise, postmenopausal estrogens, and moderate alcohol consumption increase HDL-c. It should be noted, however, that alcohol consumption appears not to increase HDL_2-c, which is epidemiologically associated with a reduction in CAD, but rather HDL_3-c, which is not clearly related to CAD (Lieber, 1984). Consequently, moderate alcohol consumption as a means of increasing HDL-c is generally not encouraged, particularly given the other adverse effects of alcohol and the potential risk of alcohol abuse.

In contrast to HDL-c, elevated LDL-c levels appear to accelerate atherogenesis, thereby increasing risk. Reducing LDL-c cholesterol or total cholesterol/HDL-c ratio has proven effective both in preventing and in slowing progression of CAD (Wenger, 1990). In addition, in patients at high risk for cardiovascular events,

TABLE 1-1. RISK FACTORS FOR CORONARY ARTERY DISEASE

Major Modifiable Risk Factors

Hypertension
Hypercholesterolemia
Cigarette smoking

Nonmodifiable Risk Factors

Heredity
Increasing age
Male sex

Contributing Risk Factors

Diabetes
Cocaine
Obesity
Sedentary life-style
Stress

intensive pharmacologic therapy to lower LDL-c has been shown not only to reduce progression but also to cause regression of coronary artery lesions (Brown et al., 1990). Hypertriglyceridemia (> 500 mg/dL) is not considered an independent risk factor for CAD. However, it is commonly present in patients with CAD and may be a useful marker of risk in women (Stone, 1990; Reaven, 1993).

Cigarette smoking is the third major modifiable risk factor for CAD. The tar, nicotine, and carbon monoxide contained in cigarettes have the following injurious physiologic effects: peripheral vasoconstriction, cardiac stimulation (increased heart rate, stroke volume, cardiac output, and contractility), increased oxygen consumption, reduced oxygen-carrying capacity, and increased arrhythmias (Yee, 1986). There is strong evidence that smoking accelerates atherosclerosis in already susceptible individuals, lowers HDL-c levels, and increases risk for MI and sudden cardiac death (SCD) in persons with CAD (Stone & Green, 1980).

Although the proportion of smokers is decreasing in the United States, 32% of men and 27% of women continue to smoke (Taylor et al., 1992). At highest risk are young men who smoke more than 40 cigarettes per day and women who smoke and also take oral contraceptives (Wenger, 1990). Nonsmokers exposed to environmental tobacco smoke also face an increased risk of CAD. The American Heart Association Council on Cardiopulmonary and Critical Care has concluded that environmental tobacco smoke is a major preventable cause of cardiovascular disease and death (Taylor et al., 1992).

Risk factors for CAD that cannot be modified include heredity, older age, and male sex. A propensity clearly exists for some family groups to develop CAD at a younger age. However, genetic factors are difficult to distinguish from environmental influences. Familial predisposition to associated risk factors for CAD, such as hypertension or hypercholesterolemia, may be determined by their intake of salt, saturated fat, or overall calories (Farmer & Gotto, 1992). Because of increased longevity in this country and the progressive nature of atherosclerosis, increased age is a risk factor for CAD. Fifty percent of individuals older than 65 years of age have evidence of cardiac disease (Kern, 1991). Elderly persons compose 55% of MI victims and have the highest cardiovascular death rate in the United States (Acinapura et al., 1988; American Heart Association, 1991).

Throughout early and middle adulthood, CAD affects men much more commonly than women. Premenopausal women have a much lower incidence of CAD than age-matched men (Farmer & Gotto, 1992). Although CAD is less common in women, those women with the combined risk factors of smoking and high cholesterol are at significant risk. Also, use of oral contraceptives increases risk in women older than 35 years of age, especially if other risk factors are also present (Wenger, 1990; Peberdy & Ornato, 1992).

After menopause, the risk in women increases markedly, approaching that of men.

Risk factors that play a lesser but still important role include diabetes, cocaine use, obesity, a sedentary life-style, and stress. Diabetes mellitus is a demonstrated risk factor for development of atherosclerosis, particularly in young and middle-aged women (Hoogwerf et al., 1991). In addition, CAD in diabetic patients tends to be of a more severe nature than in nondiabetic patients.

Increasing evidence demonstrates use of cocaine as a risk factor for myocardial ischemia and MI, even in young adults without other risk factors. Three etiologic mechanisms have been postulated: (1) increased myocardial oxygen consumption due to cocaine-induced sympathetic overstimulation, (2) a direct vasoconstricting effect, and (3) coronary artery thrombosis precipitated by increased platelet aggregation (Harris, 1987).

Individuals who are greater than 30% over ideal body weight are more likely to develop heart disease, even in the absence of other risk factors (American Heart Association, 1991). Obese persons who smoke have a 10-fold increased risk of cardiovascular events compared with nonobese, nonsmoking persons (Gottlieb, 1992). Two life-style factors contribute to progression of CAD: physical inactivity and persistently high levels of psychologic stress.

CLINICAL MANIFESTATIONS

Significant clinical symptoms of CAD typically do not develop until late middle age. Traditionally, researchers believed that excessive demand in the presence of a fixed supply was the sole etiologic mechanism for myocardial ischemia. However, more recent studies demonstrate that in some patients a reduction in supply may occur as well, owing to inappropriate vasoconstriction in response to exercise, exposure to cold, or cigarette smoking (Hillis et al., 1992a). Therefore, myocardial ischemia may represent an increase in myocardial oxygen consumption in the presence of fixed obstruction, a dynamic reduction in myocardial oxygen supply, or a combination of both (Braunwald & Sobel, 1992).

Myocardial oxygen deprivation can produce a continuum of events in the muscle, ranging from intermittent symptoms of ischemia to irreversible muscle necrosis or MI. In addition, acute pulmonary edema or ventricular tachyarrhythmias can occur. The type and severity of event is quite unpredictable; in many cases, a fatal MI or SCD is the first manifestation of CAD. In fact, SCD accounts for approximately one half of the deaths from CAD (Chung, 1988).

Myocardial Ischemia

The cardinal recurring symptom of CAD is *angina*, representing transient episodes of myocardial ischemia. Typically, angina is precipitated by exercise, stressful situations, overeating, or exposure to cold (i.e., the "four Es"—exercise, emotion, eating, exposure). It usually lasts several minutes and is relieved by rest or administration of nitroglycerin. The Canadian Cardiovascular Society Classification System is useful in categorizing angina according to conditions under which it occurs (Table 1-2).

The terms *angina* and *chest pain* are often used interchangeably. Although angina, or myocardial ischemia, is usually manifested as chest pain, it can alternatively cause a variety of other somatic sensations. Angina, therefore, describes not only chest pain but also any somatic manifestation of myocardial ischemia. The term *anginal equivalent* is sometimes used to denote ischemic symptoms other than typical chest pain. Conversely, chest pain can occur with conditions other than myocardial ischemia, such as gastroesophageal reflux or pleuritis.

Anginal chest pain is classically described as substernal, squeezing chest discomfort or pressure. Because of its similarity to epigastric distress, it is frequently mistaken for heartburn. Angina may also occur as an abnormal sensation in the chest, epigastric region, neck, back, or arms. Often patients will deny chest pain but describe a long history of tightness, fullness, numbness, or heaviness. Occasionally, the abnormal sensation is entirely outside the thorax (e.g., numbness in the wrist, elbows, throat, or jaw). Because of the wide variance in presentation, it is quite common for angina to continue unrecognized or ignored for long periods before its cardiac etiology is diagnosed and appropriate therapy is initiated. The most characteristic feature of angina is that the pattern is generally consistent for a particular person, that is, the nature of the discomfort is similar each time. Angina is sometimes accompanied by other symptoms, such as palpitations, dyspnea, weakness, or near syncope (Chung, 1988).

A variety of terms are used to categorize angina. *Exertional* and *rest angina* describe whether the discomfort occurs in the presence or absence, respectively, of physical effort. *Chronic stable angina* is defined as angina that is precipitated by exertion and that has a reasonably stable pattern over weeks to

months (Roberts & Pratt, 1991). When the anginal pattern increases in frequency, severity, or both, it is described as *accelerating. Unstable angina* is that which (1) occurs at rest and is of sufficient severity to warrant hospitalization, (2) produces transient, reversible ST-T wave abnormalities, and (3) is not associated with enzymatic evidence of MI (Goldschlager, 1988). In contrast to stable angina, episodes of unstable angina are often prolonged and do not abate with rest or sublingual administration of nitroglycerin. Unstable angina that occurs despite maximal medical therapy, yet without enzymatic evidence of MI, is often termed *preinfarction* or *crescendo* angina. The terms unstable, preinfarction, and crescendo angina all describe an *acute myocardial ischemic syndrome* and are discussed in further detail later in this chapter.

Variant or *Prinzmetal's* angina is myocardial ischemia that occurs due to spasm of the coronary arteries. The specific mechanisms that produce coronary artery spasm are not well defined. However, both smoking and use of cocaine have been implicated as etiologic factors. Although many patients with variant angina have associated severe proximal atherosclerotic lesions involving one or more major coronary arteries, others have angiographically normal arteries (Hillis et al., 1992b). In contrast to other forms of angina, variant angina typically occurs at rest and is unrelated to exertion. The natural history in patients with Prinzmetal's angina varies and spontaneous remission sometimes occurs. In the absence of significant obstructive CAD, prognosis is excellent (Rutherford & Braunwald, 1992).

Myocardial Infarction

Myocardial infarction is irreversible necrosis of cardiac muscle. It occurs when sudden cessation or prolonged reduction of blood flow severely compromises the supply of oxygenated blood to a portion of the myocardium. Acute disruption in blood flow through a coronary artery may be due to hemorrhage under or rupture into an atherosclerotic plaque, thrombus superimposed upon an atherosclerotic lesion, prolonged vasospasm, embolus to the artery, or vasculitis (Goldschlager, 1988). In 85% to 90% of cases, MI is due to thrombotic occlusion of the artery. Most MIs damage a significant portion of ventricular muscle, and many are fatal.

The subendocardium is the most distal region supplied by the coronary arterial system and is subjected to the greatest intramyocardial pressure (Chung, 1988). Consequently, it is the portion of muscle most vulnerable to infarction. An MI limited to the subendocardial layer is termed *subendocardial* or *nontransmural*. An infarction that extends through all layers of muscle is termed *transmural*. MI is also categorized by location. Most MIs involve primarily the left ventricle. However, necropsy studies provide evidence that some degree of right ventricular infarction occurs in 14% to 40% of patients, particularly in association

---

TABLE 1-2. CANADIAN CARDIOVASCULAR SOCIETY CLASSIFICATION SYSTEM FOR ANGINA PECTORIS

Class	Description
I	Angina occurs with strenuous or rapid or prolonged exertion at work or recreation
II	Slight limitation of ordinary activities by angina
III	Marked limitation of ordinary activities by angina
IV	Angina with any physical activity or at rest

(Adapted from Campeau L, 1976: Grading of angina pectoris. Circulation 54:522)

with inferior wall MI (Robison, 1987; Goldschlager, 1988).

Infarct location corresponds to the occluded coronary artery from which the affected muscle receives its blood supply (Fig. 1-2). The left anterior descending artery supplies the anterior wall of the left ventricle. Left anterior descending artery occlusion usually produces infarction of the anterior and apical portions of the left ventricle; portions of the septum, anterolateral wall, papillary muscles, and inferoapical wall of the left ventricle may also be affected (Pasternak et al., 1992). Because of the anterior wall's crucial importance to effective left ventricular contraction, an *anterior wall MI* is particularly damaging. The left circumflex artery supplies the posterior left ventricle and posterior septum. *Lateral* or *inferoposterior infarctions* result from circumflex artery occlusion. Left main coronary artery occlusion damages all muscle supplied by both the left anterior descending and circumflex arteries, producing global infarction that is invariably fatal. The inferior wall of the left ventricle, the right ventricle, and, usually, sinus and atrioventricular (AV) nodal tissue are supplied by the right coronary artery. Right coronary artery occlusion produces an *inferior* or *diaphragmatic MI* of the left ventricle, or a *right ventricular infarction.*

MI is commonly associated with severe chest pain that is unrelieved by rest or oral medications. The pain, often described as crushing, is usually substernal and may radiate to the arms, neck, or jaw. Shortness of breath, diaphoresis, anxiety, nausea, and vomiting often accompany the pain. Less common manifestations include pulmonary edema, heart block, and ventricular tachycardia. Some patients have what is termed a *silent MI,* in that the event is not accompanied by symptoms. Persons with diabetes mellitus are particularly susceptible to silent infarction.

Arrhythmias are quite common after MI. Ventricular arrhythmias of some type occur in nearly 100% of patients, bradycardia in up to one third (especially with inferior wall MI), and atrial arrhythmias in 10% to 15% (Goldschlager, 1988). First-, second-, or third-degree heart block is also common, occurring in 15% to 25% of patients hospitalized with acute MI (Hillis et al., 1992c). AV block that follows an inferior wall MI usually occurs transiently as a result of AV nodal ischemia, may require temporary pacing, and resolves after a few days. AV block after an anterior wall MI, on the other hand, usually denotes extensive myocardial necrosis that involves conducting tissue below the AV node (Kessler, 1991; Hillis et al., 1992c). It is more likely to be permanent and necessitate pacemaker implantation. Because AV block after anterior MI signifies damage to a large amount of myocardium, it is associated with a poor prognosis.

Pericarditis (inflammation of the pericardial sac) or *pericardial effusion* sometimes occurs in the early post-MI period but usually abates without sequelae. Clinical manifestations of pericarditis include a pericardial friction rub, chest pain, and low-grade fever. *Dressler's syndrome* is a more pronounced form of pericarditis that develops in some patients weeks or months after MI. It is characterized by protracted or

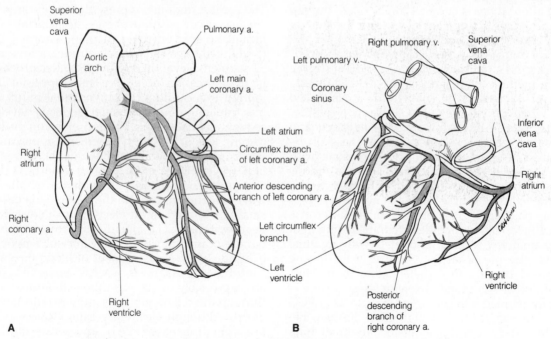

FIGURE 1-2. Anterior **(A)** and posterior **(B)** view of the heart displaying normal distribution of coronary arteries. (Porth CM, 1990: Alterations in cardiac function. In Pathophysiology: Concepts of Altered Health States, ed. 3, p. 337. Philadelphia, JB Lippincott)

recurrent fever, pericarditic chest pain, pericardial friction rub, and left pleural effusion (Morris et al., 1990).

The clinical sequelae and prognosis after MI depend not only on location of the infarct but also on the amount of damaged muscle. Small infarcts may produce no symptoms and may not be detected until an electrocardiogram (ECG) is obtained or the heart is visually inspected during a cardiac operation or post-mortem examination. On the other hand, large amounts of muscle necrosis or multiple infarcts may produce significant segmental wall motion abnormalities or global hypokinesis. Such patients may have considerable functional impairment with limited survival prognosis (Riegel, 1988). Acute MI can also lead to a number of serious and potentially lethal complications, discussed later in the chapter and including cardiogenic shock, ventricular aneurysm, systemic or pulmonary embolization, acute mitral regurgitation, and ventricular rupture.

DIAGNOSIS

Coronary Artery Disease

The first symptom of CAD is often a fatal MI or SCD. Therefore, preventive therapy, screening of individuals in high-risk categories, and early diagnosis and treatment are necessary to reduce mortality and morbidity. Individuals with known risk factors require a thorough review of clinical history and a physical examination, chest roentgenogram, and ECG. Unfortunately, severe CAD may be present despite normal physical and roentgenographic findings. The ECG also remains normal, except during episodes of angina and after MI has occurred. Angina often, but not always, produces ST segment depression in leads reflective of ischemic myocardium. Variant angina and myocardial injury produce ST segment elevation.

Exercise stress testing is the most useful noninvasive screening method for diagnosis of CAD. The study consists of exercising the patient in a controlled setting while monitoring ECG, blood pressure, and heart rate. Although both false-negative and false-positive responses limit conclusiveness of exercise stress testing, the majority of persons with hemodynamically significant atherosclerotic lesions develop signs or symptoms of myocardial ischemia during the study. Exercise testing is not always performed as part of the diagnostic evaluation. Because cardiac catheterization provides accurate definition of coronary anatomy and is associated with minimal morbidity, the physician may omit exercise testing and proceed directly to catheterization in patients with suggestive symptoms. Exercise stress testing is specifically avoided if the nature of symptoms or ECG findings are suspicious for high-grade lesions, because the study may precipitate life-threatening myocardial ischemia.

Cardiac catheterization is the definitive diagnostic study for CAD. The procedure usually includes coro-nary angiography and left ventriculography. Unless coexisting cardiac pathology is suspected, a full catheterization (with catheterization of the right chambers and measurement of intracardiac pressures) is not necessary. During *coronary angiography*, contrast material is injected selectively into the ostia of the right and left coronary arteries, the coronary anatomy is outlined, and areas of narrowing are identified. A contrast injection of the left ventricle (*ventriculography*) is performed to demonstrate the contractile status of the left ventricle and to obtain an estimation of left ventricular ejection fraction. Areas of akinesis (lack of movement), hypokinesis (diminished movement), dyskinesis (abnormal movement), or aneurysmal dilatation are also identified with this portion of the study.

Two radionuclide imaging techniques (i.e., *myocardial scintigraphy*) are useful in the diagnostic evaluation of selected patients with CAD. First, exercise testing, combined with myocardial imaging using thallium-201, is useful in patients with baseline ST segment abnormalities and in those with an inadequate heart rate response to routine exercise testing (Chung, 1988). In the second imaging technique, technetium-99m pyrophosphate is used to assess ventricular contractility and estimate ejection fraction.

Acute Myocardial Infarction

MI is diagnosed and definitively distinguished from angina by its ECG manifestations and its effect on cardiac isoenzyme levels. The evolution of a transmural MI produces specific changes in the ECG tracing. The earliest findings, representative of transmural ischemia, occur within minutes. The tracings in leads facing the area of injury display abnormal T waves (prolonged, increased in magnitude, or inverted) and ST segment elevation (Fisch, 1992). Reciprocal ST segment depression occurs in leads opposite those of injured myocardium. As myocardial injury evolves into transmural necrosis, affected leads develop subsequent changes over a period of hours or days, including loss of R wave voltage and appearance of Q waves, normalization of ST segments, and inversion of T waves (Hillis et al., 1992d). The ECG does not always provide diagnostic evidence of MI. New Q waves do not appear if the MI is subendocardial, small, or located in an electrically silent area of the heart or if the ECG is already abnormal because of left bundle branch block or left ventricular hypertrophy (Chung, 1988). Measurement of blood enzymes also contributes to diagnosis of MI. When myocardial cells are irreversibly damaged, intracellular enzymes leak through the cell membranes and are detectable in the blood. Although elevated creatine kinase (CK), lactate dehydrogenase (LDH), and serum glutamic oxaloacetic transaminase levels are all representative of cellular damage, the most sensitive indicator of myocardial damage is a CK isoenzyme, CK-MB. Be-

TABLE 1-3. ENZYME ELEVATIONS AFTER MYOCARDIAL INFARCTION

Finding	Creatine Kinase	Creatine Kinase-MB	Lactate Dehydrogenase
Rises (hours)	4–8	4–8	8–12
Peaks (hours)	12–24	12–20	72–144
Returns to normal (days)	3–4	2–3	8–14

(Adapted from Lee TH, Goldman L, 1986: Serum enzyme assays in the diagnosis of acute myocardial infarction. Ann Intern Med 105:221)

cause of its high specificity and sensitivity, elevated CK-MB is the enzymatic criterion generally relied on for diagnosis of acute MI (Sobel & Jaffe, 1993). In addition, the amount of muscle damage can be estimated by calculating the percentage of CK-MB isoenzyme (CK-MB/CK). CK-MB levels rise 4 to 8 hours after MI, peak in 12 to 20 hours, and return to normal in 2 to 3 days (Lee & Goldman, 1986) (Table 1-3). In patients evaluated more than 48 hours after onset of ischemia, the LDH isoenzyme LDH I may be measured because elevation of this enzyme may persist for 8 to 14 days.

TREATMENT

CAD is a chronic disease. Its presence mandates consistent medical supervision and periodic evaluations for the duration of the patient's life. At present, there is no known cure for CAD. Thus, goals of currently available therapy are primarily palliative: to slow progression of atherosclerosis, to effectively control current symptoms, to prevent MI and its potential consequences, and to prolong life. Treatment must be individualized, based on the presence of modifiable risk factors, location and severity of existing lesions, type and severity of symptoms, and the patient's age and life-style. Often a combination of medical (risk factor modification and medications) and invasive therapies is used. With treatment advances in the past decade, age-corrected mortality from CAD has decreased approximately 30% (Mueller, 1989).

Medical Therapy

Attempts to slow progression of atherosclerosis are focused on modification of identified risk factors. Pharmacologic treatment to lower high blood pressure is a major component of risk reduction in susceptible individuals. Beta-adrenergic blocking and calcium-channel blocking agents are used to maintain normal blood pressure in patients with hypertension. Other antihypertensive agents, including diuretics, vasodilators, and angiotensin-converting enzyme inhibitors may also be used. Dietary modifications are encouraged to lower elevated cholesterol levels. If necessary, cholesterol-lowering medications, such as cholestyramine, cholestipol, niacin, gemfibrozil, or lovastatin may be prescribed. In patients with elevated LDL-c, these agents not only slow disease progression but in fact may cause regression of existing lesions (Brown et al., 1990). A surgical procedure, partial ileal bypass, may be performed in severely affected individuals to achieve sustained lowering of LDL-c (Buchwald et al., 1990).

Cessation of smoking is imperative because of the injurious effects of cigarettes. Smoking cessation decreases the risk of ischemia due to nicotine and carbon monoxide, increases HDL-c levels, and results in improved long-term survival (Gottlieb, 1992). A consistent exercise program and weight reduction in obese patients are prescribed to improve cardiac function. Appropriate physical conditioning aids the patient in maintaining a healthier body weight, lower total serum cholesterol, higher HDL-c, improved muscle tone, and an enhanced sense of well-being (Klein, 1991). Cardiac rehabilitation programs provide a structured setting for consistent exercise and ongoing counseling about life-style modification to facilitate risk factor reduction.

Three major categories of medications are used to reduce frequency of angina and improve exercise tolerance: nitrates, beta-adrenergic blocking agents, and calcium-channel blocking agents (Roberts & Pratt, 1991). *Nitrates* have the following therapeutic actions: (1) venous vasodilatation resulting in preload reduction, (2) arterial vasodilatation resulting in afterload reduction, (3) dilatation of collateral coronary arteries or the epicardial coronary arteries from which collateral vessels arise, and (4) relaxation of smooth muscle in epicardial vessels narrowed by atherosclerotic lesions or spasm (Kadota & Burke, 1990). Short-acting nitrates (sublingual, topical, or intravenous nitroglycerin) are used for acute relief of angina. Long-acting oral nitrates (e.g., isosorbide dinitrate) are used to provide sustained drug effects and to prevent myocardial ischemia.

Beta-blocking medications decrease both heart rate and contractility, thus lowering myocardial oxygen demand so that it does not exceed the fixed supply available through obstructed coronary arteries. Beta-blocking agents have been shown to significantly decrease the risk of cardiovascular mortality in patients who have experienced an MI (Frishman et al., 1984). *Calcium-channel blocking medications* are effective principally due to vasodilation that increases coronary blood flow. To differing degrees, individual calcium-channel blocking agents also decrease myocardial oxygen consumption by reducing blood pressure, afterload, and contractility (Kutcher, 1991).

Aspirin has become a standard component of therapy in patients with CAD. It irreversibly inactivates platelet cyclooxygenase, thereby impairing platelet aggregation and reducing the release of platelet-derived vasoconstrictors (Passen & Schaer, 1991). Antiarrhythmic agents and medications to treat congestive heart failure are necessary in selected patients. Nitrates and calcium-channel antagonists are the most useful agents for treating variant angina. Thrombolytic therapy, used in treatment of acute MI, is discussed later in this chapter.

Invasive therapy may eventually be necessary to restore blood supply to cardiac muscle that is jeopardized by acute or chronic obstruction of one or more coronary arteries. Currently available invasive therapies include percutaneous transluminal coronary angioplasty (PTCA) and surgical revascularization (i.e., coronary artery bypass grafting [CABG]).

Percutaneous Transluminal Coronary Angioplasty

PTCA has become increasingly popular as a treatment modality for CAD since it was first performed by Gruentzig in 1977 (Gruentzig, 1978). More than 200,000 PTCAs are performed yearly in the United States (American Heart Association, 1991). The procedure is performed in a cardiac catheterization laboratory. A balloon-tipped catheter is inserted into one of the femoral arteries, advanced in a retrograde fashion through the aorta, and guided into the target coronary artery. With the balloon across the stenotic lesion, serial balloon inflations are performed to dilate the atheromatous segment (Fig. 1-3).

Improvements in angioplasty catheters and in the skills of interventional cardiologists have made it possible to dilate more complex coronary artery lesions. However, the procedure is suited to a particular subset of patients and is not a substitute for CABG. Factors favoring success of PTCA include age younger than 65 years, male gender, single-vessel disease, single-lesion PTCA, subtotal vessel occlusion, absence of calcification, accessibility of the lesion, and normal left ventricular function (Douglas, 1991). Data regarding value of PTCA in patients with multivessel disease are being evaluated. PTCA is not advisable in patients with left main coronary artery obstruction or in vessels with less than critical stenoses (Hurst, 1987).

Cardiothoracic surgeons, an operating room, support personnel, and equipment for rapid institution of cardiopulmonary bypass should be readily available in any setting in which PTCA or other invasive coronary artery procedures are performed. Balloon dilatation of a coronary artery can cause acute occlusion of blood flow due to spasm, dissection, or embolization of thrombotic material. Acute ischemia, infarction, cardiogenic shock, or cardiac arrest may

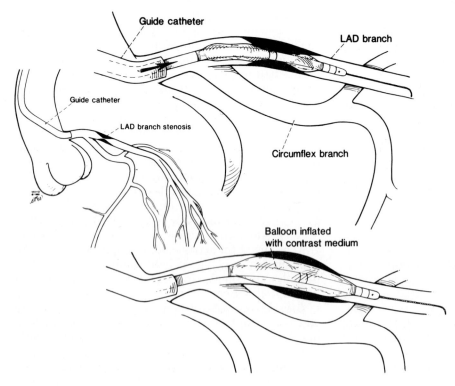

FIGURE 1-3. Diagram of percutaneous transluminal coronary angioplasty. A preformed guide catheter is positioned at left coronary artery ostium; the deflated balloon catheter is advanced over a guidewire through the stenosis in the left anterior descending artery; the balloon is then inflated. (Vlietstra RE, Holmes DR, 1988: Percutaneous transluminal coronary angioplasty. J Cardiac Surg 3:55)

result. In such cases, emergency CABG may be necessary to restore blood flow to jeopardized muscle.

In extreme cases it may be necessary to perform cardiopulmonary resuscitation while transporting a patient from the catheterization laboratory to the operating room. In this situation, every effort is made to place the patient on cardiopulmonary bypass as quickly as possible to protect jeopardized myocardium. Portable cardiopulmonary bypass, using percutaneous femoral cannulation, may be instituted in the catheterization laboratory to stabilize the patient before transportation to the operating room. Operative mortality in this group of patients is high.

In selected high-risk situations, PTCA may be performed with arterial and venous cannulas in place for rapid institution of portable cardiopulmonary bypass or with prophylactic institution of percutaneous bypass during the procedure. Such maneuvers help protect the patient in those situations in which iatrogenic arterial occlusion jeopardizes a significant amount of myocardium and is likely to have lethal consequences. However, the value of percutaneous cardiopulmonary bypass for this purpose is not established, and the practice remains controversial because of its potential complications.

Death occurs in approximately 0.5% of patients who undergo PTCA, nonfatal MI occurs in 1%, and emergency surgical revascularization is necessary in 4% (Raizner, 1991). The most significant long-term limitation of PTCA is the high restenosis rate. Re-stenosis of the dilated artery occurs in approximately 30% of patients within 3 months (Douglas, 1991).

Coronary Artery Bypass Grafting

Surgical revascularization of the coronary arteries has been performed in this country since the late 1960s. Nearly 400,000 patients undergo CABG each year in the United States (American Heart Association, 1991). The procedure consists of using internal thoracic arteries or saphenous veins as conduit material to bypass obstructed coronary arteries.

The choice of initial invasive therapy, that is, PTCA versus CABG, is based primarily on the anatomic appearance, location, number, and severity of coronary artery lesions. However, quality of ventricular function, associated medical problems, and age and life-style of the patient must also be considered. In general, PTCA may be more suitable for many patients with discrete stenosis in one or two major coronary artery branches (i.e., single- or double-vessel CAD) while CABG is usually preferable for those with triple-vessel disease or left main coronary artery stenosis (Kirklin & Barratt-Boyes, 1993a).

In some situations, either PTCA or CABG is clearly preferable. For example, patients with single-vessel disease are almost never treated with surgical revascularization, unless the lesion is in the left anterior descending artery, proximal to the first septal perforator or other branches. On the other hand, significant left main coronary artery stenosis is almost always treated with CABG because of the large amount of jeopardized left ventricular myocardium. Because of the significant restenosis rate after PTCA and the progressive nature of CAD, many patients treated with PTCA eventually require CABG. Surgical revascularization is discussed in detail in Chapter 15, Surgical Treatment of Coronary Artery Disease.

Other Invasive Therapies

Several alternative techniques for reopening obstructed coronary arteries are available in some centers for primary or adjunctive use. *Laser therapy* appears to be effective in treating chronic, total occlusions and long-length lesions; its use is limited by a significant incidence of arterial dissection. *Atherectomy* devices (high-speed rotational, low-speed rotational, and directional) are available for debulking plaque from coronary artery lesions not well treated by standard PTCA. *Stenting devices* used to brace open narrowed segments of coronary arteries are also being investigated for adjunctive use with PTCA. Long-term data are not yet available about these techniques, and thus their efficacy remains undetermined.

ACUTE MYOCARDIAL ISCHEMIC SYNDROME

DEFINITIONS

Acute myocardial ischemic syndrome is uncontrolled exacerbation of cardiac muscle ischemia or injury during which time portions of ventricular myocardium are jeopardized but not yet irreversibly damaged. The syndrome represents a continuum of myocardial pathophysiology, ranging from reversible ischemia to partial or full thickness MI with bordering areas of ischemic tissue. It occurs because of the dynamic nature of myocardial necrosis. Jeopardized muscle does not infarct simultaneously, but rather in an uneven manner surrounded by severely ischemic tissue (Morris et al., 1990). Acute myocardial ischemic syndrome includes the following conditions: (1) *unstable angina*, defined earlier, and including anginal equivalents such as acute pulmonary edema or ventricular tachycardia; (2) evolving MI; and (3) completed MI with unstable, postinfarction angina.

Evolving MI is defined as prolonged ischemia, usually lasting more than 20 minutes but less than 4 to 6 hours (Morris et al., 1990). During this period, muscle necrosis spreads from the subendocardium through ventricular muscle to the subepicardium (Fig. 1-4). After 4 to 6 hours of ischemia, 85% to 100% of necrosis is thought to be completed (Black et al., 1990).

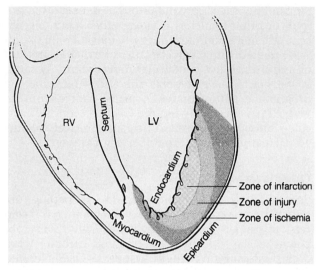

FIGURE 1-4. Diagram of dynamic nature of myocardial infarction with the potential for spread of muscle necrosis from the subendocardium through the ventricular myocardium. (Woods SL, Underhill SL, Cowan M, 1991: Coronary heart disease. In Patrick ML, Woods SL, Craven RF, et al [eds]: Medical-Surgical Nursing: Pathophysiological Concepts, ed. 2, p. 695. Philadelphia, JB Lippincott)

Postinfarction angina is unstable angina that occurs during the first 7 to 10 days after a completed MI. It indicates the presence of reversibly ischemic muscle surrounding the infarct.

Four potential mechanisms are believed to contribute to precipitation of an acute myocardial ischemic syndrome: (1) progression of atherosclerosis, (2) acute coronary thrombosis, (3) coronary artery spasm, and (4) platelet aggregation (Epstein & Palmeri, 1984). These factors may act in isolation or in combination with one another. In fact, interactions probably occur among the factors whereby the presence of one triggers the activation of another (Epstein & Palmeri, 1984). The distinction between the clinical entities that make up acute myocardial ischemic syndrome is not always clear. However, the common factor among them is the presence of jeopardized, ischemic myocardium. The delivery of oxygen and nutrients to cells in the ischemic area of muscle is compromised, altering cell metabolism and impairing both electrical conduction and ventricular contractility (Black et al., 1990). An acute myocardial ischemic syndrome that is not reversed leads either to a completed MI or, in the case of postinfarction angina, to extension of the infarct with increased muscle loss.

DIAGNOSIS AND TREATMENT

Prompt diagnostic and therapeutic interventions during the period of acute myocardial ischemia greatly increase the probability of salvaging myocardium (preventing infarct or limiting infarct size) and, in many cases, of saving the patient's life. The patient must be carefully monitored in a coronary care setting for episodes of angina. Severity of discomfort is usually measured using a 1 to 10 rating scale (1 = minimal, 10 = maximal discomfort). Duration of discomfort and any associated ECG changes or symptoms are carefully noted. ECGs are obtained daily and during episodes of suspected ischemia. CK-MB evaluation is performed after each presumed episode of angina to determine if muscle necrosis (MI) has occurred. If acute invasive therapy is likely, oral nourishment may be withheld to avoid possible induction of general anesthesia in the presence of a full stomach.

The major goal of therapy is correction of the myocardial oxygen demand–supply imbalance. Thus, treatment has two major components: (1) reducing myocardial oxygen consumption and (2) improving blood flow through compromised arteries. Complete bed rest and, if necessary, sedation are used to reduce myocardial oxygen consumption. Narcotic analgesia (morphine sulfate or meperidine) is administered for pain relief. Therapeutic doses of beta-adrenergic blocking and calcium-channel antagonistic medications are maintained.

The most dramatic advances in treatment have occurred in acute therapies for improving myocardial oxygen supply. Increased understanding of the roles that thrombosis, spasm, and platelet aggregation play in precipitating acute ischemic syndromes has broadened therapeutic options to include additional strategies. Both pharmacologic (vasodilating, thrombolytic, and anticoagulant) agents and emergency invasive procedures (PTCA and CABG) are commonly used to treat acute myocardial ischemic syndrome. The specific therapy or combination of therapies depends on a number of factors, most importantly, the extent and severity of CAD, occurrence and timing of MI, and ability to palliate ischemic symptoms.

Intravenous nitroglycerin is a standard component of therapy for acute myocardial ischemic syndrome. It improves coronary artery blood flow and also relieves coronary artery spasm, which may be a contributing factor (Epstein & Palmeri, 1984). Administered as a continuous infusion, nitroglycerin is titrated to suppress anginal episodes and maintain systolic blood pressure in the range of 100 to 110 mm Hg. Angina that persists despite maximal pharmacologic therapy may be treated with intra-aortic balloon counterpulsation (IABC). IABC is beneficial in reducing ischemia because it improves coronary blood flow and reduces afterload.

Because nonoccluding thrombus is present in most patients with unstable angina, heparin is usually administered to prevent further intracoronary thrombosis (Roberts & Pratt, 1991). Clinical trials investigating the use of heparin for treatment of unstable angina have demonstrated an 85% reduction in the risk of fatal or nonfatal MI (Theroux, 1991). Aspirin may also be administered to patients with unstable angina or after acute MI because it significantly reduces the incidence of subsequent infarction, stroke, or death (ISIS-2 Collaborative Group, 1988). The benefits of aspirin therapy must be carefully evaluated if surgical revascularization within 1 week is likely, with recognition that aspirin impairs platelet function and increases the likelihood of perioperative blood transfusions or reexploration for bleeding.

Reducing myocardial oxygen demand is palliative only. Definitive therapy for acute myocardial ischemic syndrome refractory to pharmacologic therapy is urgent PTCA or CABG to restore blood flow through severely stenosed arteries. Differentiation of ischemia from infarction and ascertaining the approximate onset of MI have profound implications for timing of therapies that reestablish blood flow. Restoring perfusion to newly infarcted muscle more than 6 hours but within 7 to 10 days after onset of MI can cause a complex pathophysiologic process called *reperfusion injury*. The cascade of biochemical cellular events that result from reperfusion of recently infarcted myocardium increases cell damage and produces significant ventricular dysfunction.

If MI has not yet occurred, coronary angiography is performed urgently to identify the severity and extent of coronary artery lesions. If an evolving MI is in progress, the probability of saving the patient and salvaging myocardium is greatly increased by aggressive therapy directed at reopening the occluded vessel (thrombolytic therapy) or bringing new blood supply (PTCA or CABG) to infarcted muscle.

Thrombolytic therapy is the most commonly used initial treatment for patients hospitalized with evolving MI. It is used specifically for evolving transmural (Q wave) MI to preserve ventricular function and decrease mortality (Black et al., 1990). Because most MIs are due to acute thrombotic occlusion of an artery, blood flow through the vessel can often be restored with a medication that lyses thrombus. Thrombolytic therapy can produce rapid recanalization of the occluded artery if given during a critical window of time after thrombotic occlusion of the vessel.

Thrombolytic agents may be given intravenously or directly into the compromised coronary artery during coronary angiography. Because of the delay involved in performing cardiac catheterization in patients with acute MI, intracoronary administration of thrombolytic therapy is generally reserved for those who develop coronary thrombosis during an angiographic procedure (Pasternak et al., 1992). Intravenous infusion is more practical because it can be initiated earlier after onset of infarction and emergency coronary angiography is not necessary.

Three thrombolytic agents are approved by the Food and Drug Administration for intravenous use in patients with acute MI: (1) streptokinase, (2) recombinant tissue-type plasminogen activator (rt-PA), and (3) anisoylated streptokinase activator complex (AP-SAC) (Pasternak et al., 1992). Data from more than 60,000 patients in the International rt-PA/Streptokinase Mortality Trial/GISSI-2 and International

Study of Infarct Survival-3 (ISIS-3) trials suggest equivalent early survival rates among these three agents (Kirshenbaum, 1992).

Because enzymatic elevation cannot be detected during the critical period of MI evolution, the decision to administer thrombolytic agents is based on a clinical and ECG diagnosis of MI. The thrombolytic agent is usually administered in the emergency department as soon as ECG evidence of acute MI is obtained. Successful recanalization is manifest initially by the combined occurrence of relief of chest pain, resolution of ST segment elevation, and appearance of arrhythmias; CK washout (i.e., early and exaggerated peaking of CK and CK-MB levels) occurs later (Black et al., 1990). An intravenous heparin infusion is initiated after administration of thrombolytic therapy to help prevent reocclusion.

If the thrombolytic agent is successful in restoring blood flow to jeopardized myocardium and if the patient remains hemodynamically stable, coronary angiography and a definitive plan of therapy for residual disease can be delayed 2 to 3 weeks. However, thrombolytic therapy is effective only in eradicating fresh thrombus and has no effect on underlying atherosclerotic lesions. PTCA or CABG to treat underlying disease is frequently necessary once the risk of reperfusion injury is no longer present.

The incidence of early reocclusion of a coronary artery successfully recanalized by thrombolytic therapy ranges from 4% to 33% (Kirshenbaum, 1992). Although reocclusion may not produce clinical symptoms, it adversely affects ventricular function. The major complication of thrombolytic medications is bleeding, most commonly at the insertion site of an invasive catheter. Bleeding can also occur during median sternotomy when urgent surgical revascularization is necessary. Intracranial hemorrhage occurs rarely but is the most serious form of bleeding complication. Patients at increased risk for bleeding complications include those older than 75 years of age or with a history of significant hypertension, recent trauma or surgery, bleeding ulcer or bleeding diathesis, aneurysm, or cerebral vascular accident (Andrein & Lemberg, 1990; Black et al., 1990).

Patients with acute MI who can be brought to a catheterization laboratory within 1 hour of hospital admission may alternatively be treated with PTCA of the infarct vessel. Emerging data demonstrate that immediate PTCA, as compared with thrombolytic therapy, lowers the combined rates of nonfatal infarction or death (Grines et al., 1993). Emergent CABG as a primary intervention for evolving MI is generally reserved for patients in whom thrombolytic therapy or immediate PTCA is contraindicated or unsuccessful. Because of the potential for reperfusion injury, PTCA or CABG is ideally delayed 7 to 10 days after a completed MI. Postinfarction angina is treated with medications and IABC to relieve ischemia. However, if the patient continues to have severe postinfarction angina that is unrelieved by medical therapy and

IABC, emergent PTCA or CABG may be necessary to prevent extension of the MI.

COMPLICATIONS OF MYOCARDIAL INFARCTION

VENTRICULAR DYSFUNCTION

MI can be associated with serious, sometimes fatal, complications. If a significant amount of myocardium is damaged by MI, a dysfunctional portion of ventricular muscle, called a *wall motion abnormality*, remains. Either hypokinesis, dyskinesis, or akinesis of the affected segment may be present, compromising the ability of the ventricle to eject an adequate stroke volume. Global or diffuse hypokinesis may be present after massive MI or after MI in a ventricle already damaged by previous infarction(s). The ventricular dysfunction can result in congestive heart failure, pulmonary edema, or cardiogenic shock. In addition, scarred endocardial tissue associated with a major wall motion abnormality can act as a focus for recurrent ventricular tachycardia or fibrillation. These patients are at increased risk for recurring, symptomatic ventricular tachyarrhythmias or SCD.

Cardiogenic shock, or inability of the myocardium to maintain cardiac output at a level necessary for adequate organ perfusion, is characterized by a cardiac index less than 2.0 L/min/m^2, systolic blood pressure less than 90 mm Hg, and urine output less than 20 mL/h. Its occurrence after MI is related to the amount of damaged myocardium, which usually exceeds 40% of left ventricular muscle mass (Becker & Alpert, 1991). Cardiogenic shock can result from massive, acute damage or from a smaller amount of acute damage in association with myocardial necrosis from a prior MI.

Cardiogenic shock after MI causes infarct extension for two reasons. First, ventricular function is compromised to such a degree that coronary blood flow is inadequate to meet myocardial oxygen demands. Second, the reduction in coronary blood flow promotes coronary artery thrombosis. Consequently, cardiogenic shock is almost certain to be fatal unless aggressive supportive therapy is instituted promptly. IABC is a major component of therapy in almost all patients, along with inotropic and, if tolerated, vasodilating agents. If the patient cannot be stabilized with these interventions, coronary angiography may be undertaken to determine if areas of reversible ischemia are present. If so, emergency PTCA or CABG may be performed with the goal of improving ventricular function by relieving ischemia. Cardiogenic shock after acute MI is commonly associated with an 80% to 90% mortality rate (Becker & Alpert, 1991).

VENTRICULAR ANEURYSM

MI can also cause formation of *ventricular aneurysm*, a discrete area of necrosed myocardium that is noncontractile or that contracts paradoxically from the rest of the ventricular muscle. Twelve to 15% of patients who survive MI develop a ventricular aneurysm (Churchwell, 1991). Aneurysms most often occur in the anterolateral wall near the apex after a large transmural infarction (Kirklin et al., 1993b) (Fig. 1-5). The presence of a ventricular aneurysm is suggested by an abnormal precordial pulsation, abnormally contoured left heart border on chest roentgenogram, and persistent ST segment elevation on the ECG after transmural MI (Chung, 1988). In some cases, the an-

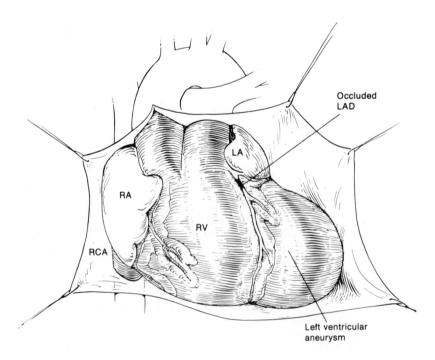

FIGURE 1-5. Typical presentation of a postinfarction left ventricular aneurysm involving the anterolateral left ventricular wall and apex. The illustration depicts the commonly associated finding of occlusion of the proximal left anterior descending (LAD) artery. (With permission from Mundth ED, 1979: Left ventricular aneurysmectomy. In Cohn LH [ed]: Modern Technics in Surgery, p. 11-4. Mount Kisco, NY, Futura Publishing)

eurysm does not produce symptoms and may not require surgical therapy. However, it can cause congestive heart failure, angina, or arrhythmias. Because ventricular aneurysms often contain thrombus, they provide a source of recurrent systemic emboli and may lead to stroke, subsequent MI, or peripheral arterial occlusion.

THROMBOEMBOLISM

Deep venous thrombosis and *pulmonary embolism* can occur, particularly in patients with congestive heart failure, cardiogenic shock, and preexisting venous disease and in those who are older than 70 years of age (Chung, 1988). In addition, thrombotic material is likely to collect along endocardial surfaces of akinetic or dyskinetic infarcted muscle. Portions of this thrombotic material, known as mural thrombus, can embolize to one of the vital organs or to the extremities. The risk for systemic embolization from mural thrombus continues, not just in the immediate postinfarction period but indefinitely (Stratton & Resnick, 1987).

ACUTE MECHANICAL DEFECTS

Acute mechanical complications of MI include mitral valve regurgitation and rupture of the left ventricular free wall or septum. All three of these defects gener-ally produce significant hemodynamic instability and often necessitate emergency operative intervention. As a group, they are estimated to account for approximately 15% of deaths resulting from acute MI (Pasternak et al., 1992).

Acute mitral regurgitation can develop due to one of several different pathophysiologic mechanisms, including papillary muscle dysfunction, papillary muscle rupture, or annular dilatation. Two papillary muscles (posteromedial and anterolateral) support the mitral valve. Because both have chordal attachments to each of the mitral valve leaflets, dysfunction or rupture of either papillary muscle can affect function of both valve leaflets (Roberts, 1980). Mitral regurgitation secondary to papillary muscle dysfunction may represent transient muscle ischemia or necrosis. Papillary muscle ischemia is sometimes successfully reversed by reestablishing blood flow to the papillary muscle with thrombolytic therapy, PTCA, or CABG. If so, valve competence is likely to be restored and surgical valve replacement may be avoided.

Actual rupture of a papillary muscle may also occur (Fig. 1-6). In 75% of cases, rupture occurs in the posteromedial papillary muscle; in 25%, the anterolateral papillary muscle is ruptured (Kirklin et al., 1993c). Most commonly, rupture involves only one or two of the apical heads of a papillary muscle. Less often, one of the papillary muscles is completely disrupted, resulting in flailing of both valve leaflets

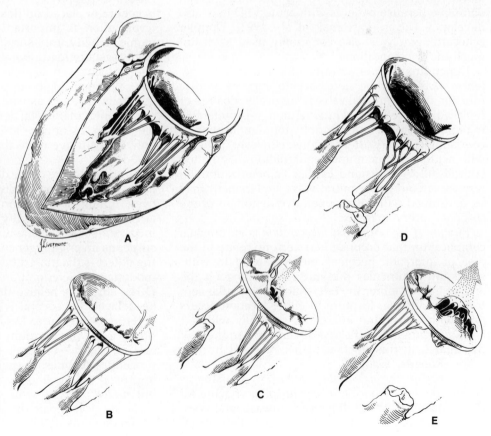

FIGURE 1-6. Disruption of mitral subvalvular apparatus. (**A**) Spatial relationships of the anatomic components of the mitral valve apparatus. (**B**) Rupture of chordae tendineae. (**C**) Partial rupture of the head of a papillary muscle. (**D**) Complete rupture of papillary muscle. (**E**) Severe mitral valve regurgitation caused by papillary muscle disruption. (Khonsari S, 1988: Surgical correction of mechanical complications of myocardial infarction. In Cardiac Surgery: Safeguards and Pitfalls in Operative Technique, p. 145. Rockville, MD, Aspen Publishers)

(Kirklin et al., 1993c). Acute annular dilatation of the mitral valve occurs less commonly for several reasons: (1) the surface area of the valve leaflets is about twice that of the orifice size and is adequate to maintain valvular competence despite some degree of annular dilatation, (2) the mitral valve annulus contracts during ventricular systole, and (3) the fibrous skeleton surrounding the annulus makes dilatation at the base of the left ventricle less than in its midportion (Roberts, 1980).

Acute mitral regurgitation is suggested by a new holosystolic murmur and progressive congestive heart failure after MI. Because these findings also occur with acute rupture of the ventricular septum, further diagnostic testing is necessary to differentiate the two complications. Often this can be accomplished with placement of a pulmonary artery catheter. Oxygen saturation levels from the proximal and distal ports of the catheter are measured to detect a "step-up" or increase in oxygen saturation between the right atrium and pulmonary artery.

Oxygen saturation levels are normally the same until blood travels through the pulmonary vasculature. In patients with acute mitral regurgitation, pulmonary artery blood samples reveal no step-up in oxygen saturation. A step-up indicates left to right shunting of oxygenated blood at the ventricular level, or the presence of a ventricular septal defect. Patients with mitral regurgitation also demonstrate large "v waves" on the pulmonary capillary wedge and pulmonary artery tracings. However, this finding is not definitive because patients with acute VSD may also develop v waves (Pasternak et al., 1992). Doppler echocardiography is also commonly used to distinguish the two conditions.

Depending on the severity of valvular incompetence, IABC may be necessary to support cardiac function until the mitral valve is surgically repaired or replaced. Before surgical intervention, it is preferable to perform coronary angiography for identification of coexisting coronary artery lesions. However, patients with acute ischemic mitral regurgitation may be too critically ill to withstand cardiac catheterization. In rare cases emergency mitral valve replacement may be performed without preoperative definition of the coronary artery anatomy.

Rupture of the ventricular myocardium is an unusual complication that occurs when necrotic tissue in the area of infarction becomes too weakened to withstand intraventricular pressure. Depending on the area of infarct, either the free wall or ventricular septum may rupture. Rupture in either location occurs only with transmural infarction, generally within 1 week of acute MI, and classically in the periphery of the infarct, at the junction of necrotic and healthy tissue (Roberts, 1980).

Ventricular free wall rupture occurs in as many as 10% of patients who die in the hospital of acute MI (Pasternak et al., 1992). It is nearly always fatal. Ventricular wall rupture is treated with immediate operative intervention. Portable cardiopulmonary bypass may be necessary to support the patient during transport to the operating room and until formal cardiopulmonary bypass is instituted. Rarely, the rupture is small and bleeding is contained by pericardium. Such a *contained rupture* forms a *pseudoaneurysm* (i.e., false aneurysm). The term pseudoaneurysm denotes that the aneurysm wall consists of pericardium and not myocardium, as would be the case with a true ventricular aneurysm. Pseudoaneurysms are also treated with surgical resection because delayed rupture can occur at any time.

Ventricular septal rupture occurs less frequently than rupture of the ventricular free wall. However, survival from septal rupture is more likely if recognition and treatment are prompt. Acute septal rupture is usually associated with extensive transmural infarction in a patient with less diffuse CAD and thus less well-developed collateral vessels (Johnson et al., 1991). Septal rupture produces an *acute ventricular septal defect*. Acute ventricular septal defect after an anterior MI is usually apical; inferior infarctions are associated with rupture of the basal septum (Pasternak et al., 1992).

The diagnosis of ventricular septal defect is suggested by a new holosystolic murmur, particularly in the presence of hypotension, congestive heart failure, or cardiogenic shock after acute MI. The diagnosis is confirmed by measurement of pulmonary artery oxygen saturation, as previously described, or by echocardiography. An intra-aortic balloon catheter is generally placed on detection of the defect. Counterpulsation is important in maintaining hemodynamic stability until surgical repair is undertaken. It decreases afterload, thereby increasing forward flow and reducing left to right shunting through the defect. Pharmacologic support of cardiac function is generally required as well. Mortality associated with acute ventricular septal defect is high; 25% of patients die within 24 hours, 50% die within 1 week, and only 20% survive more than 4 weeks (Kirklin et al., 1993d).

Surgical closure of the defect is performed immediately in hemodynamically unstable patients. However, timing of operation in relation to MI greatly affects operative mortality and remains controversial in patients who are hemodynamically stable. Many surgeons favor emergency operative repair as soon as the defect is diagnosed because precipitous, fatal hemodynamic deterioration can occur at any time. Other surgeons believe that operative repair should be delayed for several weeks unless hemodynamic deterioration occurs. Delay of the operation allows time for the myocardium to recover from the infarct and for the defect edges to strengthen, making the procedure technically easier. Waiting 6 to 8 weeks improves the likelihood of surviving the operation, but many patients who might have survived with early surgical repair die during the waiting period (Komeda et al., 1990).

REFERENCES

Acinapura AJ, Rose DM, Cunningham JN, et al, 1988: Coronary artery bypass in septuagenarians: Analysis of morbidity and mortality. Circulation 78(Suppl I):I-179

American Heart Association, 1991: 1992 Heart and Stroke Facts. Dallas, American Heart Association

Andrien P, Lemberg L, 1990: Thrombolytic therapy in acute myocardial infarction. Heart Lung 19:1

Becker RC, Alpert JS, 1991: Investigation and treatment of the patient with Q-wave myocardial infarction. In Roberts R (ed): Coronary Heart Disease and Risk Factors. Mount Kisco, NY, Futura Publishing

Black L, Coombs VJ, Townsend SN, 1990: Reperfusion and reperfusion injury in acute myocardial infarction. Heart Lung 19:3

Braunwald E, Sobel BE, 1992: Coronary blood flow and myocardial ischemia. In Braunwald E (ed): Heart Disease: A Textbook of Cardiovascular Medicine, ed. 4. Philadelphia, WB Saunders

Brown G, Albers JJ, Fisher LD, et al, 1990: Regression of coronary artery disease as a result of intensive lipid-lowering therapy in men with high levels of apolipoprotein B. N Engl J Med 323:1289

Buchwald H, Varco RL, Matts JP, et al, 1990: Effect of partial ileal bypass surgery on mortality and morbidity from coronary heart disease in patients with hypercholesterolemia. N Engl J Med 323:946

Campeau L, 1976: Grading of angina pectoris. Circulation 54:522

Chung EK, 1988: Coronary artery disease. In Chung EK: Manual of Acute Cardiac Disorders. Boston, Butterworths

Churchwell AL, 1991: Ventricular aneurysm due to myocardial infarction. In Hurst JW (ed): Current Therapy in Cardiovascular Disease, ed. 3. Philadelphia, BC Decker

Douglas JS, 1991: Coronary angioplasty. In Hurst JW (ed): Current Therapy in Cardiovascular Disease, ed. 3. Philadelphia, BC Decker

Epstein SE, Palmeri ST, 1984: Mechanisms contributing to precipitation of unstable angina and acute myocardial infarction: Implications regarding therapy. Am J Cardiol 54:1245

Farmer JA, Gotto AM, 1992: Risk factors for coronary artery disease. In Braunwald E (ed): Heart Disease: A Textbook of Cardiovascular Medicine, ed. 4. Philadelphia, WB Saunders

Fisch C, 1992: Electrocardiography and vectorcardiography. In Braunwald E (ed): Heart Disease: A Textbook of Cardiovascular Medicine, ed. 4. Philadelphia, WB Saunders

Frishman WH, Furberg CD, Friedewald WT, 1984: β-Adrenergic blockade for survivors of acute myocardial infarction. N Engl J Med 310:830

Fuster V, Badimon JJ, Badimon L, 1992: Clinical-pathological correlations of coronary disease progression and regression. Circulation 86(Suppl III):III-1

Goe MR, 1989: Hyperlipoproteinemia. In Underhill SL, Woods SL, Froelicher ES, Halpenny CJ (eds): Cardiac Nursing, ed. 2. Philadelphia, JB Lippincott

Goldschlager NF, 1988: Acute myocardial infarction. In Luce JM, Pierson DJ (eds): Critical Care Medicine. Philadelphia, WB Saunders

Gottlieb SO, 1992: Cardiovascular benefits of smoking cessation. Heart Dis Stroke 1:173

Grines CL, Browne KF, Marco J, et al, 1993: A comparison of immediate angioplasty with thrombolytic therapy for acute myocardial infarction. N Engl J Med 328:673

Gruentzig A, 1978: Transluminal dilatation of coronary artery stenosis. Lancet 1:263

Harris EA, 1987: Cardiovascular effects of cocaine use. Prog Cardiovasc Nurs 2:53

Hillis LD, Lange RA, Wells PJ, Winniford MD, 1992a: Exertional angina pectoris. In: Manual of Clinical Problems in Cardiology, ed. 4. Boston, Little, Brown & Co

Hillis LD, Lange RA, Wells PJ, Winniford MD, 1992b: Coronary arterial spasm. In: Manual of Clinical Problems in Cardiology, ed. 4. Boston, Little, Brown & Co

Hillis LD, Lange RA, Wells PJ, Winniford MD, 1992c: Atrioventricular block complicating myocardial infarction. In: Manual of Clinical Problems in Cardiology, ed. 4. Boston, Little, Brown & Co

Hillis LD, Lange RA, Wells PJ, Winniford MD, 1992d: Detection and quantitation of myocardial infarction. In: Manual of Clinical Problems in Cardiology, ed. 4. Boston, Little, Brown & Co

Hoogwerf BJ, Sheeler LR, Licata AA, 1991: Endocrine management of the open heart surgical patient. Semin Thorac Cardiovasc Surg 3:75

Hurst JW, 1987: Percutaneous transluminal coronary angioplasty: A word of caution. Circulation 75:5

ISIS-2 (Second International Study of Infarct Survival) Collaborative Group, 1988: Randomised trial of intravenous streptokinase, oral aspirin, both, or neither among 17,187 cases of suspected acute myocardial infarction: ISIS-2. Lancet 1:349

Johnson RG, Jacobs ML, Dagget WM Jr, 1991: Postinfarction ventricular septal rupture. In Baue AE, Geha AS, Hammond GL, et al (eds): Glenn's Thoracic and Cardiovascular Surgery, ed. 5. Norwalk, CT, Appleton & Lange

Kadota LT, Burke LE, 1990: Nitrates. In Underhill SL, Woods SL, Froelicher ES, Halpenny CJ (eds): Cardiovascular Medications for Cardiac Nursing. Philadelphia, JB Lippincott

Kern LS, 1991: The elderly heart surgery patient. Nurs Clin North Am 3:749

Kessler KM, 1991: Cardiac arrhythmias following myocardial infarction. In Hurst JW (ed): Current Therapy in Cardiovascular Disease, ed. 3. Philadelphia, BC Decker

Kirklin JW, Barratt-Boyes BG, 1993a: Stenotic arteriosclerotic coronary artery disease. In Cardiac Surgery, ed. 2. New York, Churchill Livingstone

Kirklin JW, Barratt-Boyes BG, 1993b: Left ventricular aneurysm. In: Cardiac Surgery, ed. 2. New York, Churchill Livingstone

Kirklin JW, Barratt-Boyes BG, 1993c: Mitral incompetence from ischemic heart disease. In Cardiac Surgery, ed. 2. New York, Churchill Livingstone

Kirklin JW, Barratt-Boyes BG, 1993d: Postinfarction ventricular septal defect. In Cardiac Surgery, ed. 2. New York, Churchill Livingstone

Kirshenbaum JM, 1992: Therapy for acute myocardial infarction: An update. Heart Dis Stroke 1:211

Klein MS, 1991: Chronic ischemic heart disease. In Roberts R (ed): Coronary Heart Disease and Risk Factors. Mount Kisco, NY, Futura Publishing

Komeda M, Fremes SE, David TE, 1990: Surgical repair of postinfarction ventricular septal defect. Circulation 82(Suppl IV):IV-243

Kutcher MA, 1991: Angina pectoris: stable. In Hurst JW (ed): Current Therapy in Cardiovascular Disease, ed. 3. Philadelphia, BC Decker

Lee TH, Goldman L, 1986: Serum enzyme assays in the diagnosis of acute myocardial infarction. Ann Intern Med 105:221

Lieber CS, 1984: To drink (moderately) or not to drink. N Engl J Med 310:846

Morris DC, Walter PF, Hurst JW, 1990: The recognition and treatment of myocardial infarction and its complications. In Hurst JW, Schlant RC, Rackley CE, et al (eds): The Heart, ed. 7. New York, McGraw-Hill

Mueller HS, 1989: Management of acute myocardial infarction. In Shoemaker WC, Ayres S, Grenvik A, et al (eds): Textbook of Critical Care, ed. 2. Philadelphia, WB Saunders

Passen EL, Schaer GL, 1991: Acute myocardial infarction. In Parrillo JE (ed): Current Therapy in Critical Care Medicine, ed. 2. Philadelphia, BC Decker

Pasternak RC, Braunwald E, Sobel BE, 1992: Acute myocardial infarction. In Braunwald E (ed): Heart Disease: A Textbook of Cardiovascular Medicine, ed. 4. Philadelphia, WB Saunders

Peberdy MA, Ornato JP, 1992: Coronary artery disease in women. Heart Dis Stroke 1:315

Raizner AE, 1991: Angioplasty and ischemic heart disease. In Roberts R (ed): Coronary Heart Disease and Risk Factors. Mount Kisco, NY, Futura Publishing

Reaven GM, 1993: Are triglycerides important as a risk factor for coronary disease? Heart Dis Stroke 2:44

Riegel B, 1988: Acute myocardial infarction: Nursing interventions to optimize oxygen supply and demand. In Kern LS (ed): Cardiac Critical Care Nursing. Rockville, MD, Aspen Publishers

Roberts R, Pratt CM, 1991: Medical treatment of coronary artery disease. In Roberts R (ed): Coronary Heart Disease and Risk Factors. Mount Kisco, NY, Futura Publishing

Roberts WC, 1980: Morphologic features of certain myocardial complications. In Moran JM, Michaelis LL (eds): Surgery for the Complications of Myocardial Infarction. New York, Grune & Stratton

Robison JS, 1987: Acute right ventricular infarction: Recognition, evaluation, and treatment. Crit Care Nurs: 7:4

Ross R, 1992: The pathogenesis of atherosclerosis. In Braunwald E (ed): Heart Disease: A Textbook of Cardiovascular Medicine, ed. 4. Philadelphia, WB Saunders

Ross R, 1990: Factors influencing atherogenesis. In Hurst JW, Schlant RC, Rackley CE, et al (eds): The Heart, ed. 7. New York, McGraw-Hill

Rutherford JD, Braunwald E, 1992: Chronic ischemic heart disease. In Braunwald E (ed): Heart Disease: A Textbook of Cardiovascular Medicine, ed. 4. Philadelphia, WB Saunders

Sobel BE, Jaffe AS, 1993: The value and limitations of cardiac enzymes in the recognition of acute myocardial infarction. Heart Dis Stroke 2:26

Stone NJ, 1990: Clinical approach to hyperlipidemia. Cardiovasc Rev Rep 90:39

Stone NJ, Green D, 1980: Sustaining factors in atherosclerosis. In Moran JM, Michaelis LL (eds): Surgery for the Complications of Myocardial Infarction. New York, Grune & Stratton

Stratton JR, Resnick AD, 1987: Increased embolic risk in patients with left ventricular thrombi. Circulation 75:5

Taylor AE, Johnson DC, Kazemi H, 1992: Environmental tobacco smoke and cardiovascular disease. Circulation 86:699

Theroux P, 1991: Management of unstable angina. In Roberts R (ed): Coronary Heart Disease and Risk Factors. Mount Kisco, NY, Futura Publishing

Wenger NK, 1990: Prevention of coronary atherosclerosis. In Hurst JW, Schlant RC, Rackley CE, et al (eds): The Heart, ed. 7. New York, McGraw-Hill

Yee BH, 1986: Coronary artery disease: Clinical sequelae. In Yee BH, Zorb SL (eds): Cardiac Critical Care Nursing. Boston, Little, Brown & Co

VALVULAR HEART DISEASE

Valvular heart disease (VHD) is a significant health problem in the United States, although it is far less common than coronary artery disease. VHD is characterized by impaired function of one or more of the four cardiac valves. Either or both of two functional abnormalities may be present: *stenosis* (impeded forward flow through an opened valve) or *regurgitation* (backward leaking of blood through a closed valve). VHD affects the left-sided valves (mitral and aortic) more commonly than those on the right (tricuspid and pulmonic). Mitral valve disease is most prevalent. Tricuspid valve disease usually occurs secondary to left-sided valvular lesions. Pulmonic valve disease is rare in adults. In some patients, more than one valve is diseased. For example, end-stage mitral regurgitation may cause right ventricular enlargement that leads to annular dilatation and regurgitation of the tricuspid valve.

ETIOLOGIES

A variety of etiologies can lead to VHD. In most cases, pathologic changes in valvular endothelium occur gradually and the heart compensates for pro-

gressively worsening valve function for many years. Less commonly, etiologic factors, such as myocardial infarction or infective endocarditis, cause acute valvular dysfunction and precipitous hemodynamic instability.

RHEUMATIC HEART DISEASE

Chronic rheumatic valvular disease is the result of an inflammatory process caused by *acute rheumatic fever*. In the United States, the incidence of rheumatic heart disease has substantially decreased in recent decades owing to widespread, effective prophylaxis against rheumatic fever in children (Spencer, 1990). However, in developing countries, which contain two thirds of the world's population, rheumatic fever is the leading cause of cardiovascular death in the first 5 decades of life (Kaplan, 1990). In these countries, a rapid and progressive form of valvular disease may follow rheumatic fever in children and young adults (John et al., 1990).

Acute rheumatic fever occurs primarily in children between 5 and 15 years of age (Kaplan, 1990). The exact mechanism for its development is not clear, but the primary etiologic factor is known to be a group A

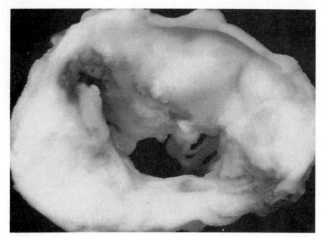

FIGURE 2-1. Resected mitral valve demonstrating scarring and leaflet retraction due to rheumatic fever. (Hurst JW, Rackley CE, Becker AE, Wilcox, BR, 1988: Valvar heart disease. In Hurst JW, Anderson RH, Becker AE, Wilcox BR [eds]: Atlas of the Heart, p. 4.37. London, Times Mirror International)

streptococcal infection of the pharynx, more commonly known as "strep throat." The syndrome is insidious, producing generalized malaise, low-grade fevers, and arthralgias. Patients in whom the diagnosis of acute rheumatic fever is suspected are treated with penicillin or another appropriate antibiotic (Kaplan, 1991). Treatment also includes aspirin, corticosteroids, and bed rest. Recurring attacks of rheumatic fever are characteristic, occurring in 30% to 50% of individuals.

Rheumatic endocarditis occurs when endothelial tissue, generally that comprising the cardiac valves, becomes inflamed, causing edema, lymphatic infiltration, and neovascularization of leaflets (Jacobs & Austen, 1990). With each subsequent bout of acute rheumatic fever, damage is compounded (Fig. 2-1). Chronic rheumatic endocarditis produces three distinct pathologic changes in valvular structures: (1) fusion of the commissures between valve leaflets; (2) fibrosis, stiffening, retraction, and calcification of leaflets; and (3) in the atrioventricular valves, fusion and shortening of chordae tendineae (Spencer, 1990). Although the interval is variable, in the United States it generally takes 2 decades or more after acute rheumatic fever for clinically significant rheumatic valve disease to develop. The mitral valve is most often affected, in isolation or with associated aortic or tricuspid valve involvement. Rheumatic endocarditis of only the aortic or tricuspid valve is less common.

INFECTIVE ENDOCARDITIS

Infective endocarditis is localized infection of one or more of the cardiac valves. It occurs when organisms (usually bacteria, but occasionally fungi) enter the bloodstream and invade cardiac valvular endothelial tissue. Although the term *subacute bacterial endocarditis*

has traditionally been used to describe this condition, infective endocarditis has more recently been adopted because the condition is usually acute and the invading pathogen may not be bacterial. Infective endocarditis most often occurs in individuals with a valve or valves that are already damaged by another disease, such as mitral valve prolapse, rheumatic endocarditis, a congenital malformation, or previous infection. However, normal cardiac valves are also susceptible to particularly virulent organisms (e.g., *Staphylococcus aureus*) or when there is repetitive blood contamination from intravenous drug abuse.

Native valve endocarditis in individuals who are not intravenous drug abusers is usually caused by streptococci (50%–70%), staphylococci (25%), or enterococci (10%); in intravenous drug abusers, *S. aureus* is the responsible pathogen in 60%, streptococci or enterococci in 20%, gram-negative bacilli in 10%, and fungi in 5% (Korzeniowski & Kaye, 1992). Bacteria or other organisms can enter the bloodstream from the mouth, gastrointestinal tract, skin, or contaminated needles used for venipuncture. Ordinary dental procedures in susceptible individuals are one of the most common sources of infection. Often, the precipitating cause of the bacteremia is never identified.

The infective process causes erosion of leaflet tissue and deposition of fibrin, leukocytes, and platelets on the leaflet, forming particulate matter known as a *vegetation* (Fig. 2-2). Leaflet perforation may occur, or, in the case of mitral or tricuspid valve endocarditis, chordae tendineae may be destroyed. The degree of valvular damage is dependent on the pathogenicity of the infecting organism, the duration of infection, and the timeliness of appropriate antibiotic therapy (Larbalestier et al., 1992). In severe cases, infection

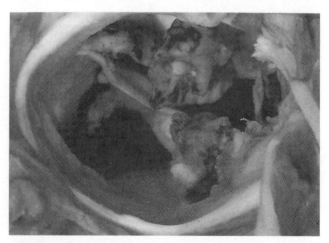

FIGURE 2-2. Infective endocarditis of this aortic valve has caused extensive destruction of leaflet tissue with resultant acute aortic regurgitation. (Hurst JW, Rackley CE, Becker AE, Wilcox BR, 1988: Valvar heart disease. In Hurst JW, Anderson RH, Becker AE, Wilcox BR [eds]: Atlas of the Heart, p. 4.18. London, Times Mirror International)

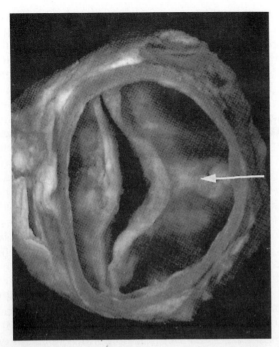

FIGURE 2-3. Bicuspid aortic valve viewed from above; note the raphe or seam (*arrow*) fusing the right and left coronary leaflets. The valve is also thickened and stenotic. (Hurst JW, Nugent EW, Anderson RH, Wilcox BR, 1988: Congenital heart disease. In Hurst JW, Anderson RH, Becker AE, Wilcox BR [eds]: Atlas of the Heart, p. 3.39. London, Times Mirror International)

CONGENITAL MALFORMATION

The most common congenital valve malformation is a *bicuspid aortic valve* (Fig. 2-3). Normally, the aortic valve is tricuspid, composed of three leaflets or cusps. If one or both of the valve commissures is absent, the valve is bicuspid or unicuspid, respectively. Bicuspid aortic valves are estimated to occur in 1% of the general population (Fuster et al., 1991). The abnormality is most common in males and may be accompanied by other congenital cardiac defects. A bicuspid aortic valve is predisposed to calcification and is susceptible to infective endocarditis (Nugent et al., 1990). The abnormal valve frequently produces no hemodynamic dysfunction during childhood. However, progressive sclerosis, thickening, and calcification may cause the valve to become increasingly stenotic as the individual ages. A bicuspid aortic valve may also become regurgitant.

Congenital pulmonic valve stenosis is another common congenital cardiac anomaly. It usually consists of a dome-shaped valve with a central opening and fused commissures (Warnes et al., 1991). Hemodynamically significant pulmonic stenosis is almost always corrected during childhood and thus is unusual in adults. *Congenital mitral valve malformation* is rare. *Marfan's syndrome*, a heritable connective tissue disorder, can produce myxomatous valvular degeneration and can be associated with aortic, mitral, or tricuspid valve regurgitation. Marfan's syndrome is discussed in more detail in Chapter 3, Disorders of the Thoracic Aorta.

OTHER ACQUIRED DISEASES

Acquired aortic valvular stenosis (aortic valve sclerosis) is the most common valvular abnormality in elderly persons (Fig. 2-4). It occurs secondary to degenera-

extends beyond endocardial tissue of the valve to form intramyocardial abscesses. In aortic valve endocarditis, the infective process may involve the adjacent aortic root, resulting in valve ring abscess or sinus of Valsalva rupture (Lindsay et al., 1990).

MITRAL VALVE PROLAPSE

Mitral valve prolapse (MVP), or *Barlow's syndrome*, is the most common valvular abnormality, occurring in an estimated 1% to 5% of the population. MVP is diagnosed most frequently in young and middle-aged adults, particularly young women (Underhill & McGregor, 1989). Although it is usually a benign condition, it comprises a continuum of degrees of valvular abnormality. In its most common form, MVP is not associated with valvular regurgitation or any significant clinical sequelae. It is detected only by the presence of an auscultatory ejection click and its characteristic echocardiographic features. On the other end of the spectrum, however, are individuals with severely myxomatous and redundant valve leaflets that prolapse into the left atrium during systole. These patients are likely to develop mitral regurgitation, which may be chronic or which may increase acutely if a chordal structure tears. Ventricular arrhythmias may occur as well and often persist despite surgical replacement of the mitral valve.

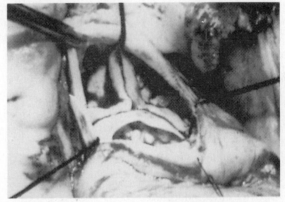

FIGURE 2-4. Severely stenotic, calcified aortic valve. The obstruction to blood flow across this valve is created by sclerotic changes in the leaflets themselves and by masses of calcium deposits on their mural surface. (Robicsek F, Harbold NB, Daugherty HK, et al, 1988: Balloon valvuloplasty in calcified aortic stenosis: A cause for caution and alarm. Ann Thorac Surg 45:519; reprinted with permission from the Society of Thoracic Surgeons)

tive calcification and fibrosis of the aortic valve. As the number of elderly persons in this country increases, severe aortic stenosis in persons in the eighth or ninth decade of life has become more commonplace. *Ischemic heart disease* can produce dysfunction or rupture of the mitral valve's supportive apparatus (chordae tendineae or papillary muscles). Diseases of the ascending aorta often lead to aortic regurgitation. For example, *aortic dissection* that extends in a retrograde fashion to the aortic valve annulus produces valvular incompetence. An *ascending aortic aneurysm* can also cause aortic regurgitation by dilating and distorting the valve annulus. *Myxomatous valvular degeneration* is fairly common, particularly in association with MVP. Rarely, damage to cardiac valves occurs secondary to *blunt* or *penetrating chest trauma.*

MITRAL VALVE DISEASE

The mitral valve is a complex structure comprising several components: leaflets, chordae tendineae, papillary muscles, and annulus. Abnormalities of any of these structures can produce functional problems. Mitral valve disease is most often caused by rheumatic fever, MVP, or coronary artery disease. Causes of mitral valve disease are listed in Table 2-1.

MITRAL STENOSIS

Mitral stenosis is narrowing of the mitral valve orifice that impedes blood flow into the left ventricle during diastole. A stenotic valve may represent one or more pathologic changes in valve structure, including (1)

TABLE 2-1. ETIOLOGIES OF MITRAL VALVE DISEASE

Mitral Stenosis

Rheumatic heart disease
Atrial myxoma
Vegetation
Annular calcification
Congenital deformity

Mitral Regurgitation

Mitral valve prolapse
Coronary artery disease
   Papillary muscle dysfunction or rupture
   Annular dilatation
   Chordae tendinae elongation or rupture
Infective endocarditis
Cardiomyopathy
Rheumatic heart disease
Connective tissue disorders
   Marfan's syndrome
   Ehlers-Danlos syndrome
Congenital deformity
Systemic lupus erythematosus
Trauma

calcification, thickening, or scarring of leaflets; (2) fusion of commissures; and (3) fusion or shortening of chordae tendineae. In adults, it is almost always due to rheumatic endocarditis, although a history of rheumatic fever is elicited in only 50% to 60% of patients (Schlant, 1991). Rare causes of mitral stenosis include atrial myxoma, vegetations, annular calcification, and congenital deformity of the valve (Rackley et al., 1990a; Schlant, 1991).

Mitral stenosis is generally diagnosed by auscultation of a characteristic low-pitched, apical diastolic murmur. Severity of valvular stenosis is described in two ways. First, an estimated valve area may be calculated. The orifice of the open mitral valve normally measures 4 to 6 cm^2. A valve opening less than 2.5 cm^2 is moderately stenotic; in severe stenosis, the valve area may measure less than 1 cm^2. Second, pressures in the chambers retrograde and antegrade to the valve may be measured. In contrast to the normal similarity of left atrial and ventricular pressures during diastole, a stenotic mitral valve produces an abnormal pressure gradient between the two chambers.

A pressure gradient as high as 30 to 40 mm Hg may develop as left atrial pressure rises to compensate for mitral valve narrowing. Because there are no valves between the left atrium and pulmonary vasculature, the elevated atrial pressure is transmitted into the pulmonary veins and capillaries. If the left atrium is poorly compliant (i.e., it does not distend in response to increased left atrial pressure), more of the pressure is transmitted to the pulmonary vascular bed and mitral stenosis is not well tolerated. More commonly, chronically elevated left atrial pressure produces left atrial enlargement (dilatation and hypertrophy). This compensatory mechanism allows the pulmonary circulation to better tolerate the increased left atrial pressure.

Chronically increased left atrial pressure eventually produces damaging changes in left atrial muscle, pulmonary vasculature, lungs, and right ventricle. Atrial muscle architecture disintegrates, leading to intractable atrial fibrillation and a resultant reduction in cardiac output and increased left atrial pressure (Kirklin & Barratt-Boyes, 1993a). Because the fibrillating atria fail to contract in an organized fashion, blood many stagnate along atrial walls and form intra-atrial thrombus. Systemic embolization may result, producing arterial occlusion at any of a variety of sites throughout the systemic circulation. Individuals at increased risk for systemic embolism, particularly a cerebral vascular accident, include those with decreased cardiac output, left atrial enlargement, or advanced age. Left atrial enlargement can also produce hoarseness due to compression of the left recurrent laryngeal nerve, dysphagia due to esophageal displacement, or cough due to bronchial irritation (Goldberger, 1982).

Ten to 20% of patients with mitral stenosis develop pulmonary vascular disease and disproportionate pulmonary hypertension (Schlant, 1991). When pulmonary artery pressure exceeds the oncotic pressure of plasma, transudation of fluid into the pulmonary interstitial tissue occurs, and the patient may develop pulmonary edema (Spencer, 1990). To compensate for chronic fluid transudation, lymphatic channels hypertrophy and drain the flooded alveoli. Chronic pulmonary congestion also causes thickening of alveolar walls and may produce areas of pulmonary infarction or hemorrhage. The right ventricle hypertrophies in response to increased pulmonary artery pressure and eventually dilates. When the distended right ventricle can no longer compensate, the patient develops debilitating symptoms of right-sided heart failure. Although the left ventricle is protected from chronic dilatation and failure by the stenotic mitral valve, it probably does not remain normal.

The most common symptom of mitral stenosis is shortness of breath, specifically dyspnea on exertion, paroxysmal nocturnal dyspnea, or orthopnea. Exertional dyspnea is most common and episodes of pulmonary edema may occur. The chronically reduced preload is thought to impair the left ventricle's capacity to increase cardiac output in response to increased metabolic demand. Attempts to increase cardiac output with exercise typically produce significant dyspnea for the patient (Spencer, 1990). Other common symptoms of mitral stenosis include cough, fatigue, and palpitations. Hemoptysis may also occur as blood enters the bronchioles from engorged pulmonary vessels that have ruptured.

Fatigue and exercise intolerance typically cause patients with mitral stenosis to adopt an increasingly sedentary life-style. With such adaptations and appropriate medical therapy, a stenotic mitral valve is usually tolerated for many years before corrective therapy becomes necessary. Often, a pregnancy, with its associated hemodynamic alterations (i.e., increased blood volume and cardiac output) precipitates a deterioration in functional status. Percutaneous balloon valvotomy, surgical commissurotomy, or valve replacement is recommended in a symptomatic patient when mitral valve area decreases to less than 1.2 cm² (Rapaport, 1993).

MITRAL REGURGITATION

Mitral regurgitation is the leakage of a portion of left ventricular stroke volume into the left atrium during ventricular systole. It is most often caused by (1) MVP, (2) scarring and retraction of leaflets due to rheumatic fever, (3) distortion of the relationship between leaflets and subvalvular apparatus secondary to left ventricular dilatation, or (4) ischemic damage to the subvalvular apparatus of the valve (see Table 2-1). Mitral regurgitation is most often chronic but can develop acutely. It may be diagnosed by a late systolic or holosystolic murmur at the apex of the heart. The severity of valvular incompetence in combination with the amount of resistance to forward flow (after-

load) determines the degree of regurgitation (Underhill & McGregor, 1989). Valvular regurgitation is categorized by angiographic techniques using a four-point grading system, ranging from 1+ (mild) to 4+ (severe).

Regurgitation of a portion of each stroke volume through the malfunctioning valve causes increased volume and pressure in the left atrium with resultant marked chamber dilatation. In contrast to mitral stenosis, the left ventricle is not protected in mitral regurgitation. Left ventricular hypertrophy develops as the ventricle pumps more forcefully to maintain adequate forward flow. If significant regurgitation continues, left ventricular hypertrophy is followed by eventual ventricular dilatation and failure. Pulmonary congestion occurs as with mitral stenosis, and eventually the right ventricle fails.

Symptoms develop late in the course of chronic mitral regurgitation and are often insidious (Raizner & Siegel, 1991). They include fatigue, dyspnea on exertion, orthopnea, palpitations, and paroxysmal nocturnal dyspnea. As with mitral stenosis, the heart's ability to increase cardiac output in response to increased demands is impeded. Therefore, limitation of activities is common. With severe mitral regurgitation, atrial fibrillation and systemic embolization may occur.

Mitral regurgitation sometimes develops acutely as a result of (1) papillary muscle or chordae tendineae dysfunction or rupture secondary to myocardial infarction; (2) infective endocarditis; or, rarely, (3) blunt trauma. Acute mitral regurgitation generally produces precipitous hemodynamic instability. Because the left atrium is poorly distensible, pulmonary venous pressure increases suddenly. As a result, pulmonary edema and left ventricular failure develop rapidly.

AORTIC VALVE DISEASE

AORTIC STENOSIS

Aortic stenosis is narrowing that obstructs left ventricular outflow into the aorta during systole. In adults, aortic stenosis is almost always due to abnormalities of the valve leaflets. Common etiologies include congenital valve malformation, calcific degeneration (aortic valve sclerosis), and rheumatic heart disease (Rackley et al., 1990b). Supravalvular (narrowing of the ascending aorta) or subvalvular (left ventricular fibrous ring or tunnel) stenosis occasionally occurs (Saenz et al., 1987) (Table 2-2).

The degree of orifice narrowing may vary from mild to severe and determines the compensatory responses and symptoms. The open aortic valve orifice normally measures 2.5 to 3.5 cm². When the orifice narrows to 0.5 to 0.75 cm², significant obstruction to left ventricular outflow exists. As left ventricular pressure increases to maintain normal systemic arte-

TABLE 2-2. ETIOLOGIES OF AORTIC VALVE DISEASE

Aortic Stenosis
Congenital deformity
Aortic valve sclerosis
Rheumatic heart disease
Supravalvular stenosis
Subvalvular stenosis

Aortic Regurgitation
Rheumatic heart disease
Syphilis
Infective endocarditis
Aortitis
Congenital deformity
Aortic dissection
Aortic aneurysm
Annuloaortic ectasia
Connective tissue disorders
   Cystic medial necrosis
   Marfan's syndrome
Trauma
Arthritic inflammatory diseases

rial pressure, a gradient develops between systolic left ventricular and aortic pressures. A gradient greater than 50 mm Hg represents clinically significant aortic stenosis, and gradients as high as 100 to 120 mm Hg may occur. Aortic stenosis is associated with a systolic ejection murmur and an ejection click. Because systolic ejection is prolonged, the arterial pulse wave has a delayed upstroke and increased duration (Jacobs & Austen, 1990).

Over time, the left ventricular muscle mass hypertrophies to generate adequate pressure to eject blood through the stenotic valve orifice. Although systolic function (contractility) is initially preserved by the compensatory hypertrophy, diastolic filling (compliance) of the ventricle is impaired (Rackley et al., 1990b). Eventually, the ventricle dilates and systolic function deteriorates as well. Left-sided failure occurs as the left ventricle is forced to work increasingly harder to eject blood into the aorta. Left ventricular end-diastolic pressure rises, cardiac output and ejection fraction decrease, and pulmonary hypertension develops (Rackley et al., 1990b).

The heart generally compensates for a stenotic aortic valve for many years, producing no symptoms until mid or late life (Ronan, 1991). However, average life expectancy is 5 years or less from the onset of clinical symptoms (Kirklin & Barratt-Boyes, 1993b). The classic symptoms of aortic stenosis are angina, dyspnea on exertion, and syncope. Angina occurs in approximately two thirds of patients with aortic stenosis (Braunwald, 1992). It is produced by the imbalance between oxygen demand and supply. Demand is increased because of left ventricular muscle hypertrophy, and supply is compromised because the stenotic valve is obstructive to left ventricular output. Diastolic filling of the coronary arteries is also impaired by the hypertrophied, poorly compliant ventricle. Angina caused by aortic stenosis may be erroneously attributed to coronary artery disease. In other cases, both aortic stenosis and coronary artery disease are present and the angina may be produced by either condition. Because both disease processes produce similar symptomatology, coronary angiography is often necessary to determine the correct etiology of the angina.

Effort dyspnea, orthopnea, paroxysmal nocturnal dyspnea, or frank pulmonary edema occurs in 30% to 40% of patients; these symptoms are associated with increased left ventricular end-diastolic pressure and systolic wall stress and decreased cardiac output and ejection fraction (Kirklin & Barratt-Boyes, 1993b). Syncopal episodes may also occur. The precise pathologic mechanism for syncope is not well understood but may be related to an inability to increase cardiac output in response to effort.

Ventricular arrhythmias and conduction disturbances are also common. Sudden cardiac death is estimated to occur in 15% to 20% of symptomatic patients with aortic stenosis and has been attributed to arrhythmias or myocardial ischemia caused by increased oxygen demands of the hypertrophied ventricle (Rackley et al., 1990b). The risk of sudden cardiac death increases markedly when the gradient across the valve is high. Ventricular tachycardia and fibrillation are easily sustained in the hypertrophic left ventricle. Consequently, patients with severe aortic stenosis are notoriously difficult to resuscitate if cardiac arrest occurs. Ventricular arrhythmias associated with aortic stenosis are thought to be related to the abnormal ventricle rather than to the valve itself. Thus, the arrhythmic disorder is generally not corrected by valve replacement and life-long antiarrhythmic therapy may be necessary. In patients with extensive calcification of a stenotic aortic valve, complete heart block occasionally develops (Kirklin & Barratt-Boyes, 1993b).

Patients with aortic stenosis are particularly sensitive to afterload reduction or hypovolemia. Because of fixed obstruction to ventricular output and poor compliance of the ventricle, vasodilating medications, volume loss, or bleeding are poorly tolerated and may lead to catastrophic hemodynamic compromise. Therapeutic maneuvers such as induction of general anesthesia or administration of diuretic or afterload-reducing agents must be performed with caution.

AORTIC REGURGITATION

Aortic regurgitation is leakage of a portion of left ventricular stroke volume from the aorta backward into the ventricle during diastole. It may result from primary disease of the aortic valve leaflets, the wall of the aortic root, or both (Braunwald, 1992). Chronic aortic regurgitation is commonly caused by rheumatic fever or, less often, a bicuspid aortic valve. Aortic diseases producing chronic aortic regurgitation include ascending aortic aneurysm, chronic aortic dissection, Marfan's syndrome, cystic medial necrosis, syphilitic aortitis, and inflammatory disorders of the aorta (see Table 2-2).

Severity of aortic regurgitation is determined by the size of the regurgitant orifice and the pressure gradient between the aorta and left ventricle during diastole (Jacobs & Austen, 1990). In the early stages of aortic regurgitation, the ventricle hypertrophies, producing an increased ventricular ejection fraction. A compensatory decrease in systemic vascular resistance occurs to facilitate forward flow. Peripheral vasodilation and regurgitation of blood into the left ventricle result in a low diastolic arterial pressure. Systolic arterial pressure, on the other hand, is high as the ventricle works to maintain an adequate ejection fraction. Eventually, chronic aortic regurgitation causes the left ventricle to dilate and lose its ability to contract effectively (i.e., systolic impairment). The combination of volume overload of the left ventricle during both systole and diastole produces marked cardiomegaly.

Patients with mild or moderate chronic aortic regurgitation may remain asymptomatic for many years. However, as ventricular contractility becomes increasingly impaired, ejection fraction decreases and symptoms of left-sided heart failure, particularly dyspnea on exertion, develop. Angina is also common owing to the increased left ventricular work and mass and decreased coronary artery perfusion pressure during diastole (Jacobs & Austen, 1990).

With severe aortic regurgitation, patients may develop awareness of an audible heartbeat, head bobbing, or tickling in the throat from pressure on the uvula. Severe aortic regurgitation is also associated with a number of signs that may be apparent during physical examination, including a widened pulse pressure (high systolic and low diastolic blood pressure), bounding or "water-hammer" peripheral pulses (rapid upstroke and descent on arterial pressure tracing), Quincke's sign (alternating paling and flushing of lightly compressed nail beds or mucous membranes), and a high-pitched, decrescendo, diastolic murmur (Hillis et al., 1992).

Acute aortic regurgitation may result from acute aortic dissection that involves the aortic valve annulus, infective endocarditis, or trauma (Treasure, 1991). In acute aortic regurgitation, the left ventricle has no time to undergo the compensatory changes associated with chronic aortic regurgitation. Consequently, acute left ventricular failure with pulmonary edema or cardiogenic shock is likely to occur.

TRICUSPID AND PULMONIC VALVE DISEASE

Tricuspid valve disease is uncommon and usually occurs secondary to left-sided valvular disease. When associated with rheumatic mitral or aortic valve disease, either regurgitation or stenosis may be present.

Tricuspid regurgitation can also result from annular dilatation secondary to right ventricular enlargement; the precipitating cause is usually severe disease of the left-sided heart valves in association with pulmonary hypertension (Kirklin & Barratt-Boyes, 1993c). Tricuspid valve endocarditis, with resultant tricuspid regurgitation, may occur secondary to intravenous drug abuse, immunodeficiency, or indwelling vascular catheters (Crawley, 1991).

Infrequently, blunt trauma produces acute tricuspid regurgitation from injury to the tricuspid valve leaflets or its subvalvular apparatus. Unusual causes of tricuspid regurgitation are myocardial infarction, carcinoid, leaflet prolapse, and congenital abnormalities such as atrial septal defect or Ebstein's anomaly (Rackley et al., 1990c) (Fig. 2-5). Tricuspid stenosis is rare; in addition to rheumatic fever, its causes include carcinoid syndrome, endocardial fibroelastosis, endomyocardial fibrosis, and systemic lupus erythematosus (Rackley et al., 1990c). Tricuspid valve disease produces elevated right atrial pressure and subsequent symptoms of right-sided heart failure.

Pulmonic valve disease is rare in adults. Pulmonic stenosis is almost always congenital. The most common causes of pulmonic regurgitation are pulmonary hypertension and infective endocarditis (Braunwald, 1992).

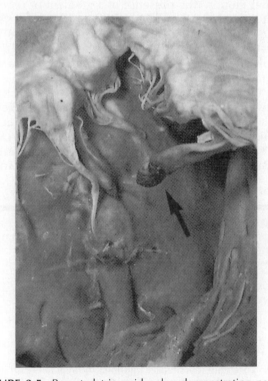

FIGURE 2-5. Resected tricuspid valve demonstrating papillary muscle rupture (*arrow*) due to myocardial infarction with resultant severe tricuspid regurgitation. (Hurst JW, Rackley CE, Becker AE, Wilcox, BR, 1988: Valvar heart disease. In Hurst JW, Anderson RH, Becker AE, Wilcox BR [eds]: Atlas of the Heart. p. 4.53. London, Times Mirror International)

DIAGNOSIS

In contrast to coronary artery disease, physical examination reveals important clues about the nature and severity of VHD. Auscultation of heart sounds may reveal a change in quality or intensity of a murmur that represents a worsening in the patient's condition. Another important diagnostic guide is clinical symptomatology produced by the dysfunctional valve. Assessment of the patient's ability to perform daily activities and of the presence and severity of associated symptoms aids in evaluating effectiveness of medical therapy and establishing optimal timing of surgical intervention.

The classic method for categorizing severity of functional impairment in patients with VHD is the New York Heart Association (NYHA) Functional Classification System (Table 2-3). A four-point scale is used to rate degree of exertion with which the classic symptoms of heart disease (i.e., chest pain, shortness of breath, palpitations, and fatigue) occur. The NYHA functional rating system is widely used because of its simplicity and usefulness in categorizing patients in a standardized fashion.

The echocardiogram, electrocardiogram, and chest roentgenogram are the primary diagnostic studies used for evaluation of VHD. Either transthoracic or transesophageal echocardiography may be performed to provide important information about valve leaflet motion, the presence of a gradient or regurgitant flow across the valve, and the presence of vegetations or thrombus. Serial electrocardiograms and chest roentgenograms are important because of the information they provide about progressive cardiac chamber hypertrophy or dilatation.

In the past, cardiac catheterization was almost performed before surgical treatment of VHD. However, the sophisticated echocardiographic and nuclear scanning techniques now available can often provide necessary diagnostic information. Therefore, cardiac catheterization is sometimes omitted if relevant information can be obtained with less invasive studies. In older adults, catheterization with coronary angiography is almost always performed to define coronary anatomy and detect coexisting coronary artery lesions that might be treated at the time of the valve surgery.

Cardiac catheterization can provide the following information about valvular abnormalities and cardiac function: (1) measurement of intracardiac pressures with calculation of valve area and pressure gradient across the valve, (2) visualization of valve leaflet appearance (e.g., abnormal thickening, redundant tissue, or presence of calcium) and movement, (3) assessment of regurgitant flow across a valve, and (4) estimation of ventricular contractility (ventriculogram).

TREATMENT

The presence of any significant valvular abnormality mandates lifelong medical supervision. Treatment varies depending on the specific valvular lesion, its etiology, and its acuity. For example, mitral stenosis is often managed medically for many years before invasive, corrective therapy is required. Conversely, early surgical correction of moderate to severe aortic stenosis in symptomatic patients is essential because of the limited life expectancy with medical therapy alone.

Management of patients with chronic mitral or aortic regurgitation varies greatly depending on severity of valvular incompetence. Asymptomatic patients with mild regurgitation may not require either pharmacologic therapy or restriction of normal activities. Moderate but asymptomatic valvular regurgitation may be adequately treated with medications and avoidance of strenuous physical activities. In patients with severe valvular regurgitation, early operative therapy may be important to avoid irreversible ventricular damage.

Acute mitral or aortic regurgitation often necessitates emergent surgical therapy to restore valve competence and correct cardiogenic shock. Intra-aortic balloon counterpulsation provides important preoperative cardiac support in patients with mitral regurgitation. However, its use is contraindicated in patients with aortic regurgitation because regurgitant flow would be worsened by balloon inflations.

PHARMACOLOGIC THERAPY

Pharmacologic treatment of VHD is aimed at improving the heart's ability to compensate for the poorly functioning valve or valves. Digitalis is used if ventricular contractility is impaired. Diuresis and sodium restriction are important in controlling congestive heart failure. Medications that reduce afterload, such as captopril, are important for mitral or aortic regurgitation. Afterload reduction enhances forward blood

---

TABLE 2-3. NEW YORK HEART ASSOCIATION FUNCTIONAL CLASSIFICATION SYSTEM

Class	Description
I	Ordinary physical activity does not cause undue fatigue, palpitation, dyspnea, or angina.
II	Ordinary physical activity causes undue fatigue, palpitation, dyspnea, or angina.
III	Less than ordinary physical activity causes undue fatigue, palpitation, dyspnea, or angina.
IV	Fatigue, palpitation, dyspnea, or angina occur at rest.

(Adapted from Criteria Committee of the New York Heart Association, 1964: Physical capacity with heart disease. In Diseases of the Heart and Blood Vessels: Nomenclature and Criteria for Diagnosis, ed. 6. Boston, Little, Brown & Co)

TABLE 2-4. EXAMPLES OF PROCEDURES REQUIRING ANTIBIOTIC PROPHYLAXIS IN PATIENTS AT RISK FOR ENDOCARDITIS

Dental procedures (e.g., cleaning, root canal)
Tonsillectomy or adenoidectomy
Urethral catheterization
Cystoscopy
Gallbladder surgery
Vaginal hysterectomy
Prostatic surgery
Incision and drainage of infected tissue

(Adapted from Dajani AS, Bisno AL, Chung KJ, et al., 1990: Prevention of bacterial endocarditis: Recommendations by the American Heart Association. JAMA 264:2919)

flow from the left ventricle, reducing regurgitant flow through the incompetent mitral or aortic valve.

Treatment of mitral valve disease often includes pharmacologic therapy for management of associated atrial fibrillation or, less commonly, atrial flutter. Medications, such as digoxin, beta-blocking agents, or calcium-channel blocking agents are used to control the rapid ventricular response to these atrial arrhythmias. However, pharmacologic agents that slow the ventricular rate when the patient is in atrial flutter may result in unacceptably slow ventricular rates with atrial fibrillation. If so, a permanent pacemaker may become necessary. Patients with atrial fibrillation also require long-term anticoagulation.

Antibiotic prophylaxis against infective endocarditis is an important component of medical therapy for all patients with valvular abnormalities. Accordingly, the American Heart Association has established recommendations to guide prophylactic antibiotic therapy (Dajani et al., 1990). Patients with valvular dysfunction due to any cause or with a valvular prosthesis require appropriate antibiotic therapy before dental procedures and instrumentation or surgery involving the respiratory, genitourinary, and gastrointestinal tissues (Table 2-4). Probably the most common source of infection is bacteremia resulting from gum disease, dental abscesses, or dental procedures. Because endocarditis can occur after even minor dental procedures, antibiotic prophylaxis is recommended in susceptible patients before all dental procedures likely to cause gingival bleeding, including routine professional cleaning (Dajani et al., 1990).

TREATMENT OF INFECTIVE ENDOCARDITIS

The increasing problem with intravenous drug abuse has made infective endocarditis a more prevalent problem. Because of the tricuspid valve's location on the right (venous) side of the heart, it is most likely to be infected by intravenous contaminants. Infective endocarditis should be suspected in any febrile patient who has a valve that is known to be abnormal,

who has a history of intravenous drug abuse, or who has been septic. Clinical manifestations of endocarditis include fever and elevated white blood cell count. If blood cultures reveal bacteremia, an echocardiogram is performed to assess valve function and to detect the presence of valvular vegetations. However, endocarditis sometimes occurs in the absence of vegetations and thus the diagnosis may be based on clinical findings alone.

Patients with confirmed infective endocarditis are treated with appropriate organism-specific intravenous antibiotics for 6 to 8 weeks. Streptococcal infections can often be cured with antibiotic therapy alone, sparing the native valve. *S. aureus* or fungal infections are more virulent, often destroying valve leaflets and producing valvular incompetence. Valve replacement may be the only effective therapy for particularly virulent or drug-resistant endocarditis.

Embolization of vegetations to the brain, abdominal viscera, or extremities is a potential threat from endocarditis of the left-sided valves and to the lungs from right-sided valves. Septic emboli are even more damaging than ordinary bland emboli. Because they contain pathogenic organisms, an additional area of infection may develop at the site of the embolus. For example, a cerebral embolus may cause a brain abscess as well as a stroke. In intravenous drug abusers, recurrent embolism of septic vegetations from the tricuspid valve to the pulmonary artery is common. The resulting pulmonary infarction can produce infection (e.g., pneumonitis or lung abscess) and atelectasis of substantial portions of lung tissue with secondary pleural effusion. Prosthetic valve endocarditis (infection of valvular prostheses) is discussed in Chapter 16, Surgical Treatment of Valvular Heart Disease.

BALLOON VALVOTOMY FOR VALVULAR STENOSIS

Balloon valvotomy, also called *balloon valvuloplasty*, is an invasive, nonsurgical procedure performed in the cardiac catheterization laboratory. It is appropriate for selected patients with valvular stenosis. Balloon valvotomy is most commonly performed in patients with mitral stenosis. It appears to be best suited to the same group of patients who benefit from surgical mitral commissurotomy, that is, those of young age and those with no previous procedure on the valve, normal sinus rhythm, absence of calcium on the valve, absence of thrombus in the left atrial appendage, and no regurgitation.

Balloon valvotomy consists of dilatation of a cardiac valve by inflation of a balloon passed by catheter technique across the valve (Fig. 2-6). For mitral balloon valvotomy, a balloon flotation catheter is inserted into the femoral vein and passed through the inferior vena cava into the right atrium. The catheter is passed through a patent foramen ovale, if present, or a hole is punctured in the atrial septum with a needle tip passed through the catheter. Once the

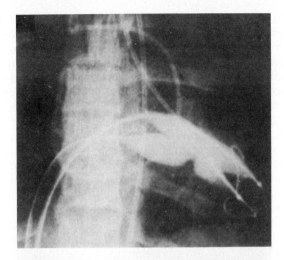

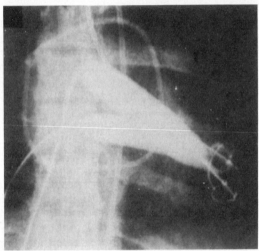

FIGURE 2-6. Balloon valvotomy of mitral valve. Cinefluoroscopy in right anterior oblique view shows two balloons during inflation. Balloons are across mitral valve, and exchange wires are curved in left ventricular apex. **(Top)** During early inflation, "waist" is apparent in balloon silhouette. **(Bottom)** After repeated inflations, both balloons maintain their position across mitral valve during inflation and no waist is seen. (McKay CR, Kawanishi DT, Rahimtoola SH, 1987: Catheter balloon valvuloplasty of the mitral valve in adults using a double-balloon technique. JAMA 257:1753–1761; American Medical Association)

catheter is in the left atrium, it is advanced until one large or two smaller balloons extend across the mitral valve orifice. The balloon is then inflated to split the fused commissures of the valve. At the conclusion of the procedure, the pressure gradient between the left atrium and ventricle is measured to assess residual stenosis and ventriculography is performed to detect new regurgitation resulting from the balloon inflations. Complications of mitral balloon valvotomy include embolic events, cardiac perforation, and development of mitral regurgitation severe enough to require operation (Braunwald, 1992).

Pulmonic stenosis occurs rarely in adults but may also be treated with balloon valvotomy. Balloon valvotomy for aortic valve stenosis has been performed with limited success. Adults with aortic stenosis usually have calcified valve leaflets, and results of valvotomy in calcified valves have been disappointing. Restenosis is a major problem, occurring in approximately 50% of patients within 6 months (Braunwald, 1992). In addition, balloon dilatation of the aortic annulus may produce aortic dissection. Therefore, aortic balloon valvotomy is generally performed only in patients considered at prohibitive risk for surgical valve replacement.

Balloon valvotomy is a relatively new procedure, with a wide range of initial results being reported. The technology is still evolving in terms of selection of patients and valvular anatomy best suited for the technique, types of catheters and balloons, and methods of catheter insertion and placement. The procedure is an important advancement for children and young adults who may face multiple surgical procedures and for patients who are too elderly or medically compromised to withstand an operation that includes general anesthesia, an incision in the thoracic cavity, use of cardiopulmonary bypass, and surgical manipulation of the heart.

SURGICAL THERAPY

Surgical therapy is a major component in the treatment of moderately severe or severe VHD. Improvements in myocardial protection techniques and cardiopulmonary bypass, successful reparative techniques for preserving native valves, and better valvular prostheses have led to performing operative therapy earlier in the course of many forms of VHD. Although valve replacement with an artificial prosthetic valve is most common, valve repair is possible for some valvular lesions. Surgical therapy is discussed in detail in Chapter 16, Surgical Treatment of Valvular Heart Disease.

REFERENCES

Braunwald E, 1992: Valvular heart disease. In Braunwald E (ed): Heart Disease: A Textbook of Cardiovascular Medicine, ed. 4. Philadelphia, WB Saunders
Crawley IS, 1991: Acquired tricuspid and pulmonary valve disease. In Hurst JW (ed): Current Therapy in Cardiovascular Disease, ed. 3. Philadelphia, BC Decker
Criteria Committee of the New York Heart Association, 1964: Physical capacity with heart disease. In Diseases of the Heart and Blood Vessels: Nomenclature and Criteria for Diagnosis, ed. 6. Boston, Little, Brown
Dajani AS, Bisno AL, Chung KJ, et al, 1990: Prevention of endocarditis: Recommendations by the American Heart Association. JAMA 264:2919
Fuster V, Warnes CA, Driscoll DJ, McGoon DC, 1991: Congenital heart disease in adolescents and adults: Congenital left-sided outflow obstruction. In Giuliani ER, Fuster V, Gersh BJ, et al (eds): Cardiology Fundamentals and Practice. St. Louis, Mosby–Year Book

Goldberger E, 1982: Valvular cardiovascular syndromes. In: Textbook of Clinical Cardiology. St. Louis, CV Mosby

Hillis LD, Lange RA, Wells PJ, Winniford MD, 1992: Chronic aortic regurgitation. In Manual of Clinical Problems in Cardiology, ed. 4. Boston, Little, Brown

Jacobs ML, Austen WG, 1990: Acquired aortic valve disease. In Sabiston DC Jr, Spencer FC (eds): Surgery of the Chest, ed. 5. Philadelphia, WB Saunders

John S, Ravikumar E, Jairaj PS, et al, 1990: Valve replacement in the young patient with rheumatic heart disease. J Thorac Cardiovasc Surg 99:631

Kaplan EL, 1990: Acute rheumatic fever. In Hurst JW, Schlant RC, Rackley CE, et al (eds): The Heart, ed. 7. New York, McGraw-Hill

Kaplan EL, 1991: Acute rheumatic fever. In Hurst JW (ed): Current Therapy in Cardiovascular Disease, ed. 3. Philadelphia, BC Decker

Kirklin JW, Barratt-Boyes BG, 1993a: Mitral valve disease with or without tricuspid valve disease. In Cardiac Surgery, ed. 2. New York, Churchill Livingstone

Kirklin JW, Barratt-Boyes BG, 1993b: Aortic valve disease. In Cardiac Surgery, ed. 2. New York, Churchill Livingstone

Kirklin JW, Barratt-Boyes BG, 1993c: Tricuspid valve disease. In Cardiac Surgery, ed. 2. New York, Churchill Livingstone

Korzeniowski OM, Kaye D, 1992: Infective endocarditis. In Braunwald E (ed): Heart Disease: A Textbook of Cardiovascular Medicine, ed. 4. Philadelphia, WB Saunders

Larbalestier RI, Kinchla NM, Aranki SF, et al, 1992: Acute bacterial endocarditis. Circ 86(Suppl II):II-68

Lindsay J Jr, DeBakey ME, Beall AC, 1990: Diseases of the aorta. In Hurst JW, Schlant RC, Rackley CE, et al (eds): The Heart, ed. 7. New York, McGraw-Hill

Nugent EW, Plauth WH, Edwards JE, Williams WH, 1990: The pathology, abnormal physiology, clinical recognition, and medical and surgical treatment of congenital heart disease. In Hurst JW, Schlant RC, Rackley CE, et al (eds): The Heart, ed. 7. New York, McGraw-Hill

Rackley CE, Edwards JE, Karp RB, 1990a: Mitral valve disease. In Hurst JW, Schlant RC, Rackley CE, et al (eds): The Heart, ed. 7. New York, McGraw-Hill

Rackley CE, Edwards JE, Wallace RB, Katz NM, 1990b: Aortic valve disease. In Hurst JW, Schlant RC, Rackley CE, et al (eds): The Heart, ed. 7. New York, McGraw-Hill

Rackley CE, Wallace RB, Edwards JE, Katz NM, 1990c: Tricuspid valve disease. In Hurst JW, Schlant RC, Rackley CE, et al (eds): The Heart, ed. 7. New York, McGraw-Hill

Raizner AE, Siegel CO, 1991: Mitral regurgitation. In Hurst JW (ed): Current Therapy in Cardiovascular Disease, ed. 3. Philadelphia, BC Decker

Rapaport E, 1993: Recognition and management of mitral stenosis. Heart Dis Stroke 2:64

Ronan JA Jr, 1991: Aortic stenosis in adults. In Hurst JW (ed): Current Therapy in Cardiovascular Disease, ed. 3. Philadelphia, BC Decker

Saenz A, Hopkins CB, Humphries JO, 1987. Valvular heart disease. In Chung EK (ed): Quick Reference to Cardiovascular Diseases, ed. 3. Baltimore, Williams & Wilkins

Schlant RC, 1991: Mitral stenosis. In Hurst JW (ed): Current Therapy in Cardiovascular Disease, ed. 3. Philadelphia, BC Decker

Spencer FC, 1990: Acquired disease of the mitral valve. In Sabiston DC Jr, Spencer FC (eds): Surgery of the Chest, ed. 5. Philadelphia, WB Saunders

Treasure CB, 1991: Aortic regurgitation. In Hurst JW (ed): Current Therapy in Cardiovascular Disease, ed. 3. Philadelphia, BC Decker

Underhill SL, McGregor MS, 1989: Acquired valvular heart disease. In Underhill SL, Woods SL, Froelicher ESS, Halpenny CJ (eds): Cardiac Nursing, ed. 2. Philadelphia, JB Lippincott

Warnes CA, Fuster V, McGoon DC, 1991: Congenital heart disease in adolescents and adults: Pulmonic stenosis with intact ventricular septum. In Giuliani ER, Fuster V, Gersh BJ, et al (eds): Cardiology Fundamentals and Practice. St. Louis, Mosby–Year Book

CHAPTER 3

DISORDERS OF THE THORACIC AORTA

ETIOLOGIES OF AORTIC PATHOLOGY

TYPES OF AORTIC PATHOLOGY

Thoracic Aortic Aneurysm

Aortic Dissection

Aortic Transection

The thoracic aortic is subject to three major types of pathology. An *aneurysm* is the localized enlargement of a segment of aorta, *dissection* is longitudinal separation of the three layers of aortic wall, and *transection* is traumatic disruption of aortic wall. Although these terms are sometimes mistakenly used synonymously, they represent three distinct entities. However, sometimes one type of pathology leads to a second (such as acute transection causing chronic aneurysm) or two types coexist (such as dissection and aneurysm).

ETIOLOGIES OF AORTIC PATHOLOGY

Pathologic conditions of the aorta can result from various diseases, iatrogenic injury, trauma, or congenital anomalies. The most common disease affecting the thoracic aorta is *atherosclerosis*. Atherosclerotic aortic pathology usually affects persons older than 50 years of age and often coexists with coronary or peripheral arterial manifestations of the disease. Atherosclerosis is discussed in more detail in Chapter 1, Coronary Artery Disease. Aortic pathology can also result from degeneration of the medial (middle) layer of the aortic wall. A certain degree of elastic and smooth muscle fiber degeneration of the media occurs with aging, causing the aorta to become dilated, elongated, and less elastic (Lindsay et al., 1990). Accordingly, aortic tortuosity and ectasia is common among elderly individuals but usually is not clinically significant (Lindsay et al., 1990).

Severe medial degeneration, known as *cystic medial necrosis*, occurs in some individuals. It can lead to aneurysm, dissection, or both as a result of loss of elastic fibers and medial weakening. Although the entire aortic root is susceptible, medial degeneration is most severe at the aortic root. Therefore, the ascending aorta and aortic valve are most likely to be affected. The term *annuloaortic ectasia* is used to denote marked dilatation of the sinuses of Valsalva and the aortic valve annulus (Kouchoukos, 1991).

The cause of cystic medial necrosis is unknown. It is commonly associated with *Marfan's syndrome*, a heritable connective tissue disorder that primarily affects the skeletal, ocular, and cardiovascular systems (Pyeritz, 1979). Physical stigmata of Marfan's syndrome include bilateral lens displacement, arachnodactyly (abnormally long and slender fingers and toes), lanky extremities, chest wall deformities, kyphosis, hyperextensibility of the joints, high arched palate, and sparse muscle mass (Fig. 3-1). Cardiovascular complications, specifically disease of the aorta or cardiac valves, are a prevalent problem in Marfan's syndrome and are responsible for a shortened life expectancy. A number of studies based on

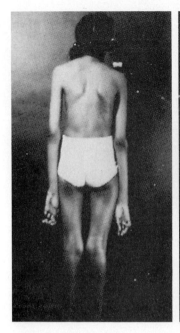
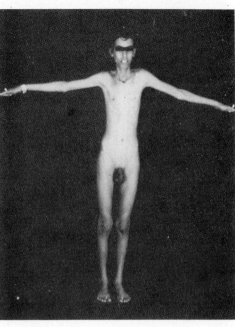

FIGURE 3-1. Typical stigmata of Marfan's syndrome; note tall stature, long extremities, arachnodactyly, and scoliosis. (Pyeritz RE, 1992: Genetics and cardiovascular disease. In Braunwald E [ed]: Heart Disease: A Textbook of Cardiovascular Medicine, ed. 4, p 1641. Philadelphia, WB Saunders)

echocardiographic findings have documented cardiovascular abnormalities in as many as 95% of persons with Marfan's syndrome (Geva et al., 1987). All portions of the aorta may be affected, as well as the aortic valve. Mitral or tricuspid valve regurgitation may also occur, caused by the same myxomatous changes that affect the aorta and aortic valve or by ventricular dilatation that occurs secondary to aortic regurgitation. Only 50% of men and women with Marfan's syndrome reach 40 and 50 years of age, respectively (Murdoch et al., 1972).

Although most patients with Marfan's syndrome have cystic medial necrosis, the converse is not true. Cystic medial necrosis may occur in persons with no physical stigmata of Marfan's syndrome. It is unclear whether cystic medial necrosis of the aorta identical to that seen in Marfan's syndrome, but in persons without skeletal or ocular manifestations of Marfan's syndrome, represents a forme fruste (atypical or incomplete form) of the syndrome or a separate disease (Lindsay et al., 1990).

Aortic pathology, particularly aneurysm, may also be caused by various forms of aortitis (inflammation of the aorta). *Granulomatous aortitis* is a rare condition in which aortic tissue has the microscopic appearance of infectious changes but no bacterial organisms are present (Kirklin & Barratt-Boyes, 1993a). It typically occurs in older persons, particularly women (Crawford, 1989). Aortitis can also occur secondary to autoimmune disorders, such as ankylosing spondylitis and Reiter's syndrome (Lindsay et al., 1990).

Bacterial aortitis occurs when bacteria invade the aortic wall. Aortic endothelium is normally quite resistant to bacterial infection; bacterial aortitis almost always occurs in a previously diseased or injured segment of aorta (Lindsay et al., 1990). *Syphilitic aortitis* is

a late complication of syphilis infection. It has become rare since the widespread availability of antibiotic therapy to treat primary syphilis infection. Nevertheless, syphilitic aortitis can occur, usually many years after the primary infection. The ascending or transverse portion of the thoracic aorta is most often affected, and aortic valve involvement is common.

Takayasu's arteritis is an unusual inflammatory arterial disease that produces stenosis or aneurysm in the aorta or its major branches and in the pulmonary and coronary arteries. The disease is characterized by degeneration of elastic fibers and proliferation of connective tissue (Peyton & Isom, 1990). All three layers of the arterial wall are affected, and the arteritis may be diffuse or segmental. The etiology of Takayasu's

---

TABLE 3-1. PROCEDURES ASSOCIATED WITH IATROGENIC AORTIC INJURY

Cardiac Surgery

Aortic cannulation
Saphenous vein–aorta anastomoses
Cross-clamping
Aortotomy

Aortic Surgery

Aortic–prosthetic graft anastomoses
Aortotomy
Aortic cannulation

Cardiac Catheterization, Intra-aortic Balloon Counterpulsation, Cardiopulmonary Bypass

Femoral artery cannulation
Retrograde perfusion

disease is unknown, although genetic and autoimmune factors are thought to play a role (Lindsay et al., 1990). Women younger than 30 years of age are most commonly affected (Crawford, 1989).

Congenital anomalies of the aorta include coarctation and anomalies of the aortic arch. Occasionally, aortic pathology results from iatrogenic injury or from trauma. *Iatrogenic aortic injury*, occurring as a complication of cardiac surgery, operations on the aorta itself, or femoral artery cannulation can lead to aneurysm formation or dissection (Table 3-1). Severe *blunt chest trauma*, especially that associated with rapid horizontal or vertical deceleration, can cause aortic transection.

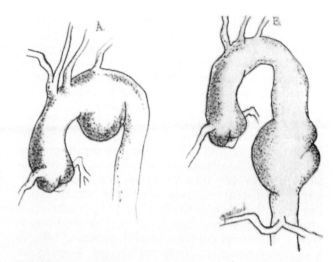

FIGURE 3-2. Thoracic aneurysms are categorized by shape as sacciform **(A)** or fusiform **(B)**. (Weiland AP, Walker WE, 1986: Thoracic aneurysms. Crit Care Q 9:21; Aspen Publishers)

TYPES OF AORTIC PATHOLOGY

THORACIC AORTIC ANEURSYM

Any condition that weakens aortic wall integrity can produce localized dilatation of the aorta, with eventual aneurysm formation. A *true aneurysm* is one in which there is transmural dilatation and thinning but all layers of the aortic wall remain intact (Weiland & Walker, 1986). The lumen of the aneurysm typically contains laminated clot (Lindsay et al., 1990). A *false aneurysm* is one in which there is partial or complete disruption of the aortic wall. Aortic blood is contained by the adventitial layer alone or by periaortic fibrous tissue (Cohn, 1990). Most thoracic aneurysms are true aneurysms. Abnormalities of the aorta that are sometimes confused with aortic aneurysm include aortic enlargement secondary to aortic regurgitation and post-stenotic dilatation in patients with aortic stenosis.

Aneurysms are described according to shape and location. An aneurysm that widens the aorta circumferentially is called *fusiform;* one that deforms only one side of the vessel is said to be *sacciform* or *saccular* (Weiland & Walker, 1986) (Fig. 3-2). Thoracic aneurysms are categorized by location as *ascending* (between aortic valve annulus and origin of innominate artery), *transverse arch* (between origins of innominate and left subclavian arteries), or *descending* (distal to origin of left subclavian artery). An aneurysm of the descending thoracic aorta that extends below the diaphragm is termed *thoracoabdominal*. Sometimes, multiple discrete aneurysms are present or the entire thoracic aorta is aneurysmal. Rarely, an aneurysm occurs in one of the sinuses of Valsalva, the three pouch-like areas of aortic wall that originate at the aortic valve annulus and extend just beyond the coronary artery ostia (DeBakey & McCollum, 1987).

The most common etiology of thoracic and thoracoabdominal aneurysms is atherosclerosis (Kirklin & Barratt-Boyes, 1993a). Although atherosclerosis primarily affects the intimal layer of arterial wall, media beneath severely diseased segments becomes weakened and prone to aneurysm formation (Lindsay et

al., 1990). Hypertension is frequently present and may accelerate the degenerative process. Although atherosclerosis is generally more severe in the abdominal aorta, aneurysms of atherosclerotic origin sometimes develop in the thoracic aorta, usually in the descending segment or arch. The ascending segment is generally spared from severe atherosclerosis, except in persons with diabetes mellitus, type II hyperlipoproteinemia, and syphilitic aortitis (Lindsay et al., 1990). Atherosclerotic aneurysms are most often fusiform.

Aortic aneurysm is also common in persons with Marfan's syndrome or cystic medial necrosis. Such aneurysms commonly begin at the aortic valve in the area of the sinuses of Valsalva and extend to the origin of the innominate artery. Aortic regurgitation is frequently present owing to annuloaortic ectasia and the resulting loss of valve leaflet coaptation (Kouchoukos, 1991).

Thoracic aneurysms can also be caused by other processes that affect the aortic wall, such as aortitis. Granulomatous aortitis is a common cause of diffuse aneurysmal disease, sometimes involving the entire thoracic segment or even the entire aorta. Syphilitic aortitis often leads to development of very large saccular aneurysms in the ascending aorta or aortic arch (Pairolero et al., 1976). The term *luetic aneurysm* describes an aneurysm that occurs secondary to syphilis.

An aneurysm caused by infective aortitis is called a *mycotic aneurysm*. Mycotic aneurysms are usually local, saccular false aneurysms. They can result from (1) septic embolism; (2) contiguous spread from recent abscesses, infected lymph nodes, or empyema; and (3) bacteremia due to trauma, intravenous injections, or surgical procedures (Cohn, 1990). Sepsis, distal embolization, and a significant threat of aortic rupture are characteristic of mycotic aneurysms (Akins, 1989).

Another cause of aneurysm formation is persistence of a false lumen after acute aortic dissection. The thin outer wall of the false lumen has a tendency to gradually weaken; as wall stress increases, an aneurysm may develop and enlarge (Kirklin & Barratt-Boyes, 1993a). An unusual cause of thoracic aneurysm formation is aortic transection due to trauma (Finkelmeier et al., 1982). If rupture resulting from aortic transection is contained by adventitia, the lesion may evolve into a chronic false aneurysm. *Chronic traumatic aneurysm* classically occurs at the thoracic isthmus (near the origin of the left subclavian artery) but may arise from tears in other locations as well. Circumferential tears usually produce fusiform aneurysms; saccular aneurysms are more likely to develop from partial tears (Ákins, 1989). Occasionally, an aneurysm develops in the thoracic aorta that is caused by iatrogenic aortic injury that occurred during previous cardiac or aortic surgery.

Aneurysms sometimes develop secondary to aortic stenosis or coarctation because of post-stenotic dilatation. The change in velocity of blood flow through an area of stenosis increases lateral pressure on the aortic wall just beyond the stenotic area, producing a *jet lesion* with eventual aneurysm formation. *Congenital aneurysms* can occur near the ligamentum arteriosum or in the sinuses of Valsalva. Etiologies of thoracic aneurysm are listed in Table 3-2.

Thoracic aortic aneurysm is often diagnosed when its appearance is noted on a chest roentgenogram. Aneurysms of the descending thoracic aorta in particular are likely to be detected before development of any symptoms because of a chest roentgenogram taken for another reason. An aortogram is performed to clearly define aneurysm location and its relationship to arteries branching from the aorta. Computed

TABLE 3-2. ETIOLOGIES OF THORACIC AORTIC ANEURYSM

Atherosclerosis
Cystic medial necrosis
Marfan's syndrome
Annuloaortic ectasia
Aortitis
  Granulomatous
  Syphilis (luetic)
  Mycotic (bacterial, fungal)
Trauma
  Aortic transection
  Iatrogenic injury
Poststenotic dilatation
Chronic aortic dissection with persisting false lumen
Congenital anomalies
  Sinus of Valsalva
  Ductus (ligamentum arteriosum)

TABLE 3-3. SIGNS AND SYMPTOMS OF THORACIC AORTIC ANEURYSM ENLARGEMENT

Sign or Symptom	Due to Compression of
Superior vena cava syndrome	Superior vena cava
Chest wall pain	Ribs
Back pain	Vertebrae, spinal nerves
Hoarseness	Recurrent laryngeal nerve
Left hemidiaphragm elevation	Phrenic nerve
Dysphagia	Esophagus
Wheezing, cough, stridor, dyspnea	Trachea or bronchi

tomographic (CT) scanning is sometimes performed as well. If the aortic valve is involved in the aneurysmal process, echocardiography and cardiac catheterization are generally obtained.

Thoracic aneurysms often expand over time. Aneurysm expansion is worrisome because of the known propensity for aortic rupture. As an aneurysm enlarges, it can also produce symptoms because of its encroachment on surrounding structures. Depending on location, aneurysmal enlargement can produce a variety of symptoms (Table 3-3). If the ascending aorta is aneurysmal, the aortic valve annulus may become distorted, leading to aortic regurgitation and congestive heart failure. Aortic regurgitation may also produce angina because low diastolic blood pressure impairs coronary artery filling and ventricular dilatation increases myocardial oxygen demand. Arch aneurysms may be associated with dyspnea, stridor, hoarseness, hemoptysis, cough, or chest pain (Crawford & Coselli, 1991). The most common symptom of descending thoracic aneurysm is upper back pain between the scapulae (Rose et al., 1991).

Likelihood of aortic rupture is directly related to aneurysm size and the development of symptoms (Eagle & DeSanctis, 1992). The more the aortic wall is stretched, the greater the wall tension (law of Laplace) and the more likely is rupture to occur (Cohn, 1990). Rupture of aortic aneurysm may occur precipitously, before development of any symptoms, and cause exsanguination into the mediastinum, pleural space, tracheobronchial tree, or esophagus (Lindsay et al., 1990). Occasionally, aortic rupture occurs without exsanguination because blood is contained by periaortic, pericardial, or pleural tissue. Patients with *contained rupture* generally experience severe chest pain and have roentgenographic evidence of a widened mediastinum or pleural effusion. Precipitous disruption of a contained rupture with rapid exsanguination can occur at any time. Rarely, a contained rupture remains intact, forming a false aneurysm.

Studies have suggested that mortality from aortic aneurysm approaches 75% at 5 years, with almost one half of deaths due to rupture (Lindsay et al., 1990). The only treatment for aortic aneurysm is operative repair. The decision to proceed with surgical aneurysm resection is based primarily on two factors: (1) any symptoms or radiographic evidence of enlargement and (2) for fusiform aneurysms, aortic diameter size. Many surgeons advocate operative repair of fusiform aneurysms, even in asymptomatic patients, when aortic diameter reaches 6 cm as measured by aortography or CT scan. Although natural history data for thoracic aortic aneurysms are somewhat limited, size is known to affect survival; aneurysms greater than 7 cm are more prone to rupture than are smaller ones (Eagle & DeSanctis, 1992). Because of the friable quality of aortic tissue associated with Marfan's syndrome, operative repair is often recommended when an aneurysm reaches 5.0 to 5.5 cm. Normal diameter of the ascending aorta is 2.5 to 3.0 cm.

The nature of the operative repair is determined primarily by location and extent of the aneurysm. The diseased segment of aorta is usually replaced with a prosthetic tubular graft. Blood flow to arterial branches supplied by the diseased segment must be preserved. Arteries are either reimplanted into the side of the tubular graft or, in the case of the great vessels, a graft designed with arch branches or a human cadaver homograft is used to replace the segment. If the aortic valve is regurgitant, valve resuspension, valvuloplasty, or valve replacement to restore competency may be necessary. Operative repair of the thoracic aorta is discussed in greater detail in Chapter 17, Surgery on the Thoracic Aorta.

AORTIC DISSECTION

Aortic dissection is the most common catastrophic illness involving the aorta, occurring two to three times more frequently than rupture of the abdominal aorta (Wolfe & Moran, 1981). The disorder is estimated to occur in as many as 60,000 persons per year in the United States; those at highest risk are men, African-Americans, and persons between 45 and 70 years of age (Wheat, 1987; Wolfe & Moran, 1981). Acute aortic dissection has a grim prognosis. Without treatment, more than 25% of patients die within 24 hours, more than 50% die within 1 week, more than 75% die within 1 month, and more than 90% die within 1 year (Eagle & DeSanctis, 1992).

Dissection of the aortic wall occurs as an acute event secondary to a disruption in the intima. Two factors promote development of an intimal tear: (1) repeated motion of the ascending and proximal descending aorta secondary to the force of cardiac contractions and (2) intraluminal hydrodynamic force of the pulse wave propagated by each cardiac contraction, particularly in the ascending aorta and exaggerated in the presence of systemic hypertension (Wheat, 1987). Intimal tears can occur anywhere in the aorta, but the two most frequent sites of origin are the ascending aorta, within 5 cm of the aortic valve and just distal to the left subclavian artery, near the ligamentum arteriosum (Eagle et al., 1989). Approximately two thirds of dissections involve the ascending aorta (Lindsay et al., 1990).

When intimal disruption occurs, blood from the true lumen of the aorta dissects the abnormal medial layer, forming a false lumen between intima and adventitia. Systemic blood pressure in the aorta causes blood to track retrograde, antegrade, or in both directions, separating intimal and adventitial layers for a variable length of the aorta. Progression of the dissection is enhanced by continued hypertension, anticoagulation, or an elevated dV/dt (i.e., the velocity of left ventricular ejection). Multiple reentry points may be present where blood in the false lumen ruptures the intima to reenter the true lumen. Alternatively, the dissection may stop at a point where further dissection is precluded by atherosclerotic changes in the aortic wall. The term *dissecting aneurysm* is frequently used to label this disorder. However, the word "aneurysm" is a misnomer because the pathologic abnormality is really a dissecting hematoma and not an aneurysm. The two conditions sometimes coexist.

A number of etiologic factors are thought to play a role in the occurrence of aortic dissection (Table 3-4). Cystic medial necrosis is present in approximately 20% of patients with acute aortic dissection (Kirklin & Barratt-Boyes, 1993b). As a result, cohesiveness of inner (intimal) and outer (adventitial) wall layers is diminished. Medial degeneration is most often related to a connective tissue disorder, such as Marfan's syndrome. Even in patients without physical stigmata of Marfan's syndrome, cystic medial degeneration is often detected on pathologic examination of the aortic tissue. Other disorders that affect aortic wall integrity, such as aortitis or the connective tissue disorder Ehlers-Danlos syndrome, are also causative factors.

Factors associated with increased risk for aortic dissection, particularly in young persons, are hypertension, pregnancy, congenital bicuspid aortic valve, and coarctation (Wheat, 1987; Wolfe & Moran, 1981). Approximately 90% of patients with aortic dissection

---

TABLE 3-4. ETIOLOGIC FACTORS IN AORTIC DISSECTION

Cystic medial necrosis
Marfan's syndrome
Aortitis
Ehlers-Danlos syndrome
Coarctation of the aorta
Bicuspid aortic valve
Pregnancy
Hypertension
Iatrogenic arterial injury
Blunt chest trauma

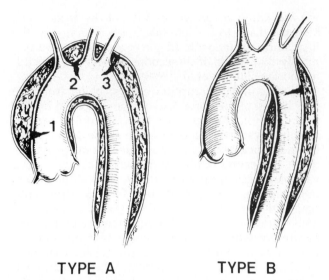

TYPE A   TYPE B

FIGURE 3-3. Stanford classification of aortic dissection. The primary intimal disruption in type A dissections can be in the ascending aorta (*1*), transverse arch (*2*), or descending aorta (*3*). (Wheat MW Jr, 1987: Acute dissection of the aorta. In McGoon DC [ed]: Cardiac Surgery, ed. 2, p. 250. Philadelphia, FA Davis)

tent bicuspid aortic valve. Occasionally, iatrogenic aortic dissection occurs secondary to femoral artery or aortic cannulation for cardiopulmonary bypass, intra-aortic balloon catheter insertion, or aortic cross-clamping during cardiovascular operations.

Aortic dissections are categorized according to location and extent. Two classification systems are commonly used. The *Stanford classification system* categorizes aortic dissection according to ascending aortic involvement, irrespective of intimal disruption origin (Fig. 3-3). Type A dissection involves the ascending aorta. The dissection may be confined only to the ascending aorta or extend beyond the aortic arch to involve the descending aorta as well. Type B dissection involves only the descending aorta, distal to the left subclavian artery. The *DeBakey classification system* also remains in common use: type I dissection extends from the ascending aorta to beyond the left subclavian artery, type II is limited to the ascending aorta, proximal to the left subclavian artery, and type III involves only the descending aorta, distal to the left subclavian artery (DeBakey & McCollum, 1987) (Fig. 3-4). Types I and II are combined in the Stanford system as type A, and type III is the same as type B. Categorization of aortic dissection according to location is important because therapy is distinctly different.

Aortic dissections are further classified as acute or chronic. Because most of the mortality from dissection occurs within 2 weeks after its onset, dissection recognized during this period is considered acute (Eagle et al., 1989). Acute dissection is a catastrophic event that can produce several life-threatening consequences. Sudden death can occur (1) when rupture causes tamponade or exsanguination or (2) when

are hypertensive at the time of presentation or have a history of hypertension (Wheat, 1987). Although hypertension has not been definitively linked to initiation of aortic dissection, it is the major factor in promoting progression of dissection (Ergin et al., 1991). Of aortic dissections in young women, 50% occur during pregnancy (Wolfe & Moran, 1981). Twenty to 25% of patients with aortic dissection have a coexis-

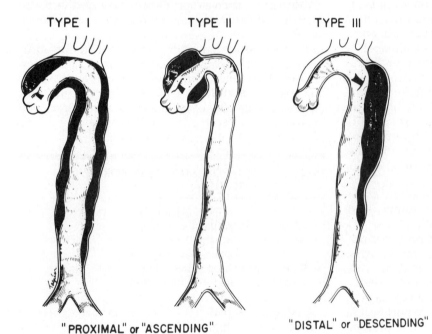

TYPE I   TYPE II   TYPE III

"PROXIMAL" or "ASCENDING"   "DISTAL" or "DESCENDING"

FIGURE 3-4. DeBakey classification of aortic dissection. (Eagle KA, Doroghazi RM, DeSanctis RW, Austen WG, 1989: Aortic dissection. In Eagle KA, Haber E, DeSanctis RW, Austen WG [eds]: The Practice of Cardiology, ed. 2, p. 1371. Boston, Little, Brown & Co) proximal extension of the dissection causes occlusion of the coronary ostia or severe acute aortic regurgitation.

Rupture of the dissected aorta, with hemorrhage into the pericardium, mediastinum, pleural space, or abdomen, is the most common cause of death. Although rupture can occur anywhere along the length of aorta, proximal dissections most commonly rupture into the pericardium and distal dissections rupture into the left pleural space (Eagle et al., 1989). Free rupture is invariably fatal owing to rapid exsanguination. Bleeding into the pericardial sac or mediastinum may cause cardiac tamponade. In some instances, the rupture is temporarily contained by periaortic fibrous, pericardial, or pleural tissue.

Type A (i.e., ascending) aortic dissection frequently extends retrograde to involve the aortic valve. Acute aortic regurgitation can occur as a result of annular dilatation, altered geometry of the aortic root, or leaflet or annular tear (Fann et al., 1991). In contrast to chronic aortic regurgitation, in which the left ventricle is able to compensate for the regurgitated stroke volume, acute aortic regurgitation produces severe congestive heart failure, pulmonary edema, or frank cardiogenic shock. The coronary ostia, particularly that of the right coronary artery, may become involved in the dissection, leading to inferior wall myocardial ischemia or infarction.

Aortic dissection can also occlude any of the other aortic branches, causing acute ischemia to organs supplied by affected branches. Thirty to 50% of patients develop signs or symptoms of acute peripheral arterial occlusion as a consequence of extrinsic compression of the arterial true lumen by the false lumen (Fann et al., 1989). Stroke, paraplegia, or peripheral neuropathy may occur secondary to compromised blood flow to the brain, spinal cord, or peripheral nerves (Fann et al., 1989). Renal failure, bowel infarction, or limb ischemia may also develop as supplying arteries become occluded by the dissection.

The most prevalent symptom associated with aortic dissection is the sudden onset of excruciating chest or back (interscapular) pain, often described as tearing, shearing, or "knife-like." Frequently, pain migrates as the dissection extends along the aorta (Eagle et al., 1989). Acute aortic dissection and myocardial infarction are sometimes difficult to differentiate, and both conditions should be considered during the evaluation of any patient with severe chest pain. Occasionally, dissection is not accompanied by pain or the pain waxes and wanes or dissipates after a short duration.

Shock may be present due to (1) loss of blood volume from the false channel into periaortic tissues and spaces, (2) acute aortic regurgitation, or (3) rupture into the pericardium with cardiac tamponade (Kirklin & Barratt-Boyes, 1993b). Other manifestations that may occur include abdominal pain, extremity weakness, acute renal failure, hematuria, hemiparesis,

hemiplegia, paraplegia, syncope, and speech or visual disturbances.

Physical examination may reveal unequal pulses or blood pressure in the extremities, a diminishing hematocrit, and a new diastolic murmur of aortic regurgitation. Hypertension may be present despite a general appearance of shock. Neurologic signs and symptoms as well as blood flow to one or several extremities can wax and wane as pressure in the dissecting hematoma (false lumen) increases or decreases (Wheat, 1987).

The diagnosis is suggested by the clinical presentation in combination with a chest roentgenogram that reveals widening of the mediastinum. Mediastinal width is difficult to interpret, however, because prior chest roentgenograms may be unavailable or may have been taken using a posteroanterior projection. A chest film taken for evaluation of acute dissection will almost always be done at the bedside and, therefore, will use an anteroposterior projection. The mediastinum will, by virtue of the anteroposterior projection, appear somewhat wider than it does on the posteroanterior film. Also, aortic dissection does not always produce radiographic evidence of mediastinal widening. The chest roentgenogram may also demonstrate pleural effusion (usually left-sided) or cardiomegaly secondary to pericardial effusion (Kirklin & Barratt-Boyes, 1993b).

Although symptoms and roentgenographic demonstration of a widened mediastinum are helpful in suggesting the presence of dissection, they should not be used to rule out the diagnosis. If there is suspicion of dissection, an aortogram or CT scan with infusion must be obtained to definitively determine whether dissection has occurred. An aortogram is the standard diagnostic study because it most effectively demonstrates the origin (intimal flap), the true and false lumens, the extent of dissection, and the involvement of major aortic branches.

In community hospitals where aortography may not be immediately available, CT scanning is often helpful in establishing the diagnosis. However, unless ultrafast scanning techniques are available, the rapidly moving, disrupted intima is not always demonstrated by CT scanning. Transesophageal echocardiography is an evolving diagnostic technique that may play an increasing role in diagnosis of aortic dissection. It is highly reliable in detecting dissection, but the passage of a probe into the esophagus in a conscious patient may exacerbate hypertension. Transthoracic echocardiography is usually not helpful in diagnosing dissection.

Because of the devastating complications and lethal nature of aortic dissection, particularly if diagnosis or treatment is delayed, the patient is monitored in a cardiothoracic surgical intensive care unit and both a cardiothoracic surgeon and cardiologist are involved in initial patient evaluation and management. The patient is at highest risk for death during the first hours after onset of dissection, particularly if hypertension is not corrected. Thorough, serial assessments are essential to monitor occurrence and progression of complications of the dissection.

Type A aortic dissection is treated in most centers as a surgical emergency, unless irreversible complications of dissection have already occurred. In contrast, the primary treatment of patients with type B (i.e., descending) aortic dissection is pharmacologic therapy to control hypertension. However, acute management of type B dissection is often directed by a cardiothoracic surgeon in a surgical intensive care setting because urgent operative intervention may become necessary if the dissection extends or rupture occurs. Persistent pain, or evidence of threatened perfusion to abdominal viscera, the spinal cord, or lower extremities indicate extension of the dissection. Operative repair of aortic dissection is discussed in Chapter 17, Surgery on the Thoracic Aorta.

Whether surgical therapy is undertaken, immediate treatment of hypertension is the most important component of medical therapy in all patients with aortic dissection. Antihypertensive therapy is essential to prevent further dissection and must be instituted as soon as the diagnosis is suspected, even before angiography. Medications that are effective in reducing systolic arterial pressure and the velocity of left ventricular ejection (dV/dt) are used. Intravenous nitroprusside is almost always the agent of choice because of its immediate and potent antihypertensive effect. However, nitroprusside alone may cause a reflex increase in dV/dt, possibly accelerating dissection progression (Eagle & DeSanctis, 1992). Therefore, a beta-blocking agent, such as esmolol or propranolol must also be used acutely to reduce dV/dt. Blood pressure is generally maintained between 90 and 100 mm Hg, or at the lowest level that continues to provide adequate organ perfusion.

With either surgical or medical treatment, long-term management of hypertension is important. An oral beta-blocking agent, such as propranolol, is often used for chronic blood pressure control. Residual aortic pathology and cardiovascular disease are significant causes of late death and morbidity in persons with aortic dissection, regardless of the mode of treatment of the disease (Glower et al., 1990).

Rarely, acute dissection remains unrecognized. Such patients, and those who have received medical therapy only, are considered to have chronic aortic dissection. In chronic aortic dissection, the false channel either thromboses and heals or remains patent and continues to enlarge, leading to aneurysmal dilatation (Ergin et al., 1991). Type A chronic dissection (i.e., type A dissection that was undetected during its acute phase) is usually treated with elective operative repair if any of the following develop: (1) significant aortic regurgitation, (2) aneurysm formation, or (3) progression of dissection (Eagle et al., 1989). Elective repair of type B chronic dissection is considered in patients in whom aortic diameter exceeds 6 cm, especially in association with uncontrolled hypertension (Neya et al., 1992).

AORTIC TRANSECTION

Acute transection of the aorta occurs as a consequence of severe blunt chest trauma. Intimal disruption almost always occurs in one of two sites: (1) in the descending aorta just distal to the origin of the left subclavian artery, and (2) in the aortic root just above the aortic valve. These two locations are classic sites of aortic injury because of the stress to which they are subjected. The heart and the descending aorta are relatively fixed in position by contiguous structures. However, the ascending and transverse aorta (aortic arch), from the aortic root to the ligamentum arteriosum, are not tethered. Therefore, these two junctures of fixation are likely injury points.

Transection just distal to the left subclavian artery is most often produced by rapid horizontal deceleration, such as occurs with high-speed motor vehicle accidents. Rapid vertical deceleration, such as occurs with a fall from a building or airplane, generally causes disruption of the ascending aorta, usually just above the aortic valve. Aortic disruption in this location is almost always immediately fatal. Aortic transection is described in more detail in Chapter 32, Cardiac and Thoracic Trauma.

REFERENCES

Akins CW, 1989: Nondissecting aneurysms of the thoracic aorta. In Eagle KA, Haber E, DeSanctis RW, Austin WG (eds): The Practice of Cardiology, ed. 2. Boston, Little, Brown & Co

Cohn LH, 1990: Thoracic aortic aneurysms and aortic dissection. In Sabiston DC Jr, Spencer FC (eds): Surgery of the Chest, ed. 5. Philadelphia, WB Saunders

Crawford ES, 1989: Replacement of the thoracic aorta. In Grillo HC, Austen WG, Wilkins EW, et al (eds): Current Therapy in Cardiothoracic Surgery. Toronto, BC Decker

Crawford ES, Coselli JS, 1991: Aneurysms of the transverse aortic arch. In Baue AE, Geha AS, Hammond GL, et al (eds): Glenn's Thoracic and Cardiovascular Surgery, ed. 5. Norwalk, CT, Appleton & Lange

DeBakey ME, McCollum CH, 1987: Diseases of the aorta. In Chung EK (ed): Quick Reference to Cardiovascular Diseases, ed. 3. Baltimore, Williams & Wilkins

Eagle KA, DeSanctis RW, 1992: Diseases of the aorta. In Braunwald E (ed): Heart Disease: A Textbook of Cardiovascular Medicine, ed. 4. Philadelphia, WB Saunders

Eagle KA, Doroghazi RM, DeSanctis RW, Austen WG, 1989: Aortic dissection. In Eagle KA, Haber E, DeSanctis RW, Austin WG (eds): The Practice of Cardiology, ed. 2. Boston, Little, Brown & Co

Ergin MA, Lansman SL, Griepp RB, 1991: Dissections of the aorta. In Baue AE, Geha AS, Hammond GL, et al (eds): Glenn's Thoracic and Cardiovascular Surgery, ed. 5. Norwalk, CT, Appleton & Lange

Fann JI, Glower DD, Miller DC, et al, 1991: Preservation of aortic valve in type A aortic dissection complicated by aortic regurgitation. J Thorac Cardiovasc Surg 102:62

Fann JI, Sarris GE, Miller C, et al, 1989: Surgical management of acute aortic dissection complicated by stroke. Circulation 80(Suppl I):I-257

Finkelmeier BA, Mentzer RM, Kaiser DL, et al, 1982: Chronic traumatic aneurysm. J Thorac Cardiovasc Surg 84:257

Geva T, Hegesh J, Frand M, 1987: The clinical course and echocardiographic features of Marfan's syndrome in childhood. Am J Dis Child 141:1179

Glower DD, Fann JI, Speier RH, et al, 1990: Comparison of medical and surgical therapy for uncomplicated descending aortic dissection. Circulation 82(Suppl IV):IV-39

Kirklin JW, Barratt-Boyes BG, 1993a: Chronic thoracic and thoracoabdominal aortic aneurysms. In Cardiac Surgery, ed. 2. New York, Churchill Livingstone

Kirklin JW, Barratt-Boyes BG, 1993b: Acute aortic dissection. In Cardiac Surgery. ed. 2. New York, Churchill Livingstone

Kouchoukos NT, 1991: Aneurysms of the ascending aorta. In Baue AE, Geha AS, Hammond GL, et al (eds): Glenn's Thoracic and Cardiovascular Surgery, ed. 5. Norwalk, CT, Appleton & Lange

Lindsay J Jr, DeBakey ME, Beall AC, 1990: Diseases of the aorta. In Hurst JW, Schlant RC, Rackley CE, et al (eds): The Heart, ed. 7. New York, McGraw-Hill

Murdoch JL, Walker BA, Halpern BL, et al, 1972: Life expectancy and causes of death in the Marfan syndrome. N Engl J Med 286:15

Neya K, Omoto R, Kyo S, et al, 1992: Outcome of Stanford Type B acute aortic dissection. Circulation 86(Suppl II):II-1

Pairolero PC, Bernatz PE, 1976: Aneurysms. In Gay WA (ed): Cardiovascular Surgery (Goldsmith Practice of Surgery—revised edition). Philadelphia, Harper & Row

Peyton RB, Isom OW, 1990: Occlusive disease of branches of the aorta. In Sabiston DC Jr, Spencer FC (eds): Surgery of the Chest, ed. 5. Philadelphia, WB Saunders

Pyeritz RE, 1979: The Marfan syndrome: Diagnosis and management. N Engl J Med 300:772

Rose DM, Laschinger JC, Cunningham JN Jr, 1991: Descending thoracic aortic aneurysms. In Baue AE, Geha AS, Hammond GL, et al (eds): Glenn's Thoracic and Cardiovascular Surgery, ed. 5. Norwalk, CT, Appleton & Lange

Weiland AP, Walker WE, 1986: Thoracic aneurysms. Crit Care Q 9:3

Wheat MW, 1987: Acute dissection of the aorta. In McGoon DC (ed): Cardiac Surgery, ed. 2. Philadelphia, FA Davis

Wolfe WG, Moran JF, 1981: Dissecting aneurysms. In Gay WA (ed): Cardiovascular Surgery (Goldsmith Practice of Surgery—revised edition). Philadelphia, Harper & Row

4

CARDIAC RHYTHM DISORDERS

ELECTRICAL ACTIVATION OF THE HEART
PATHOGENESIS OF ARRHYTHMIAS
   Abnormal Impulse Formation
   Abnormal Impulse Conduction
CLASSIFICATION OF ARRHYTHMIAS
   Bradyarrhythmias
   Tachyarrhythmias

SUDDEN CARDIAC DEATH
DIAGNOSIS
TREATMENT
   Antiarrhythmic Medications
   Catheter and Surgical Ablation
   Antitachycardia Devices

Recurring or persistent cardiac arrhythmias represent a *chronic rhythm disorder,* usually occurring secondary to underlying cardiac pathology or other abnormality. Chronic rhythm disorders likely to be treated with invasive or surgical therapies are the focus of this chapter. Cardiac arrhythmias may also occur as transient events, triggered by a specific precipitant, such as myocardial ischemia, proarrhythmic agents, or electrolyte imbalance. Characteristics and acute management of such transient arrhythmias are discussed in Chapter 25, Cardiac Arrhythmias.

ELECTRICAL ACTIVATION OF THE HEART

Electrical activation of the heart normally occurs as a coordinated, progressive excitation process by means of specialized conductive tissue. Impulses originate in the sinus node, a small group of automatic cells located just beneath the epicardial surface at the junction of the superior vena cava and right atrium. Automatic cells differ from contractile cells of the myocardium in that membrane potential does not remain constant during phase 4 depolarization but varies, leading to subsequent spontaneous depolarization. This property of *automaticity,* enables the sinus node to initiate action potentials independent of any prior impulse (Smith, 1990). Although there are automatic cells in other areas of the heart (atrioventricular [AV]

node, some atrial cells, and Purkinje fibers), the sinus node has the most rapid rate of spontaneous depolarization and, under normal conditions, acts as the dominant pacemaker. Its rich innervation with postganglionic adrenergic and cholinergic nerve terminals increase and decrease the rate of spontaneous depolarization, accounting for variations in sinus heart rate (Zipes, 1992a).

From its origin in the sinus node, the electrical wave front proceeds in a somewhat concentric fashion to excite muscle cells throughout both atria (Halpenny, 1989). Impulse conduction between the sinus and AV node does not occur at the same velocity through all parts of the atrium but instead appears to travel more rapidly by means of three preferential conduction pathways (internodal tracts) in the atria. However, despite anatomic evidence indicating the presence of such internodal pathways, they are not identifiable as histologically discrete tracts of tissue and surgical division does not block atrial conduction (Cox, 1990; Zipes, 1992a). Thus, the precise role these preferential pathways play in internodal conduction remains unclear.

The impulse passes through the AV node to the ventricles after a slight delay. The AV node functions both as the means of conducting impulses to the ventricles and as the origin of the cardiac rhythm in the presence of sinus nodal dysfunction (e.g., sinus arrest, sinus bradycardia, and sinus block) (Chung,

1989a). Except for AV nodal and bundle of His tissue, the atria and ventricles are separated by an electrically inert barrier, the fibrous skeleton. Therefore, the AV node is normally the only pathway for electrical conduction between atria and ventricles. When it is dysfunctional, the ventricles no longer receive impulses originating in the atria.

Impulses traveling through the AV node are conducted to ventricular myocardium through the bundle of His, bundle branches, and Purkinje fibers. This specialized conductive network spreads the impulse almost simultaneously to the entire right and left ventricular endocardium. Activation then spreads from the endocardium toward the epicardium, depolarizing all regions of the ventricles.

PATHOGENESIS OF ARRHYTHMIAS

Mechanisms of arrhythmogenesis can be categorized as disorders of impulse formation, disorders of impulse conduction, or a combination of both (Jacobson, 1989).

ABNORMAL IMPULSE FORMATION

The most common disorder of impulse formation is *enhanced automaticity,* a phenomenon in which either (1) the spontaneous depolarization rate of myocardial pacemaker cells becomes abnormally accelerated or (2) myocardial contractile fibers abnormally exhibit automaticity. Enhanced automaticity of sinus node cells produces sinus tachycardia. Atrial, nodal, or ventricular tachycardias may result from enhanced spontaneous depolarization of normally latent automatic cells. Clinical conditions that enhance automaticity (by accelerating spontaneous phase 4 depolarization) include ischemia, hypokalemia, digitalis administration, and beta-adrenergic receptor stimulation (Ruskin & Schoenfeld, 1989).

Alternatively, impulse formation (automaticity) may become abnormally slow. If the sinus depolarization rate still surpasses that of other automatic cardiac cells, sinus bradycardia results. Alternatively, pronounced slowing of the sinus depolarization rate allows a latent or ectopic pacemaker to initiate the cardiac rhythm. Because the AV node usually has the second fastest spontaneous depolarization rate, a nodal escape rhythm typically occurs. Causes of decreased sinus node automaticity include excessive vagal stimulation, medications, or disease of the sinus node (Jacobson, 1989).

ABNORMAL IMPULSE CONDUCTION

Two primary disorders of impulse conduction occur: slowed or blocked conduction and a phenomenon known as reentry. *Slowed* or *blocked conduction* may result in bradycardia, tachycardia, or no change in heart rate. For example, impaired AV nodal conduction may cause complete heart block with a ventricular escape rhythm (bradycardia). Alternatively, a tachycardia may result because slowed conduction provides the substrate for establishment of a reentry tachycardia. Impaired conduction through the bundle branches, on the other hand, produces prolongation of ventricular depolarization (widened QRS complex) but usually does not change the heart rate.

Reentry, or continuous circulating excitation, is the second type of abnormal impulse conduction. Reentry occurs when an impulse depolarizes an area of myocardium and then reenters and depolarizes the same area again (Jacobson, 1989). Under normal conditions, an impulse originating in the sinus node is transmitted to all cardiac cells and is extinguished when all cells have been depolarized and are completely refractory (Zipes, 1992a). However, when an area of unidirectional block is present in combination with slowed conduction through an alternative pathway, a reentry circuit is established in the following manner: in the area of unidirectional block, antegrade impulse propagation is blocked and cells distal to the area are depolarized through an alternate pathway. If conduction velocity through the alternate pathway is sufficiently slow, the electrical wave front travels retrograde through the area of unidirectional block, then reenters previously depolarized cells that have recovered and are capable of reexcitation (Fig. 4-1). Because the wave front is always preceded by excitable tissue, reentrant arrhythmias can continue indefinitely (Cox, 1990). Reentry circuits may involve anatomically large portions of myocardium or may be confined to small areas of tissue. Either premature complexes or tachyarrhythmias can result from reentry.

CLASSIFICATION OF ARRHYTHMIAS

BRADYARRHYTHMIAS

A variety of etiologic factors can produce bradyarrhythmias, including degenerative changes in the conductive system, myocardial infarction (MI), cardiac operations, hypersensitive carotid sinus syndrome, and certain medications. The need for treatment of bradyarrhythmias is based primarily on (1) presence and severity of associated symptoms, (2) ventricular rate and length of pauses between consecutive beats, and (3) clinical circumstances, specifically the presence and severity of organic heart disease (Lowe & German, 1990).

Diagnosis of bradyarrhythmias is usually accomplished with a standard 12-lead electrocardiogram (ECG) or Holter monitoring. Sometimes, an electrophysiologic study (EPS) is necessary to demonstrate sinus or AV nodal dysfunction or to precisely define the level of block in the AV node (McGregor, 1989). Results of this evaluation help determine arrhythmic risk and clarify the need for specific treatment. Except in cases in which a precipitating etiologic agent is

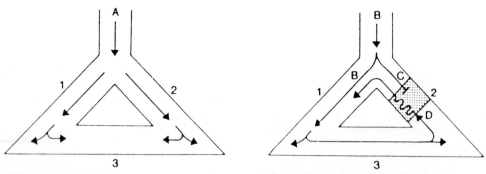

FIGURE 4-1. Schematic representation of reentry phenomenon. **(A)** Normal conduction of an impulse through cardiac muscle. **(B)** Conditions required to permit reentry: The impulse depolarizes pathway 1 normally, but antegrade conduction is blocked (*shaded area*) in pathway 2. The electrical wave front traveling through pathway 1 proceeds retrograde through the area of unidirectional block in pathway 2 and reenters myocardial cells in pathway 1 that have recovered and are capable of reexcitation. (Adapted from Rosen RM, Danilo P, 1979: The electrophysiological basis for cardiac arrhythmias. In Narula OS [ed]: Cardiac Arrhythmias: Electrophysiology, Diagnosis, and Management, p. 9. Baltimore, Williams & Wilkins)

identified and corrected, the primary treatment modality for bradyarrhythmias is artificial pacing. Bradycardia of a transient nature is treated with temporary pacing, using an external pulse generator to stimulate the myocardium through transvenous, epicardial (after cardiac surgery), or transthoracic leads. Implantation of a permanent pacing system is required for significant symptomatic bradycardia that persists or can be expected to recur. Temporary and permanent pacing systems are discussed in Chapter 26, Temporary Pacing and Defibrillation, and Chapter 20, Permanent Cardiac Pacemakers, respectively.

TACHYARRHYTHMIAS

Tachyarrhythmias can be subdivided into supraventricular and ventricular tachycardias according to whether the site of origin or perpetuation is above or below the bifurcation of the bundle of His (Guiraudon et al., 1991). Reentry is thought to cause the majority of tachyarrhythmias. However, there is increasing belief that the autonomic nervous system is also an important factor in arrhythmogenesis. Indeed, the electrophysiologic mechanism for most clinically occurring arrhythmias may be presumptive because present diagnostic methods are not sophisticated enough to unequivocally determine an etiologic mechanism (Zipes, 1992a).

A fundamental difference exists between supraventricular and ventricular tachyarrhythmias. Although the electrophysiologic mechanism in most forms of supraventricular tachycardia (SVT) is well understood, the responsible anatomic tissue cannot be distinctly visualized; in contrast, electrophysiology of ventricular tachycardia (VT) is not well understood, but the responsible anatomic tissue (areas of endocardial fibrosis) is often visually apparent (Cox, 1990).

Supraventricular Tachyarrhythmias

Supraventricular tachyarrhythmias may be caused by a variety of mechanisms. Reentry is most common although an automatic mechanism is presumed responsible for some forms of SVT. For example, ectopic foci in the left or right atrium can precipitate *ectopic atrial tachycardia* (Kirklin & Barratt-Boyes, 1993). This uncommon form of SVT, which occurs more often in children, can lead to cardiomyopathy in untreated patients (Walsh et al., 1992).

The various forms of reentry SVT are categorized by location of the reentrant circuit. *Atrial-ventricular reentry* describes a circuit within an anomalous tract of electrically active cardiac tissue extending directly from atrium to ventricle and bypassing the AV node. *AV nodal reentry* refers to a circuit located within the AV node or perinodal tissue, and *intra-atrial reentry* describes a reentrant pathway within the atrial muscle. Early data supporting a reentrant mechanism for SVT were developed in the electrophysiologic evaluation of patients with anomalous atrial-ventricular conduction, as occurs in individuals with *Wolff-Parkinson-White (WPW) syndrome* (Zipes, 1992a). The anatomic and electrophysiologic data obtained in these patients have since been successfully applied to support existence of a reentrant mechanism in AV nodal and atrial tachycardias as well.

Atrial-ventricular reentrant tachycardia associated with WPW syndrome is the supraventricular rhythm disorder most commonly treated with invasive therapy. The anomalous pathway, called a *Kent bundle*, is present at birth and may manifest itself clinically at any age. The pathway is usually categorized according to its anatomic location within the AV ring (i.e., left free wall, right free wall, posterior septum, or anterior septum) (Guiraudon et al., 1991). The Kent bundle may also be referred to as a type A or type B pathway. *Type A pathways* are generally between the left atrium and ventricle, and *type B pathways* are between the right atrium and ventricle. Twenty percent of patients have more than one accessory pathway (Hood et al., 1991).

The presence of an anomalous pathway is usually suggested by the following electrocardiographic features: a short PR interval (< 0.12 second), a prolonged QRS complex (> 0.12 second), and slurring of the ascending limb of the QRS wave (delta wave); secondary ST segment and T wave changes are almost always present (Fisch, 1992) (Fig. 4-2). An EPS is necessary to definitively confirm the presence and location of the anomalous pathway.

In patients with WPW syndrome, conduction may occur intermittently or continuously through the accessory tract and in an antegrade or retrograde direction. During sinus rhythm or any atrial arrhythmia, antegrade conduction through the accessory pathway may cause ectopic early activation of the ventricles, a phenomenon known as *ventricular preexcitation* (Waldo et al., 1991) (Fig. 4-3). When this occurs, the protection against rapid ventricular response rates normally provided by the AV node is absent. Retrograde, or concealed, conduction through the AV node or accessory tract provides the necessary alternate pathway for atrial-ventricular reentrant tachycardias.

Anomalous atrial-ventricular conduction is potentially life threatening. Although some patients with WPW syndrome have no significant tachyarrhythmias, the frequency of paroxysmal tachycardia appears to increase with age (Zipes, 1992a). Most common is a reciprocating SVT, which occurs in 80% of patients with WPW and tachyarrhythmias; atrial fibrillation occurs in 15% and atrial flutter in 5% (Kirklin & Barratt-Boyes, 1993). Rapid ventricular response rates during atrial fibrillation can result in syncope and occasionally ventricular fibrillation (VF) with sudden cardiac death (SCD).

AV nodal reentrant tachycardia arises from the presence of two anatomically or functionally distinct

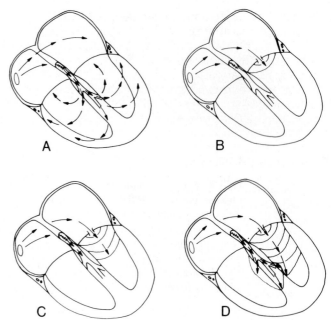

FIGURE 4-3. **(A)** Normal spread of electrical activation in the heart during sinus rhythm; the electrical impulse is delayed approximately 100 msec in the AV node. **(B** to **D)** Spread of electrical activation during sinus rhythm in Wolff-Parkinson-White syndrome with an accessory pathway in the left free wall. (Cox JL, 1990: The surgical management of cardiac arrhythmias. In Sabiston DC Jr, Spencer FC [eds]: Surgery of the Chest, ed. 5, p. 1866. Philadelphia, WB Saunders)

pathways in the region of the AV node (Guiraudon et al., 1991). These dual AV nodal conduction pathways provide the anatomic-electrophysiologic substrate for reentrant SVT (Cox et al., 1990). Usually, antegrade conduction of a premature atrial impulse blocks in the fast pathway, alternatively propagates antegrade through the slow pathway, and returns retrograde through the fast pathway (Zipes, 1992a).

Experimental and intraoperative mapping studies suggest that atrial fibrillation and atrial flutter are intra-atrial reentrant tachycardias. Atrial fibrillation appears to be caused by multiple reentrant wavelets in the atrium that are maintained by inhomogeneity of tissue refractoriness in the atrial myocardium; atrial flutter most likely arises from a large reentrant circuit in the right atrial tissue (Ferguson & Cox, 1993).

Ventricular Tachyarrhythmias

Ventricular arrhythmias arise within or distal to the bundle of His. They represent a continuum of severity that can be categorized as (1) premature ventricular complexes, (2) nonsustained VT (i.e., >100 beats per minute and <30 seconds in duration), (3) sustained VT (i.e., >100 beats per minute and ≥30 seconds in duration or requiring intervention to eradicate), and (4) VF. The most common ventricular arrhythmia requiring therapy is VT, usually due to a

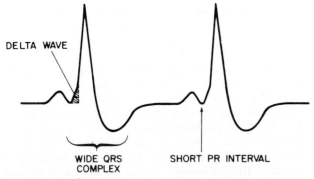

DELTA WAVE

WIDE QRS COMPLEX   SHORT PR INTERVAL

FIGURE 4-2. Characteristic electrocardiographic features during normal sinus rhythm in a patient with Wolff-Parkinson-White syndrome. (Cox JL, 1990: The surgical management of cardiac arrhythmias. In Sabiston DC Jr, Spencer FC [eds]: Surgery of the Chest, ed. 5, p. 1866. Philadelphia, WB Saunders) reentry phenomenon. Sustained VT may cause symptoms, including syncope or, in some cases, SCD. Patients who experience sustained, symptomatic VT almost always have organic heart disease, usually coronary artery disease.

Chronic ventricular rhythm disorders are generally categorized by etiology (Table 4-1). The most common etiology is coronary artery disease. Ventricular tachyarrhythmias associated with coronary artery disease almost always arise in the left ventricle or on the left ventricular side of the septum (Zipes, 1992b). These arrhythmias may be the result of either ischemia-mediated or scar-mediated electrical disorders. *Ischemia-mediated tachyarrhythmias* arise from tissue that is acutely or chronically ischemic secondary to obstructive lesions in the coronary arteries. *Scar-mediated ventricular tachyarrhythmias* are caused by changes in electrical properties of endocardial tissue that has been damaged by MI. The heterogeneity of the scar tissue provides a focus for reentrant arrhythmogenesis. Serious ventricular arrhythmias related to endocardial scar are almost always associated with major left ventricular wall motion abnormalities and often with significantly compromised left ventricular function.

Ventricular arrhythmias that occur in the absence of coronary artery disease may be associated with various other forms of organic heart disease. A congenital form of cardiomyopathy, termed *arrhythmogenic right ventricular dysplasia,* may be associated with ventricular arrhythmias that arise in the right ventricle (Cox, 1990). Both dilated and hypertrophic forms of *cardiomyopathy* are associated with serious ventricular rhythm disturbances, most likely related to pathologic changes in the ventricular myocardium. A recognized association exists between hypertrophic cardiomyopathy (also called idiopathic hypertrophic subaortic stenosis) and SCD.

Specific forms of *valvular heart disease,* particularly aortic stenosis and mitral valve prolapse are commonly associated with ventricular arrhythmias. Once present, the ventricular rhythm disorder is generally not eradicated by valve replacement. *Primary electrical*

disorder describes arrhythmias that occur in the absence of underlying structural heart disease, proarrhythmic agents, or metabolic imbalance. This entity may sometimes account for sudden, unexplained deaths that occur in presumably healthy young adults. The *prolonged QT syndrome* is a disorder in which abnormalities of ventricular repolarization occur, manifested by prolongation of the QT interval on the ECG. The condition may occur either congenitally or as an acquired disorder, such as due to medication, electrolyte imbalance, or hypothermia. Prolonged QT syndrome may be associated with *torsades de pointes,* a distinctive form of VT that is characterized by QRS complexes of changing amplitude that appear to twist around the isoelectric line and occur at rates of 200 to 250 per minute (Zipes, 1992c).

A number of medications are also known to predispose to ventricular arrhythmias. In fact, pharmacologic therapy for arrhythmic disorders is limited by the tendency for many commonly used antiarrhythmic agents to have proarrhythmic properties; that is, the drug itself may cause serious ventricular arrhythmias. Ventricular arrhythmias can also occur secondary to metabolic or endocrine abnormalities. Still other ventricular arrhythmias are related to autonomic influences and occur in the setting of stress or exertion.

SUDDEN CARDIAC DEATH

Sudden cardiac death is unexpected cardiac death preceded by no apparent symptoms or by symptoms less than 1 hour in duration (Cobb, 1990). Only 20% of SCD episodes are associated with acute MI (Myerburg & Castellanos, 1992). Instantaneous death is almost always due to a catastrophic arrhythmia. The initial documented arrhythmia is VF in 75% of SCD victims, asystole in 20%, and electromechanical dissociation in 5% (Greene, 1990). SVT in the presence of an anomalous atrial-ventricular conduction pathway can also cause arrhythmic death. SCD due to bradycardia may occur as a result of sick sinus syndrome with sinus arrest or AV block (Chung, 1988).

An estimated 300,000 persons experience SCD each year in the United States (Myerburg & Castellanos, 1992). Most episodes occur outside of hospitals during routine activities of daily living. The typical SCD survivor is male, 48 to 72 years of age, with a history of cardiovascular disease, not taking antiarrhythmic drugs, not exercising, with no distinctive warning symptoms, and no acute Q wave MI (Greene, 1990). Most individuals who experience SCD have significant coronary artery disease and a history of previous MI. Risk factors for coronary artery disease, particularly hypertension, hypercholesterolemia, and cigarette smoking are frequently present (Cobb, 1990). Etiologic factors for SCD other than coronary artery disease are the same as those responsible for ventricular arrhythmic disorders.

TABLE 4-1. ETIOLOGIES OF LIFE-THREATENING VENTRICULAR ARRHYTHMIAS

Coronary artery disease
   Ischemia-mediated
   Scar-mediated
Cardiomyopathy
Valvular heart disease
Primary electrical disorder
Prolonged QT syndrome
Medications
Metabolic disturbances
Endocrine abnormalities
Autonomic influences

Twenty to 30% of individuals who experience SCD survive (Mason & McPherson, 1992). Survival from SCD has become more common in recent years owing to widespread community awareness of cardiopulmonary resuscitation techniques and development of emergency systems that provide trained personnel capable of defibrillating victims in the field. The increased population of SCD survivors has encouraged development of new diagnostic methodologies, treatment modalities, and therapeutic devices to prevent recurrences. Survivors of SCD comprise a challenging patient population who require aggressive therapy. Unless the precipitating factor is controlled, these patients remain at increased risk for future major arrhythmic events. The probability of SCD recurrence for those who survive out-of-hospital VF is approximately 30% within 1 year (Greene, 1990; Waldo et al., 1990).

A number of factors have been identified that predispose to SCD recurrence. Arrhythmia recurrence is more likely in patients who experience SCD without associated acute MI. Arrhythmias that occur with acute MI are likely to be the result of electrophysiologic and biochemical abnormalities in the infarcted muscle. When the acute phase of the MI is over, the risk for arrhythmia recurrence decreases. Another useful predictor is left ventricular dysfunction, as demonstrated by a left ventricular ejection fraction that is less than 40% or by left ventricular wall motion abnormalities. Other markers for increased risk of SCD recurrence include history of previous MI or congestive heart failure, acute myocardial ischemia, frequent or complex ventricular ectopy, extensive coronary artery disease, advanced age, male gender, and inducibility at EPS (Greene, 1990).

DIAGNOSIS

The *electrophysiologic study* is the definitive diagnostic modality for defining arrhythmic disorders and guiding therapy. The procedure is generally performed in a laboratory setting. Intracardiac catheters are placed transvenously with the aid of fluoroscopy in various locations within the heart. These catheters are used for two purposes: (1) recordings of intracardiac action potentials and (2) programmed electrical stimulation (PES). Intracardiac recordings provide a sophisticated method of analyzing cardiac electrical activation and defining abnormalities of impulse formation and conduction (Chung, 1989b). Types of information that can be obtained during EPS are displayed in Table 4-2.

PES consists of using pacing stimuli to induce and terminate clinical arrhythmias and to identify abnormal activation sequences, thus localizing reentrant pathways. During PES, repetitive electrical stimuli are delivered at specific points in the cardiac cycle to provoke an arrhythmia that has occurred clinically. Extra stimuli can be delivered at progressively shorter

---

TABLE 4-2. PURPOSES OF ELECTROPHYSIOLOGIC STUDY

Recording of intracardiac electrograms
  Assessment of sinus node function
  Definition of atrioventricular nodal function (site of block)
  Mapping of cardiac activation during arrhythmias
Programmed electrical stimulation
  Initiation of arrhythmias
  Determination of inducibility and sustainability
  Determination of arrhythmia mechanism (reentrant versus autonomic)
  Termination of arrhythmia
Evaluation of antiarrhythmic medication or intervention effectiveness
Assessment of sensing and response by antiarrhythmic device

---

intervals until tissue refractoriness occurs. PES defines the origin and nature of the arrhythmia and reveals prognostic information about likelihood of arrhythmia recurrence. Therapy can then be more specifically directed at a particular arrhythmia, thus enhancing therapeutic efficacy. PES is also performed in the operating room during surgical procedures to ablate arrhythmogenic tissue. Electrodes are placed directly on the epicardial and endocardial surfaces of the heart to localize reentrant arrhythmic pathways or arrhythmogenic foci.

Clinically occurring arrhythmias provoked by PES are referred to as *inducible.* In general, inducible arrhythmias are thought to reflect a reentrant mechanism. A clinically occurring arrhythmia caused by an autonomic mechanism is more likely to be noninducible during PES (i.e., it cannot be provoked) (Cox, 1990). An important characteristic of an induced arrhythmia is *sustainability.* Sustained arrhythmias during PES are generally defined as those that are greater than or equal to 30 seconds in duration or that require intervention for hemodynamically compromising symptoms.

Inducibility and sustainability have important prognostic implications. For example, inducible, sustained VT correlates with a high probability of clinical arrhythmia recurrence. Similarly, inability to induce VT suggests a decreased risk of arrhythmia recurrence and, in selected patients, antiarrhythmic therapy may not be indicated. Finally, if arrhythmia provocation is reproducible, serial PES may be performed to evaluate efficacy of antiarrhythmic therapy. The effectiveness of a particular medication in preventing laboratory provocation of a clinically occurring tachyarrhythmia correlates in most cases with prognosis for clinical arrhythmia recurrence.

In SVT due to an accessory pathway (i.e., WPW syndrome) the type and location of pathway can be identified by the sequence of electrical activation through the heart after the clinical arrhythmia has been induced. The reentry circuit may be either *ortho-*

dromic (i.e., antegrade conduction over the AV node and retrograde conduction over the anomalous pathway) or *antidromic* (i.e., antegrade conduction through the anomalous pathway and retrograde conduction through the AV node) (McGregor, 1989). Tracking the pathway of electrical activation helps localize the anomalous pathway. Similar techniques are used to track the electrical activation sequence in other reentrant tachycardias.

Electrophysiologic testing has greatly enhanced understanding of a variety of rhythm disorders and provides valuable descriptive and prognostic information about cardiac rhythm disorders in individual patients. However, caution must be used in interpretation of findings. PES is not uniformly helpful in its predictive information; the ability of PES to predict arrhythmic outcome is variable based on the clinical situation. Therefore, particular consideration must be given to the clinical arrhythmia and the type and extent of underlying cardiac disease.

For example, inducible monomorphic VT (uniform QRS morphology) is often due to endocardial scar from a remote MI and is typically reproducible. Accordingly, PES is a valuable tool in defining arrhythmic risk and antiarrhythmic drug efficacy for these arrhythmias. In contrast, the induction of nonsustained, monomorphic VT or polymorphic (frequent changes in QRS morphology or axis) VT is less specific and of less clinical significance, particularly in patients with limited underlying structural heart disease. PES is also less predictive for patients with cardiomyopathic heart disease and in those with greater left ventricular dysfunction.

Before development of EPS, arrhythmia analysis and the plan of therapy were primarily based on the standard ECG, Holter monitoring, and exercise stress testing. Today, these diagnostic modalities provide valuable adjunctive information to supplement EPS. They are described in more detail in Chapter 8, Diagnostic Evaluation of Cardiac Disease.

Development of the *signal averaged electrocardiogram* (SAE) provides another noninvasive diagnostic study for evaluation of ventricular arrhythmias. In an SAE, QRS complexes are magnified and characterized by voltage and duration criteria. There is increasing evidence that patients with an abnormal SAE (prolonged QRS complex duration of predominantly low voltage activity) have an increased incidence of symptomatic ventricular tachyarrhythmias. Interpretation of SAEs in patients with a paced cardiac rhythm or complete bundle branch block is limited.

TREATMENT

Treatment of chronic cardiac rhythm disorders begins with elimination of any correctable etiologic factors, such as proarrhythmic medications. If the arrhythmia is attributed to active myocardial ischemia, coronary artery bypass grafting, percutaneous transluminal angioplasty, or antianginal medications may be indicated. In the absence of correctable precipitants, there are several forms of antiarrhythmic therapy: (1) antiarrhythmic drugs, (2) catheter or surgical ablation of arrhythmogenic foci or anomalous conduction pathways, and (3) antitachycardia devices. Often a combination of therapies is required for effective treatment of the cardiac rhythm disorder.

ANTIARRHYTHMIC MEDICATIONS

Antiarrhythmic medications are generally the initial therapeutic intervention. However, antiarrhythmic drug therapy is associated with significant problems. All currently available antiarrhythmic drugs have significant adverse effects and may not be tolerated as chronic therapy. Some antiarrhythmic drugs produce significant myocardial depression and may be contraindicated in patients with ventricular arrhythmias who typically have poor left ventricular function. Also, many antiarrhythmic agents have proarrhythmic properties. Finally, SCD recurs in a significant number of patients despite all currently available antiarrhythmic agents.

Antiarrhythmic medications are generally prescribed in patients with recurring supraventricular tachyarrhythmias that produce symptoms. An antiarrhythmic agent that is unlikely to be proarrhythmic and with a good side effect profile is selected. In patients with ventricular arrhythmias there is some controversy regarding the optimal endpoint of antiarrhythmic therapy—eradication of spontaneous ectopy during ambulatory monitoring or the suspension of inducible VT during PES. Before availability of PES techniques, suppression of spontaneous ventricular ectopy during ambulatory monitoring (Holter or exercise testing) was the primary method of determining antiarrhythmic efficacy. In selected patients at increased arrhythmic risk, PES is helpful in determining antiarrhythmic drug efficacy. Serial electrophysiologic testing with different medications may be performed to determine the most effective agent. If a patient is rendered noninducible during PES while receiving a specific antiarrhythmic drug, use of the drug is thought to have favorable prognostic implications.

Antiarrhythmic therapy is generally recommended for patients with sustained or symptomatic ventricular arrhythmias. Controversy remains about arrhythmic risk and the need for antiarrhythmic therapy in patients with nonsustained or asymptomatic tachycardia with underlying structural heart disease (Waldo et al., 1990). In the absence of structural heart disease, patients with nonsustained or asymptomatic VT are thought to be at low arrhythmic risk; specific antiarrhythmic therapy is not indicated.

A variety of medications are available for antiarrhythmic therapy. They are commonly classified into four categories, according to their mechanism of action: (1) membrane-stabilizing agents, (2) beta-adrenergic blocking agents, (3) agents that prolong repolarization, and (4) calcium-channel antagonist agents. Beta-blocking agents (e.g., propranolol) are often chosen for treatment of supraventricular tachyarrhythmias. Membrane-stabilizing agents (e.g., quinidine) or agents that prolong repolarization (e.g., sotalol) are commonly used for ventricular arrhythmias.

Amiodarone is generally considered the most effective antiarrhythmic agent in treatment of patients with ventricular rhythm disorders who have survived SCD. However, the efficacy of this potent agent must be carefully weighed against the arrhythmic risk and ongoing medical supervision is essential in patients receiving the drug. Amiodarone has many potentially serious side effects, including pulmonary, hepatic, neuromuscular, and thyroid toxicity. In addition, arrhythmia recurrence occurs in 30% to 40% of patients within 1 to 2 years and cannot be predicted (Rosenthal & Josephson, 1990).

CATHETER AND SURGICAL ABLATION

Difficulties with antiarrhythmic drug therapy have led to development of ablative therapy. *Ablative therapy* consists of catheter and open heart surgical techniques for disruption of a reentrant pathway. It is indicated for patients with either SVT or VT in whom pharmacologic therapy is not well tolerated or is ineffective in preventing frequent, disabling, or life-threatening arrhythmic episodes.

Catheter ablation, performed in the electrophysiology laboratory, is used to interrupt reentrant pathways responsible for supraventricular tachyarrhythmias. After identifying the endocardial site of earliest activation during the arrhythmia, radiofrequency energy is delivered through a transvenous, intracardiac electrode catheter positioned in the area of the reentrant pathway (Fig. 4-4). Radiofrequency ablation produces localized destruction of arrhythmogenic cardiac tissue. Because the area of tissue charge is localized, the technique is associated with few complications.

Catheter ablative techniques are most commonly performed to interrupt AV nodal reentrant pathways or anomalous atrial-ventricular connections (WPW syndrome) (Fig. 4-5). Complete AV nodal eradication may be performed in selected patients, such as those with refractory atrial arrhythmias. Radiofrequency ablative techniques have also been used to eradicate the arrhythmogenic focus in patients with ectopic atrial tachycardia (Walsh et al., 1992).

Cryoablation and *direct surgical excision* are ablative techniques performed during cardiac operations. Cryoablation is the direct application of an extremely cold (−60°C) probe to arrhythmogenic cardiac tissue to destroy it. It is increasingly used as adjunctive ablative therapy along with surgical excision. Surgical ablation to eradicate arrhythmogenic tissue or interrupt reentrant circuits is used in the treatment of both supraventricular and ventricular tachyarrhythmias.

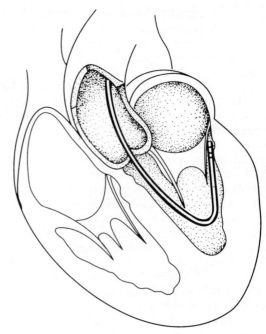

FIGURE 4-4. Retrograde catheterization of the left ventricle for radiofrequency ablation of left free wall accessory pathway. Catheter tip is positioned near mitral valve annulus in region of identified reentrant pathway. (Scheinman MM, 1991: Catheter ablation: Present role and projected impact on health care for patients with cardiac arrhythmias. Circulation 83:1492; American Heart Association)

Supraventricular tachyarrhythmias are surgically treated with mapping-directed division or cryoablation of reentrant pathways. Except for selected pathways which can be divided on the epicardial surface, most must be interrupted on the endocardial surface and therefore require atriotomy (incision into the atrium) and cardiopulmonary bypass. Surgical ablation is most commonly performed for division of atrial-ventricular pathways (e.g., Kent bundles). Surgical ablation for intra-atrial reentry arrhythmias (i.e., atrial fibrillation and atrial flutter) is evolving; initial success has been achieved with a surgical procedure called the *maze operation* (Cox et al., 1991). Selected patients with ectopic atrial tachycardia may also be treated with surgical ablative techniques.

Ventricular tachyarrhythmias are surgically treated by ventriculotomy and visually or mapping-directed excision of endocardial scar. Because ventriculotomy further damages an already compromised ventricle, the procedure is used selectively, typically in patients with a discrete anterior aneurysm, fairly good ventricular function, and frequent, monomorphic VT. Surgical resection is not possible in patients with ventricular arrhythmias due to diffuse myopathic heart disease as opposed to discrete areas of endocardial scarring. Endocardial resection may also carry a prohibitive operative risk in patients with severe left ventricular dysfunction and congestive heart failure.

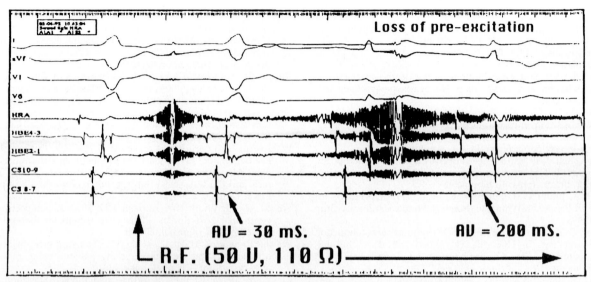

FIGURE 4-5. Loss of preexcitation during radiofrequency ablation in a patient with Wolff-Parkinson-White syndrome. Electrocardiographic tracings from top to bottom include surface leads (I, aVf, V1, and V6), and electrograms recorded from high right atrium (HRA), the region of the His bundle (HBE4-3, HBE2-1), and the coronary sinus (CS10-9), CS8-7). First *arrow* on left represents application of radiofrequency energy; second and third *arrows* demonstrate lengthening of AV internal with loss of preexcitation. (Finkelmeier BA, 1994: Ablative therapy in the treatment of tachyarrhythmias. Crit Care Nurs Clin North Am 6:106)

ANTITACHYCARDIA DEVICES

An *implantable cardioverter/defibrillator* (ICD) is the most appropriate form of therapy for some patients with ventricular tachyarrhythmias. An ICD does nothing to prevent an arrhythmia from occurring but rather provides conversion of the arrhythmia when it occurs. Therefore, it is most often used in combination with either antiarrhythmic medications or, occasionally, with endocardial resection. ICDs sense tachyarrhythmias and in response deliver one or more shocks to defibrillate the heart and restore an intrinsic cardiac rhythm. Newer programmable devices offer tiered therapy, that is, antitachycardia pacing as well as both low- and high-energy defibrillating shocks (Former et al., 1992). Defibrillator implantation is an attractive therapeutic option in patients with ventricular arrhythmias and poor left ventricular function. It can generally be performed transvenously and, in contrast to endocardial resection, does not necessitate a major thoracic operation with cardiopulmonary bypass and ventriculotomy. Availability of defibrillating devices as an additional therapeutic modality has resulted in much more selective indications for surgical endocardial resection.

Antitachycardia pacemakers are occasionally used for treatment of supraventricular tachyarrhythmias that are proven to be terminated by overdrive pacing during PES. An antitachycardia pacemaker is a device that delivers four or five pacing stimuli in succession at progressively shorter intervals. Patients receiving antitachycardia pacemakers are usually those with disabling symptoms whose arrhythmias are refractory to pharmacologic therapy. The effectiveness of catheter and surgical ablation techniques has limited the applicability of this form of therapy to a small number of patients. Surgical therapies are described in more detail in Chapter 18, Surgical Treatment of Cardiac Rhythm Disorders.

REFERENCES

Chung EK, 1988: Sudden cardiac death. In Manual of Acute Cardiac Disorders. Boston, Butterworths

Chung EK, 1989a: Some aspects of the anatomy, electrophysiology, and hemodynamics of the heart. In Principles of Cardiac Arrhythmias, ed. 4. Baltimore, Williams & Wilkins

Chung EK, 1989b: Electrophysiologic studies. In Principles of Cardiac Arrhythmias, ed. 4. Baltimore, Williams & Wilkins

Cobb LA, 1990: The mechanisms, predictors, and prevention of SCD. In Hurst JW, Schlant RC, Rackley CE, et al (eds): The Heart, ed. 7. New York, McGraw-Hill

Cox JL, 1990: The surgical management of cardiac arrhythmias. In Sabiston DC Jr, Spencer FC (eds): Surgery of the Chest, ed. 5. Philadelphia, WB Saunders

Cox JL, Ferguson TB, Lindsay BD, Cain ME, 1990: Perinodal cryosurgery for atrioventricular node reentry tachycardia in 23 patients. J Thorac Cardiovasc Surg 99:440

Cox JL, Schuessler RB, D'Agostino HJ, et al, 1991: The surgical treatment of atrial fibrillation (III). J Thorac Cardiovasc Surg 101:569

Ferguson TB, Cox JL, 1993: Surgical treatment of cardiac arrhythmias. Heart Dis Stroke 2:37

Fisch C, 1992: Electrocardiography and vectorcardiography. In Braunwald E (ed): Heart Disease: A Textbook of Cardiovascular Medicine, ed. 4. Philadelphia, WB Saunders

Fromer M, Brachmann J, Block M, et al, 1992: Efficacy of automatic multimodal device therapy for ventricular tachyarrhythmias as delivered by a new implantable pacing cardioverter-defibrillator: Results of a European multicenter study of 102 implants. Circulation 86:363

Greene HL, 1990: Sudden arrhythmic cardiac death—mechanisms, resuscitation, and classification: The Seattle perspective. Am J Cardiol 65:4B

Guiraudon GM, Klein GJ, Sharma AD, Yee R, 1991: Surgical treatment of supraventricular tachycardias. In Baue AE, Geha AS, Hammond GL, et al (eds): Glenn's Thoracic and Cardiovascular Surgery, ed. 5. Norwalk, CT, Appleton & Lange

Halpenny CJ, 1989: Cardiac electrophysiology. In Underhill SL, Woods SL, Froelicher ES, Halpenny CJ (eds): Cardiac Nursing, ed. 2. Philadelphia, JB Lippincott

Hood MA, Smith WM, Robinson C, et al, 1991: Operations for Wolff-Parkinson-White syndrome. J Thorac Cardiovasc Surg 101:998

Jacobson C, 1989: Pathophysiology of arrhythmias and conduction disturbances. In Underhill SL, Woods SL, Froelicher ES, Halpenny CJ (eds): Cardiac Nursing, ed. 2. Philadelphia, JB Lippincott

Kirklin JW, Barratt-Boyes BG, 1993: Tachycardia. In Cardiac Surgery, ed. 2. New York, Churchill Livingstone

Lowe JE, German LD, 1990: Cardiac pacemakers and cardiac conduction system abnormalities. In Sabiston DC, Spencer FC (eds): Surgery of the Chest, ed. 5. Philadelphia, WB Saunders

Mason P, McPherson C, 1992: Implantable cardioverter defibrillator: A review. Heart Lung 21:141

McGregor MS, 1989: Electrophysiologic studies. In Underhill SL, Woods SL, Froelicher ES, Halpenny CJ: Cardiac Nursing, ed 2. Philadelphia, JB Lippincott

Myerburg RJ, Castellanos A, 1992: Cardiac arrest and sudden cardiac death. In Braunwald E (ed): Heart Disease: A Textbook of Cardiovascular Medicine, ed. 4. Philadelphia, WB Saunders

Rosenthal ME, Josephson ME, 1990: Current status of antitachycardia devices. Circulation 82:1890

Ruskin JN, Schoenfeld MH, 1989: Mechanisms of ventricular arrhythmias. In Eagle KA, Haber E, DeSanctis RW, Austin WG (eds): The Practice of Cardiology, ed. 2. Boston, Little, Brown

Smith WB, 1990: Mechanisms of cardiac arrhythmias and conduction disturbances. In Hurst JW, Schlant RC, Rackley CE, et al (eds): The Heart, ed. 7. New York, McGraw-Hill

Waldo AL, Henthorn RW, Carlson MD, 1991: Electrophysiologic evaluation for the surgical management of arrhythmias. In Baue AE, Geha AS, Hammond GL, et al (eds): Glenn's Thoracic and Cardiovascular Surgery, ed. 5. Norwalk, CT, Appleton & Lange

Waldo AL, Henthorn RW, Carlson MD, 1990: A perspective on ventricular arrhythmias: Patient assessment for therapy and outcome. Am J Cardiol, 65:30B

Walsh EP, Saul JP, Hulse JE, et al, 1992: Transcatheter ablation of ectopic atrial tachycardia in young patients using radiofrequency current. Circulation 86:1138

Zipes DP, 1992a: Genesis of cardiac arrhythmias: Electrophysiological considerations. In Braunwald E (ed): Heart Disease: A Textbook of Cardiovascular Medicine, ed. 4. Philadelphia, WB Saunders

Zipes DP, 1992b: Management of cardiac arrhythmias: Pharmacological, electrical, and surgical techniques. In Braunwald E (ed): Heart Disease: A Textbook of Cardiovascular Medicine, ed. 4. Philadelphia, WB Saunders

Zipes DP, 1992c: Specific arrhythmias: Diagnosis and treatment. In Braunwald E (ed): Heart Disease: A Textbook of Cardiovascular Medicine, ed. 4. Philadelphia, WB Saunders

5

CARDIOMYOPATHY

DILATED CARDIOMYOPATHY
HYPERTROPHIC CARDIOMYOPATHY
RESTRICTIVE CARDIOMYOPATHY

The term *cardiomyopathy* is used to describe any of a group of primary disorders of the heart muscle. Although several causative agents and systemic syndromes are known to produce myocardial dysfunction, a specific etiology is not identified in most cases (Wenger et al., 1990). Therefore, pathophysiology, instead of etiology, is generally used to categorize cardiomyopathy into three major forms: (1) dilated, (2) hypertrophic, and (3) restrictive. Because of the differing anatomic and functional characteristics, each produces different hemodynamic consequences and requires different types of therapy.

DILATED CARDIOMYOPATHY

Dilated cardiomyopathy (DCM), formerly known as congestive cardiomyopathy, is the most commonly occurring form of heart muscle disorder in this country. It is a syndrome characterized by cardiac enlargement and impaired systolic function of one or both ventricles (Wynne & Braunwald, 1992) (Fig. 5-1).

The cause or causes of DCM remain unclear, but at least four conditions, if not etiologically linked, appear to lower the threshold for development of DCM: infection, alcoholism, pregnancy, and systemic hypertension (Wynne & Braunwald, 1992). Other factors may also play a role, such as familial predisposition, endocrine abnormalities, and exposure to various toxins (e.g., cocaine or cigarette smoking). In a great many cases no specific etiologic factor is identified, and the condition is termed *idiopathic dilated cardiomyopathy*.

There is considerable speculation that *infective myocarditis*, particularly *viral myocarditis*, may progress to DCM, particularly in children (Kirklin & Barratt-Boyes, 1993a). Acute myocarditis is an inflammatory process of the myocardium that can affect persons of all ages and may be caused by almost any bacterial, viral, rickettsial, mycotic, or parasitic organism (Wenger et al., 1990). Viral myocarditis is particularly difficult to diagnose because of the infrequency with which the presence of viral organisms can be histologically detected. It most often has an insidious and benign course but can produce serious cardiovascular complications. Because of the highly variable clinical presentation, myocarditis frequently remains undiagnosed until chronic cardiac dysfunction and congestive heart failure develop (Grady & Costanzo-Nordin, 1989).

DCM can also result from heavy ingestion of alcohol beverages over a prolonged period of time. The relationship between alcohol abuse and DCM is well documented, but the causative mechanism remains unclear. Many patients with DCM have a history of alcohol abuse, but others with similar alcohol consumption patterns do not develop cardiomyopathy (Hillis et al., 1992a). Alcohol-induced DCM differs from other forms in that the primary clinical manifestation, congestive heart failure, may abate during periods of abstinence and usually recurs when alcohol consumption is resumed (Wenger et al., 1990). However, myocardial damage eventually becomes irreversible, leading to a progressively downward course despite drinking patterns.

Pregnancy may also precipitate DCM. *Peripartum*

Betsy Finkelmeier: CARDIOTHORACIC SURGICAL NURSING.
© 1995 J.B. Lippincott Company.

53

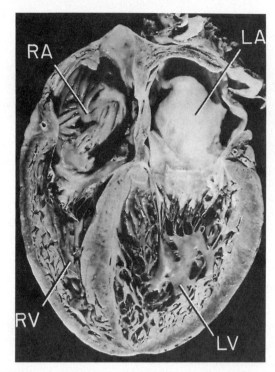

FIGURE 5-1. Autopsy specimen demonstrating dilated cardiomyopathy. Note all four cardiac chambers are dilated, particularly the left ventricle (*LV*). The ventricular walls are hypertrophied, but not disproportionately to the degree of chamber dilation. *RA,* right atrium; *LA,* left atrium; *RV,* right ventricle. (Johnson RA, Fifer MA, Palacios IF, 1989: Dilated and restrictive cardiomyopathies. In Eagle KA, Haber E, De-Sanctis RW, Austen WG [eds]: The Practice of Cardiology, ed. 2, p. 896. Boston, Little, Brown)

cardiomyopathy in this country is most common in women who are multiparous, older than 30 years of age, and African-American (Elkayam, 1992). It generally occurs during the latter part of pregnancy or in the puerperium (confinement after labor) and may recur with subsequent pregnancies (Wenger et al., 1990). Factors leading to peripartum DCM are not well understood. Systemic arterial hypertension appears to be an important etiologic factor in patients with DCM, particularly African-American men (Hillis et al., 1992a). The causative mechanism is not well defined.

Patients with DCM may remain asymptomatic for a period of time. Congestive heart failure is the major clinical manifestation. Exertional dyspnea, generalized weakness, and fatigue typically develop gradually over weeks or months (Bush & Healy, 1987). Both systemic and pulmonary embolism can occur as a result of thrombus associated with atrial fibrillation, poorly contractile ventricles, or peripheral venous stasis. As left ventricular dysfunction progresses, the propensity for malignant ventricular arrhythmias and sudden cardiac death (SCD) increases (Wenger et al., 1990).

The natural history of patients with DCM is variable but development of symptoms is generally followed by a downward course. Some patients die within 1 to 2 years of onset, and approximately 80% of patients are dead within 10 years, usually due to chronic congestive heart failure (Kirklin & Barratt-Boyes, 1993a). Indicators of a poor prognosis include age at onset greater than 55 years, New York Heart Association class IV functional status, marked cardiomegaly, ejection fraction less than 20%, cardiac index less than 3 L/min/m², left ventricular end-diastolic pressure greater than 20 mm Hg, and symptomatic ventricular tachycardia (Gay & O'Connell, 1990).

In some cases, a treatable cause of DCM is identified. However, in most cases, there is no curative therapy. Medical treatment is aimed at palliating symptoms of progressive heart failure. Inotropic agents are used to improve contractility and vasodilating agents to reduce preload and afterload. Intravenous dobutamine, administered continuously over 2 to 3 days or on a weekly basis by means of a portable infusion device, has exhibited sustained hemodynamic benefits that last weeks or months (Smith et al., 1992). In addition, specific vasodilating therapy (enalapril and hydralazine plus nitrates) has proven effective in prolonging survival (Wynne & Braunwald, 1992). Antiarrhythmic agents are used if significant ventricular arrhythmias are present. Implantation of an internal cardioverter/defibrillator may also be considered in patients with symptomatic ventricular tachyarrhythmias (Wynne & Braunwald, 1992). Anticoagulation is recommended to reduce the risk of thromboembolism.

Before development of *cardiac transplantation* as a therapeutic modality, patients with DCM faced a dismal future. Survival prognosis has been substantially increased by improvements in and availability of cardiac transplantation. However, the number of patients treated with cardiac transplantation is limited by the scarcity of donor hearts. *Dynamic cardiomyoplasty* is an alternative form of surgical therapy that is being performed in some patients in selected centers (Moreira et al., 1991).

HYPERTROPHIC CARDIOMYOPATHY

Hypertrophic cardiomyopathy (HCM) is a genetically transmitted form of cardiomyopathy. It is characterized by impaired diastolic ventricular function and hypertrophy of ventricular muscle mass (Fig. 5-2). Ventricular hypertrophy may occur in a concentric or asymmetric fashion and may or may not obstruct outflow from the left ventricle. Ventricular cavity size is small or normal, and systolic function is usually hyperdynamic (Bush & Healy, 1987). HCM has formerly been called idiopathic hypertrophic subaortic stenosis (IHSS), hypertrophic obstructive cardiomyopathy,

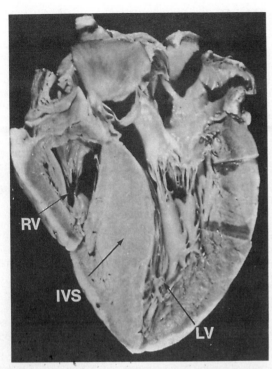

FIGURE 5-2. Autopsy specimen demonstrating hypertrophic cardiomyopathy. Ventricular walls are disproportionately thickened relative to the ventricular chambers; note massively thickened interventricular septum. *RV,* right ventricle; *IVS,* interventricular septum; *LV,* left ventricle. (Johnson RA, Fifer MA, Palacios IF, 1989: Dilated and restrictive cardiomyopathies. In Eagle KA, Haber E, DeSanctis RW, Austen WG [eds]: The Practice of Cardiology, ed. 2, p. 896. Boston, Little, Brown)

and asymmetric septal hypertrophy (Nishimura et al., 1991).

The pathophysiology of HCM is not well understood, but the process involves fibrosis of myofibrils, leading to impaired ventricular contraction and relaxation. Left ventricular hypertrophy occurs over time, reducing size and compliance of the chamber (Miracle, 1988). Abnormal anterior displacement of the mitral valve and systolic anterior motion of the anterior valve leaflet contribute to left ventricular outflow tract obstruction and the variable degree of mitral regurgitation that is usually present (Jacobs & Austen, 1990).

HCM occurs more commonly in males and is often associated with coronary artery disease. It can be manifested at any age from early infancy to the sixth or seventh decade but most commonly becomes evident in the second or third decade (Kirklin & Barratt-Boyes, 1993b). The most frequently occurring symptoms are (1) dyspnea, present in up to 90% of patients with HCM, (2) angina, occurring in 70% to 80%, and (3) syncope, in approximately 20% (Nishimura et al., 1991). Symptoms are commonly associated with exertion when ventricular contractility and oxygen demands are increased. One of the most distressing as-

pects of HCM is a propensity for sudden death. Although the etiology of SCD in these patients is not clearly established, it may be related to a primary electrical disorder, abnormality of conductive tissue, or hypotension secondary to left ventricular outflow tract obstruction.

In contrast to valvular aortic stenosis, left ventricular obstruction associated with HCM is dynamic; that is, it changes with varying hemodynamic conditions. Therefore, the intensity of the systolic murmur produced by outflow obstruction varies directly with increases or decreases in the pressure gradient between the left ventricle and aorta. Murmur intensity is increased with the Valsalva maneuver and during squatting-to-standing action; it is decreased by maneuvers such as standing-to-squatting action, passive leg elevation, and hand grip (Wynne & Braunwald, 1992).

The most important study for diagnostic evaluation of HCM is Doppler echocardiography. Medical treatment is directed at (1) reducing the degree of left ventricular outflow tract obstruction (by decreasing contractility) and (2) improving diastolic relaxation. Both calcium-channel antagonistic and beta-adrenergic blocking medications may be useful in reducing symptoms because of their negative inotropic effects. Beta-blocking agents also enhance diastolic filling by increasing ventricular compliance and lowering heart rate (Bush & Healy, 1987). Antiarrhythmic medications may be administered in patients with evidence of ventricular arrhythmias. Inotropic medications, such as digoxin, are contraindicated because they increase contractility and thereby increase the degree of obstruction. Antibiotic prophylaxis against infective endocarditis is recommended (Bush & Healy, 1987). Because SCD often occurs during exercise and is the major cause of death in patients with HCM, strenuous exercise is contraindicated, even in those without prominent symptoms (Wynne & Braunwald, 1992).

Surgical treatment of HCM is reserved for patients who remain symptomatic despite medical therapy or who are unable to tolerate medications. The most common reparative procedure is a *myectomy,* or resection of a portion of the hypertrophied ventricular septum. Mitral valve replacement may be necessary in some cases. Surgical therapy is described in detail in Chapter 21, Surgical Treatment of Other Cardiovascular Disorders.

RESTRICTIVE CARDIOMYOPATHY

Restrictive cardiomyopathy is the least common form of primary myocardial dysfunction. It is characterized by diffuse ventricular hypertrophy and impaired diastolic function with loss of compliance (Kirklin & Barratt-Boyes 1993a). Restrictive cardiomyopathy often occurs secondary to infiltration of the myocardium with an abnormal substance. Causative disorders include (1) *amyloidosis,* a disorder of unknown etiology in which eosinophilic fibrous protein is deposited in the myocardium and other tissue; (2) *hemochromatosis*, characterized by excessive deposition of iron in body tissues, including the myocardium; and (3) *glycogen deposition* in the myocardium (Hillis et al., 1992b). Restrictive cardiomyopathy may also occur secondary to mediastinal irradiation or a collagen-vascular disorder, such as scleroderma. *Endomyocardial fibroelastosis* is a form of restrictive cardiomyopathy in which the pathologic process occurs in the endocardium (Kirklin & Barratt-Boyes, 1993a). In some instances, etiology is unknown.

The restrictive process in the endocardium or myocardium produces abnormal rigidity of the ventricular chambers. The resultant inability of the myocardium to relax during diastole impedes ventricular filling and results in decreased cardiac output. Restrictive cardiomyopathy is usually associated with elevated right- and left-sided filling pressures, dilated atria, normal-sized ventricles, and well-preserved systolic function as measured by ejection fraction (Siegel et al., 1984). Restrictive cardiomyopathy secondary to endomyocardial fibrosis is characterized by the presence of a thick, fibrous, tissue layer covering the endocardial surface of the ventricles (Barretto et al., 1989). Both ventricles are likely to be affected by the process.

Exercise intolerance is commonly present in patients with restrictive cardiomyopathy because the associated reflex tachycardia that occurs to increase cardiac output further compromises ventricular filling (Wynne & Braunwald, 1992). The clinical manifestations of restrictive cardiomyopathy are frequently difficult to distinguish from constrictive pericarditis. Echocardiography may be helpful in differentiating the two conditions.

The biventricular failure that results from restrictive cardiomyopathy is difficult to treat with conventional medical therapy. In fact, digoxin, diuretics, and salt restriction may make the condition worse in some patients (Hillis et al., 1992b). Because of the systemic nature of the underlying disease process, these patients are not candidates for cardiac transplantation. A progressive downhill course is typical; most patients die within 1 or 2 years of diagnosis.

REFERENCES

Barretto ACP, da Luz PL, de Oliveira SA, et al, 1989: Determinants of survival in endomyocardial fibrosis. Circulation 80(Suppl I):I-177

Bush DE, Healy BP, 1987: Cardiomyopathies. In Chung EK (ed): Quick Reference to Cardiovascular Diseases, ed. 3. Baltimore, Williams & Wilkins

Elkayam U, 1992: Pregnancy and cardiovascular disease. In Braunwald E (ed): Heart Disease: A Textbook of Cardiovascular Medicine, ed. 4. Philadelphia, WB Saunders

Gay WA, O'Connell JB, 1990: Cardiac transplantation. In Sabiston DC Jr, Spencer FC (eds), 1990: Surgery of the Chest, ed. 5. Philadelphia, WB Saunders

Grady KL, Costanzo-Nordin MR, 1989: Myocarditis: Review of a clinical enigma. Heart Lung 18:4

Hillis LD, Lange RA, Wells PJ, Winniford MD, 1992a: Dilated cardiomyopathy. In Manual of Clinical Problems in Cardiology, ed. 4. Boston, Little, Brown

Hillis LD, Lange RA, Wells PJ, Winniford MD, 1992b: Restrictive cardiomyopathy. In Manual of Clinical Problems in Cardiology, ed. 4. Boston, Little, Brown

Jacobs ML, Austen WG, 1990: Acquired aortic valve disease. In Sabiston DC Jr, Spencer FC (eds): Surgery of the Chest, ed. 5. Philadelphia, WB Saunders

Kirklin JW, Barratt-Boyes BG, 1993a: Primary cardiomyopathy and cardiac transplantation. In Cardiac Surgery, ed. 2. New York, Churchill Livingstone

Kirklin JW, Barratt-Boyes BG, 1993b: Hypertrophic obstructive cardiomyopathy. In Cardiac Surgery, ed. 2. New York, Churchill Livingstone

Miracle VA, 1988: Idiopathic hypertrophic subaortic stenosis. Crit Care Nurse 8:3

Moreira LF, Stolf NA, Jatene AD, 1991: Benefits of cardiomyoplasty for dilated cardiomyopathy. Semin Thorac Cardiovasc Surg 3:140

Nishimura RA, Giuliani ER, Tajik AJ, Brandenburg RO, 1991: Hypertrophic cardiomyopathy. In Giuliani ER, Fuster V, Gersh BJ, et al (eds): Cardiology Fundamentals and Practice, ed. 2. St. Louis, Mosby–Year Book

Siegel RJ, Shah PK, Fishbein MC, 1984: Idiopathic restrictive cardiomyopathy. Circulation 70:165

Smith TW, Braunwald E, Kelly RA, 1992: The management of heart failure. In Braunwald E (ed): Heart Disease: A Textbook of Cardiovascular Medicine, ed. 4. Philadelphia, WB Saunders

Wenger NK, Abelmann WH, Roberts WC, 1990: Cardiomyopathy and specific heart muscle disease. In Hurst JW, Schlant RC, Rackley CE, et al (eds): The Heart, ed. 7. New York, McGraw-Hill

Wynne J, Braunwald E, 1992: The cardiomyopathies and myocarditides: Toxic, chemical and physical damage to the heart. In Braunwald E (ed): Heart Disease: A Textbook of Cardiovascular Medicine, ed. 4. Philadelphia, WB Saunders

CONGENITAL HEART DISEASE IN ADULTS

CLASSIFICATION OF DEFECTS
DEFECTS WITH LEFT TO RIGHT SHUNTS
  Atrial Septal Defect
  Ventricular Septal Defect
  Patent Ductus Arteriosus
DEFECTS WITH OUTFLOW OBSTRUCTION
  Aortic Stenosis
  Coarctation of the Aorta
  Pulmonic Stenosis
  Tetralogy of Fallot

COMPLICATIONS OF CONGENITAL HEART DISEASE
  Infective Endocarditis
  Eisenmenger's Syndrome
  Paradoxical Embolism
  Arterial Desaturation
  Aortic Aneurysm
  Complications Associated With Pregnancy

Approximately 30,000 infants are born each year with one or more congenital heart defects, and an estimated 930,000 persons with *congenital heart disease* (CHD) are currently living in the United States (American Heart Association, 1991). A combination of genetic predisposition and environmental factors is thought to cause congenital cardiac anomalies. Some defects, such as those that occur with Down's syndrome, are primarily genetic; others are caused by exposure to environmental teratogens, such as rubella, during a critical period of fetal development (Nugent et al., 1990). Innovations in surgical techniques over the past several decades have made possible correction of most congenital cardiac defects. As a result, many individuals with CHD undergo surgical correction during infancy or early childhood.

Adults with unrepaired heart defects are uncommon and can be grouped into three categories. Most common in a cardiac surgical setting are those persons with defects undiagnosed or without symptoms during childhood. The diagnosis in such patients is frequently made when, as an adult, the individual first has reason to receive a physical examination,

chest roentgenogram, or electrocardiogram. In other cases, the defect is detected when a period of increased hemodynamic demands, such as occurs with pregnancy, provokes the development of symptoms. With some defects, such as bicuspid aortic valve or mitral valve prolapse, harmful sequelae of the lesion may appear only after several decades, precipitated by degenerative tissue changes or endocarditic infection. Whereas ventricular septal defect (VSD) is the most common congenital lesion in the pediatric population, atrial septal defect (ASD) and aortic stenosis secondary to a bicuspid aortic valve are most common in adults (Henning & Grenvik, 1989).

The second group of adults with CHD are those who have already undergone surgical correction. Because many congenital heart defects are repaired during infancy or childhood, the number of adults with repaired lesions is steadily increasing. Although lifelong medical supervision for management of postoperative sequelae is necessary, treatment in a cardiac surgical setting is rarely required. However, a small number of persons with previously repaired defects require further surgical therapy as adults. Revision of

Betsy Finkelmeier: CARDIOTHORACIC SURGICAL NURSING.
© 1995 J.B. Lippincott Company.

prosthetic conduits, (e.g., those used in Rastelli or Mustard procedures) and replacement of prosthetic valves or homografts are most common.

The third group of adults with CHD are those with lesions for which no corrective surgery is available. Survival to adulthood is rare in these patients. Of those who do reach adulthood, some may have undergone a palliative procedure during childhood. Rarely, a subsequent palliative operation is performed.

CLASSIFICATION OF DEFECTS

Nearly 100 types of anatomic congenital deformities of the heart exist; most are rare or represent combinations of isolated lesions (Nolan, 1974). The anatomic and physiologic abnormalities are extensive, complex, and beyond the scope of this chapter. Adults with CHD represent only a small segment of the population of affected individuals. Similarly, with rare exceptions, untreated defects in adults consist of only a handful of the most common and least complex isolated cardiac deformities. Only those congenital heart lesions that are present most commonly in adults are included in this chapter. For an in-depth discussion of the multitude of cardiovascular deformities that constitute CHD, the reader is referred to a textbook of pediatric cardiology.

The common congenital anatomic deformities of the heart may be classified into four categories, according to the type of physiologic abnormality. Individual defects within each category differ in anatomic location of the deformity but are similar in the resulting pathophysiology (Table 6-1). The categories are (1) abnormal communication between systemic and pulmonic circulations, producing a left to right shunt, (2) valvular or vascular obstruction, with or without a right to left shunt, (3) transposition of great vessels or cardiac chambers, and (4) venous anomalies (Nolan, 1974). Almost all untreated defects in adults that require surgical intervention are in the first two categories.

DEFECTS WITH LEFT TO RIGHT SHUNTS

ASD, VSD, and patent ductus arteriosus (PDA) are the most common defects associated with left to right shunts. In each, an abnormal communication allows shunting of blood from the left side of the heart with its high systemic resistance to the right side with its low pulmonary vascular resistance. The three defects differ primarily in the anatomic level of systemic-pulmonic communication. The opening is between the atria with ASD, between the ventricles with VSD, and between the great vessels (pulmonary artery and aorta) with PDA.

The predominant hemodynamic effect of each of these lesions is left to right shunting of blood. The resultant increased blood flow through the pulmonary vasculature produces congestive heart failure and pulmonary hypertension that may evolve to pulmonary vascular obstruction, that is, an irreversible

---

TABLE 6-1. CLASSIFICATION SYSTEM FOR COMMON FORMS OF CONGENITAL HEART DISEASE

I. Left to Right Shunt

(Abnormal communication between systemic and pulmonic circuits)

Defect	Level of Communication
Atrial septal defect*	Atria
Ventricular septal defect*	Ventricles
Patent ductus arteriosus*	Great vessels (aorta to pulmonary artery)

II. Valvular or Vascular Obstruction

(With or without abnormal communication proximal to obstruction)

Defect	Level of Obstruction	Level of Communication
Aortic stenosis*	Aortic valve	None
Pulmonic stenosis	Pulmonic valve	None
Coarctation*	Aorta	None
Tetralogy of Fallot	Right ventricular outflow tract	Ventricle

III. Transposition of Great Vessels or Cardiac Chambers

Transposition of great vessels

IV. Venous Anomalies

Total or partial anomalous pulmonary venous connection

* Most common congenital heart defects in adults.
(Nolan SP, 1974: Congenital heart disease: Indications for and timing of operation. Paediatrician 3:144)

increase in pulmonary vascular resistance. Patients with chronically increased pulmonary vascular pressure may be comfortable at rest but develop such symptoms as tachypnea, dyspnea, cough, fatigue, and orthopnea with exercise (McNamara, 1989). Often, such exercise intolerance is not recognized as abnormal by the adult because it has always been present. Eventually, right-sided pressure may increase substantially, decreasing the shunt and causing a diminution in intensity of the heart murmur associated with the defect. This indicates worsening, not improvement, of the patient's condition. If pulmonary hypertension remains uncorrected, pulmonary artery pressure eventually exceeds systemic arterial pressure and the shunt direction reverses to become right to left. This condition, known as Eisenmenger's syndrome, is discussed further later in the chapter.

ATRIAL SEPTAL DEFECT

Atrial septal defects comprise nearly 50% of CHD in adults (Henning & Grenvik, 1989). The defect occurs approximately twice as commonly in females (Spencer, 1990). ASDs are classified by their location in the interatrial septum (Fig. 6-1). Most common is *ostium secundum,* or *fossa ovalis ASD,* located in the middle portion of the atrial septum.

Less common are *sinus venosus ASDs,* located at the junction of the superior vena cava. Sinus venosus ASDs are often associated with *partial anomalous pulmonary venous connection* (PAPVC), a structural abnormality in which the anomalous location of one or both right pulmonary veins causes part or all of the venous

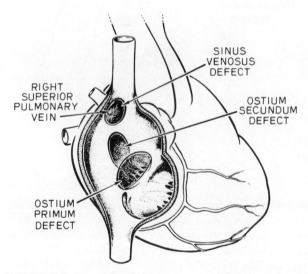

FIGURE 6-1. Location of the most common types of atrial septal defect. (Watson SP, Watson DC Jr, 1982: Anatomy, physiology, and hemodynamics of congenital heart disease. In Ream AK, Fogdall RP [eds]: Acute Cardiovascular Management: Anesthesia and Intensive Care, p. 584. Philadelphia, JB Lippincott)

(oxygenated) blood from the right lung to empty through the septal defect into the right instead of the left atrium. Rarely the left pulmonary veins drain anomalously (Liberthson, 1989a). PAPVC occasionally occurs without an ASD and, like an ASD, produces left to right shunting of blood. *Ostium primum ASDs* are located at the base of the septum. They are also referred to as *endocardial cushion* or *incomplete atrioventricular canal defects.* Ostium primum defects are often associated with defects in the mitral or tricuspid valve. If the entire septum fails to develop, a *common* or *single atrium* is said to exist.

The pressure gradient between the left and right atria is minimal and is not responsible for left to right shunting. Instead, the direction and amount of blood flow across an ASD is determined by the size of the defect and the compliance of the left and right ventricles during diastole (Kopf & Laks, 1991). Most shunting occurs during ventricular diastole when the atria are emptying blood into the ventricles. Because the thin-walled right ventricle is more compliant, blood shunts across the defect from left to right. Increased blood flow through the right ventricle and pulmonary vasculature causes right atrial enlargement, right ventricular hypertrophy and enlargement, and pulmonary hypertension. The degree of shunting is described using a ratio that compares the amount of pulmonary blood flow in relation to systemic blood flow (Qp:Qs). For example, with a 2:1 shunt, cardiac output from the right ventricle into the pulmonary artery is twice that of the left ventricle into the aorta.

In most instances, an ASD is diagnosed during childhood when a systolic ejection murmur is auscultated. Fixed splitting of the second heart sound is also common. Increased blood flow across the pulmonic valve delays its closing, causing the two components of the second heart sound (aortic and pulmonic valve closure) to be heard separately throughout the respiratory cycle. The term *fixed splitting* is used to describe this finding. Increased blood flow through the pulmonary artery may produce a palpable thrill over the pulmonic valve area.

An abnormal electrocardiogram or chest roentgenogram may also lead to diagnosis of ASD. Electrocardiographic signs associated with ASD include incomplete right bundle branch block, right axis deviation, and right ventricular hypertrophy. The chest roentgenogram may demonstrate increased pulmonary vascular markings as well as enlargement of the pulmonary artery and right atrium and ventricle.

Although many children appear asymptomatic, careful study reveals easy fatigability and dyspnea with limited endurance in as many as 50% to 60% of patients, particularly those with large shunts (Kopf & Laks, 1991). Children with ASDs may also be shorter and of slighter stature than their peers (Kirklin & Barratt-Boyes, 1993a). Occasionally, an asymptomatic ASD is not detected until adulthood. Although the young adult is often asymptomatic, symptoms develop in most persons by the third or fourth decade and are almost always present by 60 years of age (Henning & Grenvik, 1989).

An ASD in a adult may first become apparent when a condition common to older adults, such as hypertension or ischemic heart disease, decreases left ventricular compliance and thereby increases left to right shunting (Henning & Grenvik, 1989). Conversely, if right ventricular compliance is acutely decreased (e.g., due to right ventricular myocardial infarction) or pulmonary vascular resistance increases (e.g., due to pulmonary embolism), transient right to left shunting with resultant arterial desaturation may occur. Although atrial arrhythmias are unusual in children with ASDs, atrial fibrillation or flutter commonly develop in older adults with unrepaired defects.

Pulmonary embolism and paradoxical systemic embolism are also fairly common in older patients with ASDs (Liberthson, 1989a). Paradoxical embolization is the migration of venous thrombus or air into the arterial circulation through an anomalous intracardiac communication. Although flow across an ASD is predominantly left to right, some degree of right to left shunting across the defect occurs as well, allowing thrombus or air from the right atrium to enter the left side of the heart. ASD is not associated with increased risk of infective endocarditis (Spencer, 1990).

Surgical repair is recommended regardless of age in individuals with significant shunts (Qp:Qs > 1.5:1). The primary indication for operative repair is the unpredictable development of irreversibly elevated pulmonary vascular resistance that converts an ASD from an easily correctable lesion into an invariably fatal one (Spencer, 1990). Although some patients survive to old age with unrepaired ASDs, average life expectancy is estimated to be near 40 years of age and 75% of patients die by 50 years of age, usually as a consequence of pulmonary hypertension or heart failure (Henning & Grenvik, 1989; Spencer, 1990). The likelihood of atrial arrhythmias, pulmonary vascular obstruction, and right ventricular failure increases as the patient ages. Eventually, the increased pulmonary vascular resistance and decreased right ventricular compliance cause blood to shunt from right to left, producing cyanosis (Kopf & Laks, 1991). When this occurs, operative repair is no longer possible.

VENTRICULAR SEPTAL DEFECT

Ventricular septal defect occurs in 28% of infants with CHD (Nugent et al., 1990). It is, however, uncommon in adults. An estimated 40% of VSDs close spontaneously during infancy, and 60% close by 5 years of age (Warnes et al., 1991a). Although large defects rarely close, those associated with significant shunts generally produce symptoms of congestive heart failure that lead to operative repair during childhood.

Defects in the ventricular septum are categorized according to location. There are four components of the septum: the membranous septum, composed of fibrous tissue and located beneath the atrioventricular valves, and three muscular components (the inlet septum, the apical or trabecular septum, and the outlet or infundibular septum) (Pacifico et al., 1990) (Fig. 6-2). Defects in the membranous septum are most common, accounting for 70% to 80% of VSDs (Arciniegas, 1991). Often, a VSD is associated with another congenital cardiac defect.

The degree of shunting through a VSD is determined by the size of the defect and the pulmonary vascular resistance (Nugent et al., 1990). In small to moderate-sized defects, the pressure gradient between the left and right ventricles results in shunting of blood from left to right with increased blood flow into the pulmonary vasculature. In large defects, pressures in the ventricles, aorta, and pulmonary artery are essentially the same. The degree and direction of shunting are therefore determined by the relative resistances of the aortic and pulmonary vasculature (Nugent et al., 1990). VSDs are associated with a harsh, holosystolic murmur, enlargement of the left atrium and left and right ventricles, and dilatation of the pulmonary artery (DeAngelis, 1991). An unrepaired VSD with significant left to right shunting

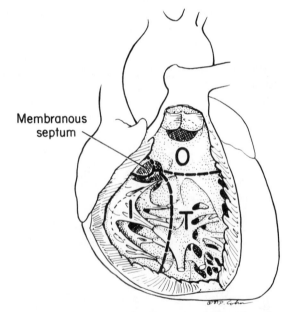

FIGURE 6-2. Ventricular septum as viewed from the right side demonstrates the four components: the membranous septum; the inlet septum (*I*), extending from the tricuspid valve to the valve's distal attachments; the trabecular septum (*T*), extending from inlet septum out to apex and up to smooth-walled outlet septum; the outlet or infundibular septum (*O*), extending to pulmonary valve. (Graham TP, Bender HW, Spach MS, 1989: Ventricular septal defect. In Adams FH, Emmanouilides GC, Riemenschneider TA [eds]: Moss' Heart Disease in Infants, Children, and Adolescents, ed 4, p. 191. Baltimore, Williams & Wilkins)

TABLE 6-2. HEMODYNAMIC SEVERITY OF VENTRICULAR SEPTAL DEFECT

Defect	Size	Ventricular Pressures	Qp : Qs	Pulmonary Pressure
Small	0.5 cm^2	Not equal	<1.75 : 1	<1/2 systemic
Moderate	0.5–1.0 cm^2	Not equal	3 : 1	1/2 systemic
Large	>1.0 cm^2	Equal	>3 : 1	Systemic

Qp : Qs = Ratio of pulmonary to systemic blood flow.
(Liberthson RR, 1989a: Congenital heart disease. In Liberthson RR [ed]: Congenital Heart Disease. Boston, Little, Brown)

(Qp:Qs > 1.8:1) eventually leads to progressive congestive heart failure and, sometimes, irreversible pulmonary vascular obstruction and right to left shunting. Table 6-2 categorizes VSDs by hemodynamic severity.

PATENT DUCTUS ARTERIOSUS

The ductus arteriosus is a vascular connection between the descending thoracic aorta and the pulmonary artery (Fig. 6-3). A normal vessel in fetal circulation, the ductus routes blood flow from the pulmonary artery into the distal aorta, bypassing the lungs. At or shortly after birth, the walls of the ductus, which contain smooth muscle fibers in the medial layer, actively contract to obliterate the lumen (Hallman et al., 1987). The residual fibrous, connective tissue is known as the ligamentum arteriosum. If the fetal ductus arteriosus fails to close, a *patent ductus arteriosus* remains. Hypoxemia is thought to contribute to failure of the ductus to close. Premature infants and those born at high altitude have a higher incidence of the defect (Hillis et al., 1992a). PDA occurs twice as often in females, is particularly common when the mother contracts rubella during the first trimester of pregnancy, and may occur in siblings (Kirklin & Barratt-Boyes, 1993b). It often coexists with other congenital cardiac defects.

Shortly after birth, systemic vascular resistance rises and pulmonary vascular resistance falls. As soon as this occurs, a PDA allows shunting of blood from the aorta to the pulmonary artery (left to right), opposite the direction of blood flow through the ductus during fetal life. This shunting of blood continues through both systole and diastole, producing a characteristic continuous murmur often described as a "machinery" murmur. Because of the easily recognized murmur, most PDAs are detected, definitively diagnosed with echocardiography, and repaired during infancy or early childhood.

The degree of shunting determines the presence and severity of symptoms. If only a small shunt exists, the patient is likely to remain asymptomatic. However, if a large shunt is present, exertional dyspnea may result from the left ventricular failure and pulmonary hypertension that occur secondary to volume overload of the left ventricle and pulmonary vasculature. Whether symptoms are present, surgical repair is recommended. Congestive heart failure, irreversible pulmonary vascular obstruction, and infective endocarditis can all occur as a consequence of the PDA. A PDA may also become markedly dilated and aneurysmal; degenerative changes in the ductal tissue occur with aging and rarely lead to aortic dissection or rupture (Liberthson, 1989a). Natural history data reveal a dramatically shortened life span, with an average age at death of only 40 years (Henning & Grenvik, 1989). If prolonged pulmonary hypertension has caused reversal of the shunt or if the patient is dependent on the PDA to compensate for other inoperable cardiac defects, operative repair is not performed (Hillis et al., 1992a).

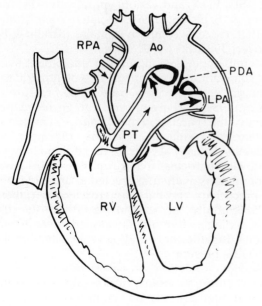

FIGURE 6-3. Patent ductus arteriosus. (Edwards BS, Edwards JE, 1987: Classification. In Roberts WC [ed]: Adult Congenital Heart Disease, p. 19. Philadelphia, FA Davis)

DEFECTS WITH OUTFLOW OBSTRUCTION

Aortic stenosis, pulmonic stenosis, and coarctation of the aorta are obstructive lesions in which no abnormal communication between cardiac chambers is present. The primary consequence of obstructive lesions is heart failure resulting from the increased work of pumping blood across an obstructed pathway. Tetralogy of Fallot (TOF), rarely seen in adults, is an example of a congenital heart defect that has an obstructive component (pulmonic stenosis) with a communication proximal to the obstruction (VSD) that allows right to left shunting of blood.

AORTIC STENOSIS

Congenital *aortic stenosis* includes lesions obstructive to left ventricular outflow that are subvalvular, valvular, or supravalvular. Subvalvular stenosis occurs in two forms: (1) type 1 (discrete), caused by a diaphragm-like membrane beneath the aortic valve and (2) type 2 (diffuse), a more extensive combination of outflow tract and valvular abnormalities that rarely permits survival beyond infancy (Liberthson, 1989a). Supravalvular stenosis is rare. Stenosis of the valve itself is most common. In 75% of individuals, congenital aortic stenosis occurs because the valve is bicuspid, instead of tricuspid (Liberthson, 1989a). Occasionally, only one cusp is present, and the valve is said to be unicuspid. A bicuspid aortic valve is often not recognized in childhood because it does not produce stenosis. However, the valve can become increasingly stenotic with aging due to fibrosis, calcification, or endocarditic infection. Congenital aortic stenosis is more common in males.

The primary hemodynamic consequence of aortic stenosis is fixed obstruction to left ventricular outflow. As a result, left ventricular pressure increases, leading to left ventricular hypertension, secondary concentric hypertrophy, and heart failure. Once symptoms develop, average life expectancy without surgical treatment is 5 years or less (Kirklin & Barratt-Boyes, 1993c). Classic symptoms of aortic stenosis include angina, dyspnea on exertion, and syncope. When severe obstruction is present, sudden cardiac death may occur. In addition, a congenitally abnormal valve is more susceptible to bacterial infection. Recurrent bouts of endocarditis may occur, further impairing valve function. Significant aortic stenosis is treated with valvotomy in children and with valve replacement in adults. Aortic stenosis and aortic valve replacement are discussed in more detail elsewhere in the text.

COARCTATION OF THE AORTA

Coarctation of the aorta, in its most common form, is a segmental narrowing of the aortic lumen, created by a discrete fibrous infolding of the aortic wall near the origin of the left subclavian artery, opposite the ligamentum arteriosum (Liberthson, 1989b) (Fig. 6-4). Coarctation may not cause significant symptoms until after 20 to 30 years of age (Perloff, 1992). As a result, it occasionally remains undiagnosed until adulthood.

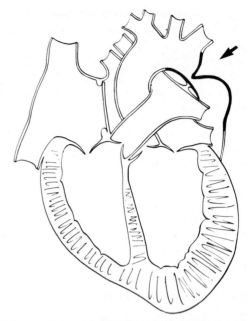

FIGURE 6-4. Coarctation of the aorta represented by focal indentation in the superior aspect of the aorta (*arrow*), which causes the aortic lumen to be eccentric and narrow. (Edwards BS, Edwards JE, 1987: Classification. In Roberts WC [ed]: Adult Congenital Heart Disease, p. 10. Philadelphia, FA Davis)

Coarctation produces arterial hypertension above the narrowing and a gradient between blood pressure in the upper and lower extremities. Significant collateral blood vessels develop over time to augment blood flow to the aorta distal to the coarctation. Aortic coarctation in children is commonly associated with other cardiac defects, particularly bicuspid aortic valve, VSD, PDA, and various mitral valve disorders (Gaynor & Sabiston, 1990). Isolated coarctation is more than twice as common in males (Kirklin & Barratt-Boyes, 1993d).

Systemic hypertension is the predominant symptom of coarctation. Occurring in 90% of individuals, it is primarily systolic with a wide pulse pressure (Liberthson, 1989a). The abnormally high blood pressure above the coarctation may produce symptoms of hypertension: headache, epistaxis, dizziness, and palpitations (Hillis et al., 1992b). In addition to hypertension, left ventricular hypertrophy is almost always present. Adults with uncorrected coarctation often have precocious coronary atherosclerosis (Liberthson, 1989b). Also, because blood flow to the distal aorta is diminished, poorly developed lower extremities, renal insufficiency, and, occasionally, claudication may be present.

Although coarctation sometimes produces congestive heart failure in infants, lesions undetected until adulthood often produce no symptoms for the first 3 decades of life. In such cases, the lesion is usually detected during a routine physical examination of peripheral pulses and blood pressure. However, symptoms and complications are almost always present by 40 years of age. Heart failure occurs in two thirds of patients; stroke, aortic dissection or rupture, and infective endocarditis are less common but can occur (Liberthson, 1989a). Aortic valve disease may also develop during adulthood. The frequently associated bicuspid aortic valve may become calcified and stenotic. In addition, aortic regurgitation may result from the association of systemic hypertension and the abnormal valve (Fuster et al., 1991). Pregnancy in a woman with unrepaired coarctation may be associated with impaired fetal development, aortic dissection or rupture, hypertension, congestive heart failure, or angina (Elkayam, 1992).

A difference in quality of upper and lower extremity pulses, the presence of severe hypertension in a child or young adult, and a gradient between upper and lower extremity blood pressure measurements are highly suggestive of coarctation. A systolic ejection murmur, suprasternal notch thrill, and fourth heart sound are typical findings, and a bruit over the left posterior thorax is common (Liberthson, 1989a). The chest roentgenogram often demonstrates erosion or notching along the inferior posterior rib edges, representing collateral arteries that have developed to enhance blood supply below the site of coarctation. These prominent collateral blood vessels may also produce visible or palpable pulsations in the scapular region.

Collateral blood vessels, which increase with the duration and severity of aortic obstruction, arise mainly from branches of the subclavian, intercostal, scapular, and internal thoracic arteries (Liberthson, 1989b). In contrast to other obstructive lesions, such as aortic stenosis, severity of obstruction is not accurately reflected by a pressure gradient across the coarcted segment because of the well-developed collateral blood vessels in adults that supply the distal aorta beyond the area of obstruction. Instead, severity of obstruction is measured by the degree of aortic narrowing and anatomic and physiologic consequences, such as hypertension and left ventricular failure (Liberthson, 1989a).

Operative repair of coarctation is the treatment of choice and has been performed since 1945. Natural history studies before that time revealed markedly reduced life expectancy in patients with unrepaired coarctation. Average age at death was approximately 35 years, and 90% of patients died before age 50, usually due to congestive heart failure, aortic rupture, intracranial hemorrhage, or infective endocarditis (Maron, 1982). In addition to reducing or preventing worsening of hypertension, coarctation repair is recommended to lessen the possibility of endocarditis or aneurysm formation at the coarctation site. Bacterial infection of the aortic wall can, in turn, lead to formation of mycotic aneurysm and aortic rupture (Lindsay et al., 1990).

Despite surgical correction of coarctation, long-term medical supervision is essential. Coexisting cardiovascular disease is prevalent; many patients have persistent hypertension after surgical repair, and, in some, the coarctation recurs. The older the child or adult at the time of repair, the less likely is hypertension to be corrected by surgical treatment. Accordingly, most persons who have undergone coarctation repair in adulthood require life-long antihypertensive therapy with angiotensin-converting enzyme inhibiting, beta-adrenergic blocking, or calcium-channel antagonist medications.

PULMONIC STENOSIS

Uncorrected *pulmonic stenosis* is rare in adults and, if present, is generally not severe enough to produce symptoms. However, severity of obstruction sometimes increases with aging. The valvular abnormality usually consists of a dome-shaped valve with a central opening and fused commissures (Warnes et al., 1991b). The defect is suggested by a systolic ejection murmur in the pulmonic area and evidence of right ventricular hypertrophy.

Moderate to severe pulmonic stenosis produces hypertrophy of the right ventricular infundibulum, which in turn can lead to right-sided heart failure, tricuspid regurgitation, and mild cyanosis due to right to left shunting across a patent foramen ovale in the presence of elevated right atrial pressure (Henning & Grenvik, 1989). Because operative repair has been performed in children since 1948, postoperative adults are much more commonly encountered than are adults with unrepaired pulmonic stenosis. Further surgical intervention is almost never required. Pulmonic stenosis is most often corrected with surgical or balloon valvotomy. Replacement of the pulmonic valve is generally not necessary because the small degree of pulmonic regurgitation that may occur secondary to valvotomy is usually well tolerated.

TETRALOGY OF FALLOT

Tetralogy of Fallot comprises 75% of cyanotic CHD in adults (Henning & Grenvik, 1989). However, the defect has become rare in adults because corrective surgery has been possible for years. TOF derives its name from its four classic components: (1) VSD, (2) aorta that overrides the VSD and communicates with both the right and left ventricles, (3) right ventricular hypertrophy, and (4) pulmonic stenosis (Fig. 6-5). The primary manifestations of TOF are cyanosis and hypoxia. Survival into adulthood without correction is unlikely. Before the development of corrective surgery, children died secondary to hypoxia, brain abscess, cerebral vascular accident, or infective endocarditis (Nolan, 1974). Correction of TOF includes closure of the VSD and widening of the right ventricular outflow tract to relieve pulmonic stenosis.

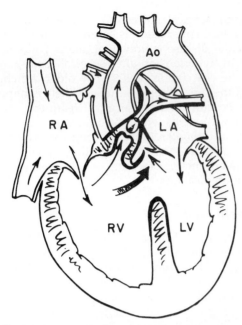

FIGURE 6-5. Classic tetralogy of Fallot. (Edwards BS, Edwards JE, 1987: Classification. In Roberts WC (ed): Adult Congenital Heart Disease, p. 24. Philadelphia, FA Davis)

COMPLICATIONS OF CONGENITAL HEART DISEASE

Congenital heart defects are associated with a number of potential complications, including infective endocarditis, pulmonary hypertension, paradoxical embolism, arterial desaturation, and aneurysm formation.

INFECTIVE ENDOCARDITIS

Almost all congenital heart defects subject an individual to an increased risk of *infective endocarditis*. The cardiac or vascular abnormality provides a potential site for deposition of pathogenic organisms and development of infection. Factors that place an individual at greatest risk are listed in Table 6-3. Adults with congenital lesions are thought to be more susceptible to infective endocarditis than are children, probably

---

TABLE 6-3. FACTORS THAT INCREASE RISK FOR ENDOCARDITIS

Turbulent blood flow
Valvular abnormalities
Prosthetic heart valves
Cyanosis and polycythemia
Aneurysmal dilatation or jet lesion of aortic wall

(McNamara DG, 1989: The adult with congenital heart disease. Curr Probl Cardiol 14:1)

---

because of two factors: (1) a longer period has elapsed for development of degenerative changes on valves, septal walls, or vessels and (2) chronic gum disease and dental abscesses (a frequent source of bacteremia) are more prevalent in adults (McNamara, 1989). TOF, VSD, and PDA are the defects associated with greatest risk for infective endocarditis (Henning & Grenvik, 1989).

Surgical correction of a congenital defect usually substantially lowers, but does not eradicate, the potential risk for endocarditis. Important exceptions (i.e., patients who continue at risk) are patients in whom prosthetic valves have been implanted and those with residual areas of turbulent flow or valvular or aortic wall abnormalities (McNamara, 1989). Prosthetic material other than cardiac valves is of lesser concern after the early postoperative period because the material becomes covered with intimal cells or fibrous tissue (McNamara, 1989) Complications of infective endocarditis include valvular destruction with resultant heart failure and septic embolization. Embolization into the pulmonic, as well as systemic, circulation can occur in those individuals with a left to right intracardiac shunt. The American Heart Association has standardized guidelines for antibiotic prophylaxis against endocarditis (Dajani et al., 1990).

EISENMENGER'S SYNDROME

A complication of defects that produce left to right shunting and chronic volume overload of the pulmonary vasculature is irreversible pulmonary vascular obstruction. Pulmonary vascular resistance becomes irreversibly elevated due to prolonged hypertension and resultant changes in the pulmonary arterioles. Severe pulmonary vascular obstruction leads to a condition known as *Eisenmenger's syndrome,* defined as a communication between the pulmonic and systemic circulations and associated obliterative pulmonary vascular disease that is severe enough to cause right to left shunting of blood through the defect (Hillis et al., 1992c). The resultant right to left shunt allows desaturated blood to enter the systemic circulation, producing arterial desaturation. Although Eisenmenger's syndrome is classically associated with unrepaired VSD, it can result from uncorrected left to right shunting at the atrial (ASD) or aortic (PDA) level as well.

Once Eisenmenger's syndrome has developed, surgical correction of the cardiac anomaly is no longer possible. Closure of the defect eliminates the right to left shunt, which has been providing compensatory decompression of the right ventricle. Profound right-sided heart failure would then result because of the irreversibly elevated right ventricular afterload (pulmonary vascular resistance). Eisenmenger's syndrome may be associated with chest pain resembling angina, exertional syncope, hemoptysis, cerebral thrombosis secondary to polycythemia, or cerebral abscess; death usually occurs by the third decade (Warnes et al., 1991a). Patients with Eisenmenger's syndrome typically succumb to arrhythmias, heart failure, embolism, or abscess (Liberthson, 1989a).

PARADOXICAL EMBOLISM

Paradoxical embolism, defined earlier, is more common with right to left shunts but can occur in the presence of defects in which shunting of blood is predominantly left to right, particularly ASD. During periods of increased right atrial pressure, such as occurs with a Valsalva maneuver, right to left shunting increases and venous thrombus or air can travel into the systemic circulation. Air or thrombus from intravenous catheters can also travel into the arterial circulation through an ASD. Particular attention must be given to handling of intravenous catheters so that no air or thrombus from the catheter is introduced into the right side of the heart.

Paradoxical embolism occasionally occurs across a patent foramen ovale, a tiny opening located in the midportion of the atrial septum. Patent foramen ovale exists normally in approximately 20% of individuals and is not considered a form of ASD. In conditions that acutely increase right atrial pressure, such as right ventricular myocardial infarction or pulmonary embolism, right to left shunting through the patent foramen ovale can occur, causing arterial desaturation or paradoxical embolism.

TABLE 6-4. RISK OF PREGNANCY IN WOMEN WITH CONGENITAL HEART DISEASE

Low Risk

Mild isolated pulmonic stenosis
Functionally normal bicuspid aortic valve
Surgically repaired atrial or ventricular septal defect or
    patent ductus arteriosus
Surgically corrected tetralogy of Fallot with NYHA I status
Congenital complete heart block

Intermediate Risk

Unrepaired:
    Ventricular septal defect
    Coarctation
    Aortic valve disease

High Risk

Cyanotic congenital heart disease
Congestive heart failure (NYHA class III or IV)
Eisenmenger's syndrome

Unknown

Following Fontan or Mustard operations (for single ventricle,
    tricuspid atresia, transposition)

NYHA, New York Heart Association.
(Canobbio MM, 1987: Pregnancy in women with congenital heart disease. Prog Cardiovasc Nurs 2:61)

ARTERIAL DESATURATION

Arterial desaturation in adults with CHD is uncommon and should become increasingly so because of the aggressive approach to surgical correction of defects in infants and children. It occurs with lesions that allow a right to left shunt primarily or with those in which a left to right shunt has reversed due to chronically elevated pulmonary vascular resistance. Desaturated blood enters the systemic circulation, producing decreased arterial saturation that can lead to hypoxemia, cyanosis, polycythemia, and clubbing. Increased blood viscosity secondary to polycythemia predisposes the individual to cerebral vascular accidents and to spontaneous hemorrhage (Nolan, 1974). The presence of right to left shunting also provides the conditions necessary for systemic embolization of venous thrombus.

AORTIC ANEURYSM

Conditions with abnormal blood flow through the aorta (turbulent flow or jetting of blood) are sometimes associated with *aortic aneurysm* formation. Coarctation, PDA, and aortic stenosis are examples of congenital defects associated with aortic aneurysm formation.

COMPLICATIONS ASSOCIATED WITH PREGNANCY

CHD can produce significant complications during pregnancy. Support of a growing fetus causes major hemodynamic alterations in the mother. Cardiac decompensation, usually in the form of congestive heart failure, may occur as physiologic demands on the heart increase. Depending on the nature of the underlying defect and severity of symptoms, abortion of the fetus and/or surgical repair of the cardiac defect in the mother may become necessary to save the life of the mother, the infant, or both. Table 6-4 (Canobbio, 1987) displays the risk of pregnancy imposed by various forms of CHD. Cardiac disease and pregnancy are discussed further in Chapter 7, Other Cardiovascular Disorders.

REFERENCES

American Heart Association, 1991: 1992 Heart and Stroke Facts. Dallas, American Heart Association

Arciniegas E, 1991: Ventricular septal defect. In Baue AE, Geha AS, Hammond GL, et al (eds): Glenn's Thoracic and Cardiovascular Surgery, ed. 5. Norwalk, CT, Appleton & Lange

Canobbio MM, 1987: Pregnancy in women with congenital heart disease. Prog Cardiovasc Nurs 2:61

Dajani AS, Bisno AL, Chung KJ, et al, 1990: Prevention of endocarditis: Recommendations by the American Heart Association. JAMA 264:2919

DeAngelis R, 1991: The cardiovascular system. In Alspach JG (ed): Core Curriculum for Critical Care Nursing, ed. 4. Philadelphia, WB Saunders

Elkayam U, 1992: Pregnancy and cardiovascular disease. In Braunwald E (ed): Heart Disease: A Textbook of Cardiovascular Medicine, ed. 4. Philadelphia, WB Saunders

Fuster V, Warnes CA, McGoon DC, 1991: Congenital heart disease in adolescents and adults: Coarctation of the aorta. In Giuliani ER, Fuster V, Gersh BJ, et al (eds): Cardiology: Fundamentals and Practice, ed. 2. St. Louis, Mosby–Year Book

Gaynor JW, Sabiston DC Jr., 1990: Patent ductus arteriosus, coarctation of the aorta, aortopulmonary window, and anomalies of the aortic arch. In Sabiston DC Jr, Spencer FC (eds): Surgery of the Chest, ed. 5. Philadelphia, WB Saunders

Hallman GL, Cooley DA, Gutgesell HP, 1987: Patent ductus arteriosus. In: Surgical Treatment of Congenital Heart Disease, ed. 3. Philadelphia, Lea & Febiger

Henning RJ, Grenvik A, 1989: Congenital heart disease in the adult. In Henning RJ, Grenvik A (eds): Critical Care Cardiology. New York, Churchill Livingstone

Hillis LD, Lange RA, Wells PJ, Winniford MD, 1992a: Patent ductus arteriosus. In Manual of Clinical Problems in Cardiology, ed. 4. Boston, Little, Brown

Hillis LD, Lange RA, Wells PJ, Winniford MD, 1992b: Coarctation of the aorta. In Manual of Clinical Problems in Cardiology, ed. 4. Boston, Little, Brown

Hillis LD, Lange RA, Wells PJ, Winniford MD, 1992c: Eisenmenger syndrome. In Manual of Clinical Problems in Cardiology, ed. 4. Boston, Little, Brown

Kirklin JW, Barratt-Boyes BG, 1993a: Atrial septal defect and partial anomalous pulmonary venous connection. In Cardiac Surgery, ed. 2. New York, Churchill Livingstone

Kirklin JW, Barratt-Boyes BG, 1993b: Patent ductus arteriosus. In Cardiac Surgery, ed. 2. New York, Churchill Livingstone

Kirklin JW, Barratt-Boyes BG, 1993c: Aortic valve disease. In Cardiac Surgery, ed. 2. New York, Churchill Livingstone

Kirklin JW, Barratt-Boyes BG, 1993d: Coarctation of the aorta and interrupted aortic arch. In Cardiac Surgery, ed. 2. New York, Churchill Livingstone

Kopf GS, Laks H, 1991: Atrial septal defects and cor triatriatum. In Baue AE, Geha AS, Hammond GL, et al (eds): Glenn's Thoracic and Cardiovascular Surgery, ed. 5. Norwalk, CT, Appleton & Lange

Liberthson RR, 1989a: Congenital heart disease. In Liberthson RR: Congenital Heart Disease. Boston, Little, Brown

Liberthson RR, 1989b: Congenital heart disease in the child, adolescent and adult. In Eagle KA, Haber E, DeSanctis RW, Austin WG (eds): The Practice of Cardiology, ed. 2. Boston, Little, Brown

Lindsay J Jr, DeBakey ME, Beall AC, 1990: Diseases of the aorta. In Hurst JW, Schlant RC, Rackley CE, et al (eds): The Heart, ed. 7. New York, McGraw-Hill

Maron BJ, 1982: Coarctation of the aorta in the adult. In Roberts WC (ed): Congenital Heart Disease in Adults, Philadelphia, FA Davis

McNamara DG, 1989: The adult with congenital heart disease. Curr Probl Cardiol 14:1

Nolan SP, 1974: Congenital heart disease: Indications for and timing of operation. Paediatrician 3:144

Nugent EW, Plauth WH Jr, Edwards JE, Williams WH, 1990: The pathology, abnormal physiology, clinical recognition, and medical and surgical treatment of congenital heart disease. In Hurst JW, Schlant RC, Rackley CE, et al (eds): The Heart, ed. 7. New York, McGraw-Hill

Pacifico AD, Kirklin JW, Kirklin JK, 1990: Surgical treatment of ventricular septal defect. In Sabiston DC Jr, Spencer FC (eds): Surgery of the Chest, ed. 5. Philadelphia, WB Saunders

Perloff JK, 1992: Congenital heart disease in adults. In Braunwald E (ed): Heart Disease: A Textbook of Cardiovascular Medicine, ed. 4. Philadelphia, WB Saunders

Spencer FC, 1990: Atrial septal defect, anomalous pulmonary veins, and atrioventricular septal defects (AV canal). In Sabiston DC Jr, Spencer FC (eds): Surgery of the Chest, ed. 5. Philadelphia, WB Saunders

Warnes CA, Fuster V, Driscoll DJ, McGoon DC, 1991a: Congenital heart disease in adolescents and adults: Ventricular septal defect. In Giuliani ER, Fuster V, Gersh BJ, et al (eds): Cardiology: Fundamentals and Practice, ed. 2. St. Louis, Mosby–Year Book

Warnes CA, Fuster V, McGoon DC, 1991b: Congenital heart disease in adolescents and adults: Pulmonary stenosis with intact ventricular septum. In Giuliani ER, Fuster V, Gersh BJ, et al (eds): Cardiology: Fundamentals and Practice, ed. 2. St. Louis, Mosby–Year Book

CHAPTER 7

OTHER CARDIOVASCULAR DISORDERS

TUMORS OF THE HEART AND PERICARDIUM

TYPES OF TUMORS

The majority of cardiac and pericardial lesions represent *secondary tumors*, that is, metastatic disease associated with lung or breast cancer, melanoma, or leukemia. These tumors can metastasize to the heart through hematogenous or lymphocytic routes or extend directly from surrounding intrathoracic structures (Schaff et al., 1991).

Primary tumors occasionally occur. Approximately 70% are benign (Kirklin & Barratt-Boyes, 1993). Most common by far is myxoma, which accounts for half of the benign primary tumors of the heart (Van Trigt & Sabiston, 1990). Other examples of benign cardiac and pericardial tumors are lipoma and papillary fibroelastoma. Nearly all primary malignant cardiac tumors are a form of sarcoma; most common is angiosarcoma (Hall et al., 1990). A list of benign and malignant primary cardiac tumors is provided in Table 7-1.

Whether benign or malignant, cardiac tumors can produce lethal complications, including arrhythmias, cardiac tamponade, pericardial constriction, valvular obstruction, or embolism (Fallon & Dec, 1989). Prog-

nosis varies greatly, depending on the nature and location of the tumor. Malignant cardiac tumors are invariably fatal unless surgical resection is possible. Unfortunately, operative removal of malignant tumors is usually precluded by extensive tumor infiltration into the myocardium, local invasion of adjacent structures, or distant metastases. The remainder of the discussion in this chapter is limited to myxoma, the most frequently occurring cardiac tumor in adults. For information on other cardiac tumors, the reader is referred to a textbook of cardiology.

MYXOMA

A *myxoma* is a soft, gelatinous, mucoid mass that is usually grayish white with areas of hemorrhage or thrombosis (Hall et al., 1990). Myxomas arise from the endocardium and extend into a cardiac chamber, most commonly the left atrium. However, they are sometimes found in the right atrium alone, in both atria, or in the right or left ventricle (Fig. 7-1). Atrial myxomas are typically attached by a pedunculated stalk to the interatrial septum near the fossa ovalis. Although myxomas occur in persons of all ages, they are most often found in the third to sixth decades of life, somewhat more frequently in women (Van Trigt

Betsy Finkelmeier: CARDIOTHORACIC SURGICAL NURSING.
© 1995 J.B. Lippincott Company.

TABLE 7-1. MOST COMMON PRIMARY NEOPLASMS OF THE HEART AND PERICARDIUM

Benign Neoplasms	Malignant Neoplasms
Myxoma	Angiosarcoma
Lipoma	Rhabdomyosarcoma
Papillary fibroelastoma	Mesothelioma
Rhabdomyoma	Fibrosarcoma
Fibroma	Malignant lymphoma

& Sabiston, 1990; Schaff et al., 1991). Two forms of myxoma occur—the more common sporadic myxoma and a familial form that predominantly affects young men (Novick & Dobell, 1991).

Myxomas are typically associated with three types of symptoms: (1) obstructive, (2) embolic, and (3) constitutional (Hall et al., 1990; Van Trigt & Sabiston, 1990). Obstructive symptoms occur when the tumor occludes or interferes with blood flow through the heart. During diastole, left or right atrial myxomas can occlude or prolapse through the mitral or tricuspid valve, respectively, creating transient obstruction to blood flow between the atrium and ventricle. As a result, patients often experience clinical manifestations of valvular stenosis. Manifestations of left atrial myxoma often mimic those of mitral stenosis except that there is no antecedent history of rheumatic fever and symptoms progress more rapidly (Novick & Dobick, 1991). Because of mobility of the tumor mass within the cardiac chamber, episodes of dyspnea, hypotension, or syncope may occur intermittently or

with positional changes. Catastrophic complications, such as sudden cardiac death or acute cardiac failure, may also be caused by tumor occlusion of outflow from a cardiac chamber.

Embolic complications occur because portions of the tumor itself or thrombus that has formed on the tumor can embolize. Systolic emboli occur in 30% to 45% of patients with left atrial myxoma (Kirklin & Barratt-Boyes, 1993). Consequently, it is not unusual for the presenting symptom of myxoma to be stroke, sudden visual loss, acute limb ischemia, or myocardial infarction (Table 7-2). Approximately 50% of emboli affect the brain, often producing major, irreversible neurologic deficits (Novick & Dobell, 1991). Peripheral emboli occasionally lead to a diagnosis of myxoma when embolic material removed from a peripheral artery is identified as myxomatous tissue on pathologic examination. Constitutional manifestations are those simulating a systemic illness, such as weight loss, fatigue, fever, and arthralgias. Systemic symptoms have been reported in as many as 90% of patients with cardiac myxomas (Schaff et al., 1991).

Echocardiography is the primary diagnostic study used to confirm the presence of myxoma. Improvements in echocardiography have greatly aided in diagnosis of myxoma and of cardiac tumors in general. Previously, diagnosis was difficult because of the transitory nature of symptoms and the absence of other objective signs of organic heart disease. It was not unusual for patients with myxomas to be treated as if symptoms were entirely psychosomatic because the diagnosis of myxoma was not suspected and other cardiac disease could not be found. Cardiac catheterization is usually not performed in patients with suspected myxomas because of the potential for catastrophic, systemic embolization of tumor fragments that might be broken off by an intracardiac catheter. However, patients at risk for coronary artery disease may undergo coronary angiography to detect the presence of significant coronary artery lesions.

Treatment of myxoma is surgical resection. Although myxomas are almost invariably benign, operative resection is necessary to eliminate the intracavitary lesion. Surgical resection of myxoma is highly successful in providing total cure. However, all myxomatous tissue must be removed to prevent tumor recurrence, particularly in those with a familial form

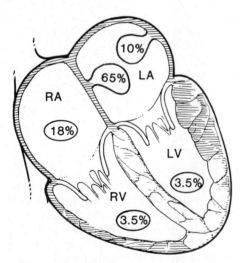

FIGURE 7-1. Percentage of myxomas occurring in the right atrium (*RA*), left atrium (*LA*), right ventricle (*RV*), and left ventricle (*LV*). (DiSesa VJ, Collins JJ Jr, Cohn LH, 1988: Considerations in the surgical management of left atrial myxoma. J Cardiac Surg 3:16)

TABLE 7-2. EMBOLIC COMPLICATIONS OF MYXOMA

Site of Embolization	Clinical Manifestation
Cerebral artery	Cerebral vascular accident
Retinal artery	Sudden visual loss
Femoral artery	Lower extremity ischemia
Coronary artery	Myocardial infarction

of myxoma. Recurrent myxomas may be benign or may become progressively more malignant with each recurrence (Novick & Dobell, 1991).

PERICARDIAL DISEASE

The *pericardium*, a sac that snugly encircles the heart, has two components: (1) parietal, with a fibrous outer coat tethered to the sternum, great vessels and diaphragm, and an inner serosal layer; and (2) visceral, comprising the epicardium and overlying serosal membrane (Shabetai, 1990) (Fig. 7-2). A small space between the visceral and parietal layers, containing 10 to 15 mL of clear, plasma-like fluid, accommodates for physiologic expansion of the heart that occurs with changes in blood volume and posture, respiration, and straining (Shabetai, 1985).

Normal cardiac function can occur in the absence of the pericardium. However, the sac has important physiologic functions, including (1) limiting acute cardiac distention and valvular incompetence secondary to high filling pressures, (2) limiting cardiac displacement, (3) protecting the heart from inflammation of nearby tissues, and (4) reducing friction associated with cardiac movement (Brandenburg et al., 1991). Although a variety of etiologic processes can affect the pericardium, pericardial disease is generally manifested as inflammatory pericarditis, constrictive pericarditis, or pericardial effusion.

INFLAMMATORY PERICARDITIS

Inflammatory pericarditis is a syndrome involving the parietal and visceral pericardium. It can result from any of a variety of causes but is most often idiopathic or due to viral or bacterial infection, uremia, acute myocardial infarction, tuberculosis, pericardiotomy, tumor, or trauma (Lorell & Braunwald, 1992) (Table 7-3). Pericarditis is associated with chest pain, low-grade fevers, a pericardial friction rub, malaise, and characteristic electrocardiographic findings. Typically, chest pain associated with pericarditis is precordial and is aggravated by movement of the trunk, cough, respiration, and recumbency; patients characteristically assume a position of sitting and leaning forward to lessen the discomfort (Brandenburg et al., 1991). Pericardial or pleural effusion may be present. Acute nonmicrobial pericarditis is treated with anti-inflammatory medications such as aspirin, indomethacin, or ibuprofen, and by correcting the underlying cause, if known. Some persons experience recurring bouts of acute pericarditis, which may require treatment with corticosteroids.

Postpericardiotomy syndrome is pericardial inflammation precipitated by pericardiotomy (surgical incision of the pericardium). It is estimated to occur in 30% to 40% of patients who undergo cardiac operations but becomes manifested clinically in less than 5% (Moreno-Cabral et al., 1988). Its onset may be as early as the third postoperative day, but more often it develops 7 days or more after cardiac surgery (Franco et

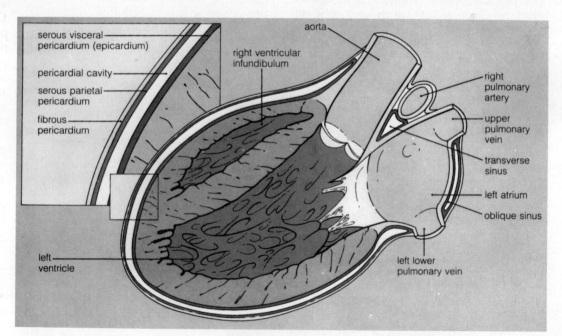

FIGURE 7-2. Diagram of the long axis of the heart demonstrates the arrangement of the pericardium. The outer (parietal) sack is firmly attached to the great arteries and veins at the base. The heart itself invaginates a second sack, the visceral pericardium. The pericardial cavity is located between the parietal and the visceral pericardium. (Anderson RH, Wilcox BR, Becker AE, 1988: Anatomy of the normal heart. In Hurst JW, Anderson RH, Becker AE, Wilcox BR [eds]: Atlas of the Heart, p. 1.2. London, Times Mirror International)

TABLE 7-3. ETIOLOGIES OF PERICARDITIS

Idiopathic
Viral infection (coxsackievirus, mumps virus)
Bacterial infection (Tuberculosis, Pneumococcus)
Fungal infection (histoplasmosis, coccidioidomycosis)
Other infections (toxoplasmosis, amebiasis)
Myocardial infarction (Dressler's syndrome)
Uremia
Neoplasm (lung cancer, breast cancer)
Mediastinal irradiation
Autoimmune disorders (acute rheumatic fever, scleroderma)
Other inflammatory disorders (sarcoidosis, amyloidosis)
Medications (hydralazine, procainamide)
Trauma (hemopericardium, surgical pericardiotomy)
Aortic dissection

(Adapted from Lorrel BH, Braunwald E, 1992: Pericardial disease. In Braunwald E [ed]: Heart Disease: A Textbook of Cardiovascular Medicine, ed. 4. Philadelphia, WB Saunders)

al., 1991). The cause of postpericardiotomy syndrome is unknown, but clinical manifestations are similar to pericarditis from other etiologies. Its course is usually one of mild symptoms that respond to a regimen of anti-inflammatory medications or a single intravenous dose of corticosteroids. Rarely, postpericardiotomy syndrome may lead to significant pericardial or pleural effusion or even cardiac tamponade. In patients who have undergone coronary artery bypass grafting, postpericardiotomy syndrome is associated with a higher incidence of saphenous vein graft closure (Horneffer et al., 1990; Smith, 1990).

Dressler's syndrome is a pronounced form of pericarditis that sometimes develops in patients weeks or months after myocardial infarction. It is characterized by protracted or recurrent fever, pericarditic chest pain, pericardial friction rub, and left pleural effusion (Morris et al., 1990).

CONSTRICTIVE PERICARDITIS

Constrictive pericarditis is the end result of chronic pericardial inflammation (Fig. 7-3). The pericardium loses its elasticity, becoming thickened, fibrotic, and adherent to the heart. Cardiac output is compromised because the noncompliant pericardium prevents cardiac chambers from filling properly. The right side of the heart and great veins are particularly compressed (Ebert & Najafi, 1990). Consequently, symptoms are basically those of systemic venous congestion: peripheral edema, ascites, and liver enlargement. Vague abdominal symptoms such as postprandial fullness, dyspepsia, flatulence, and anorexia are sometimes present (Lorell & Braunwald, 1992). The mainstay of medical therapy is diuresis. If symptoms persist, surgical removal of the pericardium (pericardiectomy) may become necessary.

PERICARDIAL EFFUSION

Pericardial effusion is abnormal accumulation of fluid (serous or purulent fluid, blood, or chyle) in the pericardial space. An unusual problem, it is most often associated with tumor, infection, postpericardiotomy syndrome, or pericarditis. The presence of pericardial effusion is generally detected when the patient develops shortness of breath or hypotension. Severity of symptoms is determined by the volume of the effusion, the rapidity with which the fluid accumulates, and the physical characteristics of the pericardium (Lorell & Braunwald, 1992). In the case of chronic pericardial effusion, gradual accumulation of fluid stretches the pericardium, accommodating as much as several liters of fluid with minimal hemodynamic effect (Ebert & Najafi, 1990).

Rapid fluid accumulation, on the other hand, is not well tolerated hemodynamically; 200 to 250 mL of fluid is likely to produce *cardiac tamponade*, a condition in which diastolic filling of cardiac chambers is im-

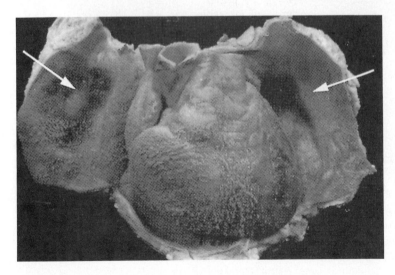

FIGURE 7-3. Resected heart demonstrating fibrinous pericarditis that is most likely of viral origin. *Arrows* point to thickened parietal surfaces of opened pericardium. (Hurst JW, Shabetai R, Becker AE, Wilcox BR, 1988: Pericardial disease. In Hurst JW, Anderson RH, Becker AE, Wilcox BR [eds]: Atlas of the Heart, p. 7.3. London, Times Mirror International)

peded by external compression. Cardiac tamponade, like constrictive pericarditis, produces equalization of intracardiac (right and left atrial and right and left ventricular end-diastolic) pressures, increased central venous pressure, and decreased cardiac output. Heart rate increases to compensate for the diminished stroke volume. Because of the similar clinical manifestations, constrictive pericarditis and pericardial effusion are sometimes difficult to differentiate.

Signs of pericardial effusion include distant heart sounds, distention of neck veins, hypotension, enlargement of the cardiac silhouette on chest roentgenogram, decreased QRS voltage on the electrocardiogram, and pulsus paradoxus. *Pulsus paridoxus* is not a paradoxical phenomenon, as the term suggests, but rather an exaggeration of a normal physiologic phenomenon. Normally, systolic arterial pressure is slightly lower during inspiration due to the decrease in left-sided heart filling as pulmonary vascular capacity increases with the decline in intrathoracic pressure (Franco et al., 1991). With cardiac tamponade, pulsus paridoxus (defined as greater than 10 mm Hg difference in arterial pressure between inspiration and expiration) may be present. Diagnosis of pericardial effusion is confirmed by echocardiographic demonstration of fluid in the pericardial sac.

Pericardiocentesis may be indicated for relief of cardiac tamponade or for cytologic examination of the fluid if etiology of the effusion is unknown. It is performed by a physician in an intensive care setting or in a laboratory in which fluoroscopic and electrocardiographic monitoring equipment is available. Using local anesthesia, a needle is inserted just distal to the xiphoid process and directed upward toward the heart. Care must be taken to aspirate the pericardial fluid without inadvertently entering one of the cardiac chambers. Particularly in the case of a bloody effusion, it can be difficult to differentiate pericardial fluid from intracardiac blood. In patients with malignant pericardial effusions, a chemotherapeutic agent, such as 5-fluorouracil or nitrogen mustard, may be injected into the pericardial space at the time of pericardiocentesis to retard reaccumulation of fluid (Franco et al., 1991). The pericardial catheter is often connected to a closed drainage system and left in place for 12 to 24 hours. Recurrent pericardial effusion may necessitate surgical drainage.

PULMONARY EMBOLISM

Pulmonary embolism is estimated to lead to 200,000 deaths each year in the United States, most often in persons not treated because the condition remains undiagnosed (Dalen & Alpert, 1990). Although pulmonary embolism is most often treated with medical therapy (i.e., systemic anticoagulation), surgical therapy may be undertaken as treatment for massive acute or chronic pulmonary embolism.

MASSIVE ACUTE EMBOLISM

Massive acute pulmonary embolism is defined as sufficient obstruction of pulmonary arterial flow to cause a substantial increase in right ventricular afterload and consequent elevation of pulmonary artery systolic pressure (Goldhaber & Braunwald, 1992). Extremely large amounts of thrombus may form a *saddle embolus,* which is a thrombus that lodges in the main pulmonary artery and extends into both the right and left pulmonary arteries. Massive pulmonary embolism produces acute *cor pulmonale,* or right-sided heart failure secondary to the abrupt rise in pulmonary vascular resistance caused by thrombotic occlusion of blood flow. When 60% to 75% of the pulmonary circulation is obstructed, the increased pulmonary vascular resistance and compensatory elevation of right ventricular pressure lead to dilatation and failure of the right ventricle, with resultant low cardiac output, hypotension, syncope, and possible cardiac arrest (Dalen & Alpert, 1990). In addition to the immediate risk of death, patients with massive pulmonary embolism are at increased risk for chronic pulmonary hypertension due to failure of the thrombus to lyse (Goldhaber & Braunwald, 1992).

The diagnosis of massive pulmonary embolism is considered in the event of an unexplained cardiac arrest, particularly in a young adult with risk factors for pulmonary embolism, such as smoking, oral contraceptives, or clotting abnormalities. Pulmonary angiography is the definitive diagnostic study. It defines pulmonary vascular anatomy and identifies location and extent of thrombus. In all but the most extreme cases, acute pulmonary embolism is treated with heparin or thrombolytic therapy. However, hemodynamically unstable patients with documented, centrally located thrombus may undergo emergent *pulmonary embolectomy.* If the patient is in cardiogenic shock or has suffered cardiac arrest, portable cardiopulmonary bypass may be used to support the patient until the embolus is surgically evacuated. Mortality for patients undergoing pulmonary embolectomy for massive acute pulmonary embolism is 30% to 50% (Dalen & Alpert, 1990). In patients who develop recurring pulmonary emboli despite anticoagulation, inferior venal caval interruption may be necessary.

CHRONIC EMBOLISM

Except in the case of massive pulmonary embolism, emboli usually resolve spontaneously as a result of intrinsic mechanisms of fibrinolysis. With appropriate anticoagulant therapy, perfusion defects are generally resolved within several weeks with no long-term sequelae. Occasionally, however, inadequate lysis or recurring emboli may lead to *chronic pulmonary embolism,* or accumulation of thrombotic material in the pulmonary arterial system. Although more often due to lack of adequate anticoagulation, chronic pulmonary embolism sometimes occurs despite therapeutic anticoagulation. The resultant chronic obstruction to blood flow through the pulmonary arteries eventually leads to pulmonary hypertension, progressive respiratory insufficiency, and right ventricular failure (Lyerly & Sabiston, 1990).

Dyspnea is the most frequently occurring symptom of the condition. Thrombophlebitis, hemoptysis, chest pain, and fatigue are also common (Lyerly & Sabiston, 1990). Chronic pulmonary embolism with cor pulmonale is associated with a poor prognosis; in patients with mean pulmonary artery pressures greater than 30 mm Hg, survival is only 30% at 5 years (Lyerly & Sabiston, 1990). In carefully selected patients, surgical *thromboendarterectomy* of the pulmonary arteries may be beneficial. The best candidates for surgical intervention are those with severe respiratory insufficiency, hypoxemia, pulmonary hypertension, proximal pulmonary artery occlusion, adequate bronchial collateral circulation, and fairly good right ventricular function (Lyerly & Sabiston, 1990). Diffuse involvement of small distal branches and severe right ventricular failure are relative contraindications to thromboendarterectomy.

CARDIAC DISEASE AND PREGNANCY

Rheumatic heart disease, usually mitral stenosis, accounts for approximately 50% of cardiac disorders in pregnant women; congenital disease is believed to comprise an additional 30% to 50% (Noller & Hill, 1991). Diseased cardiac valves or unrepaired congenital heart defects, such as atrial septal defect or coarctation, may be undetected or associated with no symptoms until the added physiologic demands of a pregnancy are imposed. Pregnancy in a woman with cardiac disease presents a number of complex and difficult issues. In addition to the survival of the mother, the health and integrity of the fetus must be considered.

Pregnancy produces major hemodynamic alterations. Blood volume increases 40% to 45%, heart rate increases 10 beats per minute, and peripheral resistance decreases (Noller & Hill, 1991). As the woman's heart and lungs take on the added burden of supporting fetal life, cardiac decompensation may occur. This is most likely to occur during the second or third trimester as increasing demands of the growing fetus strain the mother's cardiovascular system, increasing maternal cardiac output. During labor and delivery, cardiac output increases further owing to the anxiety, pain, and increased venous return to the heart associated with uterine contractions (Canobbio, 1987).

Symptoms of congestive heart failure are the most common manifestation of underlying cardiac disease. If medical therapy is unsuccessful in controlling heart failure, surgical correction of the cardiac problem may become necessary. The decision to perform an operation requiring general anesthesia and cardiopulmonary bypass with systemic anticoagulation is difficult because the risk to the fetus is high. However, recurrent congestive heart failure suggests that a woman will not be able to sustain a full-term pregnancy. In addition, as demands of the fetus increase, the mother's life is increasingly jeopardized.

Other complications of underlying cardiovascular disease can also develop. In women with aortic pathology, aortic dissection or rupture of an aortic aneurysm is more likely to occur during pregnancy. For example, women with aortic coarctation may develop aortic dissection, usually during the last trimester when connective tissue alterations occur (Liberthson, 1989). Women with unrepaired coarctation are also at risk for impaired fetal development (Elkayam, 1992).

In women with valvular heart disease who have an implanted mechanical valvular prosthesis, management of anticoagulation is complex. First, pregnancy is associated with a hypercoagulable state, and, second, warfarin sodium is contraindicated because of its teratogenic effect, which may cause fetal wastage, fetal hemorrhage, or fetal malformations (Badduke et al., 1991). Closely controlled anticoagulation with intravenous heparin is alternatively used.

Medical or surgical interventions during pregnancy to improve or correct a cardiac problem may have profound implications for viability of the fetus. Depending on severity of the mother's illness and the stage of pregnancy, abortion may be recommended. This is a difficult decision that requires input from the patient, obstetrician, and cardiologist.

REFERENCES

Badduke BR, Jamieson WR, Miyagishima RT, et al, 1991: Pregnancy and childbearing in a population with biologic valvular prostheses. J Thorac Cardiovasc Surg 102:179
Brandenburg RO, Click RL, McGoon DC, 1991: The pericardium. In Giuliani ER, Fuster V, Gersh BJ, et al (eds): Cardiology Fundamentals and Practice. St. Louis, Mosby–Year Book
Canobbio MM, 1987: Pregnancy in women with congenital heart disease. Prog Cardiovasc Nurs 2:61
Dalen JE, Alpert JS, 1990: Pulmonary embolism. In Hurst JW, Schlant RC, Rackley CE, et al (eds): The Heart, ed. 7. New York, McGraw-Hill
Ebert PA, Najafi H, 1990: The pericardium. In Sabiston DC Jr, Spencer FC (eds): Surgery of the Chest, ed. 5. Philadelphia, WB Saunders
Elkayam U, 1992: Pregnancy and cardiovascular disease. In Braunwald E (ed): Heart Disease: A Textbook of Cardiovascular Medicine, ed. 4. Philadelphia, WB Saunders
Fallon JT, Dec GW, 1989: Cardiac tumors. In Eagle KA, Haber E, DeSanctis RW, Austin WG (eds): The Practice of Cardiology, ed. 2. Boston, Little, Brown
Franco KL, Breckenridge I, Hammond GL, 1991: The pericardium. In Baue AE, Geha AS, Hammond GL, et al (eds): Glenn's Thoracic and Cardiovascular Surgery, ed. 5. Norwalk, CT, Appleton & Lange
Goldhaber SZ, Braunwald E, 1992: Pulmonary embolism. In Braunwald E (ed): Heart Disease: A Textbook of Cardiovascular Medicine, ed. 4. Philadelphia, WB Saunders
Hall RJ, Cooley DA, McAllister HA, Frazier OH, 1990: Neoplastic

heart disease. In Hurst JW, Schlant RC, Rackley CE, et al (eds): The Heart, ed. 7. New York, McGraw-Hill

Horneffer PJ, Miller RH, Pearson TA, et al, 1990: The effective treatment of postpericardiotomy syndrome after cardiac operations. J Thorac Cardiovasc Surg 100:292

Kirklin JW, Barratt-Boyes BG, 1993: Cardiac tumor. In Cardiac Surgery, ed. 2. New York, Churchill Livingstone

Liberthson RR, 1989: Coarctation of the aorta. In Congenital Heart Disease. Boston, Little, Brown

Lorell BH, Braunwald E, 1992: Pericardial disease. In Braunwald E (ed): Heart Disease: A Textbook of Cardiovascular Medicine, ed. 4. Philadelphia, WB Saunders

Lyerly HK, Sabiston DC Jr, 1990: Chronic pulmonary embolism. In Sabiston DC Jr, Spencer FC (eds): Surgery of the Chest, ed. 5. Philadelphia, WB Saunders

Moreno-Cabral CE, Mitchell RS, Miller DC, 1988: Postoperative problems. In Manual of Postoperative Management in Adult Cardiac Surgery. Baltimore, Williams & Wilkins

Morris DC, Walter PF, Hurst JW, 1990: The recognition and treatment of myocardial infarction and its complications. In Hurst JW, Schlant RC, Rackley CE, et al (eds): The Heart, ed. 7. New York, McGraw-Hill

Noller KL, Hill LM, 1991: Cardiac disease associated with pregnancy and its management. In Giuliani ER, Fuster V, Gersh BJ, et al (eds): Cardiology Fundamentals and Practice. St. Louis, Mosby–Year Book

Novick RJ, Dobell ARC, 1991: Tumors of the heart. In Baue AE, Geha AS, Hammond GL, et al (eds): Glenn's Thoracic and Cardiovascular Surgery, ed. 5. Norwalk, CT, Appleton & Lange

Schaff HV, Piehler JM, Lie JT, Giuliani ER, 1991: Tumors of the heart. In Giuliani ER, Fuster V, Gersh BJ, et al (eds): Cardiology Fundamentals and Practice. ed 2. St. Louis, Mosby–Year Book

Shabetai R, 1985: The pericardium as a source of cardiac dysfunction. In Utley JR (ed): Perioperative Cardiac Dysfunction, vol. III. Baltimore, Williams & Wilkins

Shabetai R, 1990: Diseases of the pericardium. In Hurst JW, Schlant RC, Rackley CE, et al (eds): The Heart, ed. 7. New York, McGraw-Hill

Smith PK, 1990: Postoperative care in cardiac surgery. In Sabiston DC Jr, Spencer FC (eds): Surgery of the Chest, ed. 5. Philadelphia, WB Saunders

Van Trigt P, Sabiston DC Jr, 1990: Tumors of the heart. In Sabiston DC Jr, Spencer FC (eds): Surgery of the Chest, ed. 5. Philadelphia, WB Saunders

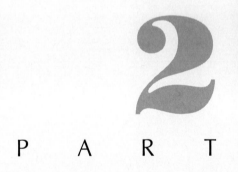

P A R T

PREOPERATIVE EVALUATION AND PREPARATION

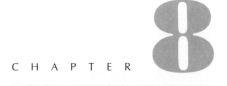

DIAGNOSTIC EVALUATION OF CARDIAC DISEASE

NONINVASIVE STUDIES
  Electrocardiogram
  Holter Monitoring
  Exercise Stress Testing
  Echocardiography
  Radionuclide Imaging

INVASIVE STUDIES
  Cardiac Catheterization
  Electrophysiologic Studies
  Endomyocardial Biopsy

For many years the principal study used in diagnosis of cardiac disease was the electrocardiogram (ECG). Although analysis of cardiac electrical activity reveals important clues about myocardial pathology, the ECG is limited in the information it provides. The development of sophisticated ultrasonic, radionuclide imaging, and cardiac catheterization techniques has greatly enhanced the accurate diagnosis of cardiac diseases. A number of diagnostic modalities, both noninvasive and invasive, are currently available. Those studies performed most commonly in patients who undergo cardiac surgical procedures are described in this chapter.

NONINVASIVE STUDIES

ELECTROCARDIOGRAM

The *electrocardiogram*, a graphic recording of cardiac electrical activity, is the most frequently used diagnostic study for patients with known or suspected cardiac disease. It documents cardiac rate and rhythm, provides information about impulse conduction and electrical axis of the heart, and reveals the presence of various pathologic conditions, such as myocardial infarction, ventricular hypertrophy, or bundle branch block. The standard, or 12-lead, ECG

records electrical cardiac activity from 12 different perspectives; six limb leads measure forces on the vertical plane, and six precordial (chest) leads measure forces on the horizontal plane (Canobbio, 1990). Because many forms of cardiac pathology produce electrocardiographic abnormalities, ECGs are obtained as part of the routine preoperative evaluation of almost all adults undergoing operations that require general anesthesia.

In patients with coronary artery disease, the ECG may reveal the presence of either myocardial ischemia or infarction. Moreover, the leads in which abnormalities are present provide information about the specific coronary artery or arteries that are obstructed. Ischemia is manifested by ST segment depression and T wave changes. Injured myocardium is evidenced by ST segment and T wave elevation. Transmural infarction produces Q waves in leads reflective of affected myocardium and reciprocal positive forces in opposite leads. Persistent ST segment elevation may indicate presence of a ventricular aneurysm.

In patients with valvular or congenital heart disease the development of irreversible ventricular damage may be detected by abnormalities in leads overlying the affected ventricle. Increased QRS amplitude occurs with right or left ventricular enlargement, and ST segment or T wave changes may indicate ventricu-

Betsy Finkelmeier: CARDIOTHORACIC SURGICAL NURSING.
© 1995 J.B. Lippincott Company.

lar strain. Atrial enlargement may be detected by changes in amplitude, width, and configuration of the P wave. The appearance and progression of right or left bundle branch block can be evaluated by width and morphology of the QRS complex in specific leads. Finally, the ECG may demonstrate changes produced by various medications or by electrolyte abnormalities. For example, a number of medications can produce hazardous prolongation of the QT interval and hyperkalemia affects the configuration of all components of depolarization and repolarization. Interpretation of ECGs is described in further detail in Chapter 24, Twelve-Lead Electrocardiography and Atrial Electrograms.

HOLTER MONITORING

Holter monitoring, or *ambulatory monitoring,* is an extended recording of the cardiac rhythm over a period of time, usually 24 hours. The recording device is contained in a portable, compact unit that the patient carries using a shoulder harness or belt. The monitoring device continuously records the electrocardiogram while the patient performs normal daily activities. The patient is asked to keep a diary of these activities, as well as medications taken and presence of any symptoms.

The recording is evaluated by computer and reviewed by a cardiologist, who characterizes heart rate and rhythm over the period of the monitoring, correlating changes or abnormalities with patient activities as documented in the accompanying diary. The number and character of supraventricular and ventricular arrhythmias are quantitated, as well as changes in heart rate or ST segments. Holter monitor recordings are typically obtained to identify and quantitate arrhythmias in persons with known or suspected arrhythmic disorders, to evaluate pacemaker function, and to identify rhythm abnormalities in persons with suggestive symptoms (e.g., syncope). In patients with life-threatening arrhythmic disorders, Holter monitor recordings are generally used as an adjunct to electrophysiologic studies. In patients with unstable angina, Holter monitoring may be helpful in detecting silent myocardial ischemia (i.e., electrocardiographic evidence of ischemia that is not accompanied by clinical symptoms) (Rutherford & Braunwald, 1992).

EXERCISE STRESS TESTING

Exercise stress testing (EST) is the observation, measurement, and recording of physiologic responses to a known amount of physical work (Froelicher & King, 1989). The study consists of monitoring the ECG, blood pressure, and heart rate while the patient walks on a treadmill or rides a bicycle ergometer and is subjected to progressively increasing, graded levels of work. The purpose of the study is to observe electrocardiographic and hemodynamic changes that occur during a dynamic state. Normal physiologic responses to exercise include increases in heart rate, stroke volume, and, usually, systolic and mean arterial pressure (Chaitman, 1992). Abnormal responses include (1) decrease or no change in systolic blood pressure, (2) excessive increase or decrease in heart rate, (3) depression of ST segments on the ECG, (4) serious arrhythmias, and (5) symptoms such as angina, dyspnea, or unusual fatigue.

The treadmill is the most commonly used device for EST in the United States (Froelicher & King, 1989). Because EST can precipitate severe ischemia or arrhythmias, the procedure is performed under supervision of a physician and with accessible emergency drugs and equipment. There are many protocols for EST; two of the most frequently used are the Bruce and modified-Bruce (low level) protocols. The *Bruce protocol* is a multistage test in which the cardiovascular workload is increased at regular intervals (Canobbio, 1990). Generally, the patient exercises to the point of fatigue or the onset of symptoms (Hudak et al., 1990). Although the Bruce protocol is widely used for screening EST in apparently healthy individuals, patients in cardiac surgical settings and those with recent myocardial infarction are more likely to undergo a *low level protocol* EST, a multistage test in which less strenuous work levels are used.

EST is most commonly used as a screening tool to detect the presence and severity of obstructive lesions in the coronary arterial circulation. Because physical exertion increases myocardial oxygen consumption and because myocardial ischemia produces typical electrocardiographic manifestations, EST often provokes and defines underlying myocardial ischemia in a controlled setting (Fig. 8-1). The magnitude of ST depression, level of exercise at which it occurs, and the persistence of ischemic changes in the recovery period provide an index of severity of coronary artery obstructive lesions (Sutherland, 1991). EST is less reliable as a screening test for coronary artery disease in women; the specificity of exercise-induced ST segment depression for obstructive coronary lesions is less in women than in men (Chaitman, 1992).

In patients with known coronary artery disease, EST may be used to assess severity of exercise-induced ischemia, as well as effectiveness of various forms of antianginal therapy. Because EST is less definitive than cardiac catheterization, the study is not always performed before cardiac catheterization in patients with signs and symptoms suggestive of significant coronary artery obstruction. Also, in patients with unstable angina or with suspected left main or other severe coronary artery lesions, EST is generally not performed since it may produce precipitous myocardial ischemia or infarction.

After myocardial infarction or coronary artery revascularization, EST is frequently performed to assess a patient's physical capabilities under monitored conditions. EST may also be used to assess heart rate response to exercise or to detect exercise-induced arrhythmias. Common indications for EST are displayed in Table 8-1.

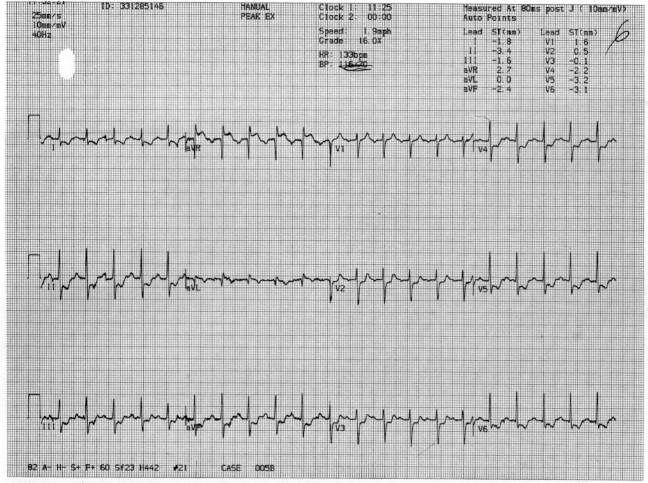

FIGURE 8-1. Twelve-lead ECG obtained at peak exercise during treadmill test in patient with a history of angina. After exercising approximately 11.5 minutes, the patient developed chest discomfort and 2- to 3-mm downsloping ST segment depression in inferior (II, AVF) and lateral (V4, V5, V6) leads consistent with myocardial ischemia. (Courtesy of James Rosenthal, MD)

ECHOCARDIOGRAPHY

Echocardiography is a noninvasive study that uses ultrasound, or sound waves of frequencies higher than the human ear can detect, to scan the heart (Hall, 1989). A transducer, which contains one or more crystals with piezoelectric properties, is used to transmit pulses of ultrasonic energy into the heart. Echos reflected back from the heart are converted into electrical impulses that provide images of cardiac structures or blood flow through the heart.

There are three types of echocardiography: motion (M) mode, two-dimensional (2-D), and Doppler. *M-mode echocardiography* provides a one-dimensional view of cardiac structures throughout the cardiac cycle (Huang et al., 1989a). In a *2-D echocardiogram*, the transducer crystal rotates through an arc or many crystals emit pulses to provide a two-dimensional display of cardiac structures during the cardiac cycle. *Doppler echocardiography* is the principal ultrasonic technique for obtaining hemodynamic data (Feigenbaum, 1992). The Doppler echocardiogram consists of recording sound waves reflected from moving red blood cells. It provides information about blood flow through cardiac chambers, across cardiac valves, and into the great vessels. Sophisticated technology now makes it possible to transform flow signals into different colors, providing a more graphic display known as a *color Doppler echocardiogram*.

TABLE 8-1. COMMON INDICATIONS FOR EXERCISE STRESS TESTING

Screen high-risk individuals for coronary artery disease

Document exercise-induced ischemia in individuals with symptoms suggestive of coronary artery disease

Evaluate functional capacity after myocardial infarction or coronary artery revascularization

Document exercise-induced arrhythmias

Determine heart rate response to exercise in individuals with a rate-programmed implantable cardioverter/defibrillator

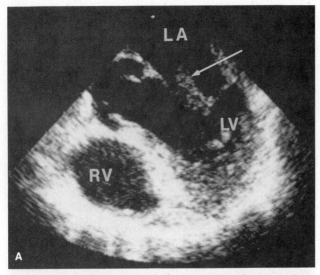

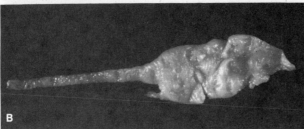

FIGURE 8-2. (A) Transesophageal echocardiogram reveals a vegetation (*arrow*) on anterior leaflet of the mitral valve. *LA,* left atrium; *RV,* right ventricle, *LV,* left ventricle. **(B)** Gross appearance of the resected vegetation. (Courtesy of David McPherson, MD)

presence of structural abnormalities, such as intracardiac shunts or intracavitary lesions; and (5) pericardial effusion or constriction. As a result, echocardiography is particularly useful in diagnosing valvular dysfunction, congenital defects, or defects caused by trauma or myocardial infarction. Cardiac chamber dilatation and abnormalities of the myocardium, such as calcification, hypertrophy, wall motion abnormalities, or ventricular aneurysm, can also be assessed. Finally, fluid collection (pericardial effusion) and abnormal masses, such as myxoma, vegetation, or thrombus, are often definitively diagnosed with echocardiography (Fig. 8-2).

In most cases, echocardiograms are obtained using a transthoracic approach; that is, the transducer is positioned on the anterior chest wall. However, a rapidly developing alternative technique is the transesophageal approach. *Transesophageal echocardiography* is performed using an ultrasound transducer on a probe that the patient swallows (Fig. 8-3). The transesophageal approach places the transducer in close proximity to the left atrium, eliminating chest wall interference and intrathoracic attenuation that occur with the conventional transthoracic approach (Matsuzaki et al., 1990). As a result, images are clearer and more accurate than those obtained with transthoracic echocardiography. Transesophageal echocardiography is particularly useful during cardiac operations because echocardiographic images can be obtained while the chest is open. It also is advantageous in clinical situations in which a transthoracic approach is unlikely to provide adequate images (Table 8-2).

These methods of echocardiography provide information about (1) characteristics, motion, and competency of cardiac valves; (2) size of cardiac chambers; (3) thickness and contractility of myocardium (left ventricular wall and interventricular septum); (4)

RADIONUCLIDE IMAGING

Radionuclide imaging (scintigraphy) is a diagnostic technique that detects pathologic cardiac conditions by tracking a small quantity of radioisotopes injected into the bloodstream. Radioisotopes are unstable at-

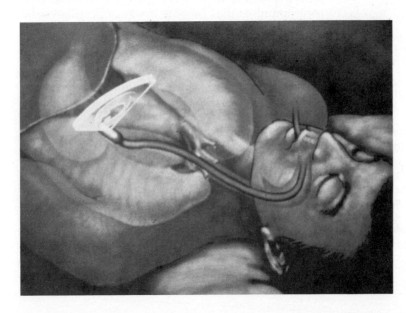

FIGURE 8-3. Transesophageal echocardiography is performed using an ultrasound transducer on a probe passed into the esophagus. (Courtesy of Hewlett-Packard, Andover, MA)

TABLE 8-2. CLINICAL SITUATIONS IN WHICH TRANSESOPHAGEAL ECHOCARDIOGRAPHY IS ADVANTAGEOUS

Obese patients
Patients with chronic obstructive pulmonary disease
Intraoperative studies
Inadequate information from transthoracic study
Patients with suspected aortic dissection
Detailed valvular anatomic assessment in infective
  endocarditis

oms that emit gamma rays as they spontaneously convert into a more stable form (Hall, 1989). Two commonly used radioisotopes are technetium-99m (^{99m}Tc) and thallium-201 (^{201}Tl). As gamma rays are emitted, a gamma-scintillation camera records the presence of the radioisotopes.

Nuclear cardiac imaging can be considered in two categories: (1) studies in which radioactive tracers remain in the intravascular space and (2) studies that visualize myocardial intracellular uptake of radioactive tracers, reflecting myocardial perfusion, metabolism, and viability (Chaitman & Fletcher, 1991). In the first group of studies, a small amount of radioisotope (usually ^{99m}Tc) is injected intravenously and the heart is scanned as tagged blood passes through it. Two techniques commonly are used: (1) *first-pass radionuclide imaging* samples a few cardiac cycles at the time of radionuclide injection, and (2) *gated blood pool imaging* analyzes several hundred cardiac cycles (Chaitman & Fletcher, 1991).

Imaging techniques in which the radionuclide remains in the intravascular space are used to assess ventricular size and volume and evaluate right and left ventricular ejection fraction (i.e., the proportion of ventricular volume ejected with each ventricular contraction). A normally functioning ventricle ejects 50% to 60% of its blood volume; a 30% to 50% ejection fraction represents a moderately impaired ventricle; and an ejection fraction that is below 30% represents severe ventricular impairment. This type of radionuclide imaging can also detect the presence of a ventricular wall motion abnormality, which is a segment of ventricular wall that contracts poorly or paradoxically in comparison to other segments. Wall motion abnormalities almost always represent ventricular damage caused by myocardial infarction and are often associated with congestive heart failure and chronic arrhythmic disorders.

The second group of radionuclide scanning techniques is used to evaluate regional myocardial perfusion and viability. *Thallium scanning* is helpful in detecting areas of ischemic or infarcted cardiac muscle. ^{201}Tl injected into the bloodstream becomes concentrated in viable myocardium in a ratio proportional to coronary blood flow to the area (Sutherland, 1991). Thus, perfusion defects ("cold spots" or areas of decreased uptake) appear in regions with diminished

coronary blood flow or that are infarcted. Subsequent scanning several hours after ^{201}Tl injection distinguishes myocardial ischemia (resolution of perfusion defect) from infarction (persistence of perfusion defect).

Thallium scanning can be performed with the patient at rest or during exercise. *Exercise thallium scanning* is particularly helpful in patients, such as women and those with baseline ST segment abnormalities, in whom conventional exercise stress testing may be inconclusive. The more severe the degree of coronary artery disease, the more likely it is that exercise ^{201}Tl images will be abnormal (Zaret et al., 1992). In patients unable to achieve adequate exercise levels, intravenous dipyridamole may be administered to increase coronary blood flow in place of exercise. This type of study is termed *dipyridamole thallium scanning*.

Another scanning technique for evaluating regional muscle viability uses the radioisotope ^{99m}Tc pyrophosphate to detect acute myocardial necrosis. Because ^{99m}Tc pyrophosphate binds with recently damaged myocardium, *technetium scanning* may be used to detect acute myocardial infarction when the clinical history is atypical, the baseline ECG is abnormal (e.g., left bundle branch block), or other reasons exist for cardiac enzyme elevation (e.g., recent defibrillation or cardiopulmonary resuscitation) (Hudak et al., 1990). "Hot spots" (areas of increased uptake), representing myocardial infarction, are most apparent 2 to 3 days after onset of necrosis (Chaitman & Fletcher, 1991).

Positron emission tomography (PET) is an imaging technique used less frequently in patients with coronary artery disease. It uses biologically active radiopharmaceuticals to distinguish dysfunctional but viable myocardium from infarcted tissue.

INVASIVE STUDIES

Invasive diagnostic studies are those in which catheters are guided into the left or right side of the heart from peripheral arteries or veins, respectively. Invasive studies used for the diagnosis of cardiac disease include cardiac catheterization, electrophysiologic studies, and endomyocardial biopsy.

CARDIAC CATHETERIZATION

Cardiac catheterization is a procedure in which catheters are placed in the heart or great vessels and used to measure intracardiac pressures and oxygen saturation and to obtain fluoroscopic angiograms. *Angiography* is radiographic visualization achieved by injection of contrast material into cardiac chambers, coronary arteries, or great vessels (Huang et al., 1989b). A full cardiac catheterization includes angiography as well as intracardiac pressure and oxygen saturation measurements from both the right and left chambers. A great deal of valuable information about the heart can be obtained during cardiac catheterization, including

(1) definition of coronary anatomy, (2) estimation of ventricular wall motion and ejection fraction, (3) measurement of intracardiac pressures and hemodynamic parameters, (4) evaluation of cardiac valve function, and (5) diagnosis of structural cardiac abnormalities, such as ventricular septal defect, ventricular aneurysm, or intracavitary mass.

Left-sided heart catheterization usually includes coronary angiography and left ventriculography. *Coronary angiography* is the most common form of cardiac catheterization procedure. It is performed in patients with suspected coronary artery disease, typically in those who have angina that has accelerated in frequency or severity or that recurs despite pharmacologic therapy or after myocardial infarction. Coronary angiography is performed by means of percutaneous cannulation of the femoral artery or cannulation of the brachial artery using a percutaneous or cutdown approach. The presence of severe aortoiliac disease may mandate use of a brachial or axillary approach.

In either case, the catheter is guided, using fluoroscopy, in a retrograde fashion through the aorta. Radiopaque contrast material is then injected selectively into the ostia of the right and left coronary arteries and fluoroscopy is used to visualize the arterial structures. *Cineangiograms* (motion pictures) of each of the coronary arteries are obtained in at least two projections: right anterior oblique and left anterior oblique. Views from other angles may also be necessary to ensure adequate visualization of the proximal and distal portion of each vessel and to better demonstrate specific coronary artery lesions (Newton, 1989; Sutherland, 1991) (Fig. 8-4).

Only a small portion of the coronary circulation is visualized (i.e., major epicardial branches and their second-, third-, and perhaps fourth-order branches); intramyocardial branches are not visualized because of their small size, cardiac motion, and limited resolution of cine imaging systems (Levin and Gardiner, 1992). Coronary artery anatomy is usually described in terms of whether the right, left, or neither coronary artery is dominant. Most common is right dominant coronary circulation, in which the posterior descending artery arises from the right coronary artery; in left dominant coronary circulation, the posterior descending artery is a branch of the left circumflex artery (Kirklin & Barratt-Boyes, 1993). From a physiologic standpoint, the term *dominance* is somewhat misleading. Despite the fact that most individuals have right dominant coronary circulation, the left coronary artery in most human hearts is of wider caliber and perfuses the largest proportion of myocardium (Halpenny & Bond, 1989).

Visualization of the major coronary arteries and their branches demonstrates vessel size, areas of narrowing or irregularity, and quality of the distal portion of the vessel. Severity of stenotic lesions can be quantitated by comparing the reduction in luminal diameter to that in a normal segment of the same artery. The percentage of luminal diameter reduction is generally categorized as (1) less than 50%, (2) 50% to 75%, or (3) greater than 75%. Lesions that reduce luminal diameter more than 50% are considered significant because they represent a 75% reduction in cross-sectional area of the artery and can decrease blood flow reserves during exercise (Remetz & Cleman, 1991). Because contrast material clears faster with higher flow rates, adequacy of perfusion is also estimated by how quickly an artery fills with and clears contrast (Newton, 1989).

Ventriculography (i.e., opacification of a ventricular chamber using contrast material) is routinely performed in association with coronary angiography. Left ventriculography is accomplished by injecting

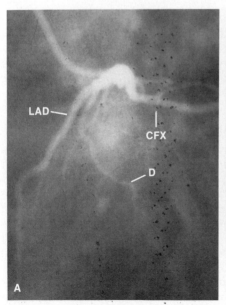
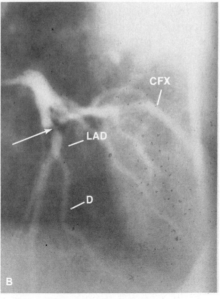

FIGURE 8-4. Two projections of the same left coronary arterial system obtained during coronary angiography. **(A)** In the left anterior oblique projection, no significant narrowings are demonstrated. **(B)** Cranially angled left anterior oblique projection demonstrates a tight stenosis in the left anterior descending (*LAD*) artery (arrow). *D*, diagonal branch of LAD; *CFX*, circumflex coronary artery. (Courtesy of Sheridan Meyers, MD)

contrast material through a catheter that has been advanced in retrograde fashion from the proximal aorta across the aortic valve into the left ventricle. A ventriculogram provides subjective demonstration of effectiveness of ventricular contractility. Wall motion abnormalities, such as areas of akinesis (lack of motion), hypokinesis (diminished motion), or dyskinesis (abnormal motion) are identified during this portion of the study. In addition, left ventriculography is used to estimate ventricular ejection fraction, to assess the mitral valve and ventricular outflow tract, and to visualize mural thrombus (Huang et al., 1989b). In hemodynamically unstable patients, a ventriculogram is more hazardous because of the adverse effects of contrast material on a poorly functioning ventricle. In these patients, the ventriculogram may be omitted.

Aortic root aortography (injection of contrast into the ascending aorta) may be performed in conjunction with coronary angiography if aortic insufficiency is suspected. Angiography of the internal thoracic arteries is occasionally performed in preoperative patients if there is a question about quality of the vessels.

Right-sided heart catheterization is performed through the cephalic or femoral vein in the same manner that a balloon-tipped flotation (pulmonary artery) catheter is inserted. Catheterization of the right side of the heart is performed for the following purposes: (1) measurement of right atrial, right ventricular, and pulmonary artery pressures and oxygen saturation levels; (2) visualization of the right atrium, right ventricle, tricuspid and pulmonic valves, or pulmonary arterial circulation; (3) measurement of cardiac output and shunt studies; and (4) access to the left atrium through transseptal cannulation (Newton, 1989; Canobbio, 1990).

Transseptal catheterization is performed by passing an intracardiac catheter from the right to left atrium. If a patent foramen ovale is present in the interatrial septum, the catheter may be passed through it. If a patent foramen ovale is not present, the septum is punctured. The catheter can then be advanced from the left atrium into the left ventricle for left ventriculography and pressure measurement (Bashore & Davidson, 1990). A transseptal approach to the left side of the heart is most often used in patients in whom it is ill advised or not possible to advance a catheter through the aortic valve, such as those with an aortic valve prosthesis or severe aortic stenosis. A transseptal approach is also used for therapeutic balloon valvotomy of the mitral valve.

Improvements in catheterization techniques, contrast material, and catheters have made cardiac catheterization quite safe and have expanded indications for the procedure. Almost all adults who undergo cardiac operations have a cardiac catheterization before surgery. The most common reason for performing catheterization of the heart is to evaluate the presence and severity of coronary artery atherosclerosis. For patients undergoing coronary artery revascular-ization, preoperative definition of the coronary anatomy is essential. Because of the prevalence of coronary artery disease in this country, coronary angiography is also important to assess coronary anatomy in high-risk patients who require other types of operative procedures. Greater numbers of both critically ill as well as ambulatory patients at risk for coronary artery disease are undergoing cardiac catheterization (Bashore & Davidson, 1990).

Patients with valvular abnormalities or structural defects of the heart may undergo heart catheterization to determine intracardiac pressures, detect abnormal communications, and assess function of the cardiac valves. However, the sophisticated echocardiographic and nuclear cardiology techniques that are available often provide sufficient diagnostic information. In young patients at low risk for coronary artery disease, cardiac catheterization is usually unnecessary.

Cardiac catheterization is performed for an increasing variety of therapeutic purposes, such as percutaneous transluminal coronary angioplasty and mitral balloon valvotomy. Therapeutic catheterization procedures are discussed elsewhere in the text.

Although cardiac catheterization is an invasive procedure, it is associated with minimal morbidity when performed by experienced angiographers. Mortality risk associated with the procedure ranges from 0.1% to 0.2% (Grossman, 1992). Patients at highest risk include those with significant left main coronary artery obstruction, poor left ventricular function, advanced age, and associated valvular disease (Bashore & Davidson, 1990).

The most common complication of cardiac catheterization is peripheral arterial injury at the site of catheter insertion. Potential clinical sequelae resulting from iatrogenic arterial injury include thromboembolism, hematoma, arterial perforation, pseudoaneurysm, and arteriovenous fistula (Finkelmeier & Finkelmeier, 1991). These complications occur more frequently in women and when a brachial artery approach is used (Bashore & Davidson, 1990). Other complications of cardiac catheterization include allergic reaction to the contrast material, severe vasovagal reflex, cardiac arrest, stroke, myocardial infarction, and arrhythmias.

ELECTROPHYSIOLOGIC STUDIES

An *electrophysiologic study* (EPS) is performed to assess the electrical conduction system of the heart. It is the definitive diagnostic modality for characterizing arrhythmic disorders and directing therapy. The procedure is similar to cardiac catheterization in that intracardiac catheters are positioned with the aid of fluoroscopy. The catheters serve two purposes. First, they are used to obtain intracardiac electrical recordings that allow sophisticated analysis of cardiac electrical activation and definition of abnormalities of impulse formation (Chung, 1989). In this portion of the study, adequacy of sinus and atrioventricular node and His bundle function can be assessed and the mechanism and characteristics of supraventricular or ventricular rhythm disorders are clarified.

The intracardiac catheters are also used to perform *programmed electrical stimulation* (PES), a method of provoking cardiac arrhythmias by delivering pacing stimuli at specific intervals during the cardiac cycle. PES makes possible induction and termination of malignant arrhythmias under controlled conditions. During PES, abnormal activation sequences are identified, thereby localizing reentrant pathways. The ability or inability to provoke an arrhythmia that has occurred clinically is termed *inducibility.* An induced arrhythmia that is sustained for 30 seconds or more or that requires intervention for hemodynamically compromising symptoms is termed a *sustained arrhythmia.* Inducibility and sustainability provide prognostic information about likelihood of clinical recurrence as well as evaluative information about efficacy of antiarrhythmic therapy. Use of EPS in guiding therapy of patients with chronic arrhythmic disorders is discussed in Chapter 4, Cardiac Rhythm Disorders.

ENDOMYOCARDIAL BIOPSY

Endomyocardial biopsy is the acquisition of a small piece of myocardium for microscopic analysis. The biopsy is obtained using a *bioptome,* which is a spe-

cially designed catheter with an externally controlled pinching mechanism at its distal end (Fig. 8-5). With the use of fluoroscopy, the bioptome is inserted through the femoral or jugular vein into the right ventricle. Endomyocardial biopsy is a valuable diagnostic technique in two categories of patients: (1) those with cardiac failure of unknown etiology and (2) those who have undergone cardiac transplantation. For adults with transplanted hearts, endomyocardial biopsy is the primary technique for detecting rejection in its early stages. Ventricular perforation is the most common complication of endomyocardial biopsy.

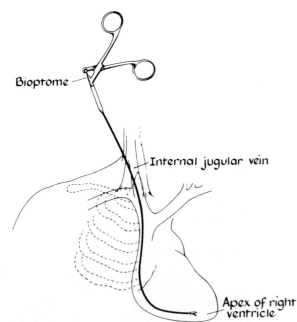

FIGURE 8-5. Bioptome is inserted through internal jugular vein and advanced through right atrium across tricuspid valve into right ventricle; a small piece of endocardial tissue is obtained from the interventricular septum. (Shinn JA, 1989: Cardiac transplantation. In Underhill SL, Woods SL, Froelicher ESS, Halpenny CJ [eds]: Cardiac Nursing, ed. 2, p. 590. Philadelphia, JB Lippincott)

REFERENCES

Bashore TM, Davidson CJ, 1990: Cardiac catheterization, angiography, and balloon valvuloplasty. In Sabiston DC Jr, Spencer FC (eds): Surgery of the Chest, ed. 5. Philadelphia, WB Saunders

Canobbio MM, 1990: Diagnostic procedures. In Cardiovascular Disorders, Mosby's Clinical Nursing Series. St. Louis, CV Mosby

Chaitman B, 1992: Exercise stress testing. In Braunwald E (ed): Heart Disease: A Textbook of Cardiovascular Medicine, ed. 4. Philadelphia, WB Saunders

Chaitman BR, Fletcher JW, 1991: Nuclear imaging in the assessment of acquired heart disease. In Baue AE, Geha AS, Hammond GL, et al (eds): Glenn's Cardiovascular and Thoracic Surgery, ed. 5. Norwalk, CT, Appleton & Lange

Chung EK, 1989: Electrophysiology studies. In Principles of Cardiac Arrhythmias, ed. 4. Baltimore, Williams & Wilkins

Feigenbaum H, 1992: Echocardiography. In Braunwald E (ed): Heart Disease: A Textbook of Cardiovascular Medicine, ed. 4. Philadelphia, WB Saunders

Finkelmeier BA, Finkelmeier WR, 1991: Iatrogenic arterial injuries resulting from invasive procedures. J Vasc Nurs 9:12

Froelicher ESS, King SC, 1989: Exercise testing. In Underhill SL, Woods SL, Froelicher ESS, Halpenny CJ (eds): Cardiac Nursing, ed. 2. Philadelphia, JB Lippincott

Grossman W, 1992: Cardiac catheterization. In Braunwald E (ed): Heart Disease: A Textbook of Cardiovascular Medicine, ed. 4. Philadelphia, WB Saunders

Hall ML, 1989: Echocardiography, radioisotope studies, magnetic resonance imaging, and phonocardiography. In Underhill SL, Woods SL, Froelicher ESS, Halpenny CJ (eds): Cardiac Nursing, ed. 2. Philadelphia, JB Lippincott

Halpenny CJ, Bond EF, 1989: Cardiac anatomy. In Underhill SL, Woods SL, Froelicher ESS, Halpenny CJ (eds): Cardiac Nursing, ed. 2. Philadelphia, JB Lippincott

Huang SH, Kessler C, McCulloch C, Dasher LA, 1989a: Echocardiography. In Coronary Care Nursing, ed. 2. Philadelphia, WB Saunders

Huang SH, Kessler C, McCulloch C, Dasher LA, 1989b: Cardiac catheterization and angiography. In Coronary Care Nursing, ed. 2. Philadelphia, WB Saunders

Hudak CM, Gallo BM, Benz JJ, 1990: Assessment: Cardiovascular system. In Critical Care Nursing: A Holistic Approach, ed. 5. Philadelphia, JB Lippincott

Kirklin JW, Barratt-Boyes BG, 1993: Anatomy, dimensions, and terminology. In Cardiac Surgery, ed. 2. New York, Churchill Livingstone

Levin DC, Gardiner GA, 1992: Coronary arteriography. In Braunwald E (ed): Heart Disease: A Textbook of Cardiovascular Medicine, ed. 4. Philadelphia, WB Saunders

Matsuzaki M, Toma Y, Kusukawa R, 1990: Clinical applications of transesophageal echocardiography. Circulation 82:709

Newton KM, 1989: Cardiac catheterization. In Underhill SL, Woods SL, Froelicher ESS, Halpenny CJ (eds): Cardiac Nursing, ed. 2. Philadelphia, JB Lippincott

Remetz MS, Cleman MW, 1991: Cardiac catheterization in the evaluation of heart disease. In Baue AE, Geha AS, Hammond GL, et al (eds): Glenn's Cardiovascular and Thoracic Surgery, ed. 5. Norwalk, CT, Appleton & Lange

Rutherford JD, Braunwald E, 1992: Chronic ischemic heart disease.

In Braunwald E (ed): Heart Disease: A Textbook of Cardiovascular Medicine, ed. 4. Philadelphia, WB Saunders

Sutherland LJ, 1991: Patient assessment: diagnostic studies. In Kinney MR, Packa DR, Andreoli KG, Zipes DP (eds): Comprehensive Cardiac Care, ed. 7. St. Louis, Mosby–Year Book

Zaret BL, Wackers FJ, Soufer R, 1992: Nuclear cardiology. In Braunwald E (ed): Heart Disease: A Textbook of Cardiovascular Medicine, ed. 4. Philadelphia, WB Saunders

9

PREOPERATIVE MANAGEMENT

PATIENT ASSESSMENT
  Patient Interview
  Physical Assessment
  Signs and Symptoms of Heart Disease
PREPARATORY INTERVENTIONS
  Diagnostic Studies
  Medications
  Blood Preparation
  Preoperative Regimen

MANAGEMENT OF HIGH-RISK PATIENTS
  Acute Myocardial Ischemic Syndrome
  Ventricular Dysfunction
  Infective Endocarditis
  Severe Aortic Stenosis

The preoperative period provides surgical, anesthesia, and nursing personnel with an opportunity to (1) interview and assess the patient; (2) review all diagnostic information, including laboratory, electrocardiographic, chest radiographic, and cardiac catheterization data; (3) prepare the patient for the planned operation and postoperative regimen; and (4) provide observation during the immediate preoperative hours.

Patients are often admitted to the hospital on the day of a planned cardiac operation. Same-day admission is appropriate for patients with low perioperative risk. It requires efficient organization of the system so that necessary evaluations can be accomplished on an outpatient basis. A disadvantage of same-day admission is that the patient is not observed during the night before operation. Myocardial ischemia or infarction, congestive heart failure, or ingestion of food may occur without detection. Also, in patients with coronary artery disease, severe preoperative anxiety that is not observed and properly treated with anxiolytic medications may cause precipitous myocardial ischemia.

For patients with greater perioperative risk, 1 or more preoperative days may be necessary. For example, patients with severe valvular heart disease may require preoperative treatment of congestive heart failure to better tolerate the operation (Behrendt &

Austen, 1985). Diuresis is performed under medical observation because of the narrow window between optimal cardiac function and congestive heart failure. Patients who undergo coronary artery revascularization for unstable angina after acute myocardial infarction may also need additional preoperative days. Operative risk is less if surgery can be delayed 7 to 10 days, and intensive monitoring is required during this time to detect the need for proceeding with emergent surgical revascularization.

Occasionally, patients with associated medical problems are hospitalized while an elective cardiac operation is postponed to allow time for interventions that decrease operative risk. Cessation of smoking and preoperative bronchodilator therapy may improve pulmonary function and lessen the likelihood of postoperative respiratory complications in patients with severe pulmonary disease. In patients with nutritional depletion secondary to severe chronic cardiac disease, preoperative nutritional supplementation may be beneficial.

PATIENT ASSESSMENT

A primary nursing intervention in the preoperative period is a thorough assessment with documentation of significant findings. The preoperative nursing as-

Betsy Finkelmeier: CARDIOTHORACIC SURGICAL NURSING.
© 1995 J.B. Lippincott Company.

sessment complements the physician's admitting history and physical examination and provides important baseline information for comparison during the postoperative period. It also allows the nurse to establish a relationship with the patient and identify problems that will require special interventions during the hospitalization. The preoperative assessment includes information elicited from the patient, family, and medical record, as well as that obtained through physical examination of the patient. The assessment is performed in a consistent and organized manner, beginning with an overall evaluation of general status and proceeding to a more detailed evaluation of cardiovascular status (Canobbio, 1990).

PATIENT INTERVIEW

The preoperative interview is used to obtain baseline information about the patient's clinical history, understanding of the illness, emotional readiness for the planned procedure, and family support system (Table 9-1). The most important features of the clinical history are (1) the history of the present illness (i.e., the type of heart disease and associated symptoms); (2) the presence of associated medical diseases, such as peripheral arterial occlusive disease, hypertension, diabetes, or chronic obstructive pulmonary disease; (3) the current medication regimen and any known allergies; and (4) the degree of functional impairment associated with the cardiac disease. Other pertinent information includes the patient's occupation and personal habits, such as smoking, alcohol use, exercise, and diet.

Information from the clinical history may reveal factors that increase perioperative risk, such as alcohol abuse, a heavy smoking history, or steroid dependency. It may also alter the planned perioperative therapy. For example, the presence of symptoms, such as transient ischemic attacks or amaurosis fugax, may necessitate further preoperative evaluation of the carotid arteries and possible combined or staged operative therapy. A history of gastrointestinal bleeding or peptic ulcer may influence the antiplatelet regimen after coronary artery revascularization or the choice of valvular prosthesis.

TABLE 9-1. PREOPERATIVE INTERVIEW: AREAS OF FOCUS

History of present illness
Functional status
Associated medical problems
Current medication regimen and drug allergies
Knowledge of cardiac disease
Understanding of illness
Emotional readiness for procedure
Family support system

TABLE 9-2. ASSESSMENT OF FUNCTIONAL STATUS IN PATIENTS WITH HEART DISEASE

Class	Description
New York Heart Association Functional Classification System*	
I	Ordinary physical activity does not cause undue fatigue, palpitation, dyspnea, or angina
II	Ordinary physical activity causes undue fatigue, palpitation, dyspnea, or angina
III	Less than ordinary physical activity causes undue fatigue, palpitation, dyspnea, or angina
IV	Fatigue, palpitation, dyspnea, or angina occur at rest
Canadian Cardiovascular Society Functional Classification System†	
I	Angina occurs with strenuous or rapid or prolonged exertion at work or recreation
II	Slight limitation of ordinary activities by angina
III	Marked limitation of ordinary activities by angina
IV	Angina with any physical activity or at rest

* Data from Criteria Committee of the New York Heart Association, 1964: Physical capacity with heart disease. In Diseases of the Heart and Blood Vessels: Nomenclature and Criteria for Diagnosis, ed. 6. Boston, Little, Brown.
† Data from Campeau, 1976: Grading of angina pectoris. Circulation 54:522.

From the patient interview, the current level of symptoms is determined. Any increase in intensity or frequency of symptoms can then be more easily identified. A baseline is also established for the degree of associated functional impairment. In the presence of cardiac disease, heart function may be adequate at rest but inadequate during exertion (Braunwald, 1992). The New York Heart Association Functional Classification system (Criteria Committee, 1964) is commonly used in patients with valvular heart disease to describe the degree of associated disability. The Canadian Cardiovascular Classification System is more applicable for patients with coronary artery disease (Campeau, 1976) (Table 9-2).

The patient's living arrangements are addressed during the interview so that appropriate discharge planning can be initiated. An increasing number of surgical patients are elderly and have limited social and financial resources. Identification of discharge needs at the beginning of or even before the hospitalization alleviates anxiety for the patient and family and makes discharge from the hospital more efficient and timely. At this time, the nurse also evaluates the patient's understanding of the underlying illness, planned course of surgical therapy, level of anxiety, and ability to comply with the postoperative regimen. Appropriate preoperative teaching and interventions to allay anxiety can then be initiated. Preoperative education and counseling of the patient are major

TABLE 9-3. PREOPERATIVE PHYSICAL ASSESSMENT: AREAS OF FOCUS

Cardiac auscultation
    Rate and rhythm
    Heart sounds
    Murmurs, clicks, rubs
Auscultation of carotid arteries
Auscultation of the lungs
    Respiratory rate
    Breath sounds
    Adventitious sounds
Palpation of peripheral pulses
Blood pressure
Weight
Temperature
Examination of extremities
    Peripheral edema
    Evidence of arterial insufficiency or venous stasis
    Evidence of prior vein ligation

components of the preoperative regimen. They are discussed in detail in Chapter 10, Education and Psychological Support for the Patient and Family.

PHYSICAL ASSESSMENT

Physical assessment of the preoperative cardiac surgical patient focuses on the heart, lungs, peripheral pulses, and extremities (Table 9-3). Heart sounds are auscultated to provide information about heart rate, rhythm, and the presence of extra sounds, murmurs, or rubs. Each of the carotid arteries is auscultated from the base of the neck to the angle of the jaw; the presence of a bruit usually represents arterial stenosis at or proximal to the site of auscultation (Fahey & White, 1994). Auscultation of the lungs provides baseline data regarding respiratory rate, breath sounds, and the presence of adventitious sounds.

Rales may indicate the need for preoperative diuresis. Rhonchi in a heavy smoker may warrant preoperative bronchodilator therapy and pulmonary hygiene measures.

Peripheral pulses are assessed as well as other indicators of peripheral perfusion (e.g., color and temperature of extremities and capillary refill). Ankle blood pressure measurements are obtained to provide baseline information about adequacy of arterial blood flow to the lower extremities (Fig. 9-1). An ankle-brachial index may be calculated by comparing systolic pedal and brachial pressures. Systolic pressure in the leg is normally equal to or slightly higher than systolic arm pressure, resulting in an ankle-brachial index of 1.0 or above (Blackburn & Peterson-Kennedy, 1994). An index of less than 0.7 is indicative of significantly compromised blood flow to the lower extremity on that side. Calculation of an ankle-brachial index detects compromised arterial flow before operation. The extremity with better arterial blood supply is used for harvesting saphenous vein or for insertion of an intra-aortic balloon catheter through the femoral artery.

Baseline blood pressure, temperature, and weight recordings are obtained. Any abnormalities, such as jugular venous distention, ascites, or peripheral edema are noted. The presence of varicose veins or thrombophlebitis is significant in patients who are to undergo coronary artery revascularization. These conditions, or previous vein ligation, may preclude availability of saphenous vein for conduit material. For the same reason, preoperative venipuncture of saphenous veins is contraindicated in patients who are to undergo coronary artery bypass grafting to avoid damaging segments of vein that might be harvested for grafting. For a more complete discussion of physical examination of the patient with cardiovascular disease, the reader is referred to a textbook of physical assessment.

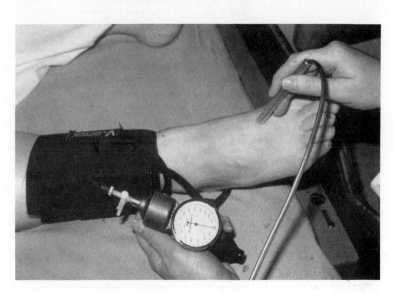

FIGURE 9-1. Measurement of ankle pressure using Doppler probe placed over the dorsalis pedis artery. (Courtesy of Victora A. Fahey, RN, MS)

SIGNS AND SYMPTOMS OF HEART DISEASE

Special consideration is given during the preoperative assessment to the presence of signs and symptoms of organic heart disease. The most frequently occurring abnormalities are described below. Of these, recognition of acute ischemia and acute congestive heart failure are particularly important.

The majority of patients who undergo cardiac operations have coronary artery disease. Thus *angina pectoris*, its cardinal manifestation, is probably the most frequently encountered symptom in preoperative cardiac surgical patients. Angina pectoris indicates transient myocardial ischemia or evolving infarction owing to an imbalance in myocardial oxygen demand and supply. It generally produces a sensation of substernal discomfort or pressure. However, it may also occur as an abnormal sensation in the throat, jaw, or arms (Fig. 9-2). Although angina may be manifested as a variety of somatic abnormalities, the pattern for a particular patient is generally consistent; that is, the nature of the discomfort is similar during each episode. Severity of pain is usually quantified using a scale from 1 to 10, with 1 being barely noticeable pain and 10 the most severe pain (Underhill, 1989).

Characteristics of the angina (e.g., how frequently it occurs, what precipitates its occurrence, its duration, and what relieves it) are used to characterize the patient's anginal pattern. Typically, angina is precipitated by one of the "four Es"—exercise, emotion, eating, or exposure to cold. Because the anginal threshold is lower in the morning than at other times throughout the day, patients commonly report that activities that may cause angina in the morning or when first undertaken do not do so later in the day (Braunwald, 1992).

Angina is generally categorized as stable or unstable. *Chronic stable angina* usually lasts less than 5 minutes and is relieved by rest or sublingual nitroglycerin. *Unstable angina* is that which (1) occurs at rest and is of sufficient severity to warrant hospitalization; (2) produces transient, reversible ST-T wave abnormalities on the electrocardiogram; and (3) is not associated with enzymatic evidence of myocardial infarction (Goldschlager, 1988). Episodes of unstable angina that are prolonged and refractory to usual medical therapy are often termed *preinfarction* or *crescendo angina*. Angina that is accelerating is discussed further later in the chapter.

Chest pain due to other etiologies can also occur, but in preoperative patients all chest pain is assumed ischemic until proven otherwise. Probably most difficult to distinguish from angina is chest pain caused by gastroesophageal reflux. Pain due to reflux frequently follows eating and is relieved by antacids. Pleuritis secondary to pleural inflammation can also cause chest pain. However, unlike angina, pleuritic pain increases on inspiration when the pleura is stretched. Musculoskeletal chest pain differs from angina in that it is usually well localized and the painful area is tender to palpation. Also, in contrast to an-

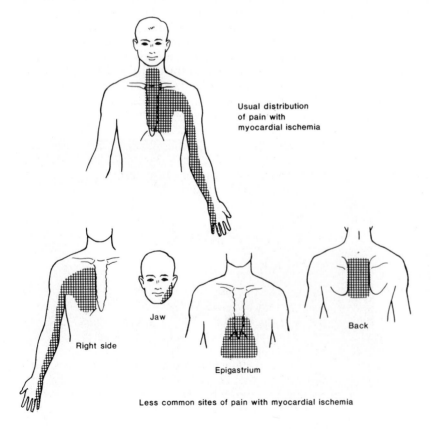

Usual distribution
of pain with
myocardial ischemia

Right side

Jaw

Epigastrium

Back

Less common sites of pain with myocardial ischemia

FIGURE 9-2. Pain patterns with myocardial ischemia. Most common distribution is referral to all or part of the sternal region, left side of the chest, neck, and down the ulnar side of the left forearm and hand. With severe ischemic pain, the right chest and right arm are often involved as well, although isolated involvement of these sites is rare. Less commonly involved, either alone or together with other sites, are the jaw, epigastrium, and back. (Horwitz LD, 1985: Chest pain. In Horwitz LD, Groves BM [eds]: Signs and Symptoms in Cardiology, p. 9. Philadelphia, JB Lippincott) gina, musculoskeletal pain is usually provoked by movement, such as jarring, coughing, or sneezing, and is relieved by massage, heat, or manipulation. Chest pain caused by anxiety may assume any form, although it frequently occurs as a dull ache in the left inframammary hemithorax. It is persistent and is often associated with fleeting sharp pains or a sensation of anxiety or breathlessness.

Dyspnea is a second common symptom of organic heart disease. Dyspnea is a gasping sensation provoked by effort that previously did not produce an awareness of breathing. Dyspnea occurs normally with strenuous exercise in healthy, well-conditioned individuals and with moderate exercise in those unaccustomed to exercise; it should be regarded as abnormal only when it occurs at rest or with a level of activity not expected to produce dyspnea (Braunwald, 1992). Paroxysmal nocturnal dyspnea, orthopnea, and dyspnea on exertion are terms used to categorize the various forms of dyspnea.

Paroxysmal nocturnal dyspnea or that which awakens the patient from sleep most commonly represents left-sided heart failure. *Orthopnea* is dyspnea that necessitates elevation of the head with more than one pillow to breathe comfortably while lying down. As cardiac disease worsens, orthopnea typically increases. *Dyspnea on exertion* signifies that the patient breathes comfortably at rest but becomes dyspneic with activity. Dyspnea is most common in patients with valvular heart disease. It may also be present in patients with ventricular dysfunction due to prior myocardial infarction. Occasionally, dyspnea occurs as an *anginal equivalent*, that is, as a manifestation of acute myocardial ischemia.

Other manifestations of cardiac disease in adults include syncope, palpitations, cough, hemoptysis, hoarseness, nocturia, fatigue, cyanosis, and peripheral edema. *Syncope,* defined as a transient loss of consciousness, may be caused by an arrhythmia, pacemaker malfunction, aortic stenosis, hypersensitive carotid sinus syndrome, or a vasovagal response. Cardiac syncope is usually of rapid onset and not associated with convulsive movements, urinary incontinence, or a postictal state (Braunwald, 1992).

Palpitations are an unpleasant awareness of the heartbeat while at rest or basal activities. Patients usually describe the sensation as fluttering, pounding, flopping, or skipping a beat. It is important to determine if the palpitating sensation represents simply an awareness of a forceful heartbeat or if it is produced by an arrhythmia. *Cardiac arrhythmias* are common in patients with organic heart disease. Many patients have chronic *premature ventricular contractions,* and often no treatment is necessary. However, documentation of their presence in the preoperative period provides useful information to formulate an appropriate response to postoperative arrhythmias. Preoperative *ventricular tachycardia* may represent acute myocardial ischemia or an underlying chronic rhythm disorder that requires electrophysio-

logic evaluation before surgical intervention. *Atrial fibrillation* is another frequently occurring arrhythmia, particularly in patients with mitral valve disease. Because chronic atrial fibrillation generally necessitates anticoagulation, its presence is an important factor in determining the type of prosthesis selected for cardiac valve replacement.

Cough associated with cardiac disease is generally nonproductive and occurs at night when the patient is lying down. It may represent an early manifestation of pulmonary edema or occur due to compression of the tracheobronchial tree by an enlarged left atrium or an aortic aneurysm. *Hemoptysis* associated with heart disease is most likely in patients with mitral stenosis. It occurs due to elevated pulmonary vascular pressure with resultant bleeding into alveoli. *Hoarseness* is unusual but may be present due to pressure on the recurrent laryngeal nerve from an enlarged left atrium or a thoracic aortic aneurysm. *Nocturia* is defined as the passage of abnormally large amounts of urine at night; it may represent congestive heart failure. *Fatigue* is a difficult symptom to evaluate since it is entirely subjective. Although it is rarely the first or only symptom of organic heart disease, it is helpful in evaluating the degree of functional impairment imposed by cardiac disease. *Central cyanosis,* a bluish discoloration of the skin and mucous membranes, is rare in adults. It represents chronic hypoxemia and may occur in patients with severe pulmonary disease or in those with unrepaired, cyanotic congenital heart defects. Localized *peripheral cyanosis* may occur due to low cardiac output or arterial occlusive disease.

Peripheral edema is unusual except in those conditions associated with right-sided heart failure, such as tricuspid valve disease or severe mitral stenosis. In ambulatory patients, edema due to cardiac disease develops bilaterally in the lower extremities. It is symmetrical, generally preceded by a 7- to 10-pound weight gain, and may progress to involve the thighs, genitalia, and abdominal wall (Braunwald, 1992). In bedridden patients, edema is likely to develop in the sacral area or back. Other signs indicative of right-sided heart failure include liver enlargement, ascites, and neck vein distention.

PREPARATORY INTERVENTIONS

DIAGNOSTIC STUDIES

Diagnostic studies performed routinely during the preoperative period include a complete blood cell count, blood clotting studies (prothrombin time, partial thromboplastin time, and bleeding time), blood chemistry survey, urinalysis, electrocardiogram, and chest roentgenogram. These baseline studies are important to detect any abnormalities that may increase risk of the operation or necessitate further preoperative evaluation. Abnormalities that may alter the timing or plan of therapy include such things as a bleeding disorder or pulmonary lesion.

Many patients, especially those with coronary artery disease have associated peripheral arterial occlusive disease. A noninvasive *carotid ultrasound study* is obtained if the patient has a carotid bruit or a history of a transient ischemic attack or cerebral vascular accident. A *Doppler arterial blood flow study* may be obtained in patients with claudication or evidence of limb ischemia. In patients with pulmonary disease, a preoperative *arterial blood gas study* on room air may be obtained to establish a baseline for the patient. *Pulmonary function testing* provides additional useful information in patients with severe pulmonary disease. If vital capacity or FEV_1 (volume of air expired at 1 second) is reduced, prolonged weaning from postoperative mechanical ventilation can be anticipated (Antman, 1992).

Before cardiac valve replacement, patients generally undergo a *dental evaluation* with *dental roentgenograms* (Fig. 9-3). Because dental infection is a common source of bacterial endocarditis, infected teeth are extracted and oral abscesses drained before implantation of a valvular prosthesis. Any dental work performed during the preoperative period is preceded by appropriate antibiotic prophylaxis according to American Heart Association guidelines (Dajani et al., 1990).

Sometimes, cardiac surgery is delayed because of diagnostic studies. If an operation is to follow within several days of a cardiac catheterization, consideration is given to nephrotoxic effects of angiographic contrast material used during the catheterization. Evidence of renal insufficiency (e.g., elevated blood urea nitrogen and creatinine values) after catheterization usually leads to postponement of the operation until renal function improves.

Occasionally, a patient becomes febrile between the time of admission and the planned operation. A temperature greater than 38.5°C (101.3°F) is suggestive of infection. The planned operation is usually postponed because of increased risk of wound contamination from a preexisting infection. Similarly, an operation is delayed if the screening urinalysis reveals the presence of a urinary tract infection. If an unsuspected malignancy is diagnosed, the cardiac operation may be postponed or canceled, depending on the urgency of the cardiac problem and the nature and extent of the malignancy.

MEDICATIONS

Most medications are continued during the preoperative period, particularly those used for control of hypertension, angina, or arrhythmias. Withdrawal of antihypertensive medications can lead to rebound hypertension or intraoperative blood pressure lability. Acute discontinuation of beta-adrenergic blocking agents is likely to precipitate myocardial ischemia or infarction or arrhythmias (Sethna et al., 1990). However, if the patient is receiving large doses or a long-acting form of beta-blocking medication, the surgeon may elect to taper the dosage or substitute a short-acting beta-blocking medication to avoid potential intraoperative myocardial depression.

Unless significant congestive heart failure is present, diuretics and digoxin are usually discontinued for several preoperative days. Diuretics are withheld to avoid loss of potassium and magnesium and marked hypovolemia (Friedman & Sethna, 1990).

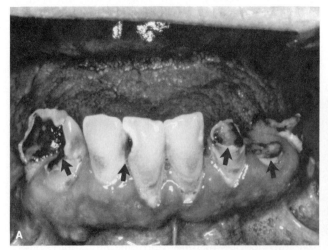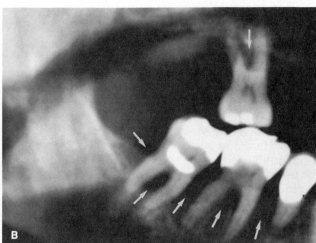

FIGURE 9-3. **(A)** The preoperative oral examination may reveal significant dental decay. In this patient, severe dental caries (*arrows*) and associated abscesses necessitated multiple dental extractions before cardiac valve replacement. **(B)** Although the gingival area surrounding these teeth appeared clinically healthy, the radiograph illustrates significant bone loss (*radiolucent areas*) around and in between the roots of the molars (*arrows*), consistent with chronic periodontal disease. (Courtesy of William Friedrich, DDS)

Preoperative digoxin administration is undesirable because the drug has a low therapeutic index and intraoperative potassium shifts may lead to digoxin toxicity (Wong, 1991).

Medications that affect hemostasis are also discontinued. Warfarin sodium (Coumadin) is generally withheld for 4 to 5 days before a planned operation so that the prothrombin time gradually decreases toward a normal level (Moreno-Cabral et al., 1988). Depending on the indication for warfarin, it may be necessary to administer heparin intravenously during this period to prevent serious thrombotic or thromboembolic complications. Because of its short half-life, heparin is usually continued until shortly before the patient is transported to the operating room.

Many patients who will undergo coronary artery revascularization are receiving aspirin because it decreases mortality and subsequent myocardial infarction in patients with unstable angina or acute myocardial infarction (Gay, 1990). Aspirin irreversibly inhibits platelet function, and aspirin ingestion within a week preceding surgery is associated with excessive perioperative bleeding that may necessitate blood transfusions or surgical reexploration. Therefore, aspirin or any aspirin-containing compound is usually discontinued a full week before an elective cardiac operation. Aspirin administration is resumed in the early postoperative period in patients who receive coronary artery bypass grafts.

Oral hypoglycemic agents are generally withheld from diabetic patients on the day of surgery. In insulin-dependent patients, the insulin dosage is adjusted because food and fluids are withheld for 8 to 12 hours before operation. A reduced dose (e.g., one-half the usual dose) is given on the morning of operation, and intravenous glucose-containing crystalloid is administered to prevent hypoglycemia. Frequent blood glucose determinations are obtained intraoperatively, and regular insulin is administered as needed. Patients who have been taking a protamine-based insulin (e.g., isophane [NPH] or protamine zinc insulin [PZI]) are at increased risk for a sensitivity reaction to protamine given intraoperatively to reverse the effects of heparin at the termination of cardiopulmonary bypass (Sather-Levine, 1990). Abrupt cessation of corticosteroids in patients who have been on chronic steroid therapy can lead to acute adrenal insufficiency (Gotch, 1991). Parenteral steroids are administered just before the operation and postoperatively until oral steroid therapy is resumed.

Patients who undergo cardiac operations almost always receive antibiotic prophylaxis despite a lack of supportive data demonstrating that it significantly lowers the incidence of postoperative wound infections. Wound contamination is most likely during the operation itself. Potential sources of pathogenic microorganisms include a preexisting infection within the patient's body, the patient's skin, and operating room personnel and equipment. Infection of the sternal wound is particularly ominous because of the significant morbidity associated with sternal dehiscence, mediastinitis, and osteomyelitis of the sternum.

Staphylococcus aureus and *S. epidermis* are the most frequently encountered causative pathogens for infection of clean wounds; enteric gram-negative rods are less common (Doebbeling et al., 1990). Although numerous clinical trials have compared a variety of antimicrobial agents, no one antibiotic has emerged as the optimal choice for prophylaxis (Miedzinski et al., 1990). Cephalosporins (e.g., cefamandole nafate or cefazolin sodium) are often chosen for prophylaxis because of demonstrated effectiveness against staphylococcal, streptococcal, and the most frequently encountered gram-negative organisms (van der Starre et al., 1988). In penicillin-allergic patients, an alternative antibiotic, such as vancomycin, must be selected (Bojar, 1989). Vancomycin and gentamicin may be used as prophylactic agents in patients at higher risk for perioperative endocarditis, such as those undergoing implantation of a valvular prosthesis. The preoperative dose of antibiotics is given intravenously in the operating room as soon as an intravenous catheter is placed or intramuscularly just before the patient is transferred to the operating room.

BLOOD PREPARATION

Blood preparation for cardiac operations has become more complex because of the risk of transmitting hepatitis B, hepatitis C (non-A, non-B hepatitis), or acquired immunodeficiency syndrome through homologous blood transfusions. Despite testing of donor blood for these agents, transmission of infection occurs in a small number of patients. The risk of transmitting infectious agents through blood product transfusion varies depending on the number of donors per recipient and the prevalence of undetected, contaminated blood in the tested blood supply (Kolins & Kolins, 1990). In addition to infection, homologous blood transfusions may also cause allergic reactions and sensitization to blood products (Scott et al., 1990).

If it is possible to schedule the operation several weeks in advance and if the patient's medical condition permits, *autologous donation* may be performed. One or 2 units of blood is donated by the patient, stored, and used as necessary during the perioperative period. Three to 4 weeks are usually necessary for recovery from anemia after collection of 400 mL of autologous whole blood and about 2 months is necessary after collection of 800 mL (Watanabe et al., 1991). Iron supplementation is usually prescribed to enhance red blood cell replenishment. In some centers, recombinant human erythropoietin is also being used. Erythropoietin, a hematopoietic hormone, is the primary regulator of erythropoiesis, or the formation of red blood cells (Levine et al., 1991).

Autologous donation is more hazardous in the presence of coronary artery disease because removal of red blood cells impairs oxygen-carrying capacity and therefore can worsen myocardial ischemia. However, safety of autologous donation in such patients has been demonstrated when performed under close physician supervision and with simultaneous saline infusion (Scott et al., 1990). Unfortunately, coronary artery revascularization procedures are often performed in patients who have recently experienced myocardial infarction, who have just undergone cardiac catheterization, who require another operative procedure after coronary bypass grafting, or who require surgery urgently. Autologous donation is usually not desirable and may be contraindicated in these situations.

Alternatively, family and friends with compatible blood types may donate blood to be used specifically for the patient. Generally, several days are needed for processing of these so-called *directed donations*. Although patients often prefer directed blood donations, it is not clear that they are safer than other exogenous blood stores because it may be difficult for family and friends, under pressure to help the patient, to be candid about possible past exposure to hepatitis or human immunodeficiency virus infection.

Because of the limited supply and associated infectious risks of homologous blood, blood products are transfused judiciously. Improved mechanisms for hemostasis and blood conservation in the operating room and intensive care unit have reduced the rate of transfusion in patients who undergo elective, primary cardiac operations. However, even in patients at low risk for blood transfusion, excessive bleeding may occur and necessitate transfusion. Appropriate preoperative testing of potential recipient and donor blood and close coordination with the local blood bank is important so that adequate type specific blood is available as needed. In some institutions, typing of recipient blood and screening for the presence of antibodies is sufficient in low risk patients to ensure adequate availability of blood for intraoperative transfusion. Alternatively, specific units of donor blood (usually two) are cross-matched and held in reserve for potential intraoperative use. In addition, fresh-frozen plasma and platelets should be readily available for all cardiac operations.

Patients at higher risk for bleeding and homologous blood transfusion include those who (1) undergo redo or combined procedures, (2) require ventriculotomy (e.g., ventricular aneurysmectomy or endocardial resection), (3) are elderly or debilitated, (4) have preoperative anemia or abnormal bleeding studies, or (5) have taken aspirin products within 1 week of operation. Two to 4 units of cross-matched blood are generally reserved for patients with increased risk for transfusion.

PREOPERATIVE REGIMEN

Preoperative showers or baths with an antibacterial soap are routinely prescribed to reduce the potential for wound infection. The most effective regimen for diminishing staphylococcal skin flora is showering both the evening before and the morning of the planned operation (Kaiser et al., 1988). The patient is instructed to thoroughly cleanse the chest, axillae, groins, and legs. Shaving of the chest, groins, and legs may be performed the evening before but is preferably done when the patient arrives in the operating room. A preoperative enema is generally not necessary because the abdominal cavity is not opened during cardiac operations and because patients return to a regular diet and ambulation within several days. In patients with unstable angina, a preoperative enema is contraindicated because it may precipitate myocardial ischemia.

A sleeping medication may be prescribed the night before surgery to help allay anxiety and to ensure that the patient is able to sleep comfortably. Caution should be exercised in patients who are elderly, are frail, or have underlying dementia; a very mild preparation or no sleeping medication is used in this group of patients. A sedative medication is administered before transporting the patient to the operating room. Preoperative sedation facilitates patient cooperation in the operating room when invasive catheters are placed. It also suppresses physiologic stress responses so that baseline hemodynamic parameters may be accurately measured. The type and dosage are generally prescribed by the anesthesiologist, based on patient age, type of cardiac disease, level of anxiety, and associated medical problems, specifically pulmonary disease. Morphine is commonly used. Scopolamine may be given adjunctively to provide perioperative amnesia and enhance the central nervous system effects of morphine (Barash & Kopriva, 1991).

Accurate timing of sedative administration is important so that the patient arrives in the operating room with minimal apprehension, yet is hemodynamically stable and alert enough to cooperate with preparatory interventions (Lake, 1985). Because sedating medications produce some degree of hypoxemia, oxygen by means of nasal cannula may be administered during transportation of the premedicated patient to the operating room, particularly in the presence of ischemic heart disease. In unstable patients, preoperative sedation is withheld until the patient arrives in the operating room and is under direct observation. Unstable patients are transported to the operating room by medical and nursing personnel with appropriate monitoring and resuscitative equipment.

MANAGEMENT OF HIGH-RISK PATIENTS

ACUTE MYOCARDIAL ISCHEMIC SYNDROME

It is essential to identify those patients who have special needs for closer observation or intervention during the preoperative period. For example, particular attention must be given to patients with coronary artery disease who experience an accelerating anginal pattern or who develop angina at rest. An increase in intensity or frequency of angina represents an *acute myocardial ischemic syndrome,* in which portions of ventricular myocardium are ischemic but not yet irreversibly damaged. The syndrome occurs because jeopardized muscle tissue does not infarct simultaneously but in an uneven manner surrounded by severely ischemic tissue (Morris et al., 1990). One of three conditions may be present: (1) unstable angina, (2) *evolving myocardial infarction* (i.e., prolonged ischemia over 4 to 6 hours during which muscle necrosis spreads from the subendocardium through the ventricular myocardium), or (3) a completed myocardial infarction with unstable *postinfarction angina.*

Patients with an acute myocardial ischemic syndrome are moved to a closely monitored setting, cardiologic consultation is obtained, and appropriate interventions are initiated to limit ischemia. Intravenous nitroglycerin is administered by continuous infusion if oral medications fail to eradicate anginal pain while the patient is at rest. Arterial blood pressure monitoring is performed to allow continuous observation of the drug's effect on systolic blood pressure. A continuous intravenous heparin infusion is usually initiated and continued until shortly before the patient is transported to the operating room. Heparin prevents extension of intracoronary thrombus, which is presumed to be present in most patients with unstable angina (Roberts & Pratt, 1991). Pain that continues despite maximal doses of pharmacologic agents may be treated with intra-aortic balloon counterpulsation. Alternatively, a decision may be made to proceed with urgent surgical revascularization.

Occasionally, ventricular tachycardia or pulmonary edema occurs as a manifestation of acute myocardial ischemic syndrome. Patients with these symptoms are generally operated on urgently. Intravenous lidocaine or other antiarrhythmic medication is administered to suppress ventricular arrhythmias until the heart is revascularized. In patients with pulmonary edema, a pulmonary artery catheter may be inserted to better assess intravascular preload and afterload and guide diuretic and vasodilating therapy, respectively. Preoperative intubation and mechanical ventilation may also be necessary to support the patient.

Because angina that is accelerating or that occurs at rest may represent myocardial infarction, it is important that it is detected promptly and reported to the cardiac surgeon. Electrocardiograms taken during episodes of chest pain and serial measurement of isoenzyme levels help determine whether acute myocardial infarction has occurred. A completed myocardial infarction that occurs during the immediate preoperative period significantly increases risk of operative death. Restoring perfusion to recently infarcted muscle can cause a complex pathophysiologic cellular process, termed *hemorrhagic reperfusion injury,* that produces significant ventricular dysfunction. If enzy-matic or electrocardiographic evidence of myocardial infarction is present, every attempt is made to delay operation, typically for 7 to 10 days. Urgent revascularization may become necessary if postinfarction angina persists despite pharmacologic antianginal therapy and balloon counterpulsation or if counterpulsation is contraindicated. Operative risk is considerably higher in these patients.

VENTRICULAR DYSFUNCTION

Patients with significant acute or chronic ventricular dysfunction also require special management in the preoperative period. *Acute ventricular dysfunction* (i.e., *cardiogenic shock*) can occur in preoperative patients with acute valvular dysfunction, postinfarction ventricular septal defect, aortic dissection, or infective endocarditis. Although left ventricular failure is more common, isolated right ventricular failure is sometimes present, such as in patients with acute tricuspid regurgitation secondary to infective endocarditis. Often it is impossible to correct cardiogenic shock with medical therapy alone, and emergent surgical therapy may be essential.

Severe *chronic ventricular dysfunction* occurs most often in patients with long-standing mitral or aortic valve disease and in those with prior myocardial infarction. Although these disorders initially affect left ventricular function, producing left-sided heart failure, manifestations of right-sided heart failure eventually develop as well (Braunwald & Grossman, 1992) (Fig. 9-4). Patients with long-standing ventricular dysfunction can generally be identified by the physical stigmata of chronic illness. Cardiac cachexia describes the appearance of such a patient who is emaciated, often with anasarca (generalized body edema), ascites, and jaundice secondary to prolonged passive congestion of the liver (Kennedy, 1988). Less common cardiac disorders sometimes associated with preoperative, refractory congestive heart failure include ventricular aneurysm, cardiac tumor, endomyocardial fibrosis, and constrictive pericarditis without calcification (Smith et al., 1992).

The presence of congestive heart failure at the time of admission may necessitate postponement of the operation to improve cardiac function and thereby lessen operative risk. Because of the narrow window between maintaining adequate preload and precipitating congestive heart failure in such patients, closely titrated pharmacologic therapy is necessary. A pulmonary artery catheter may be placed to guide therapy. Diuresis and fluid and salt restriction are primary components of treatment. Intravenous inotropic and afterload reduction (vasodilating) agents may be necessary to treat congestive heart failure refractory to oral pharmacologic therapy.

Recognition of the precarious hemodynamic status in this group of patients is essential. Although independence in self-care activities and intermittent ambulation is important in most preoperative patients to maintain strength and avoid complications of immo-

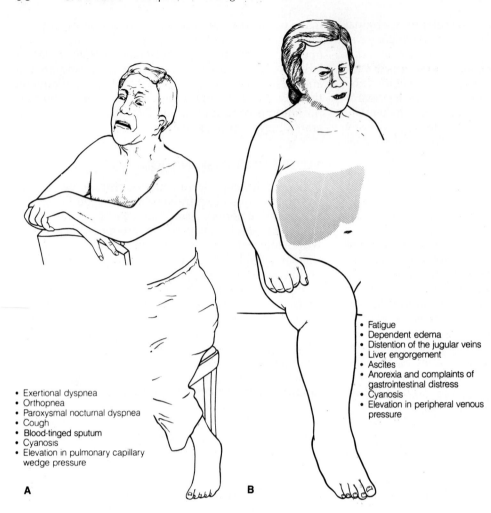

- Exertional dyspnea
- Orthopnea
- Paroxysmal nocturnal dyspnea
- Cough
- Blood-tinged sputum
- Cyanosis
- Elevation in pulmonary capillary wedge pressure

A

- Fatigue
- Dependent edema
- Distention of the jugular veins
- Liver engorgement
- Ascites
- Anorexia and complaints of gastrointestinal distress
- Cyanosis
- Elevation in peripheral venous pressure

B

FIGURE 9-4. Manifestations of left-sided **(A)** and right-sided **(B)** heart failure. (Porth CM, 1990: Heart failure. In Pathophysiology: Concepts of Altered Health States, ed. 3, pp. 381, 383. Philadelphia, JB Lippincott)

bility, such activities in patients with severely compromised ventricular function can have lethal consequences. These patients legitimately need assistance with daily care and may not be able to ambulate safely. If a preoperative patient is unable to perform daily activities independently or is unable to ambulate, the physician is consulted regarding advisability of increasing the patient's level of activity during the preoperative period.

INFECTIVE ENDOCARDITIS

Another group of preoperative patients who require close observation are those with *infective endocarditis.* Eighty to 90% of patients with infective endocarditis of native cardiac valves are effectively treated medically with an extensive course of organism specific antimicrobial therapy (Hendren et al., 1992). However, depending on the extent of valvular damage and virility of the organism, emergent surgical therapy is sometimes necessary.

Patients with infective endocarditis are often gravely ill with hemodynamic instability and multisystem organ failure (Larbalestier et al., 1992). Close

observation is essential to detect findings that indicate a deterioration in the patient's condition, including (1) a new or changed heart murmur, (2) manifestations of congestive heart failure, (3) evidence of systemic (left-sided infective endocarditis) or pulmonary (right-sided infective endocarditis) embolism, (4) persistence of fevers despite antibiotic therapy, and (5) the development of complete heart block representing intramyocardial extension of the infection. Indications for proceeding urgently with surgical therapy include acute valvular regurgitation secondary to leaflet or chordae tendineae destruction, persistent sepsis despite organism-specific antimicrobial therapy, recurrent embolization from the infected valve, or evidence of intramyocardial abscess.

SEVERE AORTIC STENOSIS

Patients with *severe aortic stenosis* also require close preoperative monitoring. Because of the fixed obstruction to left ventricular outflow, cardiac output cannot increase appropriately in response to increased metabolic demands. Hypovolemia and vasodilatation are poorly tolerated and may precipitate cardiac arrest. The patient with severe aortic stenosis who suffers cardiac arrest can seldom be successfully resuscitated.

REFERENCES

Antman EM, 1992: Medical management of the patient undergoing cardiac surgery. In Braunwald E (ed): Heart Disease: A Textbook of Cardiovascular Medicine, ed. 4. Philadelphia, WB Saunders

Barash PG, Kopriva CJ, 1991: Anesthesia for cardiac surgery. In Baue AE, Geha AS, et·al. (eds): Glenn's Cardiovascular and Thoracic Surgery, ed. 5. Norwalk, CT, Appleton & Lange

Behrendt DM, Austen WG, 1985: Preparation for operation. In Patient Care in Cardiac Surgery, ed. 4. Boston, Little, Brown

Blackburn DR, Peterson-Kennedy LK, 1994: Noninvasive vascular testing. In Fahey VA (ed): Vascular Nursing, ed. 2. Philadelphia, WB Saunders

Bojar RM, 1989: Preoperative considerations. In Manual of Perioperative Care in Cardiac and Thoracic Surgery. Boston, Blackwell Scientific Publications

Braunwald E, 1992: The history. In Braunwald E (ed): Heart Disease: A Textbook of Cardiovascular Medicine, ed. 4. Philadelphia, WB Saunders

Braunwald E, Grossman W, 1992: Clinical aspects of heart failure. In Braunwald E (ed): Heart Disease: A Textbook of Cardiovascular Medicine, ed. 4. Philadelphia, WB Saunders

Campeau L, 1976: Grading of angina pectoris. Circulation 54:522

Canobbio MM, 1990: Assessment. In Cardiovascular Disorders (Mosby's Clinical Nursing Series). St. Louis, CV Mosby

Criteria Committee of the New York Heart Association, 1964: Physical capacity with heart disease. In Diseases of the Heart and Blood Vessels: Nomenclature and Criteria for Diagnosis, ed. 6. Boston, Little, Brown

Dajani AS, Bisno AL, Chung KJ, et al., 1990: Prevention of endocarditis: Recommendations by the American Heart Association. JAMA 264:2919

Doebbeling BN, Pfaller MA, Kuhns KR, et al., 1990: Cardiovascular surgery prophylaxis. J Thorac Cardiovasc Surg 99:981

Fahey VA, White SA, 1994: Physical assessment of the vascular system. In Fahey VA (ed): Vascular Nursing, ed. 2. Philadelphia, WB Saunders

Friedman AS, Sethna DH, 1990: Hemodynamic manipulation of the patient during anesthesia. In Gray RJ, Matloff JM (eds): Medical Management of the Cardiac Surgical Patient. Baltimore, Williams & Wilkins

Gay WA Jr, 1990: Aspirin, blood loss and transfusion. Ann Thorac Surg 50:345

Goldschlager NF, 1988: Acute myocardial infarction. In Luce JM, Pierson DJ (eds): Critical Care Medicine. Philadelphia, WB Saunders

Gotch PM, 1991: The endocrine system. In Alspach JG (ed): Core Curriculum for Critical Care Nursing, ed. 4. Philadelphia, WB Saunders

Hendren WG, Morris AS, Rosenkranz ER, et al., 1992: Mitral valve repair for bacterial endocarditis. J Thorac Cardiovasc Surg 103:124

Kaiser AB, Kernodle DS, Barg NL, Petracek MR, 1988: Influence of preoperative showers on staphylococcal skin colonization: A comparative trial of antiseptic skin cleansers. Ann Thorac Surg 45:35

Kennedy G, 1988: Clinical cardiac assessment. In Kern LS (ed): Cardiac Critical Care Nursing. Rockville, MD, Aspen Publishers

Kolins J, Kolins MD, 1990: Informed consent, risk, and blood transfusion. J Thorac Cardiovasc Surg 100:88

Lake CL, 1985: Preoperative evaluation and preparation of cardiac surgical patients. In Cardiovascular Anesthesia. New York, Springer-Verlag

Larbalestier RI, Kinchla NM, Aranki SF, et al., 1992: Acute bacterial endocarditis. Circulation 86 (Suppl II):II-68

Levine EA, Rosen AL, Sehgal LR, et al., 1991: Erythropoietin deficiency after coronary artery bypass procedures. Ann Thorac Surg 51:764

Miedzinski LJ, Callaghan JC, Fanning EA, et al., 1990: Antimicrobial prophylaxis for open heart operations. Ann Thorac Surg 50:800

Moreno-Cabral CE, Mitchell RS, Miller DC, 1988: Postoperative problems. In Manual of Postoperative Management in Adult Cardiac Surgery, Baltimore, Williams & Wilkins

Morris DC, Walter PF, Hurst JW, 1990: The recognition and treatment of myocardial infarction and its complications. In Hurst JW, Schlant RC, Rackley CE, et al. (eds): The Heart, ed. 7. New York, McGraw-Hill

Roberts R, Pratt CM, 1991: Medical treatment of coronary artery disease. In Roberts R (ed): Coronary Heart Disease and Risk Factors. Mount Kisco, NY, Futura Publishing

Sather-Levine B, 1990: Perioperative agents. In Underhill SL, Woods SL, Froelicher ES, Halpenny CJ (eds): Cardiovascular Medications for Cardiac Nursing. Philadelphia, JB Lippincott

Scott WJ, Kessler R, Wernly JA, 1990: Blood conservation in cardiac surgery. Ann Thorac Surg 50:843

Sethna DH, Moffitt EA, Hackner EL, 1990: Anesthetic techniques for cardiac surgery. In Gray RJ, Matloff JM (eds): Medical Management of the Cardiac Surgical Patient. Baltimore, Williams & Wilkins

Smith TW, Braunwald E, Kelly RA, 1992: The management of heart failure. In Braunwald E (ed): Heart Disease: A Textbook of Cardiovascular Medicine, ed. 4. Philadelphia, WB Saunders

Underhill SL, 1989: History taking and physical examination. In Underhill SL, Woods SL, Froelicher ES, Halpenny CJ (eds): Cardiac Nursing, ed. 2. Philadelphia, JB Lippincott

van der Starre PJ, Trienekens PH, Harinck-de Weerd JE, et al., 1988: Comparative study between two prophylactic antibiotic regimens of cefamandole during coronary artery bypass surgery. Ann Thorac Surg 45:24

Watanabe Y, Fuse K, Konighi T, et al., 1991: Autologous blood transfusion with recombinant human erythropoietin in heart operations. Ann Thorac Surg 51:767

Wong CA, 1991: Physiologic responses to anesthesia. In Shekleton ME, Litwack K (eds): Critical Care Nursing of the Surgical Patient. Philadelphia, WB Saunders

10

EDUCATION AND PSYCHOLOGICAL SUPPORT FOR THE PATIENT AND FAMILY

PREOPERATIVE EDUCATION
  Content
  Teaching Strategies
PSYCHOLOGICAL SUPPORT

Cardiothoracic surgical nurses play a major role in preparing patients and families for operations. In facilities where cardiac surgery is performed routinely, preoperative instruction and psychological support are an integral component of nursing care. Ideally, nurses who will provide care in the postoperative period perform preoperative teaching and counseling. This allows the designated nurse to assess the patient preoperatively, plan for any special postoperative needs, and communicate information to other nursing staff. In addition, the nurse demonstrates to the patient the knowledge and skill of those who will be providing postoperative care and establishes a relationship with the patient and family before surgery.

Preparation of the patient for surgery is commonly referred to as "preoperative teaching," but the focus is actually as much on providing psychological support to the patient and family as on educational needs. As much as possible families should be included in preoperative teaching. Family members are almost always the patient's greatest source of support (Barr, 1989). In addition, family members who have been instructed about the perioperative course can reinforce teaching with the patient who may be too ill or anxious to retain information presented during the preoperative teaching session.

PREOPERATIVE EDUCATION

Patient teaching is known to have many positive effects, including increased knowledge retention, decreased anxiety, improved pain management, decreased length of hospitalization, and improved patient adherence with the medical regimen (Barr, 1989). Preoperative education is one type of patient teaching in which the patient is instructed about a planned operative procedure and the projected postoperative course. Just as the surgeon discusses with each patient the objective of an operation and its potential benefits and risks, the nurse describes to the patient and family the planned perioperative events and what will be expected of the patient in the postoperative period.

Preoperative education differs from other forms of patient teaching in that it is necessary to provide in a short time span a body of specific information that is relevant only to the period of hospitalization. In addition, the instruction must be accomplished during a time when patients are adjusting to hospital admission and impending surgery. When patients move into a "sick role," anxiety, worry, or depression are likely to interfere with concentration and learning (Hudak et al., 1990).

Betsy Finkelmeier: CARDIOTHORACIC SURGICAL NURSING.
© 1995 J.B. Lippincott Company.

The acuity of illness and the brevity of hospitalization before surgery necessitate a preoperative teaching program with realistic guidelines and standard content, teaching materials, and methods of documentation (Ruzicki, 1989). Such a program ensures that every patient receives adequate preparation for surgery and that the nurses' interventions and patients' responses are communicated appropriately. Evaluation and continued improvement of the preoperative preparation program can be achieved by soliciting feedback from postoperative patients and their families about their own recent experiences.

Before initiating preoperative teaching, the nurse reviews the patient's cardiac history, associated medical problems, planned surgical procedure, and operative risk as assessed by the surgeon. This is followed by an assessment of the patient's current level of understanding, capacity and motivation for learning new information, and emotional status, particularly the level of anxiety. Through the assessment, barriers to learning are identified (Table 10-1) (Murdaugh, 1988). The teaching plan is formulated with these limitations in mind. Principles of adult education are also taken into consideration. Guiding assumptions for preoperative teaching of adults include (1) adults want to be active participants in the learning process, (2) past experiences have an impact on learning, (3) major life events stimulate a desire to learn, and (4) information that is immediately applicable is of most interest (Gessner, 1989).

A continuum of learning needs and emotional responses is represented in preoperative cardiac surgical patients. Some patients, such as those undergoing elective valve replacement, have known and planned for the operation for months. On the other end of the

---

TABLE 10-1. BARRIERS TO LEARNING IN CARDIAC PATIENTS

Physiologic

Severity of illness
Age of patient
Prognosis

Psychological

Anxiety
Denial
Depression

Environmental

Loss of privacy
Separation from loved ones

Iatrogenic

Fragmentation of teaching
Behaviors of the teacher

(Adapted from Murdaugh C, 1988: The nurse's role in education of the cardiac patient. In Kern LS [ed]: Cardiac Critical Care Nursing. Rockville, MD, Aspen Publishers)

TABLE 10-2. SCOPE OF INFORMATION FOR PREOPERATIVE TEACHING

Basic anatomy and pathologic condition
Description of operative procedure
Common diagnostic and preoperative studies
Description of perioperative course
    Assistive catheters and tubes
    Visiting procedures
    Pulmonary hygiene
    Progression of activity
    Appetite, emotional responses, physical stamina
    Pain and pain control
Information about valve prostheses or pacemakers
Available resources
    Support personnel
    Insurance or financial concerns
    Community services after discharge

---

spectrum are patients operated on urgently, such as those with unstable angina. The latter group of patients may have had no knowledge of a heart problem before the present hospitalization. In this situation, the patient must, within a matter of hours, adjust not only to the presence of a life-threatening health problem but also to the need for a major operation.

Despite variability in learning needs, most patients are principally focused on implications of the operation itself. Also, because almost all patients are admitted to the hospital on the morning of or 1 day before the operation, teaching time is limited. Therefore, content should be relevant to the patient's current problem (i.e., the need for information about the perioperative course). Usually, a generalized description of the projected course is given to the patient, including the preoperative regimen, various units in which the patient will stay, the number of days in each unit, and what the patient's condition will be like during each phase. Interventions that require active participation from the patient, such as coughing and deep breathing exercises, are highlighted. However, the need to individualize content to individual learning needs cannot be overemphasized. Providing content that exceeds the patient's ability or desire to learn may cause the patient to become confused or increasingly anxious. Information commonly included in preoperative teaching is discussed below (Table 10-2).

CONTENT

Components of the preoperative regimen that may be discussed with the patient include evaluations by members of the surgical team, preoperative diagnostic studies, antibacterial showers, preoperative sedation, withholding of food and drink after midnight, and shaving of the chest, groin, and legs. Patients are informed that they will spend the first 24 to 48 postoperative hours in an intensive care unit and the remainder of the hospitalization (4 to 5 days) on a cardiothoracic surgical unit. Basic information about monitoring and supportive catheters and devices is given. However, the patient generally does not need a detailed description of all the various invasive catheters and tubes. By the time the patient is alert enough to examine the attached devices, most will have been removed. In addition, catheters and tubes are placed in the operating room, so the patient will have no memory of their insertion, and once in place, they are usually not uncomfortable or bothersome.

It is usually best to specifically discuss the need for intubation and assisted ventilation. The presence of an endotracheal tube and mechanical ventilation are almost always the most discomforting aspects of the early postoperative period. Although the tube is not painful, the patient is unable to talk or take fluids by mouth. In addition, the sensation of assisted mechanical ventilation may be frightening. For these reasons, it is reassuring to explain to the patient in advance that a nurse will be readily available during the period of intubation to interpret and assist with basic needs. It is also helpful to prepare the patient for the presence of a urinary drainage catheter. Often patients are unaware that urine drains freely from the bladder while a catheter is in place. Particularly in men, the catheter causes a sensation of needing to urinate.

A frequent concern of patients is separation from family during the operation and early postoperative period. Usually the family may visit during the immediate preoperative hours and accompany the patient during transfer to the operating room. It is helpful to inform the patient and family that family members will be able to stay in a comfortable area near the operating room and that the surgeon will discuss the operation with them as soon as it is completed. In addition, many cardiothoracic surgical services have clinical nurse specialists who act as liaisons to facilitate communication with the family during the operation and the postoperative period. Family members usually wish to visit patients as soon as possible after the operation, and this can be arranged in most cases. Often patients are quite concerned about being able to have dentures, glasses, or a hairpiece in place as soon as possible. Although these requests may seem minor, they can take on unusual significance for some patients, and accommodating the patient's wishes provides a great deal of comfort.

The patient is also instructed about the anticipated progression of recovery during the postoperative period (e.g., initiation of bathroom privileges and resumption of a regular diet). Particular attention is given to preparing the patient to participate with pulmonary hygiene measures and progressive ambulation. Incentive spirometry, or other assistive device for prevention of atelectasis, may be demonstrated and the patient given an opportunity to practice using it. Expectations for progressive ambulation in the corridors should also be communicated to the patient. Patients who understand the rationale will be better prepared to actively cooperate with deep breathing and coughing exercises as well as early and progressive ambulation.

Excessive fatigue, depression, insomnia, and anorexia are almost universal complaints after a cardiac operation, and it is beneficial for the patient to understand that these may occur during the recovery process. Patients may be reassured that these are expected, transient problems that should gradually diminish and resolve. Often patients fear the pain that will accompany cardiac surgery. Although pain tolerance varies greatly among individuals, patients may be reassured that postoperative pain is generally not significant after sternotomy and that adequate analgesic agents will be available.

Beyond the provision of essential information, the nurse is guided by assessment of the patient's readiness to learn. Patients will usually ask questions that reveal what information will be most useful to them. In most instances, patients request information that will lessen anxiety about the loss of control and uncertain outcome associated with a major operation. Attempts to educate patients about the underlying disease process, risk factor modification, or chronic medical therapies are usually best deferred until after the operation. However, reference material should be available for patients who do want to learn more about the underlying disease during the preoperative period.

TEACHING STRATEGIES

In hospitalized patients, preoperative teaching is typically performed the evening before the planned operation. Unfortunately, this is usually the period of highest anxiety for the patient. Although motivation for learning is high because of the life-threatening nature of cardiac surgery, learning capacity is often inversely diminished by anxiety. Alternatively, an initial preoperative teaching session may be performed before the hospital admission when the patient's anxiety level is lower. Significantly higher preoperative knowledge levels, more positive postoperative mood states, and more favorable physiologic recoveries have been demonstrated in patients who receive both preadmission and postadmission preoperative education as compared with patients who receive only postadmission preoperative education (Cupples, 1991).

Preoperative teaching is also more efficacious if an individual's learning style can be matched with an appropriate teaching technique (Lindsay et al., 1991). In some facilities, group teaching sessions are performed. Although this provides patients with a forum to share concerns and support one another, it has the distinct disadvantage that individual needs for information and support are sometimes compromised by the needs of other group members. If group teaching is used, it should not replace an individualized session during the preoperative period in which a nurse devotes full attention to providing counseling to each patient and family.

A written brochure is an excellent supplement to preoperative teaching and is used in most facilities. Use of a teaching booklet enhances consistency of information and provides a reference for both the patient and family. If a booklet specific to the institution is developed, lay terminology should be used and information should be presented in a supportive fashion. During preparation of a teaching booklet, content is evaluated to ensure that the reading level is appropriate for the majority of individuals who will be receiving it. Alternatively, a commercially prepared patient teaching booklet for cardiac surgical patients may be used.

Audiovisual aids, such as instructional videotapes, are also helpful. They are thought to increase knowledge retention because they involve more than one sense in the learning process (Scalzi & Burke, 1989). They also provide a creative supplement to preoperative teaching and, like written materials, enhance consistency of information presented to the patient.

Opportunities for informal teaching, incorporated in performance of routine preoperative nursing interventions, allow repetition of important information. In addition, interventions and their rationale are explained as they are performed. A tour of the postoperative nursing unit is helpful for some patients.

PSYCHOLOGICAL SUPPORT

Almost all patients experience some fear and anxiety when facing a cardiac operation. In fact, moderate anxiety is considered indicative that a patient is emotionally ready for an operation and is thought to enable the patient to cope with postoperative stress and discomfort (Gregersen & McGregor, 1989). Sources of anxiety for preoperative patients include physical discomfort, socioeconomic problems, a feeling of helplessness, fear of disability, uncertainty of the outcome, separation from family, and the possibility of death (Rocey, 1990). Anxiety may be manifested by a variety of psychophysiologic symptoms, such as increased tension, increased helplessness, decreased self assurance, sympathetic stimulation, and focusing on the perceived object of fear (Carty, 1991).

Although the provision of factual information is effective in reducing anxiety, preoperative teaching is not the only nor the most important method of supporting patients before surgery. In fact, the need for psychological support far outweighs the need for information in many patients. One study of patients scheduled for cardiac catheterization demonstrated that, once patients had been given adequate information to allow informed consent for the procedure, the presence of a caring person who interacted socially was as effective as repetition of information in reducing anxiety (Peterson, 1991).

Interventions to provide psychological support include allowing verbalization of concerns and providing reassurance about the commitment of the nurses and physicians to the patient's well being. Scheduling one nurse to work consistently with the patient allows more thorough assessment of the patient's psychological needs and provides the setting for development of rapport between the nurse and patient (Burke & Scalzi, 1989). In addition to the patient's primary nurse, other resources also play an important role. A clinical nurse specialist who works with the patient and family throughout the hospitalization may assist the staff nurses in assessing the patient's need for psychological support and also may have more flexibility in scheduling consistent time to spend with the patient and family. Patients who have undergone similar operative procedures also can provide support to the preoperative patient. Often, a visit from a convalescing patient is reassuring. In some facilities, individuals who have previously undergone heart surgery are permitted to visit preoperative patients and provide supportive information.

Occasionally, preoperative patients are nearly incapacitated by anxiety. Severe anxiety during the preoperative period warrants close observation and special nursing interventions. It is often these severely anxious patients who develop disorientation or frank psychosis after surgery. Severe anxiety may be manifested either overtly or in a more insidious fashion. If the patient is able to acknowledge the fear and anxiety, it is easier for the nurse to intervene by talking with the patient, allowing verbalization of concerns, and providing reassurance. An anxiolytic medication, such as diazepam, is usually administered as well, particularly in patients with ischemic heart disease.

Occasionally, patients are both severely anxious and unable to acknowledge the anxiety. The resulting manifestation may be hostile, demanding, or controlling behaviors. The patient tends to alienate staff by these behaviors, which may reduce the amount of emotional support that is given when in fact more is needed. Another manifestation may be inordinate concern by the patient regarding one aspect of the perioperative care. In attempting to establish a sense of control, the patient may magnify its importance out of proportion. For example, the patient may threaten to leave if not given a private room or insist that medical or nursing students not be allowed to participate in the care.

Most often, it is the nurse at the bedside who deals with the brunt of these behaviors. Effective methods of providing support to severely anxious patients include (1) listening to the patient's concerns and requests; (2) making special accommodations if they are reasonable and do not compromise the ability of the team to care for the patient safely; (3) providing rationale when special accommodations are not possible; and (4) throughout all interactions, maintaining an air of confidence in the team's ability to provide safe care and an attitude of concern for making the situation as comfortable as possible for the patient. If the patient's need for support is beyond what the cardiac surgical team can realistically provide, psychiatric consultation is obtained.

REFERENCES

Barr WJ, 1989: Teaching patients with life-threatening illnesses. Nurs Clin North Am 24:639

Burke LE, Scalzi CC, 1989: Behavioral responses of the patient and family: Myocardial infarction and coronary artery bypass grafting. In Underhill SL, Woods SL, Froelicher ES, Halpenny CJ (eds): Cardiac Nursing, ed. 2. Philadelphia, JB Lippincott

Carty JL, 1991: Psychosocial aspects. In Alspach JG (ed): Core Curriculum for Critical Care Nursing, ed. 4. Philadelphia, WB Saunders

Cupples SA, 1991: Effects of timing and reinforcement of preoperative education on knowledge and recovery of patients having coronary artery bypass grafting. Heart Lung 20:654

Gessner BA, 1989: Adult education. Nurs Clin North Am 24:589

Gregersen RA, McGregor MS, 1989: Cardiac surgery. In Underhill SL, Woods SL, Froelicher ES, Halpenny CJ (eds): Cardiac Nursing, ed. 2. Philadelphia, JB Lippincott

Hudak CM, Gallo BM, Benz JJ, 1990: Patient and family teaching. In Critical Care Nursing: A Holistic Approach, ed. 5. Philadelphia, JB Lippincott

Lindsay C, Jennrich JA, Biemolt M, 1991: Programmed instruction booklet for cardiac rehabilitation teaching. Heart Lung 20:648

Murdaugh C, 1988: The nurse's role in education of the cardiac patient. In Kern LS (ed): Cardiac Critical Care Nursing. Rockville, MD, Aspen Publishers

Peterson M, 1991: Patient anxiety before cardiac catheterization: An intervention study. Heart Lung 20:643

Rocey DL, 1990: Preparation of the patient and family. In Gray RJ, Matloff JM (eds): Medical Management of the Cardiac Surgical Patient. Baltimore, Williams & Wilkins

Ruzicki DA, 1989: Realistically meeting the educational needs of hospitalized acute and short-stay patients. Nurs Clin North Am 24:629

Scalzi CC, Burke LE, 1989: Education of the patient and family: In-hospital phase. In Underhill SL, Woods SL, Froelicher ES, Halpenny CJ (eds): Cardiac Nursing, ed. 2. Philadelphia, JB Lippincott

PART 3

INTRAOPERATIVE CONSIDERATIONS

CHAPTER 11

ANESTHESIA FOR CARDIAC OPERATIONS

PREOPERATIVE EVALUATION AND
   PREPARATION
INTRAOPERATIVE MONITORING AND
   PREPARATION

GENERAL ANESTHESIA
   Anesthetic Agents
   Stages of Anesthesia
TRANSFER TO THE INTENSIVE CARE UNIT

PREOPERATIVE EVALUATION AND PREPARATION

Anesthetic management of the cardiac surgical patient begins with a thorough preoperative evaluation. Assessment of cardiovascular and pulmonary status and a review of the current medication regimen are of particular importance in the clinical history. The preoperative physical examination focuses on the heart, lungs, blood pressure, peripheral pulses, extremities, and abdomen (Lake, 1985). The patient is also examined for any potential difficulties with intubation or vascular cannulation. The chest roentgenogram and electrocardiogram are reviewed as well as information obtained from available diagnostic studies, such as cardiac catheterization, stress testing, and echocardiography. Pertinent preoperative laboratory studies include serum electrolytes, blood urea nitrogen, and creatinine; complete blood cell count; liver enzyme analysis; coagulation studies; and urinalysis. Correctable abnormalities that might increase morbidity, such as hypokalemia, congestive heart failure, or infection, are identified and treated before the operation.

The anesthetic approach is formulated based on the specific type of cardiac disease and estimated complexity of the operative procedure. Patient age and associated medical problems, such as previous myocardial infarction, hypertension, congestive heart failure, or cerebral vascular disease, must be taken into consideration. Noncardiac conditions, such as severe obstructive or bronchospastic pulmonary disease, renal insufficiency, diabetes mellitus, and bleeding disorders, also influence the planned anesthetic management (Schneider, 1989). In unstable patients, such as those with acute myocardial ischemia, cardiogenic shock, or severe aortic stenosis, special anesthetic techniques are planned to avoid precipitous perioperative complications.

Oral intake is withheld for 6 to 8 hours before the operation to reduce the potential for aspiration during and after anesthesia induction. Most medications, particularly antianginal and antiarrhythmic agents, are continued during the preoperative period to avoid precipitous myocardial ischemia or arrhythmias. Aspirin, digoxin, and diuretics are usually discontinued in the preoperative period. Aspirin impairs platelet function and increases the likelihood of excessive perioperative bleeding. Digoxin has a low therapeutic index and intraoperative potassium shifts may lead to digoxin toxicity (Wong, 1991). Diuretics can cause potassium and magnesium depletion and hypovolemia (Friedman & Sethna, 1990).

Oral hypoglycemic agents are generally withheld in diabetic patients. In insulin-dependent patients, a reduced dose of insulin is given on the morning of the operative day and intravenous, glucose-containing crystalloid is administered to prevent preoperative hypoglycemia. In patients who are steroid-dependent, abrupt withdrawal of corticosteroid therapy

Betsy Finkelmeier: CARDIOTHORACIC SURGICAL NURSING.
© 1995 J.B. Lippincott Company.

107

can cause acute adrenal insufficiency (Gotch, 1991). Therefore, patients who have been on chronic steroid therapy receive parenteral steroids before operation and during the perioperative period until an oral diet is resumed.

Prophylactic antibiotics are almost always prescribed for prevention of perioperative wound infection and are administered by intramuscular injection before the patient leaves the nursing unit or intravenously on arrival in the operating room. Preoperative diagnostic evaluation and preparation of the cardiac surgical patient are described in greater detail in Chapter 9, Preoperative Management. Psychological preparation of the patient is an integral component of preoperative patient preparation and is discussed in Chapter 10, Education and Psychological Support for the Patient and Family.

Preoperative medication is usually administered before the patient leaves the nursing unit to suppress anxiety and induce sedation. Preoperative sedation facilitates patient cooperation during the preparatory period in the operating room when invasive procedures must be accomplished. In addition, it suppresses physiologic stress responses so that baseline hemodynamic parameters may be accurately measured.

The anesthesiologist prescribes the specific agents and dosage for a given patient based on a number of factors, including age, level of anxiety, type of cardiac disease, and associated medical conditions, particularly pulmonary disease. Morphine, scopolamine, and diazepam are commonly used to reduce preoperative anxiety, produce perioperative amnesia, and facilitate smooth anesthesia induction (Sather-Levine, 1990). Accurate timing of administration is important to achieve the desired effects. The goal is for the patient to arrive in the operating room with minimal apprehension yet hemodynamically stable and alert enough to cooperate with preliminary intraoperative preparations (Lake, 1985).

Because preoperative medications may decrease arterial oxygen tension, supplemental oxygen is sometimes ordered for the period of transport to the operating room, particularly in patients with ischemic heart disease. In unstable patients, preoperative medication is omitted to avoid hemodynamic alterations during patient transfer. Instead, sedatives are given in the operating room under direct observation of the anesthesiologist. Unstable patients are transported to the operating room by medical and nursing personnel with appropriate monitoring and resuscitation equipment.

INTRAOPERATIVE MONITORING AND PREPARATION

During cardiac operations, any evidence of cardiac, respiratory, neurologic, or renal dysfunction must be detected and treated promptly to prevent irreversible organ damage. Accordingly, a multitude of catheters and devices are used to monitor the function of all major organ systems. As soon as the patient arrives, electrocardiographic, noninvasive blood pressure, and pulse oximetry monitoring are initiated to allow rapid identification of ischemic changes, arrhythmias, hypotension, or hypoxemia.

Ongoing *electrocardiographic monitoring* is performed using leads that allow adequate assessment of ST segment changes, particularly in the anterolateral (lead modified V_5) and inferior (lead II) myocardial wall (Friedman & Sethna, 1990). An esophageal lead may be used in selected patients to detect right ventricular and posterior wall ischemia and to aid in diagnosis of arrhythmias. Intraoperative arrhythmias are most likely during insertion of the pulmonary artery catheter, intubation, surgical manipulation of the heart, reperfusion after release of the aortic cross-clamp, and episodes of myocardial ischemia (Friedman & Sethna, 1990).

Arterial, pulmonary artery, and central venous pressure monitoring are instituted before cardiac operations that involve extracorporeal circulation. Because the patient is vulnerable to myocardial ischemia or low cardiac output during anesthesia induction, these catheters are generally inserted after sedation but before induction. Myocardial ischemia is most likely in patients with coronary artery disease but can also occur in patients with valvular or congenital heart disease. Hypovolemia secondary to diuretic therapy or angiographic dye (e.g., administered during a recent cardiac catheterization) may require fluid infusion before or during anesthesia induction.

An indwelling arterial cannula is placed for *arterial pressure monitoring* and intermittent arterial oxygen tension measurements. The radial artery is almost always used for this purpose after ulnar artery patency is confirmed with the Allen test. In addition, oxygen saturation is monitored continuously using *pulse oximetry.* If the need for intra-aortic balloon counterpulsation is anticipated, a femoral artery catheter or sheath may be placed to make percutaneous balloon catheter insertion easier.

A *pulmonary artery catheter* is inserted through the jugular or subclavian vein. It allows continuous monitoring of intracardiac pressures (pulmonary artery and right atrial pressures). Cardiac output and mixed venous oxygen saturation measurements are also obtained using the pulmonary artery catheter. Pulmonary artery diastolic pressure is used to guide perioperative fluid management. Right atrial pressures provide information about right ventricular function. Some pulmonary artery catheters have pacing electrodes that can be used for temporary cardiac pacing before application of epicardial pacing wires. A separate triple-lumen central venous catheter may be inserted for preoperative autologous blood donation or plasmapheresis and to provide ports for continuous infusion of medications. A large-bore peripheral intravenous catheter is placed for administering fluids and blood products. A urinary drainage catheter is placed to monitor adequacy of urine output in the anesthetized patient.

Core body temperature is monitored using a blood (pulmonary artery catheter), urethral (urinary catheter), or esophageal thermistor. Nasopharyngeal or rectal temperature is often monitored as well. Ongoing temperature monitoring is essential to evaluate the status of patient cooling and rewarming, the degree of myocardial protection, the adequacy of peripheral perfusion, and the presence of malignant hyperthermia. In some institutions, a myocardial probe is also placed by the surgeon to directly monitor myocardial temperature during the period of aortic cross-clamping.

An esophageal stethoscope is inserted and used by the anesthesiologist to monitor heart sounds and effectiveness of ventilation throughout the operation. *Intraoperative echocardiography*, using transesophageal or epicardial transducers, provides important information regarding intraoperative myocardial performance, valve function, regional myocardial function, anatomic shunting, intrachamber air, and effectiveness of venting (Reves et al., 1990). In some centers, an *electroencephalogram* is used to monitor cerebral function. Electroencephalographic monitoring is thought by some to more promptly detect evidence of acute (and potentially reversible) brain injury or ischemia. However, postoperative neurologic deficits occasionally occur even in the absence of detectable changes in the intraoperative electroencephalogram (Barash & Kopriva, 1991).

GENERAL ANESTHESIA

The goals of general anesthesia are to achieve (1) unconsciousness, (2) amnesia, (3) analgesia, (4) muscle relaxation, and (5) attenuation of stress responses. Ideal general anesthesia for cardiac operations would accomplish these goals without producing hemodynamic instability or myocardial ischemia. However, because no single agent produces all of the desired effects, multiple drugs are administered to achieve general anesthesia (Table 11-1). Each anesthetic drug has a unique spectrum of actions; careful titration of drug doses and combining drugs minimizes or counteracts the deleterious effects of individual agents (Hensley et al., 1991).

ANESTHETIC AGENTS

Two major categories of anesthetic agents are commonly used for cardiac operations: volatile anesthetics (i.e., inhalation agents) and narcotics (Table 11-2). The primary difference in the two types of anesthesia is that inhalation agents more effectively provide amnesia and analgesia but also cause significant myocardial depression and vasodilatation when used in concentrations sufficient to block sympathetic responses to noxious stimuli (Warner & Warner, 1989).

TABLE 11-1. CATEGORIES OF ANESTHETIC AGENTS

Amnesic Agents	Hypnotic Agents
Diazepam	Diazepam
Lorazepam	Etomidate
Midazolam	Ketamine
	Midazolam
Analgesic Agents	Thiopental
Alfentanil	
Fentanyl	**Muscle-Relaxing Agents**
Meperidine	Atracurium
Morphine	d-Tubocurarine
Sufentanil	Metocurine
	Pancuronium
	Succinylcholine
	Vecuronium

Inhalation agents are volatile liquids administered with oxygen, nitrous oxide, or air in various concentrations that the patient inspires through a face mask or endotracheal tube. They are absorbed from alveoli into pulmonary capillary blood (Litwack, 1991). Inhalation agents include isoflurane, enflurane, and halothane. Halothane is less commonly used in adults because in a very small percentage of patients it has been associated with severe hepatic dysfunction (Tinker, 1989; Barash & Kopriva, 1991). The three agents are otherwise similar in that they rapidly induce anesthesia, allow early emergence, and act as potent myocardial depressants and peripheral vasodilators (Barash & Kopriva, 1991). In patients with myocardial ischemia, the negative inotropic effect is beneficial in reducing myocardial oxygen consumption; however, it may exacerbate heart failure in those with poor left ventricular function (Hensley et al., 1991). The bronchodilating effects of inhalation agents make them useful in patients with obstructive or bronchospastic pulmonary disease (Schneider, 1989).

Although inhalation agents have analgesic actions, the associated myocardial depression and vasodilation contraindicates using them in doses large enough to provide adequate analgesia. Therefore,

---

TABLE 11-2. PRIMARY CHARACTERISTICS OF INHALATION AND NARCOTIC AGENTS

Inhalation Agents (Isoflurance, Enflurane, Halothane)

Dose-dependent myocardial depression
Vasodilatation
Rapid induction
Early emergence

Narcotic Agents (Fentanyl, Sufentanil, Morphine)

Potent anesthesia and analgesia
Minimal hemodynamic effects
Slow emergence

---

narcotics or tranquilizers are used as supplements to provide adequate anesthesia (i.e., blocking of pain perception and physiologic responses to noxious stimuli). Even in the unconscious patient who is unaware of pain, it is important to prevent autonomic responses, such as tachycardia and hypertension (Hensley et al., 1991).

Narcotics or *opioids,* such as fentanyl, sufentanil, and morphine, comprise the second category. They are given intravenously directly into the bloodstream. Narcotic agents rapidly produce profound analgesia and anesthesia without significantly affecting cardiovascular hemodynamics, particularly during induction (Stanley, 1989). Most narcotic actions are dose dependent: the larger the dose, the greater is the level of analgesia, respiratory depression, and anesthesia (Warner & Warner, 1989).

A *high-dose narcotic technique* is used extensively in cardiac operations. With a high-dose technique, narcotic agents are used both to induce and to maintain the anesthetized state. Disadvantages of high-dose narcotic anesthesia are that it produces prolonged respiratory depression and it may not completely prevent hypertension in patients with good left ventricular function (Hensley et al., 1991).

Also, opioids do not provide hypnosis or amnesia reliably. Recall of intraoperative events, especially conversations, can occur. Supplementation with hypnotic or inhalation agents is therefore required when opioids are used as the primary anesthetic agent (Reves et al., 1990). The period of highest risk for incomplete amnesia is during rewarming before termination of cardiopulmonary bypass; the anesthetic effect of hypothermia is removed, inhalational agents are discontinued, and intravenous agents have been diluted by the perfusate (circulating blood volume in cardiopulmonary bypass circuit) (Hensley et al., 1991).

The synthetic narcotics (i.e., fentanyl and sufentanil) are used most often. Morphine is less commonly used because it produces prolonged postoperative respiratory depression and because vasodilation and decreased peripheral resistance increase perioperative blood and fluid requirements (Sethna et al., 1990). Morphine is also less effective in suppressing patient awareness and recall of intraoperative events and may fail to attenuate cardiovascular responses to stress (Barash & Kopriva, 1991).

Although inhalational and narcotic agents produce different perioperative hemodynamic effects, both forms of anesthesia are comparable with respect to incidence of postoperative myocardial infarction and death (Slogoff & Keats, 1989). A *balanced technique* (i.e., a combination of inhalation and narcotic agents) is most often used. Balanced anesthesia, using multiple agents, allows lower doses of individual agents to be used, thus reducing unwanted adverse effects.

Other agents used adjunctively during cardiac operations include barbiturates, benzodiazepines, and neuromuscular blocking agents. *Barbiturates* (e.g., thiopental) are drugs that produce hypnosis and amnesia but not analgesia. They are commonly used to induce the anesthetized state. *Benzodiazepines* (e.g., diazepam, lorazepam, and midazolam) have hypnotic, amnesic, anxiolytic, anticonvulsant, and muscle relaxant effects (Ruff et al., 1989). *Neuromuscular blocking agents* (i.e., muscle relaxants) facilitate tracheal intubation, provide intercostal muscle paralysis that makes sternal retraction less traumatic, prevent muscle movement during light levels of anesthesia, eliminate diaphragmatic movement, and allow controlled mechanical ventilation (Stanley, 1989). Metocurine and pancuronium are long-acting muscle relaxants suitable for cardiac procedures. Succinylcholine is used infrequently; its short duration of action limits its usefulness to providing neuromuscular blockade for induction and intubation (Warner & Warner, 1989). Muscle relaxants do not provide analgesia, sedation, or amnesia (Reves et al., 1990).

STAGES OF ANESTHESIA

General anesthesia consists of three phases: (1) induction, (2) maintenance, and (3) reversal, or emergence. *Induction* is the transition period from the awake to the anesthetized state. The *maintenance* period continues until near completion of the procedure. *Emergence* describes the phase when anesthetic agents are discontinued and the patient is allowed to return to the conscious state.

Before induction the patient is preoxygenated because hypoxemia and hypercarbia from premedications or intravenous sedatives can lead to hypertension and tachycardia (Friedman & Sethna, 1990). Induction is performed after monitoring is established and just before intubation. It is accomplished using either *hypnotics* (i.e., pharmacologic agents that produce sleep) or narcotics (e.g., fentanyl). Most commonly used is thiopental, an ultra-short-acting barbiturate that rapidly blocks wakefulness centers within the cerebral cortex and reticular activating system (Litwack, 1991). Other induction agents include droperidol, ketamine, diazepam, and midazolam (Kirklin & Barratt-Boyes, 1993). Intubation is carried out as soon as the induction agents are administered. A muscle relaxant is used to facilitate intubation by causing temporary paralysis of the jaw, diaphragm, and other skeletal muscles (Hoffer, 1991). Stressful intubation can produce release of catecholamines with resultant hypertension, tachycardia, and increased systemic vascular resistance, all of which affect myocardial blood flow adversely. Low doses of fentanyl or thiopental given intravenously at the time of induction may help attenuate these responses. Topical anesthetics or vasodilating agents may also be used (Hensley et al., 1991). Fiberoptic bronchoscopy is occasionally necessary to facilitate intubation.

Special induction techniques are necessary to gain rapid control of the airway in patients with increased risk of aspiration. Patients more likely to aspirate during induction and intubation include (1) those with recent oral intake who undergo emergent operation, (2) those with gastroesophageal reflux, (3) diabetic patients with gastroparesis, and (4) those with other conditions associated with delayed gastric emptying. After intubation, mechanical ventilation is instituted. Oxygenation and ventilation are carefully monitored throughout the operation. Airway management can be complicated at any point in the perioperative period by airway obstruction, aspiration of gastric contents, laryngeal or tracheal injury, or cardiovascular stimulation during airway manipulation (Hensley et al., 1991). During the period of extracorporeal circulation, ventilation of the lungs is discontinued.

Throughout the operative procedure, general anesthesia is maintained at a level to ensure unconsciousness, analgesia, muscle relaxation, and attenuated stress responses. The anesthesiologist uses knowledge of the hemodynamic effects of each agent and its interactions with other drugs to anticipate and correct hemodynamic changes throughout the procedure (Warner & Warner, 1989). Administration of anesthetic agents, fluids, and vasoactive medications is titrated according to heart rate, arterial and pulmonary artery pressures, and cardiac output. Increases in blood pressure or heart rate and patient movement may indicate an inadequate depth of anesthesia (Stanley, 1989). During cardiopulmonary bypass, inhalational agents must be administered through the cardiopulmonary bypass circuit because the lungs are not ventilated. Intravenous agents can be given directly into the patient's bloodstream.

Maintenance of anesthesia is designed to prevent myocardial ischemia and dysfunction and to treat them if they do occur (Wynands & O'Connor, 1989). Careful regulation of blood pressure is essential. Hypotension decreases subendocardial blood supply; hypertension, on the other hand, increases afterload and left ventricular oxygen demand. Intraoperative hypotension is treated with decreased amounts of anesthetic agents, volume replacement if preload is low, and inotropic agents. Nitroglycerin or sodium nitroprusside infusions are most commonly used to control hypertension.

Throughout the intraoperative period, special consideration is given to the type of underlying cardiac pathology. For example, coronary artery disease and ventricular hypertrophy significantly reduce the capacity of subendocardial vessels to dilate to increase blood flow (Buckberg, 1991). The left ventricular subendocardium is at greatest risk because compression of intramyocardial blood vessels prevents blood flow during systole.

In addition, many patients who undergo coronary artery revascularization have been on beta-blocking or calcium-channel antagonist agents. Beta-adrenergic blockers depress myocardial contractility and lower heart rate; some calcium-channel antagonists produce vasodilatation in addition to depressing contractility. These drugs in combination with volatile anesthetic agents can produce significant myocardial depression, hypotension, bradycardia, and heart block (Conahan, 1985). Bradycardia can lower cardiac output, which is the product of stroke volume times heart rate. In patients with aortic regurgitation, bradycardia increases regurgitant flow (Buckberg, 1991).

Tachycardia is particularly detrimental in patients with coronary artery disease; it further impairs coronary artery blood flow by shortening diastole when coronary artery filling occurs. Tachycardia is also poorly tolerated in patients with aortic stenosis. In the presence of a stenotic aortic valve, diastolic filling time is already reduced because ejection through the narrowed valve orifice prolongs systole (Buckberg, 1991). Aortic stenosis also poses special concerns for the anesthesiologist because myocardial depression, vasodilatation, or arrhythmias may precipitate cardiac arrest that is refractory to resuscitation (Schneider, 1989).

TRANSFER TO THE INTENSIVE CARE UNIT

As the operation is concluded, the anesthesiologist informs nursing staff in the postoperative intensive care unit (ICU) of the patient's condition, prescribed ventilator settings, and any currently infusing intravenous medications. The transfer is postponed if the patient is hemodynamically unstable. Therapeutic manipulations are instituted in the operating room, and the patient is cared for there until hemodynamic stability is achieved.

The patient is transported to the ICU using portable equipment for monitoring cardiac rhythm and arterial pressure. Ventilation is provided manually using a self-inflating bag and 100% oxygen. Vigilant observation and attention to detail are necessary during the transport period. Hemodynamic instability may be precipitated by the patient's emergence from anesthesia or physiologic changes that occur with moving the patient from the operating table to the bed (Barash & Kopriva, 1991). Potential problems during transport include sudden hypotension due to fluid shifts that occur as the patient is moved, acute hypertension due to sympathetic stimulation, and extubation or undesirable reflex responses caused by traction on the endotracheal tube (Hendren & Higgins, 1991). In addition, intravenous infusions of medications may be interrupted or the dosage changed as intravenous tubing is manipulated and equipment exchanged. Momentary lapses in monitoring may occur unless protocols are well established for the transfer process.

The anesthesiologist accompanies the patient to the ICU and remains until all monitoring equipment and intravenous infusions are safely reestablished and the patient's hemodynamic stability is confirmed. During this period, a summary of pertinent information is given to the ICU nurse regarding the patient's intraoperative course and current rates of fluid and medication infusion. The patient is allowed to slowly emerge from the anesthetized state. Administration of morphine or diazepam may be helpful to provide analgesia and reduce agitation as the patient awakens. Sedation is maintained until chest tube drainage is at an acceptable level and the patient is fully rewarmed, hemodynamically stable, and ready for weaning from mechanical ventilation (Coyle, 1991).

Residual anesthetic effects can have a major influence on the cardiovascular, respiratory, and central nervous systems and must be taken into account during the early postoperative hours (Wong, 1991). If opioid-induced narcosis resolves before neuromuscular blocking agents have been eliminated or metabolized, the patient may awaken but remain paralyzed. Aggressive pharmacologic intervention with nitrates, alpha- and beta-blocking agents, and calcium-channel antagonist medications may be necessary to suppress autonomic stress responses (Hendren & Higgins, 1991). In a patient who is slow to awaken, naloxone, a narcotic antagonist, may occasionally be given to eliminate residual narcosis. However, naloxone can produce hypertension, tachycardia, and myocardial ischemia owing to an induced release of catecholamines (Reves et al., 1990).

REFERENCES

Barash PG, Kopriva CJ, 1991: Anesthesia for cardiac surgery. In Baue AE, Geha AS, Hammond GL, et al. (eds): Glenn's Thoracic and Cardiovascular Surgery, ed. 5. Norwalk, CT, Appleton & Lange

Buckberg GD, 1991: Myocardial protection during adult cardiac operations. In Baue AE, Geha AS, Hammond GL, et al. (eds): Glenn's Thoracic and Cardiovascular Surgery, ed. 5. Norwalk, CT, Appleton & Lange

Conahan TJ, 1985. Anesthetic considerations in coronary artery disease. In Utley JR (ed): Perioperative Cardiac Dysfunction. Baltimore, Williams & Wilkins

Coyle JP, 1991: Sedation, pain relief, and neuromuscular blockade in the postoperative cardiac surgical patient. Semin Thorac Cardiovasc Surg 3:81

Friedman AS, Sethna DH, 1990: Hemodynamic manipulation of the patient during anesthesia. In Gray RJ, Matloff JM (eds): Medical Management of the Cardiac Surgical Patient. Baltimore, Williams & Wilkins

Gotch PM, 1991: The endocrine system. In Alspach JG (ed): Core Curriculum for Critical Care Nursing, ed. 4. Philadelphia, WB Saunders

Hendren WG, Higgins TL, 1991: Immediate postoperative care of the cardiac surgical patient. Semin Thorac Cardiovasc Surg 3:3

Hensley FA, Larach DR, Martin DE, 1991: Intraoperative anesthetic complications and their management. In Waldhausen JA, Orringer MB (eds): Complications in Cardiothoracic Surgery. St. Louis, Mosby–Year Book

Hoffer JL, 1991: Anesthesia. In Meeker MH, Rothrock JC (eds): Alexander's Care of the Patient in Surgery, ed. 9. St. Louis, Mosby–Year Book

Kirklin JW, Barratt-Boyes BG, 1993: Anesthesia for cardiovascular surgery. In Cardiac Surgery, ed. 2. New York, Churchill Livingstone

Lake CL, 1985: Preoperative evaluation and preparation of cardiac surgical patients. In Cardiovascular Anesthesia. New York, Springer-Verlag

Litwack K, 1991: Anesthetic agents. In Post Anesthesia Care Nursing. St. Louis, Mosby–Year Book

Reves JG, Greeley WJ, Leslie J, 1990: Anesthesia and supportive care for cardiothoracic surgery. In Sabiston DC Jr, Spencer FC (eds): Surgery of the Chest, ed. 5. Philadelphia, WB Saunders

Ruff R, Reves JG, Croughwell ND, Brusino FG, 1989: The cardiovascular effects of benzodiazepines. In Estafanous FG (ed): Anesthesia and the Heart Patient. Boston, Butterworths

Sather-Levine B, 1990: Perioperative agents. In Underhill SL, Woods SL, Froelicher ES, Halpenny CJ (eds): Cardiovascular Medications for Cardiac Nursing. Philadelphia, JB Lippincott

Schneider RC, 1989: Anesthesia for cardiac surgery. In Grillo HC, Austen WG, Wilkins EW Jr, et al. (eds): Current Therapy in Cardiothoracic Surgery. Toronto, BC Decker

Sethna DH, Moffitt EA, Hackner EL, 1990: Anesthetic techniques for cardiac surgery. In Gray RJ, Matloff JM (eds): Medical Management of the Cardiac Surgical Patient. Baltimore, Williams & Wilkins

Slogoff S, Keats AS, 1989: Randomized trial of primary anesthetic agents on outcome of coronary artery bypass operations. Anesthesia 70:179

Stanley TH, 1989: Opiates and cardiovascular anesthesia. In Estafanous FG (ed): Anesthesia and the Heart Patient. Boston, Butterworths

Tinker JH, 1989: Controversies surrounding the use of inhalation agents. In Estafanous FG (ed): Anesthesia and the Heart Patient. Boston, Butterworths

Warner MA, Warner ME, 1989: Anesthetic agents for cardiac surgery. In Tarhan S (ed): Cardiovascular Anesthesia and Postoperative Care, ed. 2. Chicago, Year Book Medical Publishers

Wong CA, 1991: Physiologic responses to anesthesia. In Shekleton ME, Litwack K (eds): Critical Care Nursing of the Surgical Patient. Philadelphia, WB Saunders

Wynands JE, O'Connor JP, 1989: Anesthesia for coronary artery surgery. In Estafanous F (ed): Anesthesia and the Heart Patient. Boston, Butterworths

CHAPTER 12

CARDIOPULMONARY BYPASS

COMPONENTS OF CARDIOPULMONARY
   BYPASS
   Venous and Arterial Cannulae
   Oxygenator, Reservoir, and Heat
     Exchanger
   Arterial Pump
   Left Ventricular Vent
   Cardiotomy Suction

EXTRACORPOREAL CIRCULATION
   Initiation
   Maintenance
   Weaning
CONSEQUENCES OF CARDIOPULMONARY
   BYPASS
   Physiologic Effects
   Clinical Sequelae

Cardiopulmonary bypass (CPB) describes a system used to temporarily perform the functions of the heart (circulation of blood) and lungs (gas exchange) during operative procedures on the heart or great vessels. Development of CPB was largely due to pioneering research by Dr. John Gibbon and heralded the beginning of the modern era of cardiac surgery (Blanche et al., 1990). For the first time, prolonged interruption of normal circulation became possible, providing a decompressed, noncontracting heart and a bloodless field within which the surgeon could work.

CPB is called *extracorporeal circulation* because blood is diverted from the vascular system and circulated through a circuit of plastic tubing outside the body. Venous cannulae are used to drain blood from the right side of the heart into the CPB circuit. As blood is pumped through the circuit, it is oxygenated, filtered, cooled or warmed, and returned by means of an arterial cannula to the systemic circulation. In this fashion, body tissues, particularly that of the brain and other vital organs, are perfused and remain viable despite temporary cessation of heart and lung function.

CPB may be either total (essentially all venous blood is diverted into the extracorporeal circuit) or partial (some venous blood returns to the heart and is ejected into the aorta) (Kirklin & Kirklin, 1990). In most cardiac operations, total CPB is used and the ascending aorta is cross clamped, excluding the coronary arteries from the extracorporeal circuit. Cardioplegic solution is separately infused into the coronary circulation to induce and maintain cardiac arrest. Any cardiac operation that involves use of CPB is correctly termed an *open heart operation* whether or not a cardiac chamber is opened during the procedure.

Extracorporeal circulation is sometimes used in situations other than during cardiac or great vessel surgery. Temporary circulatory support may be used to treat postoperative cardiogenic shock or as a bridge to emergent cardiac surgery in patients with sudden, profound ventricular failure. *Extracorporeal membrane oxygenation* (ECMO) is a form of CPB sometimes used to treat severe respiratory failure in infants and children. Temporary circulatory support of the heart outside the operating room is discussed in Chapter 30, Mechanical Assist Devices.

COMPONENTS OF CARDIOPULMONARY BYPASS

The following components comprise the CPB system: (1) venous and arterial cannulae; (2) oxygenator, reservoir, and heat exchanger; (3) arterial pump; (4) left ventricular vent; and (5) cardiotomy suction catheter (Fig. 12-1).

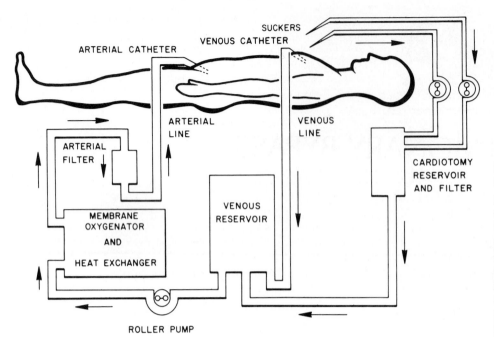

FIGURE 12-1. Diagram of a typical cardiopulmonary bypass setup with a membrane oxygenator. (Stephenson LW, Edmunds LH Jr, 1991: Cardiopulmonary bypass for open heart surgery. In Baue AE, Geha AS, Hammond GL, et al. [eds]: Glenn's Thoracic and Cardiovascular Surgery, ed. 5, p. 1402. Norwalk, CT, Appleton & Lange)

VENOUS AND ARTERIAL CANNULAE

Venous blood is diverted into the CPB circuit using one or two large-bore cannulae. Most commonly, venous blood is drained through a single cannula that is inserted through a small incision in the anterolateral aspect of the right atrium (Fig. 12-2). Single right atrial cannulation is suitable for most cardiac operations, despite the fact that a small amount of venous blood continues to enter the right atrium through the coronary sinus and thebesian veins.

Alternatively, two venous cannulae may be positioned in the superior and inferior vena cavae to totally divert venous return from the heart. Separate cannulation of the superior and inferior vena cava must be used in operations that necessitate opening the right atrium (atriotomy) or ventricle (ventriculotomy) (Blanche et al., 1990). A third technique for diverting venous return into the CPB circuit is cannulation of the femoral vein with retrograde advancement of the cannula into the inferior vena cava.

In most cases, oxygenated blood is returned to the systemic circulation by means of a cannula inserted into the ascending aorta, just proximal to the origin of the innominate artery (see Fig. 12-2). The ascending aorta is most commonly used because (1) it is easily accessible through the median sternotomy incision, (2) it eliminates the need for groin dissection and femoral artery repair, and (3) it reduces the potential for arterial dissection, which is more likely with retrograde perfusion through the femoral artery (Behrendt & Austen, 1985). Complications of ascending aortic cannulation include intimal damage that can lead to aortic dissection, disruption and embolization of intimal plaque into cerebral vessels, and inappropriate

placement of the cannula tip in the innominate artery (Blanche et al., 1990).

Alternatively, the femoral artery may be cannulated. Femoral artery cannulation provides distinct advantages in selected situations. First, cannulation of the femoral artery may be preferable in reoperations because it can be performed before opening the chest. In patients who have had one or more previous

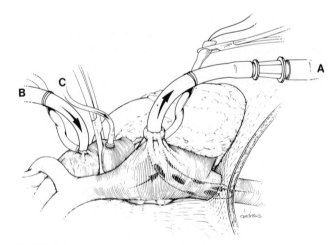

FIGURE 12-2. Cannulation for cardiopulmonary bypass. In this drawing, a single cannula has been positioned in the right atrium for venous drainage (A). The arterial cannula has been positioned in the ascending aorta (B), and a cardioplegia catheter (C) has been placed proximal to the aortic cross-clamp. (Cooley DA, 1984: Cannulation for temporary bypass. In Techniques in Cardiac Surgery, ed. 2, p. 84. Philadelphia, WB Saunders)

operations through a median sternotomy, internal scarring from prior procedures may result in adherence of the anterior surface of the heart to the posterior table of the sternum. Laceration of the right ventricle can occur as the sternum is divided. Without the ability to promptly initiate extracorporeal circulation in this situation, exsanguination and death can occur within minutes. The presence of femoral artery and vein cannulae allows rapid institution of CPB while the surgeon controls the resulting hemorrhage and repairs the injured structure.

Similarly, in unstable or high-risk patients who might experience hemodynamic deterioration with induction of anesthesia, CPB can be rapidly instituted by means of femoral vessel cannulation before the median sternotomy has been performed. Femoral arterial cannulation may also be used if the ascending aorta is heavily calcified. In such patients, embolization of calcium or atheromatous material into the cerebral circulation can occur during manipulation and cannulation of diseased tissue in the ascending aorta.

In patients who have undergone previous coronary bypass surgery with multiple saphenous vein anastomoses to the proximal aorta, there may be no remaining area to insert the arterial cannula without disrupting existing vein graft anastomoses. Femoral artery cannulation is also necessary during operative repair of the ascending aorta or aortic arch. The femoral artery and vein are routinely cannulated when a lateral thoracotomy incision is used for cardiac operations because the ascending aorta and right atrium are not accessible with this approach.

Studies have demonstrated that ascending aorta and femoral artery cannulation are similar with respect to organ perfusion (Kirklin & Kirklin, 1990). With availability of percutaneous cannulae developed for portable CPB systems, a cutdown technique may not be needed for femoral vessel cannulation; percutaneous cannulae can be quickly inserted and used with a standard CPB system (Hartz et al., 1990). The primary complication associated with femoral artery cannulation is aortic dissection, which may not be recognized until retrograde perfusion is initiated and irreversible damage has occurred. As a result, the complication is often fatal. Femoral artery cannulation can also cause limb ischemia. Aortic dissection and limb ischemia are most likely in patients with atherosclerotic peripheral arterial occlusive disease.

OXYGENATOR, RESERVOIR, AND HEAT EXCHANGER

The oxygenator is the device that oxygenates blood and facilitates carbon dioxide exchange. Two types of oxygenators are used: bubble and membrane. In a *bubble oxygenator* there is direct contact between blood and fine bubbles of oxygen. Oxygen diffuses into the blood; carbon dioxide diffuses in the reverse direction. Blood and bubbles are separated by defoaming and settling in an arterial reservoir (Stephenson &

Edmunds, 1991). A *membrane oxygenator* consists of a semipermeable membrane through which oxygen and carbon dioxide diffuse. Membrane oxygenators may be preferable for longer periods of perfusion because the absence of bubbling reduces trauma to blood elements.

The CPB system contains a *reservoir* that holds 500 to 3000 mL of blood. Its purpose is to reserve a volume of blood in the extracorporeal circuit, to allow escape of air from the blood, and to allow the rate of blood return to the patient to be manipulated somewhat independently of the patient's venous return. The reservoir contains an entry port through which blood products, crystalloids, and medications can be added to the perfusate (i.e., the circulating blood volume). The location of the reservoir varies with the type of oxygenator used. With a membrane oxygenator, blood is collected in a venous reservoir until it is pumped through the oxygenator. With a bubble oxygenator, the blood is first oxygenated and then collected in an arterial reservoir before being returned to the patient (Blanche et al., 1990).

A *heat exchanger*, which is usually incorporated in the oxygenator, is used to precisely adjust temperature of the blood and thereby the patient's body during the period of extracorporeal circulation. The heat exchanger warms or cools by exposing the blood-filled tubing to water at a selected temperature.

ARTERIAL PUMP

A primary component of the CPB system is the *arterial pump*, which propels oxygenated blood into the patient's arterial circulation. Arterial flow during CPB can be either nonpulsatile or pulsatile. Nonpulsatile pumps are most often used and may be one of two types (Fig. 12-3). Most common is a *roller pump*, which propels blood by external compression of the tubing and produces continuous flow. Roller pumps are relatively simple to operate, reliable, and provide accurate perfusion rates (Blanche et al., 1990).

Less commonly used is a *centrifugal pump*, a disposable unit that propels blood by a whirling, circular motion. Centrifugal pumps are thought to produce less hemolysis because blood elements are not subjected to compression by a roller. Additionally, air in the tubing is less likely to be propelled into the patient's arterial circulation. Instead, the centrifugal force of the pump propels minute quantities of air, which is lighter than blood, toward the center of the pump. Centrifugal pumps are often used when longer than normal periods of extracorporeal circulation are anticipated, particularly when circulatory support is necessary beyond the duration of the cardiac operation.

Pulsatile blood flow may be achieved by (1) a pulsatile arterial pump, (2) using intra-aortic balloon counterpulsation during CPB, (3) partial CPB (i.e., allowing left ventricular ejection to augment systemic blood flow), or (4) temporarily increasing arterial in-

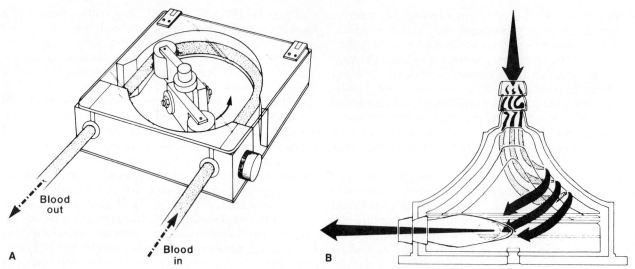

FIGURE 12-3. Types of arterial pumps. **(A)** Roller pump. (Milan JD, 1983: Blood transfusion in heart surgery. Surg Clin North Am 63:1130) **(B)** Centrifugal pump. (Kern FH, Giesser WG, Farrell DM, 1993: Extracorporeal circulation and circulatory assist devices in the pediatric patient. In Lake CL [ed]: Pediatric Cardiac Anesthesia, ed. 2, p. 154. Norwalk, CT, Appleton and Lange)

flow to the patient over venous return from the patient (Kirklin & Kirklin, 1990). The superiority of pulsatile versus nonpulsatile flow has been debated since the development of CPB and remains controversial. Although pulsatile flow is intuitively more attractive because it more closely simulates physiologic blood flow, it actually could be more damaging to blood elements. At this time, pulsatile pumps are used infrequently.

An *arterial filter* is used to trap particulate matter or air that inadvertently enters the circuit before blood is returned to the arterial system (Blanche et al., 1990). The CPB circuit also has safety devices that detect air bubbles, low flow, and low oxygen delivery.

LEFT VENTRICULAR VENT

Some cardiac operations necessitate placement of a vent in the left ventricle (Fig. 12-4). The purpose of a *left ventricular vent* is to prevent distention of the ventricle when it is not ejecting blood, that is, when the aorta is cross-clamped or when the ventricles are fibrillating. Generally the catheter is inserted into the superior pulmonary vein and directed through the left atrium and across the mitral valve into the left ventricle. Alternatively, the catheter may be inserted through the left atrial wall and directed into the ventricle or through the aortic root and advanced in retrograde fashion across the aortic valve. These techniques avoid the injurious consequences of direct insertion through the ventricular muscle. However, some surgeons prefer inserting the vent through the apex of the left ventricle.

The necessity of venting the left ventricle during

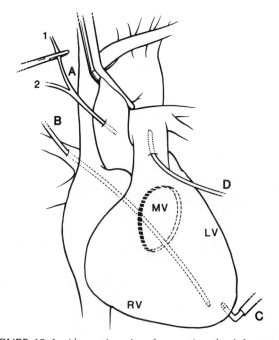

FIGURE 12-4. Alternative sites for venting the left ventricle (*LV*). **(A)** Aortic root cannula; one limb (*1*) is connected to the cardioplegia administration system and the other (*2*) to suction for venting the left ventricle. **(B)** Cannula is inserted at junction of right superior pulmonary vein and left atrium and advanced through left atrium and mitral valve (*MV*) into the left ventricle. **(C)** Cannula is inserted directly into apex of the left ventricle. **(D)** Cannula is inserted into the pulmonary artery. *RV*, right ventricle. (Hessel EA, 1993: Cardiopulmonary bypass circuitry and cannulation techniques. In Gravlee GP, Davis RF, Utley JR [eds]: Cardiopulmonary Bypass: Principles and Practice, p. 78. Baltimore, Williams & Wilkins)

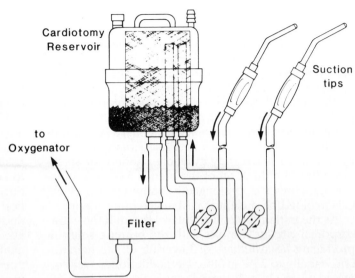

Cardiotomy
Reservoir

Suction
tips

to
Oxygenator

Filter

FIGURE 12-5. Cardiotomy aspiration system. (Milan JD, 1983: Blood transfusion in heart surgery. Surg Clin North Am 63:1130)

all cardiac operations is controversial, and some surgeons use left ventricular vents only selectively. However, if ventricular distention occurs during a procedure in which a vent has not been placed or is not functioning properly, vent insertion or correction of the problem must be performed rapidly. Distention of the left ventricle, even for a limited period, has two serious consequences: (1) damage to the lungs caused by elevated pulmonary venous pressure and (2) severe, sometimes irreversible damage to the ventricle itself due to overstretching of myocardial fibers (Behrendt & Austen, 1985; Robicsek, 1985).

CARDIOTOMY SUCTION

The *cardiotomy suction catheter* is a specially designed catheter used to aspirate blood from the operative field. During bypass, while the blood is heparinized, a cardiotomy suction catheter is placed in the opened heart or mediastinum. Aspirated blood is directed through suction tubing into the extracorporeal circuit. Because the suctioned blood contains air and particulate matter, it is filtered and defoamed before being emptied into the extracorporeal blood volume to be oxygenated, cooled, and returned to the arterial circulation (Fig. 12-5).

EXTRACORPOREAL CIRCULATION

CPB is a highly sophisticated life support system. Its operation is directed and monitored by a trained perfusionist, who regulates the device, monitors all hemodynamic and metabolic parameters, and corrects any functional problems that occur. Because the CPB system provides total cardiopulmonary support for the patient, there is a potential for catastrophic complications should system malfunction occur.

INITIATION

In preparation for CPB, the patient is given an intravenous bolus of heparin (e.g., 3 mg/kg). Systemic anticoagulation is mandatory throughout the period of extracorporeal circulation as the blood is circulated outside the body and exposed to nonbiologic surfaces. Heparin blocks the intrinsic clotting cascade by interfering with conversion of prothrombin to thrombin and fibrinogen to fibrin (Christopherson & Froelicher, 1990).

The CPB tubing is filled or "primed" with approximately 2 L of a crystalloid solution, similar in electrolyte composition to plasma. Albumin may be added to the priming solution to maintain colloidal osmotic pressure and reduce extravasation into the interstitial space (i.e., "third spacing"). Fluid is circulated through the system for several minutes to filter air and particulate matter and to ensure proper functioning. Great care is taken to remove all air from the arterial side of the circuit to prevent delivering an air embolus into the systemic circulation. This preparatory phase usually requires 30 to 40 minutes, although it can be done more quickly if emergent initiation of CPB is necessary.

After the surgeon has inserted the cannulae, they are connected to the tubing of the CPB circuit. To begin CPB, the perfusionist initiates venous drainage and activates the arterial pump. As soon as CPB is initiated, the blood is purposefully cooled and returned to the patient to lower body temperature and thus lower tissue metabolism and oxygen demand. Adjusting perfusate temperature to induce hypothermia, termed *core cooling*, enhances myocardial protection, minimizes ischemic damage to organs, and allows specific target organs to tolerate markedly reduced flow rates or transient interruption of circulation. Core cooling must be performed slowly to cool body tissues efficiently without regional temperature differences. Moderate hypothermia (e.g., 28°C to 30°C) is used for most cardiac operations.

Some complex operations require decreasing the rate of flow to very low levels or completely interrupting circulation for a period of time, a technique called *circulatory arrest*. For example, blood flow through the aortic arch and great vessels must be interrupted to perform operative repair of aneurysms of the transverse thoracic aorta. *Profound or deep hypothermia* (approximately 18°C) is used in these situations. Deep hypothermia is the only available method for safely extending the duration of the brain's tolerance to ischemia. However, prolonged hypothermia below 15°C is avoided because it may damage brain tissue.

As the patient's blood circulates through the extracorporeal circuit, it mixes with the priming solution producing *hemodilution*, or lowering of the hematocrit, usually to 25% to 30%. Hemodilution is well tolerated during hypothermia because tissue oxygen demands are reduced. A lower hematocrit is in fact advantageous in that it lowers blood viscosity (which increases during hypothermia), thereby facilitating blood flow to the microcirculation of peripheral tissues (Whitman, 1987). In addition, hemodilution reduces the need for exogenous blood, decreases trauma to blood elements, and increases urine flow and excretion of sodium, potassium, and creatinine (Stephenson & Edmunds, 1991).

MAINTENANCE

During CPB, the perfusionist controls systemic blood flow based on arterial and central venous pressures to provide adequate oxygenation of the microcirculation. While the heart is inactive, the flow rate is adjusted to deliver 4 to 5 L/min, or a cardiac index equivalent to 2.2 to 2.5 L/min/m^2. Lower flow rates may be used during the period that the patient is hypothermic. A low flow rate is advantageous in some situations because it decreases noncoronary collateral flow, which can facilitate a drier operative field and prevent rewarming of the heart (Utley, 1989).

Although the ideal flow rate is unclear, a flow rate during normothermia less than 1.6 L/min/m^2 may result in cardiogenic shock (Kirklin & Kirklin, 1990). Excessive flow rates, on the other hand, may produce more trauma to blood elements, higher gradients across the arterial cannula, and a greater risk of gaseous emboli when a bubble oxygenator is used (Kirklin & Barratt-Boyes, 1993). Mean arterial pressure is generally maintained between 50 and 70 mm Hg (Stephenson & Edmunds, 1991).

Volume, in the form of blood, other colloid, or crystalloid solution, may be added to the reservoir to increase the flow rate, particularly when there is a major bleeding problem. Flow may be lowered by reserving volume in the reservoir. Vasoconstricting or vasodilating drugs may be added to the circulating blood volume to adjust systemic vascular resistance. If an intra-aortic balloon catheter is in place, a standby mode is generally used during the period of CPB. Because the patient is systemically anticoagulated, thrombus formation along the catheter does not occur. If a nonpulsatile pump is being used, some surgeons prefer to maintain counterpulsation during CPB in the belief that it might provide a pulsatile quality to the blood flow.

Central venous and pulmonary artery pressures are maintained at or near 0 mm Hg to minimize interstitial fluid accumulation in the lungs and peripheral tissue. There appears to be no physiologic advantage to keeping central venous pressure above 0 mm Hg during CPB (Kirklin & Barratt-Boyes, 1993). In addition to interstitial fluid accumulation, increased venous pressure reduces circulating volume and may necessitate additional priming volume. An adequately sized venous cannula and unimpaired venous drainage are essential to achieve low venous pressures. A left ventricular vent may also be helpful. Excessive negative venous pressure must also be avoided because it may result in collapse of the thin-walled vena cavae and limit venous return to the CPB circuit (Stephenson & Edmunds, 1991). For this reason, most CPB systems drain venous blood by gravity.

Oxygen at an Fio$_2$ of 95% to 100% is used to oxygenate venous blood as it circulates through the pump. Because blood is oxygenated in the CPB system, it is not necessary to ventilate the lungs during the period of extracorporeal circulation. When CPB is initiated, the anesthesiologist turns off the ventilator. Leaving the lungs in a deflated state during the procedure makes the operative work technically easier by avoiding encroachment of the inflated lungs on the operative field. Sustained hypoinflation of the lungs, however, is a contributing factor toward atelectasis that routinely occurs in patients after cardiac operations.

Serial arterial blood gas measurements are obtained to assess adequacy of oxygenation and hemoglobin concentration of the perfusate. Continuous monitoring of arterial blood gases may also be performed, using a sensor placed in the arterial tubing distal to the oxygenator (Mark et al., 1991). Arterial oxygen pressure is usually maintained in the range of 200 to 250 mm Hg during CPB to ensure adequate tissue perfusion without producing oxygen toxicity or bubble formation. Arterial carbon dioxide levels are maintained in the normal physiologic range with appropriate adjustments for temperature.

Venous oxygen measurements are also obtained. Abnormally low venous oxygenation may indicate arterial hypoxemia or an inadequate perfusion rate; adjustment of arterial oxygenation or the arterial flow rate may be necessary to correct the problem. In addition to arterial and venous oxygen measurements, the perfusionist monitors acid–base status, potassium, and hematocrit. Because sensitivity to and metabolism of heparin varies among patients, activated clotting time is measured intermittently to assess the degree of anticoagulation (Stephenson & Edmunds, 1991). Periodic boluses of heparin are administered as necessary.

During cardiac operations, blood shed from the operative field may be salvaged to lessen the need for transfusion of homologous blood. Although suctioning of mediastinal blood reduces blood loss, the suction catheters are known to be one of the major causes of trauma to blood elements because of the air–blood interface and turbulence required to aspirate blood (Blanche et al., 1990; Stephenson & Edmunds, 1991).

WEANING

As reparative work on the heart or great vessels is nearing completion, the blood is rewarmed and the aortic cross-clamp is removed in preparation for weaning from CPB. Rewarming is performed slowly (0.2°C to 0.5°C per minute) to prevent decreased blood solubility with resultant bubble formation. The patient's venous blood temperature is warmed to 37° C; blood temperature is not allowed to exceed 40°C to avoid damaging blood proteins.

When the aortic cross-clamp is removed, catastrophic stroke or myocardial infarction can result if air is ejected from the left ventricle into the cerebral or coronary circulation. A number of technical maneuvers are performed by the surgeon before removing the aortic cross-clamp to prevent this complication. If the left atrium, left ventricle, or aorta has been opened during the procedure, vigorous attempts are made to ensure that all air is evacuated from inside the chambers before removing the aortic cross-clamp and allowing the heart to eject blood. In addition, the table is adjusted so that the patient is in Trendelenburg position when the clamp is removed; any residual air will thus be directed into the descending aorta.

Pump reservoir volume is adjusted to ensure adequate volume if transfusion is needed. Arterial blood gases, hematocrit, potassium, and acid–base status are measured and corrected if necessary (Conahan, 1985). Delivery of anesthetic agents is discontinued, and the lungs are ventilated with 100% oxygen and positive pressure to allow air in the pulmonary veins to escape (Behrendt & Austen, 1985; Blanche et al., 1990).

When the operative repair is completed and the heart has warmed sufficiently to resume a spontaneous cardiac rhythm, weaning from CPB is begun. The patient is weaned by slowly reducing the flow rate through the CPB circuit. The venous cannula is gradually occluded, decreasing the volume of blood diverted to the CPB circuit and increasing the volume traveling normally through the heart (i.e., partial CPB). When the heart is functioning effectively enough to sustain an adequate arterial pressure, arterial perfusion is discontinued.

Successful weaning requires complete washout of cardioplegic solution, rewarming, a stable cardiac rhythm, and adequate right and left ventricular function (Blanche et al., 1990). The surgeon uses monitored hemodynamic parameters and visual observation of the heart to assess cardiac rhythm and adequacy of right and left ventricular function. If ventricular function is good and myocardial damage has not occurred during the perioperative period, the heart usually resumes normal function quickly.

If ventricular function is impaired and low cardiac output ensues, two or three attempts at weaning CPB may be necessary. Various combinations of cardiotonic and vasodilating medications may be administered. Commonly used inotropic agents include dopamine, dobutamine, and epinephrine. Vasodilating agents, such as nitroglycerin or nitroprusside, may be administered for afterload reduction. Occasionally, lidocaine or other antiarrhythmic medication is required to treat ventricular ectopy. Temporary pacing may be used to increase heart rate, maintain the atrial contribution to cardiac output, or ensure an adequate ventricular rate. In some patients, intra-aortic balloon counterpulsation is necessary to augment left ventricular function.

When the patient is clearly able to sustain an adequate arterial pressure and cardiac output without support from the CPB system, protamine sulfate is given to reverse the heparin-induced anticoagulation. One of the cannulae (usually the venous cannula) is removed. The remaining cannula is left in place for a short while longer and used to infuse blood remaining in the CPB reservoir as needed. Boluses of 100 to 200 mL of blood can be rapidly infused through the remaining cannula. After the cannula is removed, residual blood in the CPB system is transferred into blood bags and may be infused in the intensive care unit if the patient requires blood volume in the early postoperative hours.

CONSEQUENCES OF CARDIOPULMONARY BYPASS

PHYSIOLOGIC EFFECTS

During CPB, blood is exposed to artificial, nonendothelial surfaces of the oxygenator, heat exchanger, filters, debubbling devices, and tubing. Exposure to these nonphysiologic surfaces is detrimental to the blood elements (i.e., platelets, red blood cells, white blood cells, and plasma proteins). After CPB, the number of platelets in circulating blood is only about 60% of the prebypass level, platelet survival time is reduced, and platelet function is altered (Kirklin & Barratt-Boyes, 1993).

Blood elements (particularly red and white blood cells) are further damaged by shear stresses that occur as a result of circulation through the arterial pump, suctioning forces, and turbulent flow at cannula insertion sites. The blood also incorporates abnormal substances, such as bubbles, fibrin particles, and platelet aggregates, which can embolize into the microcirculation (Kirklin & Kirklin, 1990).

Extracorporeal circulation also produces a systemic inflammatory response, causing the release of biologically active substances that impair coagulation and the immune system. As a result, capillary permeability increases, plasma may be lost through the capillary membranes, and fluid accumulates in the interstitial space. Consequently, a certain degree of extravasation of fluid into interstitial tissues occurs in all patients despite maintaining low central venous pressure during CPB. Body weight increases as a result of fluid infusion that is necessary to replete intravascular volume.

A number of other physiologic changes occur as well. Systemic vascular resistance decreases profoundly at the onset of CPB, then progressively increases, particularly as hypothermia is induced. CPB causes an increase in circulating catecholamines. Epinephrine levels rise dramatically after initiation of CPB, and, in some patients, norepinephrine levels rise as well. Venous compliance is also affected. CPB causes an increase in venous tone that continues for several hours after CPB is terminated (Kirklin & Barratt-Boyes, 1993). Since 70% to 80% of the patient's blood volume is contained in the venous capacitance bed, medications that adjust venous compliance may be necessary to control venous return.

CLINICAL SEQUELAE

The altered physiology induced by CPB may contribute to many of the clinical problems typically observed in the early postoperative hours after cardiac surgery, including fluid, electrolyte, and metabolic imbalances; hypertension; bleeding; and low cardiac output (Weiland & Walker, 1986). *Postperfusion syndrome* is the combination of adverse physiologic effects imposed by CPB. Although most patients demonstrate minimal clinical evidence of the syndrome, some patients experience a severe form of postperfusion syndrome, characterized by pulmonary and renal dysfunction, an abnormal bleeding diathesis, increased susceptibility to infection, increased interstitial fluid, leukocytosis, fever, vasoconstriction, and hemolysis (Kirklin & Kirklin, 1990). Patients subjected to a prolonged duration of CPB are most likely to experience postperfusion syndrome.

Complications of CPB are unusual but can occur. The most commonly recognized complication is air embolization. Accordingly, numerous safety features are incorporated into the CPB system to prevent infusion of air into the arterial circulation. Similarly, a number of maneuvers (venting, positioning, aspiration, lung ventilation) are routinely performed by the surgeon and anesthesiologist before discontinuing

CPB. Malfunction of the CPB system occurs rarely due to tubing disconnection or rupture, air lock (entry of a large amount of air into the venous cannula), tubing obstruction, or oxygenator or pump failure.

Occasionally, administration of protamine causes a severe adverse reaction, characterized by profound vasodilatation and hypotension. A protamine reaction is treated with rapid volume infusion, vasoconstricting medication, and corticosteroids (Kirklin & Kirklin, 1990). Protamine reactions are most likely in diabetic patients who have been sensitized to protamine from chronic use of a protamine-base insulin (e.g., isophane [NPH] or protamine zinc insulin [PZI]) (Sather-Levine, 1990). Severe protamine reactions can be fatal. Other rare complications of CPB include hematologic disorders, gastrointestinal bleeding, pancreatitis, and bowel infarction.

REFERENCES

Behrendt DM, Austen WG, 1985: Intraoperative management. In Patient Care in Cardiac Surgery. Boston, Little, Brown

Blanche C, Matloff JM, MacKay DA, 1990: Technical aspects of cardiopulmonary bypass. In Gray RJ, Matloff JM (eds): Medical Care of the Cardiac Surgical Patient. Baltimore, Williams & Wilkins

Christopherson DJ, Froelicher ES, 1990: Anticoagulant, antithrombotic, and platelet-modifying drugs. In Underhill SL, Woods SL, Froelicher ES, Halpenny CJ (eds): Cardiovascular Medications for Cardiac Nursing. Philadelphia, JB Lippincott

Conahan TJ, 1985: Anesthetic considerations in coronary artery disease. In Utley JR (ed): Perioperative Cardiac Dysfunction. Baltimore, Williams & Wilkins

Hartz RS, LoCicero J III, Sanders JH Jr, et al., 1990: Clinical experience with portable cardiopulmonary bypass. Ann Thorac Surg 50:437

Kirklin JW, Barratt-Boyes BG, 1993: Hypothermia, circulatory arrest, and cardiopulmonary bypass. In Cardiac Surgery, ed. 2. New York, Churchill Livingstone

Kirklin JK, Kirklin JW, 1990: Cardiopulmonary bypass for cardiac surgery. In Sabiston DC Jr, Spencer FC (eds): Surgery of the Chest, ed. 5. Philadelphia, WB Saunders

Mark JB, FitzGerald D, Fenton T, et al., 1991: Continuous arterial and venous blood gas monitoring during cardiopulmonary bypass. J Thorac Cardiovasc Surg 102:431

Robicsek F, 1985: Reanimation of the heart. In Utley JR (ed): Perioperative Cardiac Dysfunction. Baltimore, Williams & Wilkins

Sather-Levine B, 1990: Perioperative agents. In Underhill SL, Woods SL, Froelicher ES, Halpenny CJ (eds): Cardiovascular Medications for Cardiac Nursing. Philadelphia, JB Lippincott

Stephenson LW, Edmunds LH Jr, 1991: Cardiopulmonary bypass for open heart surgery. In Baue AE, Geha AS, Hammond GL, et al. (eds): Glenn's Thoracic and Cardiovascular Surgery, ed. 5. Norwalk, CT, Appleton & Lange

Utley JR, 1989: Cardiopulmonary bypass in the adult. In Grillo HC, Austen WG, Wilkins EW, et al. (eds): Current Therapy in Cardiothoracic Surgery. Toronto, BC Decker

Weiland AP, Walker WE, 1986: Physiologic principles and clinical sequelae of cardiopulmonary bypass. Heart Lung 15:34

Whitman G, 1987: Cardiac surgery. In Talkington S, Raterink G (eds): Every Nurses' Guide to Cardiovascular Care. New York, Fleshner Publishing

MYOCARDIAL PRESERVATION

PRINCIPLES OF MYOCARDIAL PRESERVATION
TECHNIQUES OF MYOCARDIAL PRESERVATION
Hypothermia
Cardioplegia
Alternative Techniques

Recognition of the relationship between intraoperative myocardial ischemia and postoperative outcome was a major advancement in the development of cardiac surgery. As cardiac surgeons gained experience in the early years of using cardiopulmonary bypass (CPB), it became increasingly apparent that inadequate oxygenation of myocardial tissue during CPB results in myocardial necrosis and is the major cause of perioperative myocardial infarction and death. With this knowledge came the recognition that protection of the myocardium from ischemic injury is essential to success of operations on the heart or great vessels.

Myocardial preservation may be defined as the specific intraoperative techniques designed to protect the heart from tissue damage that would otherwise result from the ischemic state associated with extracorporeal circulation. Improved techniques to protect the ischemic myocardium have had a substantial impact on lowering mortality rates associated with cardiac surgery. Because the heart can now be better protected, cardiac operations of a more complex nature have become possible and patients with significant ventricular impairment are able to withstand cardiac surgery.

Nevertheless, perioperative myocardial damage remains the leading cause of morbidity and mortality in patients undergoing heart surgery. Combinations of gross, microscopic, or histochemical evidence of myocardial necrosis are present at autopsy in as many as 90% of patients who die during the peri-

operative period after cardiac operations (Buckberg, 1991). In addition, damage from global myocardial ischemia may result in *myocardial stunning,* or myocardial *hibernation,* a condition characterized by a variable, sometimes prolonged, period of both systolic and diastolic dysfunction without muscle necrosis (Kirklin & Barratt-Boyes, 1993).

The focus of this chapter is myocardial preservation during CPB. However, preoperative titration of cardiac medications and fluids, careful induction of general anesthesia with proper monitoring, and vigilant control of hemodynamic parameters in the early postoperative hours also play an important role in perioperative myocardial protection and are addressed elsewhere in the text.

PRINCIPLES OF MYOCARDIAL PRESERVATION

A great deal of clinical and laboratory investigation has focused on how to best protect the heart during cardiac operations. Current techniques of myocardial preservation are based on the results of these investigations and an understanding of certain physiologic principles of myocardial function.

First, the amount and distribution of blood flow to the heart is regulated under normal conditions by changes in aortic pressure, tension in the various myocardial layers, and coronary vascular resistance; these protective regulatory factors are altered during

CPB (Kirklin & Barratt-Boyes, 1993). Second, ischemia (reduced blood flow) is more damaging to myocardial tissue than is hypoxia (normal blood flow and reduced oxygen content) (Hartz & Michaelis, 1985). Both conditions result in increased anaerobic metabolism that produces hydrogen ions and lactate. However, because flow is also compromised during ischemia, these harmful metabolites accumulate instead of being washed out as occurs with the normal flow that is present during hypoxia.

Third, the left ventricular subendocardium is most vulnerable to ischemic damage. Although the left ventricular subepicardium and right ventricle are perfused throughout the cardiac cycle, the subendocardium of the left ventricle receives oxygenated blood only during diastole. During systole, increased myocardial tension in the well-developed left ventricular muscle mass compresses intramyocardial branches of the coronary arteries that supply the subendocardium (Buckberg, 1987; Kirklin & Barratt-Boyes, 1993). Blood flow is further compromised if the ventricle is hypertrophied or if coronary artery disease is present (Buckberg, 1991). Ischemic tissue injury increases exponentially with time. Even with current methods of myocardial preservation, expeditious performance of a cardiac operation is essential (Rankin & Sabiston, 1990).

Finally, hypothermia diminishes the harmful consequences of ischemia. Use of hypothermia during cardiac operations reduces metabolic activity and thereby allows existing energy stores to maintain cell viability. Within limits, the lower the body temperature, the longer the ischemic time that can be endured without tissue damage. The mechanism by which hypothermia protects tissue is not fully understood. The oxygen consumption reduction that occurs with moderate to deep hypothermia does not fully explain the significant increase in myocardial tolerance to ischemia (Swain et al., 1991). Although hypothermia reduces myocardial oxygen demand, the demand is not zero even with deep hypothermia (Siwek & Daggett, 1989).

TECHNIQUES OF MYOCARDIAL PRESERVATION

Almost all cardiac operations are performed with cardioplegia and a period of aortic cross-clamping (Fig. 13-1). This technique provides the surgeon with a still, bloodless field within which to perform precise technical maneuvers. If no cross-clamp is applied, blood flows into the coronary arteries from the CPB circuit; the heart is perfused and continues to beat. Although many cardiac operations can technically be performed in this fashion, that is, with an empty, perfused, and beating heart, the myocardium is more vulnerable to ischemic damage. Induction of electromechanical arrest greatly reduces myocardial energy demands and in combination with profound myocar-

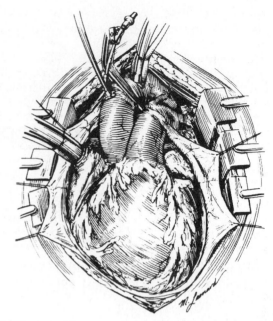

FIGURE 13-1. After cannulation of the right atrium and ascending aorta for cardiopulmonary bypass perfusion, the aorta is clamped proximal to the aortic cannula and cardioplegia is administered to induce electromechanical arrest of the heart. (Rankin JS, Newman GE, Muhlbaier LH, et al, 1985: The effects of coronary revascularization on left ventricular function in ischemic heart disease. J Thorac Cardiovasc Surg 90:820)

dial hypothermia increases the time that the heart can tolerate a globally ischemic state.

Although the aortic cross-clamp isolates the coronary circulation from the blood volume circulating through the CPB circuit, not all blood flow to the myocardium is eliminated. Noncoronary collaterals in the pericardial attachments and pulmonary vein walls continue to provide some blood flow during the period of aortic cross-clamping. Blood flow through these vessels, which are more abundant in patients with most forms of cardiac disease, produce an ischemic, rather than anoxic, state in the myocardium. Therefore, further measures are necessary to protect the heart from global myocardial ischemia. The most commonly used regimen includes (1) moderate systemic hypothermia, (2) profound myocardial hypothermia, and (3) infusion of cardioplegic solution into the coronary arteries.

HYPOTHERMIA

A combination of three techniques is used to achieve moderate systemic and profound myocardial hypothermia: (1) systemic cooling of blood as it passes through the tubing of the CPB circuit, (2) intermittent topical bathing of the heart with a cold saline solution placed in the pericardial well, and (3) infusion of the coronary arteries with chilled cardioplegic solution (Hartz & Michaelis, 1985). *Systemic hypothermia*, or core cooling of the body to 28°C to 30°C, is performed at the onset of CPB to reduce cellular metabolic demands of the myocardium and other vital organs. Before application of the aortic cross-clamp, myocardial temperature is lowered as the chilled perfusate (circulating blood volume) flows into the coronary arterial circulation. When systemic hypothermia has been achieved, an occlusive clamp is applied to the proximal aorta, just distal to the coronary artery ostia. Once the aortic cross-clamp is applied, further temperature reduction and maintenance of myocardial hypothermia is accomplished with topical bathing of the heart and infusion of cold cardioplegic solution. With these measures, myocardial temperature is lowered to approximately 15°C.

Topical (or surface) *cooling of the heart* contributes to myocardial protection by minimizing rewarming between doses of cardioplegic solution (Siwek & Daggett, 1989). It is performed by bathing the heart continuously or intermittently with ice-cold saline or Ringer's lactate solution that is dripped over the anterior surface of the heart. Care is taken to avoid exposing the left side of the pericardium containing the phrenic nerve to the iced solution to avoid nerve injury. An isolating pad may also be placed between the heart and the left side of the pericardium for this purpose (Kirklin & Barratt-Boyes, 1993). As an alternative to bathing the heart with a cold solution, a cooling pad or "jacket" may be wrapped around the heart. Ventricular temperature and effectiveness of cooling may be measured using a thermistor probe placed in the left ventricular myocardium.

In addition to active induction of hypothermia, the administration of muscle relaxants, narcotics, and sedatives preoperatively and of anesthetic agents intraoperatively inhibits the body's normal temperature regulating mechanisms, producing a state of poikilothermia in which body temperature is environmentally controlled (Whitman, 1991). Therefore, the temperature of ambient air, infused intravenous solutions, and topically applied materials contribute to maintaining a hypothermic state.

CARDIOPLEGIA

Cardioplegia is the induction and maintenance of the heart in an arrested state using a chilled solution infused into the coronary arterial circulation. The significant components of cardioplegic solutions are (1) an ingredient (usually potassium) to depolarize the cell membrane and induce rapid diastolic arrest, (2) solution temperature of 4°C to 8°C to induce profound hypothermia of myocardial tissue, (3) a substrate that provides a source for anaerobic or aerobic energy production, (4) a buffering agent to maintain appropriate pH, (5) a membrane-stabilizing ingredient, and (6) appropriate osmolarity and colloid oncotic pressure to prevent myocardial edema (Buckberg, 1987). Hypothermia is considered by many to be the most effective metabolic inhibitor and therefore the most important component of cardioplegic

solution in inducing and maintaining safe arrest of the heart.

The merits of specific ingredients of cardioplegic solutions remain controversial. Optimum concentrations of various agents and the nature of additives have not yet been standardized (Mankad et al., 1991). As a result, the exact composition of cardioplegic solution varies among surgeons. However, all cardioplegic solutions are designed with specific goals: arrest of the heart, continued energy production by the myocardium, and avoidance of ischemia (Buckberg, 1991). Generally, a standard cardioplegic solution based on the previously mentioned principles is selected for routine use.

There are two basic kinds of cardioplegic solution: *autologous blood* and *crystalloid cardioplegic solution*. Because myocardial metabolic processes and oxygen consumption are not entirely inhibited by hypothermia and cardiac arrest, cold blood or oxygenated crystalloid solutions are generally used to provide some degree of oxygen to myocardial tissue. The presence of oxygen in the solution allows increased aerobic and decreased anaerobic metabolism (Steinberg et al., 1991). The more efficient aerobic metabolism reduces the likelihood of global or regional myocardial cellular injury due to energy demand outweighing energy supply (Hartz & Michaelis, 1985). The superiority of blood or crystalloid cardioplegic solution in preserving myocardium remains controversial.

Several techniques are used for administration of cardioplegic solution. Most common is *antegrade infusion*; the solution is infused through a catheter placed proximal to the aortic cross-clamp in the aortic root. With a competent aortic valve and the aorta clamped distal to the catheter, the cardioplegic solution passes directly into the coronary arteries. Aortic root pressure is often measured simultaneously during infusion of the cardioplegic solution through a separate catheter (Fig. 13-2).

The initial volume of cardioplegic solution is generally 1 to 1.5 L. The rate of administration is adjusted to maintain aortic root pressure between 80 and 100 mm Hg to ensure effective delivery of the solution and to achieve rapid diastolic arrest. Global cardiac arrest usually occurs within 30 seconds of cardioplegia infusion but may take 1 to 2 minutes in the presence of stenotic or occluded coronary arteries that impede distal distribution of the solution (Buckberg, 1991). Since blood flow from noncoronary collateral arteries washes away infused cardioplegic solution and gradually rewarms the heart, intermittent infusions of 300 to 500 mL of cardioplegic solution may be administered every 15 to 20 minutes during the period of aortic clamping.

In addition to antegrade delivery of cardioplegic solution into the aortic root, several alternative techniques are available for selected situations. In patients with aortic valvular regurgitation, aortic root delivery of cardioplegia is ineffective because the solution escapes through the incompetent valve into

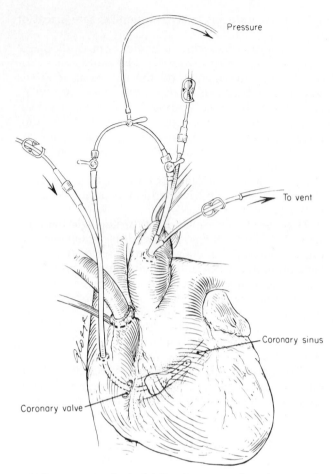

Pressure

To vent

Coronary sinus

Coronary valve

FIGURE 13-2. Method of delivering antegrade and retrograde cardioplegia. The catheter in the ascending aorta, proximal to the aortic cross-clamp, is used for antegrade delivery; the coronary sinus has been cannulated transatrially for retrograde delivery. (Drinkwater DC, Laks H, Buckberg GD, 1990: A new simplified method of sampling cardioplegic delivery without right heart isolation. J Thorac Cardiovasc Surg 100:61)

the left ventricle. If aortic regurgitation is suspected before the operation, an aortic root aortogram may be obtained during the preoperative cardiac catheterization to assess valve competence. In patients with an incompetent aortic valve or in those who undergo aortic valve replacement, the cardioplegic solution can be administered through small individual cannulae placed directly into the ostia of the right and left coronary arteries (Kirklin & Barratt-Boyes, 1993).

In patients with coronary artery disease, effective cardioplegia is limited by nonhomogeneous distribution of coronary blood flow (Buckberg, 1987). Areas of myocardium supplied by vessels with obstructive lesions are not as well cooled and display persistent electromechanical activity (Buckberg, 1987). Thus, areas of muscle already jeopardized by compromised blood flow are not well protected by cardioplegic solution.

Cardiac operations, especially coronary artery by-

pass grafting, are designed by the surgeon with this limitation in mind. Bypass grafts to areas of myocardium at most jeopardy are usually performed first. If distal anastomoses (vein to coronary artery) are performed before proximal anastomoses (vein to aorta), cardioplegic solution can be injected directly into the proximal end of each vein graft after completion of the distal anastomosis. If proximal anastomoses are performed first, cardioplegic solution delivered into the aortic root after cross-clamping the aorta will flow through a graft to the myocardium it supplies as soon as the distal anastomosis is constructed. Administration of cardioplegic solution through the graft is not possible when an internal thoracic artery is used and its proximal attachment to the subclavian artery is left intact (i.e., internal thoracic artery pedicle graft).

Antegrade delivery to myocardium beyond arterial stenoses or occlusions may thus be limited by the following factors: (1) solution cannot be delivered to jeopardized muscle until the distal anastomosis to the supplying artery is constructed; (2) muscle supplied by an artery receiving an internal thoracic artery pedicle graft is not revascularized until the end of the cross-clamp period; and (3) jeopardized muscle supplied by diseased, but not graftable, arteries is unprotected (Menasche et al., 1991). An antegrade technique for cardioplegia delivery is particularly limited in patients with diffuse distal disease and multiple totally occluded arteries. Antegrade cooling is also less effective in areas of collateral vessels and in the presence of ventricular hypertrophy (Blanche et al., 1990). Collateral blood flow, which continues despite aortic cross-clamping, is considerably warmer than the cardioplegic solution and thus interferes with the cooling provided by the chilled cardioplegic solution.

Alternatively, a retrograde technique may be used for cardioplegia administration. *Retrograde coronary sinus infusion* consists of perfusing the myocardium with cardioplegic solution infused in a retrograde fashion through the coronary sinus and coronary veins (see Fig. 13-2). The coronary venous system is an extensive and unobstructed network that provides an effective conduit to deliver cooling and cardioplegic additives throughout the thickness of the myocardium (Menasche et al., 1991).

Most commonly, the catheter is introduced through the right atrial wall and guided by digital manipulation into the coronary sinus. However, this is sometimes not easily accomplished. Also, direct cannulation can cause coronary sinus rupture or atrioventricular block and may not provide adequate protection of the right ventricle, which is thought to receive little cardioplegic solution from the coronary sinus (Diehl et al., 1988). Based on these considerations, the surgeon may instead perform retrograde coronary sinus infusion by positioning the catheter in the right atrium, with simultaneous occlusion of the pulmonary artery and vena cavae cannulae.

Retrograde administration has gained popularity because of limitations associated with antegrade cardioplegia delivery. Proponents of retrograde coronary sinus infusion believe it provides more homogeneous distribution and better myocardial cooling distal to diseased arteries, resulting in improved postischemic myocardial function (Menasche et al., 1991). Consequently, some surgeons routinely use retrograde coronary sinus infusion, either exclusively or to supplement the initial cardioplegia dose delivered by the conventional antegrade technique into the aortic root. Clinical studies have failed to demonstrate superiority of either the antegrade or the retrograde technique in preserving myocardial function.

The surgeon ceases to administer cardioplegia doses when the reparative work on the heart is nearly completed. Topical myocardial cooling is discontinued, the perfusionist begins rewarming the circulating blood volume, and the aortic cross-clamp is removed. When the myocardium has warmed sufficiently to resume a spontaneous electrical rhythm, venous return to the CPB circuit is gradually decreased, allowing blood to flow through the heart normally.

ALTERNATIVE TECHNIQUES

Certain types of operations on the heart and great vessels require special techniques in addition to those already described. For example, operations on the aortic arch necessitate interruption of circulation through the ascending aorta for an extended period. This is achieved by using the techniques of *profound hypothermia* and *circulatory arrest*. In contrast to the moderate hypothermia used in most cardiac operations, the body is systemically cooled to approximately 18°C and CPB circulation is stopped. With the body cooled to this extreme degree, perfusion of vital organs can be interrupted for as much as 60 minutes while the aortic reconstruction is performed.

In patients with active ischemia at the onset of the operation, induction of cardioplegic arrest at normal temperatures has been advocated. An oxygenated cardioplegic solution at normothermic temperature is given as the initial dose to induce cardiac arrest. This so-called *warm cardioplegia* increases myocardial oxygen uptake and is thought to provide additional ben-

efit in patients with acute ischemia (Buckberg, 1991). Warm cardioplegia is followed by cold cardioplegia administration to prevent myocardial ischemia during subsequent aortic clamping. Some surgeons routinely use warm cardioplegia for the last dose of cardioplegia.

REFERENCES

Blanche C, Matloff JM, MacKay DA, 1990: Technical aspects of cardiopulmonary bypass. In Gray RJ, Matloff JM (eds): Medical Care of the Cardiac Surgical Patient. Baltimore, Williams & Wilkins

Buckberg GD, 1987: Recent progress in myocardial protection during cardiac operations. In McGoon DC (ed): Cardiac Surgery, ed. 2. Philadelphia, FA Davis

Buckberg GD, 1991: Myocardial protection during adult cardiac operations. In Baue AE, Geha AS, Hammond GL, et al. (eds): Glenn's Thoracic and Cardiovascular Surgery, ed. 5. Norwalk, CT, Appleton & Lange

Diehl JT, Eichhorn EJ, Konstam MA, et al., 1988: Efficacy of retrograde coronary sinus cardioplegia in patients undergoing myocardial revascularization: A prospective randomized trial. Ann Thorac Surg 45:595

Hartz RS, Michaelis LL, 1985: Intraoperative protection of the myocardium. In Utley JR (ed): Perioperative Cardiac Dysfunction, Vol. 3. Baltimore, Williams & Wilkins

Kirklin JW, Barratt-Boyes BG, 1993: Myocardial management during cardiac surgery with cardiopulmonary bypass. In Cardiac Surgery, ed. 2. New York, Churchill Livingstone

Mankad PS, Chester AH, Yacoub MH, 1991: Role of potassium concentration in cardioplegic solutions in mediating endothelial damage. Ann Thorac Surg 51:89

Menasche P, Subayi JB, Veyssie L, et al., 1991: Efficacy of coronary sinus cardioplegia in patients with complete coronary artery occlusions. Ann Thorac Surg 51:418

Rankin JS, Sabiston DC Jr, 1990: Physiology of coronary blood flow, myocardial function, and intraoperative myocardial protection. In Sabiston DC Jr, Spencer FC (eds): Surgery of the Chest, ed. 5. Philadelphia, WB Saunders

Siwek LG, Daggett WM, 1989: Myocardial protection. In Grillo HC, Austen WG, Wilkins EW Jr, et al. (eds): Current Therapy in Cardiothoracic Surgery. Toronto, BC Decker

Steinberg JB, Doherty NE, Munfakh NA, et al., 1991: Oxygenated cardioplegia: The metabolic and functional effects of glucose and insulin. Ann Thorac Surg 51:620

Swain JA, McDonald TJ Jr, Balaban RS, Robbins RC, 1991: Metabolism of the heart and brain during hypothermic cardiopulmonary bypass. Ann Thorac Surg 51:105

Whitman GR, 1991: Hypertension and hypothermia in the acute postoperative period. Crit Care Nurs Clin North Am 3:661

14

BLOOD CONSERVATION

PREOPERATIVE TECHNIQUES
INTRAOPERATIVE TECHNIQUES
POSTOPERATIVE TECHNIQUES

Blood conservation may be defined as the set of techniques used to reduce perioperative bleeding, salvage shed blood, and reduce the need for homologous (i.e., from another human donor) transfusion. It is an integral feature of cardiac operations. Perioperative bleeding is more pronounced in cardiac than in other types of surgical procedures because of the extracorporeal circulation of blood using a cardiopulmonary bypass (CPB) system. Two factors inherent to CPB increase the propensity for bleeding. First, extracorporeal circulation exposes blood to nonphysiologic surfaces and shear stresses that damage platelets and clotting factors. Second, it is necessary to administer systemic anticoagulation before CPB to prevent massive thrombosis as blood is circulated through the system.

With the many less invasive forms of therapy now available for treatment of heart disease, the population of patients who undergo cardiac operations are older and have more advanced heart disease and poorer ventricular function. Preoperative anemia is more likely to be present and is less well tolerated postoperatively. Reoperations, associated with more intraoperative blood loss, have also become more common. The increasingly complex population referred for cardiac operations has resulted in a steady increase in the number of patients who require transfusion of homologous blood (Jones et al., 1991). In addition to packed red blood cells to replete hemoglobin, plasma or platelets are sometimes necessary to replace damaged clotting factors (Table 14-1). Factors that increase the risk for perioperative blood transfusion include advanced age, preexisting bleeding abnormalities, preoperative aspirin ingestion, intra-aortic balloon counterpulsation or thrombolytic therapy, and the performance of reoperations or complex procedures.

Appropriate transfusion of homologous blood products is essential. First, blood transfusion is associated with several risks. Infectious agents, specifically hepatitis B virus, hepatitis C (non-A, non-B) virus, and human immunodeficiency virus, can be transmitted through blood transfusion despite the fact that donor blood is routinely tested for these agents. The risk of transmitting an infectious agent through blood or blood product transfusion, albeit small, varies depending on the number of donors per recipient and the prevalence of undetected, contaminated blood in the tested blood supply (Kolins & Kolins, 1990). The serious consequences of these infections have heightened efforts to avoid blood transfusion. In addition to infection, transfusions can cause allergic reactions and sensitization to blood products (Scott et al., 1990).

Blood conservation is also important because homologous blood is a relatively scarce and expensive commodity. The supply of blood products is limited by the ongoing demand, as well as by the difficulty and expense in securing suitable donors and maintaining adequate stores of the various blood types and components. Certain patients, specifically those of the Jehovah's Witness faith, are forbidden by church law to receive transfusion of blood or blood derivatives. In this group of patients, blood conservation techniques are essential to lowering operative risk (Lewis et al., 1991). Because of these factors, a

TABLE 14-1. BLOOD COMPONENT THERAPY

Component	Purpose
Packed red blood cells	Increases oxygen-carrying capacity
Fresh frozen plasma	Replaces clotting factors
Platelets	Replaces destroyed or damaged platelets
Cryoprecipitate	Provides factor VIII, von Willebrand's factor, fibrinogen

variety of techniques are used before, during, and after cardiac operations to minimize homologous transfusion (Table 14-2).

PREOPERATIVE TECHNIQUES

Methods of blood conservation in the preoperative period include (1) avoiding aspirin and aspirin-containing products and (2) autologous blood donation. Many patients with heart disease, specifically those with coronary artery disease, take aspirin for its therapeutic antiplatelet effect. However, the impaired platelet function induced by aspirin increases perioperative bleeding. Because of its long half-life, aspirin ingestion within 7 to 10 days of operation increases the likelihood of blood transfusion and postoperative reexploration for bleeding. Consequently, if coronary artery revascularization is planned electively, aspirin is generally discontinued 1 to 2 weeks before the planned operative date, especially in those undergoing reoperation.

In the presence of significant coronary artery obstruction and unstable angina, it is generally considered preferable to proceed with surgical revascularization despite recent aspirin ingestion. After coronary artery bypass grafting, aspirin is routinely administered to promote long-term vein graft patency. In fact, many surgeons begin aspirin administration through a rectal route in the early postopera-

TABLE 14-2. FEATURES OF BLOOD CONSERVATION IN CARDIAC SURGERY

Avoid preoperative aspirin ingestion
Autologous donation
Platelet-rich plasmapheresis
Priming CPB circuit with crystalloid solution
Cell saver blood processing device
Hemofiltration
Cardiotomy suction
Adequate heparin reversal
Surgical hemostasis
Postoperative autotransfusion
Hemostatic agents
Tolerance of postoperative anemia

tive hours. Patients hospitalized with unstable angina may receive intravenous heparin infusions in the preoperative period. Because of its short half-life, heparin is usually continued until shortly before the operation and does not significantly increase perioperative bleeding.

Preoperative autologous donation is phlebotomy of the patient's own blood or blood components for later transfusion. This technique has been widely used in other surgical specialties but had been avoided in cardiac surgery, specifically in patients with coronary artery disease. It was feared that decreasing oxygen-carrying capacity of the blood by reducing hemoglobin would place the patient at risk for acute ischemia or infarction in the preoperative period. Recently, a number of centers have demonstrated that autologous donation can be performed safely in patients with significant but stable heart disease.

The cardiac surgeon determines which patients should donate blood preoperatively. Autologous donation is best suited for those patients whose procedures can be scheduled several weeks or months in advance, who have a normal hemoglobin value, and who are medically stable enough to withstand a phlebotomy blood loss. Adults with valvular or congenital heart disease in whom surgery is not urgently required are ideal candidates. In patients with coronary artery disease, autologous donation is performed in a monitored setting under direct physician supervision. Intravenous saline is infused simultaneously to avoid hypovolemia. Autologous donation is contraindicated in patients with severe aortic stenosis or active myocardial ischemia (i.e., unstable angina).

Commonly, 2 units of blood may be harvested on separate occasions at least 1 week apart and several weeks before the planned operation. A period of 3 to 4 weeks is usually necessary for recovery from anemia after collection of 400 mL of autologous whole blood and about 2 months after collection of 800 mL (Watanabe et al., 1991). Phlebotomy within 1 week of operation is counterproductive because the patient comes to operation anemic and thus at higher risk for homologous transfusion. Iron supplementation is generally instituted after preoperative autologous donation to enhance red blood cell replenishment. Recombinant human erythropoietin (rHuEPO), a hematopoietic hormone, is also administered in some centers. Erythropoietin is the primary regulator of erythropoiesis (i.e., the formation of red blood cells) (Levine et al., 1991). Adjunctive use of rHuEPO and iron restores hemoglobin levels to normal within 10 days of collection of 400 mL of autologous blood (Watanabe et al., 1991).

INTRAOPERATIVE TECHNIQUES

Autologous donation may also be performed in the operating room. *Platelet-rich plasmapheresis* is a special type of autologous donation that is being performed in some centers. It is attractive because it preserves those factors most susceptible to damage during extracorporeal circulation. Phlebotomy is performed in the operating room before initiating CPB. The blood is then separated, and the red blood cells are returned to the patient so that the red blood cell count, and thus oxygen-carrying capacity, is not diminished. The 2 or 3 units of withdrawn plasma, which contains platelets and other clotting factors, are kept warm until termination of CPB. The plasma is then reinfused, replenishing platelets and clotting factors damaged during extracorporeal circulation.

Another blood-conserving technique used in adults undergoing cardiac operations is priming of the CPB circuit with a crystalloid solution. Crystalloid priming hemodilutes the perfusate (i.e., blood circulating through the CPB circuit) to a hematocrit of 25% to 30%. Blood diluted to this level still has adequate oxygen-carrying capacity, and homologous blood need not be used to fill the CPB circuit.

Intraoperative blood conservation also includes salvage of shed blood. The two most common techniques of blood salvage are use of a cell saver and hemofiltration (Boldt et al., 1991). A *cell-saver blood processing device* is used to salvage shed blood before and after CPB when the patient is not anticoagulated. Blood is suctioned from the mediastinum into tubing that has an additional arm through which heparinized solution is added. The anticoagulated blood is returned to the cell-saver device where the red blood cells are separated out and washed with lactated Ringer's solution to remove heparin and hemolyzed red blood cells (Fig. 14-1). The washed red blood cells are then stored for transfusion in the early postoperative hours when volume replacement is needed.

Hemofiltration is performed during CPB. Shed blood that accumulates in the cardiotomy reservoir is pumped through a hemofiltration device in which it is concentrated. The primary difference between a cell-saver device and hemofiltration is that hemofiltration effectively removes excess water while conserving and concentrating blood components and red blood cells; with a cell-saver device the plasma fraction is removed (Boldt et al., 1991). Even if a hemofiltration device is not used, anticoagulated blood shed into the mediastinum during CPB is suctioned into a cardiotomy suction catheter, drained into the extracorporeal circuit, filtered, and added to the perfusate in the cardiotomy reservoir for return to the patient. When CPB is discontinued, blood remaining in the reservoir can be reinfused.

By using intraoperative blood salvaging techniques, it is generally possible to salvage 2 or 3 units of red blood cells that would otherwise be lost. Although shed mediastinal blood is hemostatically abnormal owing to exposure to the CPB circuit, injured tissue, air, and the collection system, salvage and retransfusion may reduce use of homologous blood by as much as 50% (Czer, 1990).

Other important components of intraoperative

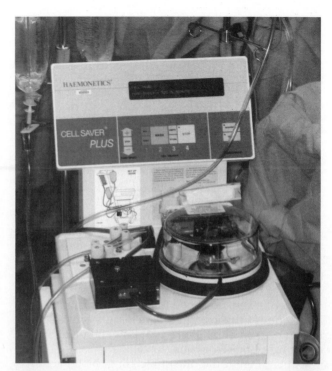

FIGURE 14-1. Haemonetics cell saver blood processing device. (Haemonetics, Braintree, MA)

blood conservation are adequate reversal of systemic anticoagulation and achievement of surgical hemostasis. At the conclusion of CPB, systemic anticoagulation is reversed using protamine sulfate. Activated clotting time is measured to ensure adequate reversal. Surgical hemostasis is assessed as body temperature is rewarmed and with the heart generating a normal blood pressure. The surgeon examines the mediastinum to detect sources of mechanical bleeding that require suture repair. Areas that are carefully inspected before closing the chest incision include anastomotic suture lines; cannulation sites; conduit side branches; the internal thoracic artery bed; and thymic, epicardial, sternal wire, and chest tube sites (Mahfood et al., 1991).

Hemostatic agents may be used to decrease diffuse bleeding. Aprotinin is a potent antifibrinolytic agent that is being evaluated in clinical trials. It is administered intraoperatively through intravenous infusion and by addition to the priming volume in the extracorporeal circuit. Perioperative bleeding and transfusion requirements are significantly reduced in patients who receive aprotinin (Blauhut et al., 1991; Havel et al., 1991). Its effectiveness in reducing blood loss may make aprotinin particularly suitable for use in patients at increased risk for bleeding, such as those undergoing reoperations or bilateral harvesting of internal thoracic arteries (Cosgrove et al., 1992: Schonberger et al., 1992). Other hemostatic agents include desmopressin acetate (DDVAP) and epsilon-aminocaproic acid (Amicar). These pharmacologic agents and topical fibrin glue are often used in the presence of significant postoperative coagulopathy or in patients who adamantly refuse homologous blood transfusion (e.g., those of the Jehovah's Witness faith).

POSTOPERATIVE TECHNIQUES

The principal blood conservation technique of the postoperative period is *autotransfusion,* which is reinfusion of shed mediastinal blood that is defibrinated by contact with the pleura and pericardium (Mahfood et al., 1991). Because average blood loss after cardiac operations is approximately 1 L, autotransfusion represents a significant source of blood replacement (Scott et al., 1990). In most centers, all blood shed through the chest tubes is routinely filtered and returned to the patient's venous system using a chest drainage system designed for autotransfusion and an intravenous infusion pump. A closed system is used to reduce the risk of blood contamination and subsequent infection (Sympson, 1991).

Depending on the rate of bleeding, blood is transfused hourly or every 2 to 4 hours. Usually postoperative bleeding subsides within 6 hours of operation and autotransfusion is discontinued at this time. However, it can be continued in the presence of active bleeding. Even if the patient has a postoperative coagulopathy and clotting factors are impaired, many surgeons choose to reinfuse shed blood to salvage red blood cells. Blood that has accumulated in the reservoir for more than 4 hours is not transfused.

Blood conservation also includes tolerance of postoperative anemia. With iron supplementation, most otherwise healthy adults can tolerate a hematocrit level of 25% or greater without untoward symptoms. In fact, many patients are extremely reticent to receive homologous blood and prefer to rebuild a normal red blood cell count with time, diet, and iron supplementation. Homologous transfusion, in the absence of active bleeding, is generally reserved for patients with a hematocrit level less than 25%, symptomatic anemia, or advanced age.

With a comprehensive blood conservation program throughout the perioperative period, use of homologous blood can be substantially reduced. However, it is not possible to eliminate blood transfusions in all patients. Indeed, transfusion of banked blood is an essential and sometimes lifesaving form of therapy for hemorrhage and postoperative coagulopathy. These conditions are discussed in Chapter 28, Complications of Cardiac Operations.

REFERENCES

Blauhut B, Gross C, Necek S, et al., 1991: Effects of high-dose aprotinin on blood loss, platelet function, fibrinolysis, complement, and renal function after cardiopulmonary bypass. J Thorac Cardiovasc Surg 101:958

Boldt J, Zickman B, Fedderson B, et al., 1991: Six different hemofiltration devices for blood conservation in cardiac surgery. Ann Thorac Surg 51:747

Cosgrove DM, Heric B, Lytle BW, et al., 1992: Aprotinin therapy for reoperative myocardial revascularization: A placebo-controlled study. Ann Thorac Surg 54:1031

Czer LS, 1990: Mediastinal bleeding, blood conservation techniques, and transfusion practices. In Gray RJ, Matloff JM (eds): Medical Management of the Cardiac Surgical Patient. Baltimore, Williams & Wilkins

Havel M, Teufelsbauer H, Knobl P, et al., 1991: Effect of intraoperative aprotinin administration on postoperative bleeding in patients undergoing cardiopulmonary bypass operation. J Thorac Cardiovasc Surg 101:968

Jones JW, Rawitscher RE, McLean TR, et al., 1991: Benefit from combining blood conservation measures in cardiac operations. Ann Thorac Surg 51:541

Kolins J, Kolins MD, 1990: Informed consent, risk, and blood transfusion. J Thorac Cardiovasc Surg 100:88

Levine EA, Rosen AL, Sehgal LR, et al., 1991: Erythropoietin deficiency after coronary artery bypass procedures. Ann Thorac Surg 51:764

Lewis CT, Murphy MC, Cooley DA, 1991: Risk factors for cardiac operations in adult Jehovah's Witnesses. Ann Thorac Surg 51:448

Mahfood SS, Higgins TL, Loop FD, 1991: Management of complications related to coronary artery bypass surgery. In Waldhausen JA, Orringer MB (eds): Complications in Cardiothoracic Surgery. St. Louis, Mosby–Year Book

Schonberger JP, Everts PA, Ercan H, et al., 1992: Low-dose aprotinin in internal mammary artery bypass operations contributes to important blood saving. Ann Thorac Surg 54:1172

Scott WJ, Kessler R, Wernly JA, 1990: Blood conservation in cardiac surgery. Ann Thorac Surg 50:843

Sympson GM, 1991: CATR™: a new generation of autologous blood transfusion. Crit Care Nurse 11:60

Watanabe Y, Fuse K, Konighi T, et al., 1991: Autologous blood transfusion with recombinant human erythropoietin in heart operations. Ann Thorac Surg 51:767

4

P A R T

CARDIOVASCULAR OPERATIONS

CHAPTER 15

SURGICAL TREATMENT OF CORONARY ARTERY DISEASE

CORONARY ARTERY REVASCULARIZATION
  Indications for Surgical Revascularization
  Target Vessels
  Conduit for Bypass Grafting
  The Operative Procedure
  Special Considerations
  Results of Surgical Revascularization

SURGERY FOR COMPLICATIONS
  OF MYOCARDIAL INFARCTION
Ventricular Aneurysm
Acute Mitral Regurgitation
Ventricular Rupture

CORONARY ARTERY REVASCULARIZATION

Surgical revascularization of the heart has been a major component in the treatment of *coronary artery disease* (CAD) for more than 20 years. It continues to be one of the most common operative procedures performed in the United States. The objectives of surgical revascularization are threefold: (1) control of ischemic symptoms, (2) prevention of myocardial infarction (MI), and (3) prolongation of life.

Coronary artery bypass grafting (CABG) is the principal method of surgical revascularization and may be combined with coronary artery endarterectomy in selected patients. Rarely, intraoperative angioplasty or laser techniques are also used. CABG consists of using autologous artery or vein as conduit to bypass stenotic lesions in the coronary arterial circulation (Fig. 15-1). Bypass grafting of coronary arteries is technically feasible because atherosclerotic lesions typically develop in proximal portions of the major coronary artery branches. These branches course through epicardial tissue on the surface of the heart for some distance before becoming embedded deep in the myocardium.

Target vessels for bypassing are identified preoperatively on the coronary angiogram, a contrast study that defines coronary artery anatomy. Any of the three major coronary arteries—left anterior descending (LAD), circumflex, or right—may be grafted, as well as branches of these arteries. As with other forms of therapy for CAD, CABG is not curative. Operative therapy must be accompanied by concomitant treatment of and counseling about modifiable risk factors that are associated with disease progression. A significant percentage of patients require more than one CABG procedure.

INDICATIONS FOR SURGICAL REVASCULARIZATION

Several large, randomized, prospective studies have investigated the benefits of medical versus surgical treatment of CAD. Specifically, the European Cooperative Study, Coronary Artery Surgery Study (CASS), and Veterans Administration Cooperative Study have helped define those patients most likely to benefit from surgical therapy (European Coronary Surgery Study Group, 1982; CASS Principal Investigators, 1983; Veterans Administration Coronary Artery Bypass Group, 1984). However, since completion of these studies, treatment of CAD has continued to evolve with increasingly effective anti-

Betsy Finkelmeier: CARDIOTHORACIC SURGICAL NURSING.
© 1995 J.B. Lippincott Company.

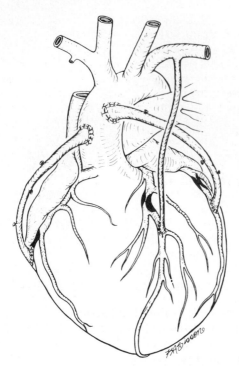

FIGURE 15-1. Typical coronary artery bypass grafting operation. In this illustration, the left internal thoracic artery has been used to construct a pedicle graft to the left anterior descending coronary artery; saphenous vein grafts have been constructed to bypass lesions in the right and circumflex coronary arteries. (Preparing for Cardiac Surgery. Division of Cardiothoracic Surgery and Department of Nursing, Northwestern Memorial Hospital)

anginal medications, thrombolytic therapy, and percutaneous transluminal coronary angioplasty (PTCA). Laser and atherectomy procedures that can be performed adjunctively to PTCA are also being introduced into clinical use. As a result, indications for surgical revascularization continue to be revised as the roles of less invasive forms of treating CAD are refined.

CABG and PTCA are the two major invasive revascularization therapies. Both procedures are designed to restore adequate blood flow to jeopardized myocardium in patients with myocardial ischemia. Information obtained from natural history studies and clinical trials has been used to identify patients who will benefit most from invasive revascularization procedures. They include individuals with significant coronary artery lesions associated with (1) stable angina refractory to adequate medical therapy and interfering with the patient's ability to function at an acceptable level of activity, (2) exercise-induced hypotension or ventricular arrhythmias secondary to myocardial ischemia, (3) demonstrated reversible ventricular dysfunction and clinical evidence of congestive heart failure, (4) unstable angina, or (5) evolving MI.

The decision to recommend CABG as the initial revascularization therapy is based primarily on anatomic findings during cardiac catheterization. Surgical therapy remains the treatment of choice in two categories of patients: (1) those with triple-vessel disease with left ventricular dysfunction or complex lesions not well suited to balloon dilatation and (2) those with significant (≥75%) left main coronary artery stenosis. In patients with double-vessel disease, either CABG or PTCA may be recommended, depending on the specific anatomy and status of the left ventricle. CABG is rarely the initial invasive intervention if only one coronary artery has significant narrowing (i.e., single-vessel disease). Other considerations also influence the choice of revascularization therapy, including age, general health status, associated cardiac disease, and associated medical problems.

A great deal of judgment and consideration of relevant data goes into the decision-making process about which form of treatment is most appropriate for a given patient since each of the options involves some risk. For some patients, it remains unclear which of the various therapies provides the best benefit–risk ratio. Ideally, in cases in which optimal therapy is controversial, the decision is made by the managing cardiologist with input from both an invasive cardiologist (who would perform PTCA) and a surgeon.

PTCA offers the distinct advantage of avoiding a major operation and is associated with a 90% success rate (Block, 1990). Improvements in angioplasty balloon catheters and increased skill of cardiologists performing PTCA have significantly increased the use of this form of therapy; in some centers, nearly one half of patients with significant coronary artery lesions undergo PTCA as the initial revascularization procedure (King & Talley, 1989). However, the procedure can result in a number of complications, including acute MI and the need for emergency surgical revascularization (King, 1990). In addition, PTCA is associated with a 25% to 35% incidence of re-stenosis of the dilated artery within 6 to 8 months (Block, 1990; Faxon et al., 1990). For this reason, and because of the progressive nature of CAD, many patients who initially undergo PTCA are eventually treated with surgical intervention.

TARGET VESSELS

A number of characteristics of a diseased coronary artery determine its suitability for grafting, including (1) degree of narrowing of the arterial lumen, (2) size of the artery distal to the stenosis, (3) presence of diffuse disease in the distal portion of the artery, and (4) viability of muscle supplied by the artery. Because lesions that produce greater than 75% narrowing of the arterial lumen significantly compromise arterial blood flow, arteries with this degree of narrowing are considered primary targets for revascularization.

However, the currently recommended strategy for CABG is complete revascularization. Therefore, all arterial trunks and branches with greater than 50% narrowing are usually bypassed as well, except those of trivial size (Kirklin & Barratt-Boyes, 1993a). The native coronary artery at the site of a planned distal anastomosis should be at least 1 mm in diameter and relatively free of atherosclerotic disease. In vessels of smaller caliber, blood flow through the graft is likely to be too low to support graft patency. Arteries with diffuse narrowing throughout the length of the vessel are not suitable for bypass grafting.

A coronary artery that is totally occluded, but distally patent and perfused by collateral circulation, may be bypassed depending on viability of muscle supplied by the vessel. Most often, total occlusion of a coronary artery causes acute MI and necrosis of muscle supplied by the artery. If so, revascularizing the necrotic muscle provides no benefit. However, when adequate collateral circulation to an area of muscle has prevented infarction at the time of coronary artery occlusion, it may be beneficial to bypass the artery. The ventriculogram, obtained during preoperative cardiac catheterization, provides an indication of muscle viability by demonstrating contractility of the various myocardial segments. A totally occluded artery may also be bypassed when surgical revascularization is performed during evolution of an MI (within 4 to 6 hours of onset) and muscle damage is judged to be reversible. Noninvasive techniques for determining reversibility of myocardial injury (i.e., differentiating "stunned" or "hibernating" from necrotic myocardium) are the focus of intense research that may revise future therapy for evolving MI.

CONDUIT FOR BYPASS GRAFTING

Bypass grafting of the coronary arteries is performed in the vast majority of patients using *internal thoracic artery* (ITA) (also called internal mammary artery), saphenous vein, or a combination of the two.

Internal Thoracic Artery

The left and right ITAs lie on the undersurface of the anterior chest wall, on either side of the sternum. In most elective revascularization procedures, one of the ITAs is harvested for use in bypassing one or two stenosed coronary arteries. The ITA has become the preferred conduit because its long-term patency rates have proven superior to those of saphenous veins. Its intrinsic qualities make it relatively immune to the three biologic modes of graft failure affecting venous conduits: early thrombosis, subintimal fibrosis, and late atherosclerosis (Galbut et al., 1991). Patency rates of 90% or greater at 10 years after operation have been demonstrated with ITA grafts in contrast to 25% to 50% patency rates with saphenous vein grafts (Rankin & Smith, 1990; Spencer, 1990). Use of ITA

conduit significantly lowers risk of late death, MI, and reoperation (Morris et al., 1990).

Factors thought to contribute to superior long-term patency of ITA grafts include the following: (1) the ITA's smaller size more closely approximates coronary artery diameter; (2) flow may be less turbulent because of similarities in ITA and coronary artery geometry; (3) ITA grafts have no valves or varicosities as do vein grafts; and (4) the ITA retains the biologic processes of an intact arterial vessel (Morris et al., 1990). Consequently, an ITA is generally used to bypass the LAD artery or, alternatively, the vessel that is judged to be most critical to myocardial function.

An ITA can be used either as a pedicle or a free graft. When used as a *pedicle graft*, the vessel is harvested from the undersurface of the chest wall in its fat pedicle. The origin of the ITA is left intact at its connection to the subclavian artery, and the distal end is attached to the target coronary artery by constructing an end-to-side anastomosis (Fig. 15-2). After construction of an ITA pedicle graft, oxygenated blood travels from the ascending aorta through the subclavian artery, ITA graft, and constructed distal anastomosis into the target coronary artery. Because of the anterior location of the LAD artery, the left ITA is most often harvested as a pedicle graft and almost always reaches the distal portion of the vessel without tension. If the ITA is to be used as a *free graft*, it is excised at its proximal as well as its distal end. An ITA free graft is anastomosed proximally to the aorta in the same fashion as a vein graft and its distal end can be used for a target coronary vessel on the side or back wall of the heart. ITA free and pedicle grafts appear to have similar long-term patency rates.

Bilateral ITA grafting is generally reserved for selected situations, such as absence of venous conduit, very young patients with accelerated atherosclerosis, and reoperation for failed vein grafts (Morris et al., 1990). Candidates for bilateral ITA grafting who lack venous conduit include patients who have undergone lower extremity amputations, previous saphenous vein ligation for varicosities, or vein harvesting for coronary or peripheral arterial bypass procedures and those who have severe and extensive varicosities. Some surgeons believe the excellent patency rates associated with ITA grafts warrant elective use of both in preference to vein grafting. However, bilateral as opposed to unilateral ITA grafting has not been shown to increase long-term patient survival (ACC/AHA Task Force, 1991). It does appear that bilateral ITA grafting lessens the likelihood that reoperation will be required (Lytle & Cosgrove, 1992).

ITA grafting of vessels with less than 75% stenoses is controversial. In contrast to a vein graft, the ITA is a muscular reactive conduit. Many surgeons believe that competitive flow through the native coronary artery (as would occur in a mildly stenosed artery) leads to low flow through the ITA graft with subsequent closure. Questions also remain regarding the influence of ITA harvesting on perioperative morbidity

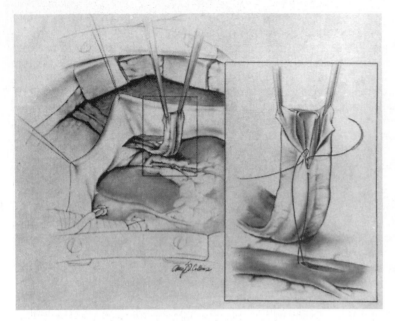

FIGURE 15-2. One technique of internal thoracic artery (ITA) grafting. In this example the left ITA pedicle has been separated from the chest wall, mobilized, and brought through a pericardial incision to reach the left anterior descending (LAD) coronary artery. An incision is made in the LAD artery (*dashed line*). The inset shows the inception of the ITA to LAD anastomosis. (Pacifico AD, Sears NJ, Burgos C, 1986: Harvesting, routing, and anastomosing the left internal mammary artery graft. Ann Thorac Surg 42:709; Society of Thoracic Surgeons)

associated with CABG. Concerns related to harvesting one or both ITAs include (1) whether the more extensive intraoperative dissection required to harvest the ITA produces increased perioperative bleeding and (2) whether diversion of a portion of the anterior chest wall blood supply increases the incidence of sternal wound infection or dehiscence, particularly in patients who are obese, diabetic, or receiving chronic steroid therapy.

Early reoperation for bleeding and postoperative blood loss may be somewhat increased with ITA harvesting (Rankin & Smith, 1990). However, current blood conservation techniques and long-term superiority of ITA grafts favor routine unilateral ITA grafting despite a tendency for more bleeding. Especially in diabetic patients, sternal wound complications may occur more frequently when both ITAs are harvested (Grossi et al., 1991). Because the ITAs provide the major source of blood supply to the sternum, mobilization of an ITA significantly devascularizes the sternal half from which it was harvested (Ulicny & Hiratzka, 1991). Unfortunately, bilateral ITA grafting is particularly suited to diabetic patients because of the diffuse nature of coronary artery atherosclerosis associated with diabetes mellitus (Lytle et al., 1986).

A higher incidence of respiratory insufficiency is sometimes reported in patients undergoing ITA grafting. It may be related to phrenic nerve dysfunction from ITA harvesting or topical hypothermia (Rankin & Smith, 1990; Lytle & Cosgrove, 1992). Postoperative anterior chest wall discomfort or paresthesia also appears to be increased when ITA harvesting is performed. However, it is almost always transient and rarely interferes with routine postoperative recovery. A very small number of patients have persistent, pronounced discomfort or paresthesias in the chest wall overlying the area of ITA dissection.

Saphenous Vein

The majority of patients who undergo surgical revascularization require three or more bypass grafts, and most surgeons prefer to use only one of the ITAs in routine CABG procedures. Because there are more target vessels for grafting than can be accomplished with ITAs alone, the greater *saphenous vein* from one or both legs is almost always harvested (Fig. 15-3). Saphenous vein is expendable, is of comparable size to coronary arteries, is pliable enough to allow easy suturing, and can usually be harvested as free grafts of sufficient length to bypass whichever arteries are stenosed (ACC/AHA Task Force, 1991). The presence of one-way valves that occur naturally inside veins makes it necessary for the surgeon to reverse the vein segments, attaching the distal end of vein to the aorta and proximal end to the coronary artery.

The rapidity with which saphenous vein can be harvested makes it the conduit of choice in emergency situations in which the myocardium is acutely ischemic, such as failed PTCA or evolving MI, or if the patient is hemodynamically unstable. Revascularization exclusively with saphenous vein grafts is also common in patients older than 75 years of age. In these elderly patients, long-term superiority of the ITA is not as important and the operation can be shortened, presumably making it safer, by using only vein grafts.

Removal of saphenous vein from one or both legs is associated with minimal morbidity if the procedure is meticulously planned and performed. Since there is redundant venous drainage from the legs, loss of the saphenous vein does not pose any long-term problems. Preoperative assessment of arterial blood flow to the lower extremities is important; if peripheral arterial occlusive disease is present, wound healing may be compromised. Vein is harvested from the

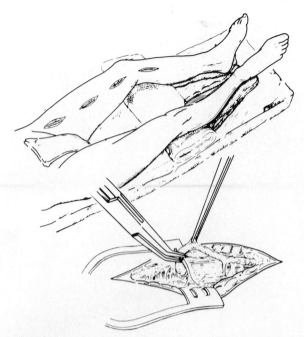

FIGURE 15-3. The greater saphenous vein is harvested from one or both legs using multiple short incisions and meticulous technique to avoid damaging the vein segments. (Loop FD, 1979: Saphenous vein bypass graft. In Cohn LH [ed]: Modern Technics in Surgery, p. 10-2. Mount Kisco, NY, Futura Publishing)

leg with the least degree of arterial disease. Also, because lymphatic drainage from the leg is interrupted at the time of vein harvest, almost all patients develop some degree of edema in the affected leg. The edema can be expected to resolve within weeks or, occasionally, months after the operation. In patients who are immobilized for a prolonged period after surgery the propensity for deep venous thrombosis may be increased because of the absent vein.

Significant morphologic changes and development of atherosclerosis have been well documented in saphenous vein grafts (Grondin et al., 1979). Diffuse intimal hyperplasia is universally present in vein grafts that have been in place more than 1 year (ACC/AHA Task Force, 1991). Postoperative coronary angiography of patients who have undergone CABG reveals the magnitude of the problem: 12% to 20% of vein grafts are no longer patent after 1 year and there is a 2% annual occlusion rate thereafter (Fitzgibbon et al., 1986). Graft closure is more likely in vein grafts with poor distal runoff and resultant low flow (e.g., grafts to coronary arteries of small caliber or arteries supplying muscle that is heavily scarred) (ACC/AHA Task Force, 1991).

Alternative Conduits

If the saphenous veins or ITAs have been previously harvested or are of poor quality, there may be insufficient conduit material for necessary grafts. In these situations, use of the *right gastroepiploic artery*, the *inferior epigastric artery*, or the *cephalic vein* as conduit material may be necessary (Fig. 15-4). Recently available *cryopreserved autologous vein* has provided good early results, but long-term data are not yet available. Artificial conduits have extremely poor long-term patency rates and are rarely used.

THE OPERATIVE PROCEDURE

Operations to revascularize the heart are performed through a median sternotomy incision. After an incision is made through the skin and soft tissue from the supraclavicular notch to the xiphoid process, the sternum is divided longitudinally using a special saw or scissors designed for this purpose. The pericardium is opened and the pericardial edges are tacked against retractors that separate the sternal halves. The median sternotomy incision provides excellent exposure of the heart and great vessels. If an ITA is to be used, it is mobilized from the undersurface of the anterior chest wall before cannulation for cardiopulmonary bypass to allow adequate exposure of the arterial bed. Most often, the left ITA is harvested as a pedicle graft

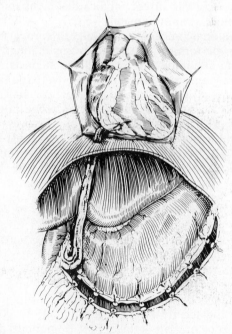

FIGURE 15-4. Diagrammatic representation of coronary artery bypass using an in situ right gastroepiploic graft. The distal portion of the right gastroepiploic artery has been mobilized from the greater curvature of the stomach, leaving intact its proximal origin from the gastroduodenal artery. In this example, the gastroepiploic artery pedicle has been routed anterior to the stomach and liver through the diaphragm and pericardium for anastomosis to the right coronary artery. (Lytle BW, Cosgrove DM, Ratliff NB, Loop FD, 1989: Coronary artery bypass grafting with the right gastroepiploic artery. J Thorac Cardiovasc Surg 97:828)

with preservation of its proximal attachment to the subclavian artery.

Great care is taken during harvest to avoid injury to the ITA or phrenic nerve, which lies medial and posterior to the artery pedicle (Jones, 1991). Because the ITA is a reactive conduit, it is vulnerable to spasm from mishandling or surgical instrumentation. For this reason, many surgeons routinely inject the harvested ITA graft with papaverine to produce intraluminal dilatation and reduce the likelihood of technical anastomotic errors caused by arterial spasm (Mills, 1991). Saphenous vein for the remainder of the grafts is harvested simultaneously by a second member of the surgical team. An atraumatic technique in procuring the saphenous vein is essential. Undue traction or avulsion of small branches at the time of harvest may damage the vein wall and lead to graft failure (Mills & Rigby, 1991).

When these steps have been accomplished, the right atrium and ascending aorta are cannulated and cardiopulmonary bypass is initiated. Core body temperature is cooled to approximately 28°C. After cross-clamping the aorta, chilled cardioplegic solution is administered into the coronary circulation to produce cardiac arrest and provide additional myocardial protection. To maintain cellular viability during the period of ischemic arrest, myocardial temperature is maintained at approximately 15°C.

Distal anastomoses (i.e., grafts to coronary arteries) are performed in the following manner. After selecting a suitable site beyond the stenosis for the distal anastomosis, the epicardium overlying the coronary artery is incised and the anterior wall of the artery is opened longitudinally. A probe is passed into the artery to measure its size and to assess proximal and distal patency (Kirklin & Barratt-Boyes, 1993a). The beveled end of the vein segment or ITA is then sewn to the coronary artery (Fig. 15-5). The remainder of the distal anastomoses are performed in similar fashion.

Sometimes one ITA or vein graft can be used to bypass two obstructed arteries in close proximity. This type of graft is called a *tandem* or *sequential graft.* The single piece of conduit is grafted with a side-to-side anastomosis between the side of the ITA or vein and one target coronary artery and an end-to-side anastomosis between the end of the conduit and the side of the second target artery (Fig. 15-6). Another special type of graft is the *Y graft.* Sometimes a bifurcated piece of saphenous vein can be harvested and each of the two limbs can be grafted to a separate target artery, with one proximal anastomosis. If a Y graft is desirable and donor vein with a natural Y is unavailable, the surgeon may fashion a Y vein graft using two separate pieces of vein.

The aorta remains cross-clamped while distal graft anastomoses are performed. Because the heart gradually rewarms and collateral blood flow washes away the cardioplegic solution, repeated doses are given every 15 to 20 minutes. Most commonly, the solution

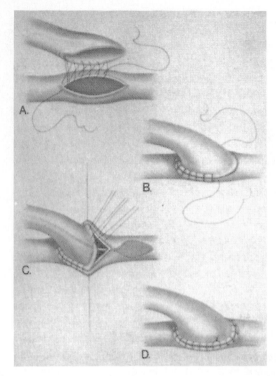

FIGURE 15-5. One technique of saphenous vein to coronary artery end-to-side anastomosis. The anastomosis begins at the heel of the beveled end of the vein graft **(A)** and is continued for three-fourths the length of the arteriotomy on either side **(B).** Traction is placed on both ends of the continuous suture, which opens the toe of the anastomosis **(C),** allowing excellent visualization. Interrupted sutures are used to secure the toe of the anastomosis **(D).** (Ochsner JL, 1980: Current operative techniques for myocardial revascularization. In Moran JM, Michaelis LL [eds]: Surgery for the Complications of Myocardial Infarction, p. 152. New York, Grune & Stratton)

is administered into the coronary arteries in antegrade fashion through a small catheter in the aortic root. Effective distribution of the solution through significantly stenosed or occluded coronary arteries is limited. Myocardium supplied by such vessels is not as well cooled and displays persistent electromechanical activity (Buckberg, 1987).

Coronary revascularization procedures are designed by the surgeon to minimize intraoperative myocardial injury. Because ischemic injury to myocardial tissue increases exponentially with time, it is important that the operative procedure is performed in an expedient manner (Rankin & Smith, 1990). Distal anastomoses to vessels that supply muscle at most risk of ischemic injury are performed first. After construction of a distal saphenous vein graft anastomosis, cardioplegic solution can be injected directly into the proximal opening of the vein graft to cool myocardium beyond the obstructed portion of the coronary artery.

Administration of cardioplegic solution through an ITA pedicle graft is not possible. Some surgeons alter-

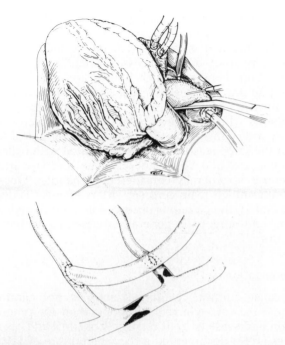

FIGURE 15-6. (Top) Operative exposure for sequential grafting of parallel branches of the left circumflex artery. **(Bottom)** A side-to-side anastomosis is constructed between a saphenous vein segment and the first coronary arterial branch; an end-to-side anastomosis is constructed between the distal end of the vein and the second arterial branch. (Loop FD, 1979: Saphenous vein bypass graft. In Cohn LH [ed]: Modern Technics in Surgery, p. 10-9. Mount Kisco, NY, Futura Publishing)

natively use a retrograde technique of cardioplegia administration. Cardioplegic solution is delivered into a catheter placed through the right atrium into the coronary sinus to perfuse the myocardium in a retrograde fashion. Detailed description of cardiopulmonary bypass and myocardial preservation techniques is provided elsewhere in the text.

Proximal vein graft anastomoses to the aorta are performed either before or after release of the aortic cross-clamp as rewarming of the patient is begun. Some surgeons alternatively perform proximal vein anastomoses (vein to aorta) before distal anastomoses. With this technique, proximal anastomoses are performed before initiating cardiopulmonary bypass, thus reducing the duration of cardiopulmonary bypass time. If proximal anastomoses are performed first, doses of cardioplegic solution administered into the aortic root after completion of a distal anastomosis flow through the newly constructed graft (Siwek & Daggett, 1989). The merits of performing distal or proximal anastomoses first remain controversial, and choice of technique is primarily determined by surgeon preference (Mills & Rigby, 1991).

After grafting has been completed, a flow probe may be used to measure blood flow through each of the vein grafts. Graft flow greater than 100 mL/min is considered desirable. Measurement of graft flows provides the surgeon with valuable information about quality of the vein graft and likelihood of its long-term patency. If flow is less than 100 mL/min, the vein graft may be infused with a vasodilating agent, such as papaverine, to ascertain if the problem is due to vasospasm. If a technical problem is compromising graft flow, it can be corrected before concluding the operation. At the present time, probes for measuring flow through ITA grafts are not available for clinical use.

When bypass grafting is completed and the myocardium has warmed sufficiently to resume a spontaneous electrical rhythm, the patient is weaned from cardiopulmonary bypass. Cannulae are removed, and hemostasis is achieved. Generally, the pericardial sac is left open or closed loosely to avoid kinking or occluding grafts that lie on the anterior surface of the heart. The sternum is reapproximated and fastened with heavy suture material or wire, and the skin incision is closed.

SPECIAL CONSIDERATIONS

Emergency Operation

Emergency CABG is performed to revascularize portions of myocardium that are thought to be in imminent danger of irreversible damage. It may be a primary intervention or may follow less invasive interventions (PTCA or thrombolytic therapy). The most common reasons for emergency CABG are (1) complications of PTCA, (2) ischemia that is uncontrolled by medical therapy (i.e., unstable angina), and (3) evolving MI.

PTCA can cause acute MI as a result of acute coronary artery occlusion, dissection of a coronary artery, or embolization of thrombus or atherosclerotic debris into the distal portion of a coronary artery. Each of these complications compromises antegrade flow through the artery. Chest pain, electrocardiographic manifestations of ischemia or infarction, and hemodynamic instability may result.

Unstable angina, or ischemic symptoms refractory to control with medical therapy, may be categorized as preinfarction or postinfarction depending on whether there is electrocardiographic or enzymatic evidence of acute MI. The most common manifestation of preinfarction ischemia is chest pain accompanied by characteristic electrocardiographic changes. Uncommonly, ventricular tachycardia or pulmonary edema occurs as a manifestation of acute ischemia. If symptoms cannot be controlled with intensive medical therapy (e.g., nitroglycerin, heparin, beta-blocking and calcium-channel antagonist agents, and intra-aortic balloon counterpulsation), CABG may be undertaken to preserve myocardium that is presumed to be reversibly injured.

Ischemia may also be present in the early period after MI has occurred. Postinfarction angina indicates that there is muscle in which blood supply is jeopardized but damage remains reversible. Such patients, if treated medically, have a substantial risk of another infarction that may lead to progressive left ventricular dysfunction or death (Hochberg et al., 1984). On the other hand, early surgical intervention is avoided if possible. Revascularization performed more than 4 to 6 hours but less than 1 week after MI is associated with significantly increased operative mortality owing to hemorrhagic reperfusion injury. Consequently, intravenous nitroglycerin and intra-aortic balloon counterpulsation are the mainstays of therapy for postinfarction ischemia during the first week after acute MI. However, if postinfarction angina is not relieved by intensive medical therapy, emergent surgical therapy may be necessary.

The third category of patients requiring emergency surgery are those with evolving MI, defined as a period of 4 to 6 hours from MI onset during which muscle damage may be reversible. The availability of thrombolytic therapy and PTCA as effective methods of reestablishing blood flow through the infarct artery (artery responsible for the MI) has dramatically lessened the need for emergency surgical revascularization as an initial form of therapy. More often, CABG for evolving MI is performed as an alternative therapy when PTCA or thrombolytic therapy is contraindicated or fails to reopen the infarct vessel. Surgical therapy is best suited for patients with suitable anatomy in whom recent coronary angiography has already been performed or in whom it can be performed within 1 to 2 hours after onset of the infarct.

Surgical revascularization under emergency conditions differs in character from procedures planned and performed electively. When active ischemia is present, the primary goal is prompt restoration of blood flow to the jeopardized portion of myocardium. The vessel supplying ischemic myocardium is grafted first so that it can be perfused with cardioplegic solution while other vessels are grafted. Use of the ITA, with its long-term superiority in patency, must usually be abandoned in the interest of restoring flow quickly by use of a saphenous vein graft. Additional time is necessary to harvest an ITA before cardiopulmonary bypass, and thus more time elapses before ischemic muscle can be protected and revascularized. Particularly in a young patient, it is disappointing when revascularization is done emergently and only saphenous vein grafts, with lower patency rates, must be used.

Operative mortality of emergency CABG is not always higher than that of elective procedures. However, it increases profoundly, approaching 100%, if the patient is in cardiogenic shock or if cardiac arrest has occurred and the operation is initiated during cardiopulmonary resuscitation or after institution of emergency femorofemoral cardiopulmonary bypass. Patients who require emergency surgical revascularization after thrombolytic therapy are at higher risk for perioperative bleeding. However, the risk is generally not prohibitive unless large doses of thrombolytic agents have been administered.

Patients with severe narrowing of the left main coronary artery do not necessarily require emergency operation. However, such lesions are usually operated on urgently because of the tremendous amount of muscle at jeopardy if the vessel occludes. Those patients who suffer occlusion of the left main coronary artery invariably die of the ensuing global MI. For the same reason, the risk associated with balloon angioplasty of a significant left main coronary artery stenosis is generally considered prohibitive. Once a significant left main coronary artery stenosis is demonstrated, the patient is observed in a monitored setting and surgery is generally performed within 24 hours.

Reoperation

Because surgical revascularization is not curative, some patients will require reoperation for progression of disease or graft closure. Cosgrove and associates (1986) documented a reoperation rate of 11% at 10 years in a retrospective analysis of 8000 patients. Young age at initial operation was the most important predictor for reoperation and the incidence of reoperation was twice as high in patients with only vein grafts as opposed to those with ITA grafts. Persons who have undergone CABG may also occasionally require reoperation for a separate cardiac problem, such as a valvular abnormality or ascending aortic aneurysm.

Reentry into the chest during reoperation must be performed cautiously because of the presence of adhesions (fibrous tissue) from the previous operation. This internal scar tissue causes the heart to adhere to surrounding tissues. The grafts on the anterior surface of the heart and the heart muscle itself (right ventricle) become adherent to the posterior table of the sternum. Division of the sternum can be complicated by inadvertent laceration of one of the grafts, particularly an ITA pedicle graft, or by entry into the right ventricular chamber. Acute MI due to graft injury or massive hemorrhage due to right ventricular laceration can ensue.

Emergency institution of cardiopulmonary bypass may be necessary to prevent death of the patient. Consequently, in high-risk reoperations, the femoral artery and vein are often cannulated before opening the chest so that cardiopulmonary bypass can be immediately instituted if necessary. Internal adhesions also blur tissue planes, making dissection during reoperations more tedious and prolonged. As a result, blood loss and need for transfusion can be expected to be greater.

At the time of a reoperative procedure, the surgeon must determine if any revision of original bypass grafts is indicated. An occluded graft is not necessarily revascularized if there is good collateral circulation to the muscle it supplies or if the muscle is necrotic. The surgeon must also determine whether to replace patent vein grafts that have been in place for a number of years. A judgment must be made as to whether it is more prudent to leave a viable but old graft alone or to replace it with a new graft that may or may not be as good as the original graft. Another consideration in determining whether to revise vein grafts is the degree of difficulty in freeing the heart from adhesions to surrounding tissues. Regrafting coronary arteries is particularly difficult if target vessels are on the lateral or posterior surface of the heart. Patent ITA grafts are almost never revised.

Reoperation is associated with a somewhat higher risk than a first operation, and risk increases substantially with a second or third reoperation. Patients undergoing reoperation tend to be older, usually have more diffuse disease, and may have sustained further myocardial damage between the initial and subsequent operations. As compared with a primary operation, risk of death during repeat CABG is approxi-

mately 3.5 times greater; perioperative MI, 8 times greater; stroke, 2.6 times greater; and reexploration for bleeding, 2 times greater (Mills & Rigby, 1991).

Diffuse Coronary Artery Disease

Sometimes, diffuse disease of one or more coronary arteries precludes complete revascularization of all areas of viable myocardium. Incomplete revascularization adversely affects relief from symptoms, freedom from repeat operation, and survival (Johnson et al., 1989). In such patients, *coronary endarterectomy* of diffusely diseased arteries is thought to be beneficial. Coronary endarterectomy consists of removing atheromatous material from the lumen of an artery that is diffusely diseased (Fig. 15-7). It is always accompanied by bypass grafting of the vessel.

Most common is endarterectomy of the right coronary artery. Left coronary artery endarterectomy remains controversial because it is associated with increased operative mortality and reduced graft pa-

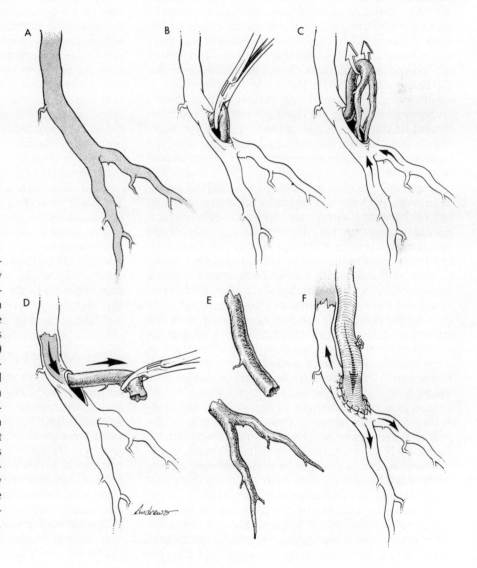

FIGURE 15-7. Technique for endarterectomy of right coronary artery (RCA). **(A)** An occluded RCA is considered for endarterectomy. **(B)** An arteriotomy is performed just above the crux and atheromatous core is brought out through the incision. **(C)** The distal vessels are cleared individually of plaque. **(D)** The proximal portion is removed by gentle traction until it breaks free. **(E)** The atheromatous specimen after extraction from the artery. **(F)** A saphenous vein graft is anastomosed to the RCA to bypass atheromatous material in the proximal portion of the vessel. (Cooley DA, 1984: Revascularization of the ischemic myocardium. In Techniques in Cardiac Surgery, ed. 2, p. 232. Philadelphia, WB Saunders)

tency in the endarterectomized vessel (Livesay & Cooley, 1991). The primary complication of endarterectomy is postoperative MI due to residual obstruction, creation of an intimal flap, or thrombosis (Livesay & Cooley, 1991).

Associated Peripheral Atherosclerosis

Atherosclerosis affects arteries throughout the body, and many patients with CAD also have atherosclerotic lesions in peripheral arteries. It is not unusual for a patient who undergoes CABG to have significant carotid artery disease, an aortic aneurysm, or occlusive lesions in the arteries supplying the lower extremities. In patients who require operative therapy for peripheral as well as coronary arterial disease, the sequence of necessary procedures is critical. Several reports have documented that after abdominal aortic aneurysm resection and extracranial or lower extremity revascularization, MI occurs with predictable frequency and accounts for approximately half of postoperative deaths (Hinkamp et al., 1991). Consequently, coronary artery revascularization is usually performed before the peripheral vascular procedure.

In patients with combined, significant coronary and carotid artery disease, the sequence and timing of procedures remains somewhat controversial (Johnsson et al., 1991). The underlying question is whether there is greater risk for MI during carotid endarterectomy or stroke during coronary revascularization. If the patient has critical, symptom-producing stenoses in both coronary and carotid vessels, the two revascularization procedures may be performed concomitantly.

The most common method for a combined procedure is to perform the carotid endarterectomy just before coronary artery revascularization. Preparations are made so that cardiopulmonary bypass can be instituted within moments should myocardial ischemia become evident. The carotid endarterectomy is then performed with careful hemodynamic monitoring, either before sternotomy, or after sternotomy but before initiating cardiopulmonary bypass. As soon as the carotid endarterectomy is completed, the patient is placed on cardiopulmonary bypass and the cardiac portion of the procedure is undertaken.

Less commonly, the carotid endarterectomy is performed with the patient on cardiopulmonary bypass. Those who favor performing endarterectomy before bypass believe the changes in perfusion pressure associated with initiation of bypass may increase the risk of stroke; those favoring endarterectomy during bypass believe the controlled perfusion pressure, hypothermia, and hemodilution present during cardiopulmonary bypass provide better protection against cerebral ischemia (Newman & Hicks, 1988).

In patients requiring surgical treatment for both CAD and an abdominal aortic aneurysm, the coronary artery revascularization is usually performed first. MI as a complication of aneurysm repair is considered a more likely risk than aneurysm rupture complicating CABG. However, rupture is a potential risk during the perioperative period, and some surgeons advocate performing elective CABG and aneurysm repair as a combined procedure (Hinkamp et al., 1991). CABG is almost always performed before peripheral arterial bypass procedures.

Occasionally, patients who undergo coronary artery revascularization have a significant degree of atherosclerosis in the ascending aorta. Calcification, atheromatous deposits, or ulcerated lesions in the ascending aorta are worrisome because they increase the risk of intraoperative stroke due to embolism. They also limit available sites for clamping, cannulation, and anastomosis of vein grafts to the aorta. Aortic atherosclerosis is more likely in patients who have associated atherosclerosis in the carotid arteries or abdominal aorta. In such patients, a preoperative chest roentgenogram or computed tomographic scan of the chest may detect aortic wall irregularity or calcification.

In the presence of severe ascending aortic calcification or atherosclerosis, special care is taken during the operation to reduce the possibility of cerebral embolism from debris in the ascending aorta. The surgeon uses various techniques to decrease manipulation, clamping, or cannulation of the ascending aorta. Instead of the usual method of myocardial protection that includes aortic cross-clamping and cardioplegic arrest, profound hypothermia with ventricular fibrillation may be used to preclude the necessity of applying a cross-clamp to the diseased aorta (Peigh et al., 1991). The femoral artery or distal ascending aorta may be used for arterial cannulation.

An ITA pedicle graft avoids the need for a proximal vein-to-aorta anastomosis. In fact, some surgeons advocate using one or both ITAs as the sole inflow conduit in this group of patients; proximal saphenous vein graft anastomoses are constructed in end-to-side fashion to the proximal portion of the ITA graft (Peigh et al., 1991). If saphenous vein grafts are anastomosed to the aorta, soft, noncalcified sites on the undersurface of the transverse arch or distal ascending aorta may be selected.

Revascularization in Young and in Elderly Adults

Patients younger than 40 years of age who require surgical revascularization appear to have a premature and more rampant form of coronary artery atherosclerosis. Both long-term survival and freedom from symptoms are decreased in these patients in comparison to older patients with similar disease at the time of surgical revascularization (Lytle et al., 1984). Subsequent revascularization procedures are likely to be necessary. Accordingly, use of one or both ITAs is particularly important because of the superiority of ITA over vein grafts in long-term patency.

Increased longevity in the United States and the epidemic and progressive nature of CAD have re-

TABLE 15-1. FACTORS ASSOCIATED WITH INCREASED OPERATIVE MORTALITY AND MORBIDITY IN PATIENTS UNDERGOING CORONARY ARTERY BYPASS GRAFTING

Ejection fraction < 30%
Perioperative myocardial infarction
Age > 70 years
Diabetes mellitus
Left ventricular end-diastolic pressure > 25 mm Hg
Female sex
Failed percutaneous transluminal coronary angioplasty
Associated mitral valve disease
Previous cardiac procedure
Emergent operation
Associated peripheral arterial occlusive disease

sulted in greater numbers of septuagenarians and octogenarians undergoing CABG. Revascularization in the elderly differs in that complete revascularization and long-term benefits of ITA grafting are less important than shortening operative time. Numerous studies have demonstrated that while CABG can be safely performed in elderly patients, mortality, morbidity, and associated costs are greater (Salomon et al., 1991).

RESULTS OF SURGICAL REVASCULARIZATION

A decade ago improvements in myocardial preservation and other intraoperative techniques had reduced operative mortality associated with CABG to less than 1%. However, the profile of patients undergoing CABG has changed since then. Increases have been noted in the mean age of patients, the percentage of women and patients older than 70 years of age, and the number of patients with triple-vessel disease, left ventricular dysfunction, peripheral arterial occlusive disease, and diabetes (Loop, 1990; Jones et al., 1991). Average ventricular ejection fraction in patients undergoing CABG has decreased, and patients with single-vessel disease are almost never treated with surgical revascularization (King & Talley, 1989). Reoperations and emergency operations are more common.

As a result, most centers, particularly those with higher risk patients, are observing higher (1%–5%) operative mortality rates associated with CABG. The most important predictor of operative mortality appears to be the status of left ventricular function. Perioperative complications occur in approximately 15% of patients undergoing CABG; risk factors for morbidity include previous cardiac surgery, emergent operation, and peripheral arterial occlusive disease (Hammermeister et al., 1990). Common factors associated with an increased mortality or morbidity risk are displayed in Table 15-1.

The most common early complications of CABG are postoperative bleeding and transient low cardiac

output syndrome. Approximately 5% of patients have significant *postoperative bleeding* that necessitates operative reexploration within the first 24 hours. Usually, bleeding is diffuse and represents impaired clotting. Postoperative coagulopathy is more likely with cardiac than with other types of operations because of the use of cardiopulmonary bypass. Extracorporeal circulation of blood damages platelets and other clotting factors. Also, the patient must be systemically anticoagulated during the period of cardiopulmonary bypass. Bleeding related to a technical problem, such as a disrupted suture line, is unusual but can also occur, particularly if the patient becomes hypertensive in the early postoperative hours.

Because some bleeding is inevitable, the chest is not closed until adequate hemostasis is achieved and drainage tubes are placed in the thorax. Blood conservation techniques, such as a cell-saver system and autotransfusion, are important to lessen the need for transfusion of homologous blood and are discussed in Chapter 14, Blood Conservation.

Low cardiac output syndrome may represent perioperative MI or transient depression of ventricular function secondary to effects of cardiopulmonary bypass and hypothermia. Low cardiac output syndrome is usually treated by intravenous infusion of inotropic and vasodilating medications. Occasionally, intra-aortic balloon counterpulsation is necessary. Rarely, frank cardiogenic shock occurs that is refractory to pharmacologic and counterpulsation therapy. In such cases, mechanical support of the heart may become necessary. Other complications of CABG, including early graft closure, arrhythmias, cerebral vascular accident, wound infection, and respiratory failure are described in Chapter 28, Complications of Cardiac Operations.

Long-term follow-up studies reveal that most patients do quite well after CABG with freedom from myocardial ischemia for many years (Table 15-2). However, although CABG is quite effective in revascularizing the myocardium, it does not cure atherosclerosis. Consequently, symptoms of myocardial ischemia eventually return in most patients and often

TABLE 15-2. LONG-TERM RESULTS OF CORONARY ARTERY BYPASS GRAFTING

Outcome	Percent at	
Freedom from:	5 Years	10 Years
Death	88	75
Angina	83	63
Myocardial infarction	95	85
Sudden cardiac death	95	

(American College of Cardiology/American Heart Association Task Force on Assessment of Diagnostic and Therapeutic Cardiovascular Procedures, 1991: ACC/AHA guidelines and indications for coronary artery bypass graft surgery. Circulation 83:1125)

lead to the patient's death. Return of angina is the most common postoperative ischemic event. Early return of angina is usually due to graft closure or incomplete revascularization; late return generally represents graft stenosis or occlusion, progression of atherosclerosis, or a combination of the two (ACC/AHA Task Force, 1991).

Most surgeons prescribe antiplatelet therapy to augment vein graft patency. Aspirin is generally regarded as the most effective agent for this purpose (Goldman et al., 1990). Antiplatelet drugs are usually not used in the immediate preoperative period to avoid associated bleeding complications. However, aspirin therapy, alone or in combination with dipyridamole, is routinely initiated in the early postoperative period and continued indefinitely.

SURGERY FOR COMPLICATIONS OF MYOCARDIAL INFARCTION

MI can produce several mechanical complications that may require surgical intervention. These include ventricular aneurysm, acute mitral regurgitation, and ventricular free wall or septal rupture.

VENTRICULAR ANEURYSM

A *ventricular aneurysm* is a discrete area of necrosed myocardium that is noncontractile or that contracts paradoxically from other ventricular segments. An aneurysm develops in 12% to 15% of patients who survive transmural MI (Churchwell, 1991). The most common location is in the anterolateral wall of the left ventricle near the apex (Kirklin & Barratt-Boyes, 1993b). Right ventricular aneurysms are rare; they may be congenital or result from MI or blunt chest trauma (Harken, 1990).

The mere presence of a ventricular aneurysm does not necessitate surgical therapy. However, specific associated problems may warrant operative intervention. Most common is congestive heart failure. Necrotic muscle and fibrous tissue that comprise the aneurysm move paradoxically, "stealing" stroke volume and decreasing cardiac output (Harken, 1990). The impaired ventricular function may also produce angina. The increased ventricular cavity size increases wall tension, which can result in higher oxygen consumption in the remaining normal myocardium and decreased oxygen supply during diastole (Jatene, 1991).

Frequently, the endocardial surface of an aneurysm contains thrombus that accumulates secondary to the endothelial injury that accompanies MI. This so-called mural thrombus can embolize from the left ventricle into the systemic circulation and cause stroke, MI, or mesenteric or limb ischemia. Finally, scar tissue on the endocardial surface of the aneurysmal segment may provide an arrhythmogenic focus. The mixture of necrotic, fibrous, and viable tissue

that constitutes the aneurysm and its adjacent border has different electrophysiologic properties of conduction and refractoriness that predispose to reentrant arrhythmias (Harken, 1990).

Ventricular aneurysmectomy consists of resecting the fibrotic, aneurysmal muscle. It is technically easier if it can be performed at least 6 weeks after acute MI because the myocardial tissue is less friable than immediately after the event. Aneurysmectomy is performed through median sternotomy using cardiopulmonary bypass. When the heart is decompressed during extracorporeal circulation, the aneurysm collapses while the remaining viable ventricular myocardium remains firm (Harken, 1990). After making a linear incision in the aneurysm, the fibrotic tissue is excised, leaving a rim of fibrous tissue. Thrombus is evacuated from the ventricle, and the cavity is irrigated. The edges of the defect are reapproximated and closed by direct suture technique using large strips of prosthetic material to buttress the reconstruction (Fig. 15-8).

In patients with large aneurysms, reapproximation of the fibrotic edges may cause inordinate distortion of ventricular geometry (Jatene, 1991). Decreased ventricular volume and diastolic function result and may cause significant ventricular dysfunction. Therefore, it may be preferable in such patients to close the defect with a prosthetic patch. Small aneurysms may sometimes be repaired by plicating, or folding, and suturing the fibrotic tissue without opening the ventricular cavity. Resection of a ventricular aneurysm is sometimes performed concomitantly with coronary artery revascularization. In patients with associated ventricular rhythm disorders, aneurysm resection alone does not ensure arrhythmia eradication. Concomitant intraoperative mapping and endocardial resection are required to treat the arrhythmic disorder. Surgical treatment of ventricular arrhythmias is discussed in Chapter 18, Surgical Treatment of Cardiac Rhythm Disorders.

ACUTE MITRAL REGURGITATION

Acute mitral regurgitation may develop secondary to MI by one of several pathophysiologic mechanisms, including papillary muscle dysfunction, papillary muscle rupture, or annular dilatation. Pulmonary edema or cardiogenic shock often accompanies acute mitral regurgitation because, in contrast to chronic mitral regurgitation, compensatory mechanisms to protect the heart have not developed. A vasodilating agent, such as nitroprusside, is generally administered to reduce afterload and facilitate forward flow. Intra-aortic balloon counterpulsation is often instituted, and emergent therapy to restore mitral valve competence may be necessary.

Ischemic papillary muscle dysfunction is sometimes successfully reversed by revascularization of the ischemic muscle with thrombolytic therapy, PTCA, or CABG. If a papillary muscle has ruptured

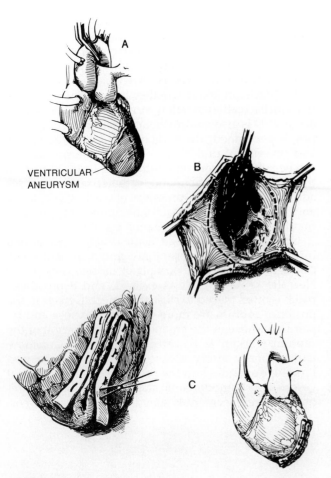

VENTRICULAR
ANEURYSM

FIGURE 15-8. One technique of left ventricular aneurysm repair. **(A)** Operation is performed through a median sternotomy incision, using cardiopulmonary bypass and cardioplegic arrest. The heart is elevated from the pericardial sac and the center of the collapsed aneursym wall is identified. **(B)** The central portion of the aneurysm is incised and any intramural clot is carefully removed. The lateral walls of the aneurysm are excised. **(C)** The edges of the defect are approximated and sutured using Teflon felt strips to reinforce the closure. (Waldhausen JA, Pierce WS, 1985: Repair of ventricular aneurysms and ventricular septal defects after myocardial infarction. In Johnson's Surgery of the Chest, ed. 5, p. 485. Chicago, Year Book Medical Publishers)

or if myocardial necrosis at the base of the papillary muscles has produced annular dilatation, surgical reconstruction or replacement of the mitral valve is required. Mitral valve repair and replacement are discussed in Chapter 16, Surgical Treatment of Valvular Heart Disease.

VENTRICULAR RUPTURE

Rupture of the ventricular myocardium occurs when necrotic tissue becomes too weakened to withstand intraventricular pressure. Rupture may occur in either the free wall or the septum of the ventricle, de-

pending on location of the MI. *Ventricular free wall rupture* occurs in as many as 10% of patients who die in the hospital after acute MI (Pasternak et al., 1992). The lesion is usually fatal but if detected before the patient's death is treated with emergent surgical intervention to restore ventricular wall integrity.

Sometimes, ventricular rupture is small and is contained by pericardium. If sufficient pericardial inflammation and adhesions are present to localize and contain the rupture, death from pericardial tamponade is evaded and the contained rupture creates a pseudoaneurysm (Cooley & Walker, 1980). A *pseudoaneurysm* or *false aneurysm* differs from a true ventricular aneurysm in that its wall consists of fibrous pericardium only. In contrast to true aneurysms, surgical resection of a false aneurysm is almost always performed to prevent repeated myocardial rupture. In addition to precipitous rupture, a pseudoaneurysm can produce the same clinical consequences as a true ventricular aneurysm.

Resection of a true aneurysm or pseudoaneurysm in the early period after MI is technically difficult because of the fragility of tissue in the area of infarction. Also, in the case of pseudoaneurysm, the pericardium may be acting to contain the rupture. The surgeon may cannulate the aorta and right atrium through the intact pericardium so that cardiopulmonary bypass can be initiated before opening the pericardium.

Rupture of the ventricular septum is estimated to occur in 1% to 2% of patients with acute MI (Komeda et al., 1990). Although less common than free wall rupture, the condition is more commonly diagnosed before the patient's death. It usually occurs in patients with extensive transmural infarction, less diffuse CAD, and thus less well-developed collateral circulation (Johnson et al., 1991). Septal rupture produces a *ventricular septal defect* (VSD). In most cases, acute VSD occurs in the anterior or apical portion of the septum, caused by a transmural infarction in the distribution of the LAD artery. VSDs due to inferior infarction occur in the basal portion of the septum (Pasternak et al., 1992).

The presence of an acute VSD is usually suggested by auscultation of a new holosystolic murmur in association with congestive heart failure or cardiogenic shock after MI. The differential diagnosis between acute VSD and acute mitral regurgitation is difficult from clinical criteria alone; echocardiography or right-sided heart catheterization is performed to distinguish between the two conditions. When a VSD with a hemodynamically significant shunt is present, prognosis for survival is dismal unless surgical repair is performed. The defect allows shunting of blood from left to right, resulting in acute congestive heart failure in a left ventricle already impaired by acute MI. Death occurs due to progressive cardiogenic shock and secondary organ failure. Approximately 25% of patients with acute VSD die within 24 hours, 50% die within the first week, and only 20% of patients with unrepaired defects survive more than 4 weeks (Kirklin & Barratt-Boyes, 1993c).

Intra-aortic balloon counterpulsation is usually necessary to support the patient until operative intervention can be performed. Counterpulsation decreases afterload, thereby promoting forward flow from the left ventricle and reducing left to right shunting. Inotropic and vasodilating medications are commonly administered as well. Surgical closure of the defect is performed emergently in hemodynamically unstable patients.

Timing of operative repair in hemodynamically stable patients is controversial. Operative repair of the defect is made technically easier if performed 1 to 2 months after the infarct when the defect edges have become fibrotic, making the tissue firmer and easier to secure with sutures. In the early period after infarction, the tissue is quite friable. Suturing is difficult and disruption of the repair is more likely. In addition, the risk of myocardial dysfunction is greater if the operation is performed within a week of MI.

Conversely, if surgical repair of the defect is delayed, precipitous, irreversible hemodynamic deterioration can occur at any time. Accordingly, many surgeons believe the risk of death to the patient during a 6- to 8-week waiting period warrants immediate repair of a postinfarction VSD once it has been diag-nosed. Although survival is generally better in those patients for whom surgical repair is delayed, patients who remain hemodynamically stable for 6 to 8 weeks are not comparable with those who require early operation because of cardiogenic shock.

The decision about whether to perform preoperative cardiac catheterization in unstable patients with acute VSD is also controversial. If coronary angiography is performed, the surgeon will know the nature and severity of underlying CAD. Significant lesions can be bypassed concomitantly with surgical repair of the VSD. On the other hand, catheterization imposes additional risk in the presence of cardiogenic shock and delays operative repair of the immediate problem that is producing hemodynamic instability.

Operative repair of an acute VSD is performed through a median sternotomy and ventriculotomy through the infarcted portion of muscle (Fig. 15-9). Necrotic septal muscle is excised, and a prosthetic patch is often placed to close the defect. Defects in the posterior septum are more difficult to expose and repair than those in the anterior or apical portion of the septum (Kirklin & Barratt-Boyes, 1993c). Concomitant coronary artery revascularization may be performed, depending on the presence of suitable target vessels and hemodynamic stability. Concomitant mitral valve replacement is sometimes necessary to cor-

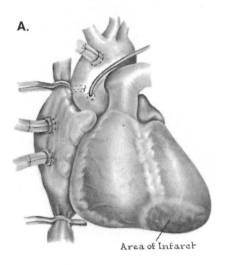

A.

Area of Infarct

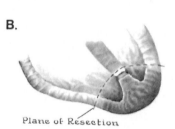

B.

Plane of Resection

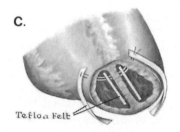

C.

Teflon Felt

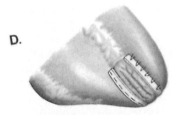

D.

FIGURE 15-9. One technique of acute VSD repair. **(A)** Apical myocardial infarction has resulted in rupture of the ventricular septum. **(B)** The infarcted muscle is excised, including the area of the septum containing the defect and adjacent areas of right and left ventricular myocardium. **(C)** Prosthetic material is used to reinforce the closure as sutures are placed through viable myocardium surrounding the area of resection. **(D)** The apex is securely closed. (Kouchoukos NT, 1979: Infarction ventricular septal defect. In Cohn LH [ed]: Modern Technics in Surgery, p. 9-4. Mount Kisco, NY, Futura Publishing) rect significant mitral regurgitation associated with acute VSD, particularly in patients with posterior MIs (Kirklin & Barratt-Boyes, 1993c).

REFERENCES

American College of Cardiology/American Heart Association Task Force on Assessment of Diagnostic and Therapeutic Cardiovascular Procedures, 1991: ACC/AHA guidelines and indications for coronary artery bypass graft surgery. Circulation 83:1125

Block PC, 1990: Restenosis after percutaneous transluminal coronary angioplasty: Anatomic and pathophysiological mechanisms. Circulation 81(Suppl IV):IV-2

Buckberg GD, 1987: Recent progress in myocardial protection during cardiac operations. In McGoon DC (ed): Cardiac Surgery, ed. 2. Phildadelphia, FA Davis

CASS Principal Investigators and Their Associates, 1983: Coronary Artery Surgery Study (CASS): A randomized trial of coronary artery bypass surgery: Survival data. Circulation 68:939

Churchwell AL, 1991: Ventricular aneurysm due to myocardial infarction. In Hurst JW (ed): Current Therapy in Cardiovascular Disease, ed. 3. Philadelphia, BC Decker

Cooley DA, Walker WE, 1980: Surgical treatment of postinfarction ventricular aneurysm: Evolution of technique and results in 1533 patients. In Moran JM, Michaelis LL (eds): Surgery for the Complications of Myocardial Infarction. New York, Grune & Stratton

Cosgrove DM, Loop FD, Lytle BW, et al., 1986: Predictors of reoperation after myocardial revascularization. J Thorac Cardiovasc Surg 92:811

European Coronary Surgery Study Group, 1982: Long-term results of prospective randomised study of coronary artery bypass surgery in stable angina pectoris. Lancet 2:1173

Faxon DP, Ruocco N, Jacobs AK, 1990: Long-term outcome of patients after percutaneous transluminal coronary angioplasty. Circulation 81(Suppl IV):IV-9

Fitzgibbon GM, Leach AJ, Keon WJ, et al., 1986: Coronary bypass graft fate: Angiographic study of 1179 vein grafts early, one year and five years after operation. J Thorac Cardiovasc Surg 91:773

Galbut DL, Traad EA, Dorman MJ, et al., 1991: Bilateral internal mammary artery grafts in reoperative and primary coronary bypass surgery. Ann Thorac Surg 52:20

Goldman S, Copeland J, Moritz T, et al., 1990: Internal mammary artery and saphenous vein graft patency. Circulation 82 (Suppl IV):IV-237

Grondin CM, Lesperance J, Solymoss BC, et al., 1979: Atherosclerotic changes in coronary grafts six years after operation. J Thorac Cardiovasc Surg 77:24

Grossi EA, Esposito R, Harris LJ, et al., 1991: Sternal wound infections and the use of internal mammary artery grafts. J Thorac Cardiovasc Surg 102:342

Hammermeister KE, Burchfiel C, Johnson R, Grover F, 1990: Identification of patients at greatest risk for developing major complications at cardiac surgery. Circulation 82 (Suppl IV):IV-380

Harken AH, 1990: Left ventricular aneurysm. In Sabiston DC Jr, Spencer FC (eds): Surgery of the Chest, ed. 5. Philadelphia, WB Saunders

Hinkamp TJ, Pifarre R, Bakhos M, Blakeman B, 1991: Combined myocardial revascularization and abdominal aortic aneurysm repair. Ann Thorac Surg 51:470

Hochberg MS, Parsonnet V, Gielchinsky I, et al., 1984: Timing of coronary revascularization after acute myocardial infarction. J Thorac Cardiovasc Surg 88:914

Jatene AD, 1991: Surgical treatment of left ventricular aneurysm. In Baue AE, Geha AS, Hammond GL, et al. (eds): Glenn's Thoracic and Cardiovascular Surgery, ed. 5. Norwalk, CT, Appleton & Lange

Johnson RG, Jacobs ML, Daggett WM Jr, 1991: Postinfarction ventricular septal rupture. In Baue AE, Geha AS, Hammond GL, et al. (eds): Glenn's Thoracic and Cardiovascular Surgery, ed. 5. Norwalk, CT, Appleton & Lange

Johnson WD, Brenowitz JB, Saedi SF, Kayser KL, 1989: Diffuse coronary artery disease. in Grillo HC, Austen WG, Wilkins EW, et al. (eds): Current Therapy in Cardiothoracic Surgery. Toronto, BC Decker

Johnsson P, Algotsson L, Ryding E, et al., 1991: Cardiopulmonary perfusion and cerebral blood flow in bilateral carotid disease. Ann Thorac Surg 51:579

Jones EL, 1991: Preparation of the internal mammary artery for coronary bypass surgery. J Cardiac Surg 6:326

Jones EL, Weintraub WS, Craver JS, et al., 1991: Coronary artery bypass surgery: Is the operation different today?. J Thorac Cardiovasc Surg 101:108

King SB, Talley JD, 1989: Coronary arteriography and percutaneous transluminal coronary angioplasty. Circulation 79(Suppl I):I-19

King SB, 1990: Prediction of acute closure in percutaneous transluminal coronary angioplasty. Circulation 81(Suppl IV):IV-5

Kirklin JW, Barratt-Boyes BG, 1993a: Stenotic arteriosclerotic coronary artery disease. In Cardiac Surgery. ed. 2. New York, Churchill Livingstone

Kirklin JW, Barratt-Boyes BG, 1993b: Left ventricular aneurysm. In Cardiac Surgery, ed. 2. New York, Churchill Livingstone

Kirklin JW, Barratt-Boyes BG, 1993c: Postinfarction ventricular septal defect. In Cardiac Surgery, ed. 2. New York, Churchill Livingstone

Komeda M, Fremes SE, David TE, 1990: Surgical repair of postinfarction ventricular septal defect. Circulation 82 (Suppl IV):IV-243

Livesay JJ, Cooley DA, 1991: The role and results of coronary endarterectomy. In Baue AE, Geha AS, Hammond GL, et al. (eds): Glenn's Thoracic and Cardiovascular Surgery, ed. 5. Norwalk, CT, Appleton & Lange

Lytle BW, Cosgrove DM, 1992: Graft patency and revascularization strategies. Curr Probl Surg 24:769

Lytle BW, Cosgrove DM, Loop FD, et al., 1986: Perioperative risk of bilateral internal mammary artery grafting: Analysis of 500 cases from 1971 to 1984. Circulation 74 (Suppl III):III-37

Lytle BW, Kramer JR, Golding LR, et al., 1984: Young adults with coronary atherosclerosis: 10 year results of surgical myocardial revascularization. J Am Coll Cardiol 4:445

Loop FD, 1990: Repeat coronary artery bypass grafting for myocardial ischemia. In Sabiston DC, Spencer FC (eds): Surgery of the Chest, ed. 5. Philadelphia, WB Saunders

Mills NL, 1991: Preparation of the internal mammary artery graft with intraluminal papaverine. J Cardiac Surg 6:318

Mills NL, Rigby CS, 1991: Techniques of coronary artery operations and reoperation. In Baue AE, Geha AS, Hammond GL, et al. (eds): Glenn's Thoracic and Cardiovascular Surgery, ed. 5. Norwalk, CT, Appleton & Lange

Morris JJ, Smith R, Glower DD, et al., 1990: Clinical evaluation of single versus multiple mammary artery bypass. Circulation 82 (Suppl IV):IV-214

Newman DC, Hicks RG, 1988: Combined carotid and coronary artery surgery: A review of the literature. Ann Thorac Surg 45:574

Pasternak RC, Braunwald E, Sobel BE, 1992: Acute myocardial infarction. In Braunwald E (ed): Heart Disease: A Textbook of Cardiovascular Medicine, ed. 4. Philadelphia, WB Saunders

Peigh PS, Disesa VJ, Collins JJ, Cohn LH, 1991: Coronary bypass grafting with totally calcified or acutely dissected ascending aorta. Ann Thorac Surg 51:102

Rankin JS, Smith LR, 1990: Utilization of the internal mammary arteries for coronary artery bypass. In Sabiston DC, Spencer FC (eds): Surgery of the Chest, ed. 5. Philadelphia, WB Saunders

Salomon NW, Page US, Bigelow JC, et al., 1991: Coronary artery bypass grafting in elderly patients. J Thorac Cardiovasc Surg 101:209

Siwek LG, Daggett WM, 1989: Myocardial protection. In Grillo HC, Austen WG, Wilkins EW Jr, et al. (eds): Current Therapy in Cardiothoracic Surgery. Toronto, BC Decker

Spencer FC, 1990: Bypass grafting for coronary artery disease. In Sabiston DC, Spencer FC (eds): Surgery of the Chest, ed. 5. Philadelphia, WB Saunders

Ulicny KS Jr, Hiratzka LF, 1991: The risk factors of median sternotomy infection: A current review. J Cardiac Surg 6:338

Veterans Administration Coronary Artery Bypass Surgery Cooperative Study Group, 1984: Eleven-year survival in the Veterans Administration Randomized Trial of Coronary Bypass Surgery for stable angina. N Engl J Med 311:133

16

SURGICAL TREATMENT OF VALVULAR HEART DISEASE

INDICATIONS FOR SURGICAL THERAPY
   Mitral Stenosis
   Mitral Regurgitation
   Aortic Regurgitation
   Aortic Stenosis
   Tricuspid Regurgitation
   Acute Valvular Dysfunction
TYPES OF SURGICAL PROCEDURES
   Valve Repair
   Valve Replacement

TYPES OF VALVULAR PROSTHESES
   Mechanical Prostheses
   Bioprostheses
POSTOPERATIVE CONSIDERATIONS
   Results of Valve Replacement
   Valve-Related Morbidity

Significant progress has occurred in surgical treatment of *valvular heart disease* (VHD). Most patients who undergo repair or replacement of damaged cardiac valves achieve increased survival and improved quality of life. Factors that have improved operative results include (1) refined techniques for repairing valves, (2) better design of valvular prostheses, (3) improved myocardial protection during cardiopulmonary bypass, (4) earlier operative intervention, (5) more sophisticated perioperative management, and (6) more closely controlled long-term anticoagulant therapy. Still, surgical therapy remains palliative, substituting a new disease state for the old. At 15 years after valve replacement, fewer than 50% of patients remain free of valve-related morbidity (Burdon et al., 1992).

Common causes of VHD include rheumatic endocarditis, infective endocarditis, congenital anomalies, and myxomatous degeneration. The functional abnormality of a diseased valve is either stenosis (narrowing of the orifice when the valve is open), regurgitation (incompetence when the valve is closed), or a combination of the two. Mitral valve disease is most prevalent, followed by aortic valve disease. The tricuspid valve is occasionally affected, usually secondary to mitral valve disease. Pulmonic valve disease is rare in adults. Mitral or aortic valve replacement comprise the majority of surgical procedures. Etiology, types of valvular lesions and their consequences, and nonsurgical therapies for VHD are discussed in detail in Chapter 2, Valvular Heart Disease.

INDICATIONS FOR SURGICAL THERAPY

In most forms of VHD, pathologic deterioration of the valve occurs gradually and the heart compensates for many years before surgical intervention is considered necessary. Optimal timing for repairing or replacing a cardiac valve depends on several factors, especially the specific valvular abnormality. With some lesions, signs and symptoms that warrant surgical intervention are well defined. With others, appropriate timing for surgical therapy is difficult to assess. It is advantageous to avoid operation and delay implantation of a prosthesis as long as possible. However, it is equally

Betsy Finkelmeier: CARDIOTHORACIC SURGICAL NURSING.
© 1995 J.B. Lippincott Company.

important to intervene early enough to avoid irreversible damage to the heart or pulmonary vasculature.

Most commonly, surgical therapy is prompted by evidence that valve dysfunction has begun to irreversibly damage one or both ventricles. For example, severe mitral or aortic regurgitation eventually produces irreversible left ventricular enlargement and failure. Less often, operative repair is recommended because the nature of the valvular lesion places the patient at risk for catastrophic consequences, such as sudden cardiac death from severe aortic stenosis or septic embolization from infected valvular vegetations. Indications for surgical correction of the most common valvular lesions are discussed below.

MITRAL STENOSIS

Mitral valve stenosis, which results predominantly from rheumatic fever, obstructs blood flow from the left atrium into the left ventricle. As a result, left atrial pressure becomes chronically elevated and the left atrium enlarges. Ten to 20% of patients develop pulmonary arterial hypertension (Schlant, 1991). Although the mechanism is not fully understood, it is thought to be related both to chronically elevated left atrial pressure and degenerative changes in the pulmonary arterioles. The time required for development of pulmonary artery hypertension and its severity vary greatly from patient to patient (Duran, 1991). In severe cases, systolic pulmonary artery pressure may be equal to or even greater than systolic arterial pressure. Right ventricular hypertrophy develops because of the elevated pulmonary vascular resistance or the afterload against which the ventricle must eject. Eventually, right-sided heart failure may occur.

Dyspnea is the most characteristic symptom of mitral stenosis, and episodes of pulmonary edema are common. Chronic atrial fibrillation, or less commonly atrial flutter, usually develops secondary to atrial enlargement. Stasis of blood along the walls of the fibrillating left atrium predisposes to thrombus formation and the possibility of systemic embolization. Although the left ventricle is protected against volume or pressure overload by the stenotic mitral valve, it probably does not remain normal. Characteristic symptoms of fatigue and progressive exercise intolerance are typically attributed to increased pulmonary blood flow, but they may also be related to the left ventricle's inability to appropriately increase cardiac output in response to increased metabolic demand.

Invasive therapy for relief of mitral stenosis is prompted by the degree of disabling symptoms. A procedure to relieve stenosis is usually recommended when the patient's New York Heart Association (NYHA) functional status deteriorates to class II or III or if symptoms of right-sided heart failure develop. However, systemic embolism, particularly to the brain, is a serious potential consequence of left atrial enlargement. Because its occurrence cannot be pre-

dicted, it is the primary reason for early invasive treatment to relieve mitral stenosis (Spencer, 1990).

It may also be preferable to correct mitral stenosis while the patient is still in normal sinus rhythm. Because atrial fibrillation reduces cardiac output and increases left atrial pressure, it accelerates the patient's downward course (Kirklin & Barratt-Boyes, 1993a). Symptoms are exacerbated, and the risk of systemic thromboembolism increases (Duran, 1991). After years of atrial distention and atrial fibrillation, a return of normal sinus rhythm is unlikely even after valvular repair or replacement. The increased pulmonary vascular resistance often associated with mitral stenosis is usually at least partially reversible after valve repair or replacement. Accordingly, pulmonary hypertension in adults with mitral stenosis is not a contraindication to surgical therapy (Spencer, 1990).

MITRAL REGURGITATION

Chronic *mitral regurgitation* may result from rheumatic endocarditis, left ventricular dilatation, ischemic damage to the subvalvular apparatus, or mitral valve prolapse. Regurgitation of blood through the incompetent valve during systole causes increased volume and pressure in the left atrium with resultant left atrial enlargement. As the ventricle pumps more forcefully to maintain adequate forward flow, left ventricular hypertrophy and dilatation develop as well. Symptoms, which are similar to those of mitral stenosis, develop late in the course of mitral regurgitation.

Ideally, surgical intervention to correct mitral regurgitation is performed early enough to preserve normal left ventricular function. Once the ventricle undergoes substantial dilatation, muscle function becomes permanently damaged despite correction of the valvular abnormality. Precise timing of operation to achieve this goal is difficult because the onset of irreversible muscle damage is not predictable. Medications, such as captopril, that reduce afterload and promote forward flow from the left ventricle may produce symptomatic improvement in patients with mitral regurgitation. However, they may not protect the ventricle from progressive dilatation. Therefore, the ventricle may become irreversibly damaged despite the lack of disabling symptoms.

AORTIC REGURGITATION

Aortic regurgitation is most often due to rheumatic endocarditis, but it may also develop secondary to conditions that dilate the valve annulus or damage valve leaflets, such as ascending aortic aneurysm, aortic dissection, or Marfan's syndrome. Aortic regurgitation subjects the left ventricle to increased volume and pressure as a portion of each stroke volume is regurgitated during diastole. Initially, the left ventricle hypertrophies and systemic vascular resistance decreases to maintain adequate forward flow. Eventually, however, the left ventricle dilates and loses the ability to contract effectively. Ejection fraction decreases, and symptoms of left-sided heart failure develop.

Because of the irreversible left ventricular damage that eventually occurs, there is a trend toward earlier valve replacement for aortic regurgitation. Surgical therapy is recommended for aortic regurgitation that produces symptoms (e.g., dyspnea on exertion or angina) (Massimiano & Hammond, 1991). In asymptomatic patients with moderate or severe aortic regurgitation, operative therapy is considered when left ventricular enlargement is suggested by radiographic evidence (an enlarged cardiac silhouette) or electrocardiographic changes (increased voltage and a strain pattern in left ventricular leads).

AORTIC STENOSIS

Aortic stenosis, defined as obstruction to left ventricular outflow, can occur at a subvalvular, valvular, or supravalvular level. In adults, it is nearly always due to a valvular abnormality, often a congenitally bicuspid valve or one that has undergone calcific degeneration. Typical features of aortic stenosis in adults are calcification of the valve, a diminished valve area, and a significant transvalvular gradient that is necessary to maintain adequate forward flow (Massimiano & Hammond, 1991). The left ventricle hypertrophies to generate sufficient pressure to eject blood through the narrowed valve orifice. As a result, left ventricular damage is a prominent feature of severe aortic stenosis. Diastolic filling of the ventricle is impaired, and the ventricle eventually dilates, leading to systolic impairment and symptoms of left-sided heart failure. In addition, severe aortic stenosis is associated with an increased incidence of ventricular arrhythmias, conduction disturbances, and sudden cardiac death.

Characteristic symptoms of aortic stenosis (i.e., angina, dyspnea, and syncope) occur late in the course of the disease. Onset of symptoms is associated with a limited life expectancy unless the valvular stenosis is relieved. Therefore, surgical intervention is undertaken when significant aortic stenosis begins to produce symptoms. Even in elderly (eighth and ninth decade) patients, aortic valve replacement is often recommended because prognosis with medical therapy is so poor. Because of the risk of sudden cardiac death, valve replacement may also be recommended for severe aortic stenosis (valve area less than 0.7 cm^2 or gradient greater than 80 mm Hg) in patients without symptoms.

TRICUSPID REGURGITATION

Isolated *tricuspid regurgitation* is uncommon. However, acquired tricuspid regurgitation develops in 22% to 30% of patients with mitral valve disease (Abe et al., 1989). Less commonly, it occurs secondary to aortic valve disease. Right ventricular enlargement and progressive symptoms of right-sided heart failure result from an incompetent tricuspid valve. Surgical intervention is usually undertaken when diagnostic studies suggest impending irreversible right ventricular failure. However, surgical treatment for tricuspid regurgitation is not straightforward. Although tricuspid regurgitation, like other types of valvular incompetence, tends to progress, deleterious effects of ventricular volume overload on the right side of the heart develop more slowly than on the left side (Kirklin & Barratt-Boyes, 1993b). Controversy exists about the necessity of correcting tricuspid regurgitation, whether valve repair or replacement is preferable, and which type of repair or prosthesis is optimal (McGrath et al., 1990).

ACUTE VALVULAR DYSFUNCTION

Most forms of VHD are associated with slowly progressive valvular dysfunction. However, in some forms, valve dysfunction can develop precipitously. *Acute mitral regurgitation* occurs most often secondary to ischemic heart disease. Dysfunction or rupture of a papillary muscle or annular dilatation associated with myocardial infarction may lead to acute valvular incompetence. In contrast to chronic mitral regurgitation, compensatory mechanisms to protect the heart have not developed. Pulmonary edema or frank cardiogenic shock typically occur as a manifestation of acute left ventricular failure. Intra-aortic balloon counterpulsation is frequently necessary to support cardiac function. Papillary muscle ischemia is sometimes effectively treated with revascularization therapies (thrombolytic therapy, percutaneous transluminal coronary angioplasty, or coronary artery bypass grafting). Papillary muscle rupture or annular dilatation usually requires emergent valve repair or replacement to restore valvular competence.

Acute aortic regurgitation may also occur, most often related to aortic dissection. The sudden volume and pressure overload of the left ventricle produces acute left ventricular failure. In contrast to cardiogenic shock from other causes, that due to acute aortic regurgitation cannot be treated with intra-aortic balloon counterpulsation because balloon inflations would increase regurgitant flow through the incompetent aortic valve. Emergent surgical intervention is usually necessary if the patient is to survive.

Acute dysfunction of any of the cardiac valves may be caused by *infective endocarditis*. In individuals who abuse intravenous drugs, it is the right-sided tricuspid valve that is most commonly infected by venous contamination. Most cases of infective endocarditis in intravenous drug abusers are due to *Staphylococcus aureus;* in individuals who are not drug abusers, infective endocarditis is most commonly caused by streptococci (Korzeniowski & Kaye, 1992).

In 80% to 90% of cases, infective endocarditis of native cardiac valves can be effectively treated with an extensive course of organism specific antibiotic therapy (Hendren et al., 1992). However, surgical therapy may be the only effective treatment in patients infected by particularly virulent organisms or with extensive valvular damage. For example, severe ventricular failure may result from leaflet or chordae tendineae destruction. Survival is unlikely unless valvular competence is restored. In addition, vegetations may form on valvular tissue and provide a source of recurring septic emboli. Although the mere presence of a vegetation is not an indication for surgical intervention, embolization of vegetative tissue is common. Twenty to 40% of patients with infective endocarditis of left-sided cardiac valves develop embolic neurologic complications (Ting et al., 1991).

Optimal timing for surgical therapy in patients with infective endocarditis is difficult to determine. Patients are usually gravely ill with hemodynamic instability and multisystem organ dysfunction (Larbalestier et al., 1992). Ideally, a full course (usually 6 weeks) of antibiotic therapy is given preoperatively. Sterilization of the native valve before implantation of prosthetic material substantially increases the likelihood of curing the infection, which is extremely difficult to eradicate once a valvular prosthesis is implanted. However, depending on virulence of the organism, the degree of valvular destruction, and the development of vegetations, it may become necessary to perform urgent valve replacement before completion of the antibiotic course.

Indications for proceeding urgently with removal of an infected valve and implantation of a valvular prosthesis include congestive heart failure due to acute valvular regurgitation, persistent fevers or septic shock despite appropriate antibiotic therapy, or evidence of recurrent embolization from the infected valve. Most surgeons also advocate prompt surgical intervention in patients who develop complete heart block because it suggests intramyocardial extension of the infection. Extension of infection beyond the valve may lead to frank abscess formation, false aneurysm, fistula, or ventricular septal defect (Haydock et al., 1992).

If septic cerebral embolization has occurred, determining timing of operative therapy is particularly challenging. Although removal of the infected valve is desirable to avoid recurrent embolization, cardiopulmonary bypass with systemic anticoagulation in a patient with recent stroke imposes the risk of cerebral hemorrhagic infarction. The major risk factor for perioperative stroke in such patients appears to be the preoperative presence of a hemorrhagic as opposed to an ischemic cerebral infarction (Ting et al., 1991).

TYPES OF SURGICAL PROCEDURES

The decision about whether to repair or replace a diseased valve depends most importantly on the specific nature of valve pathology. However, other fac-

TABLE 16-1. SURGICAL THERAPY FOR VALVULAR HEART DISEASE

Valvular Lesion	Corrective Procedure
Mitral stenosis*	Commissurotomy
	Mitral valve replacement
Mitral regurgitation	Valvuloplasty
	Mitral valve replacement
Aortic stenosis†	Aortic valve replacement
Aortic regurgitation	Aortic valve replacement
Tricuspid regurgitation	Valvuloplasty
	Tricuspid valve replacement

* Also treated with balloon valvotomy.
† Rarely treated with balloon valvotomy.

tors, such as the patient's age, clinical status, and associated medical problems must also be taken into consideration. A variety of techniques are available for repairing and replacing cardiac valves. Available options for the surgical management of common valvular lesions are displayed in Table 16-1.

VALVE REPAIR

The repair of cardiac valves dates to the beginning of the surgical treatment of heart disease. Salvage of a native cardiac valve is attractive because currently available valvular prostheses are associated with significant long-term complications. Also, valve repair usually obviates the need for chronic anticoagulation, which is necessary with all mechanical valvular prostheses.

An additional advantage of reparative procedures that salvage the mitral valve is preservation of the subvalvular apparatus. The chordae tendineae anchor the anterior and posterior leaflets of the mitral valve to the papillary muscles arising from the ventricular endocardium. This supportive apparatus exerts tension during ventricular relaxation, allowing the valve to actively open during diastole. Subvalvular structures are also thought to augment ventricular contraction during systole. Thus, mitral valve repair is less compromising to left ventricular function than is mitral valve replacement.

Types of reparative procedures are balloon valvotomy, commissurotomy, and surgical valvuloplasty. *Balloon valvotomy* (also called *balloon valvuloplasty*) and *commissurotomy* are performed to correct pure valvular stenosis. Both involve splitting open fused valve commissures to widen a stenotic valve orifice and are performed most often in patients with mitral stenosis. They are appropriate only in specific situations, determined by the particular anatomy and degree of damage to a native cardiac valve. Factors that favor successful repair of a stenotic mitral valve include young age, no previous procedure on the valve, normal sinus rhythm, absence of calcium on the valve, absence of thrombus in the left atrial appendage, and no regurgitation. Cardiac valves that are heavily calcified or that are both stenotic and insufficient are not suitable for these procedures. Balloon valvotomy is not a surgical procedure but rather is performed during cardiac catheterization. Although it offers several advantages, larger clinical trials are necessary to better define its role in treatment of VHD. It is described in more detail in Chapter 2, Valvular Heart Disease.

A commissurotomy is the surgical incision of valve commissures to relieve stenosis. *Mitral commissurotomy* has been performed for more than 30 years and remains a mainstay in treatment of mitral stenosis throughout the world. Before development of adequate cardiopulmonary bypass, mitral commissurotomy was performed as a "closed" procedure without the aid of extracorporeal circulation. The surgeon inserted a finger through a small opening in the left atrium and, guided only by palpation of the valve, blindly fractured the commissures with a finger or with an instrument inserted through the left ventricle. Mitral commissurotomy is now routinely performed as an "open" procedure. After initiating cardiopulmonary bypass, the left atrium is opened and the valve is repaired under direct visualization. When performed as an open procedure, the results are quite predictable and operative risk is low. Surgical repair of mitral stenosis sometimes includes more than simple division of the commissures. In complex cases, the procedure is more appropriately called a *surgical valvuloplasty*. In addition to the commissurotomy itself, it may be necessary for the surgeon to free or tease apart scarred chordae tendineae, split papillary muscles, or implant a supportive prosthetic ring in the valve annulus.

More often, surgical valvuloplasty describes a reparative procedure to correct mitral regurgitation. Early attempts to repair regurgitant valves were rarely successful. However, Carpentier, Duran, and others have introduced techniques that result in more satisfactory and predictable results. Because of the prevalence of mitral valve disease, most surgical experience is with mitral valvuloplasty.

Feasibility of valve repair for mitral regurgitation is dependent on underlying valvular pathology. Mitral regurgitation secondary to degenerative disease is most suited to a reparative procedure because, in contrast to rheumatic pathology, pure regurgitation is often present. In centers where mitral valvuloplasty is routinely performed, repair may be possible in as many as 95% of patients with degenerative valve disease, 75% of those with ischemic valvular disease, and 70% of those with rheumatic valvular disease (Deloche et al., 1990). Although valves damaged by infective endocarditis usually require replacement, recent success has been reported with reconstruction of mitral valves for treatment of mitral valve endocarditis (Hendren et al., 1992).

Satisfactory valvuloplasty necessitates thorough intraoperative assessment of functional pathology of the native valve. The mitral valve is a complex, dynamically integrated structure, and incompetence may be due to abnormalities of the leaflets, chordae

tendineae, papillary muscles, annulus, or a combination of these. Intraoperative transesophageal echocardiography is used to quantify the degree of regurgitation and determine the precise functional anatomy. Valvular regurgitation may be due to increased leaflet motion (i.e., leaflet prolapse) or restricted leaflet movement. The subvalvular structures (the chordae tendineae and papillary muscles) may be elongated, redundant, or ruptured. Dilatation of the annulus is also common.

Valve reconstruction is tailored to the identified problems. Techniques have been designed to restore normal anatomy and function to all components of the valve apparatus. For example, excessive leaflet tissue may be resected. Elongated chordae may be shortened by incising a papillary muscle and imbricating it with the elongated chordae (Fig. 16-1). In the case of posterior leaflet chordal rupture, a portion of the leaflet may be resected (Fig. 16-2). Annular dilatation is treated by tightening the annulus, usually with placement of a supportive ring to remodel annular shape without reducing orifice size.

Although these procedures can be more technically complex and necessitate longer operative time than valve replacement, many surgeons prefer to attempt valve repair. Operative results, late survival, and late valve durability obtained with mitral valve reconstruction are equal or superior to those obtained with mitral valve replacement (Galloway et al., 1988). Cardiothoracic surgeons experienced in valvuloplasty have been able to salvage native mitral valves with increasingly innovative techniques (David et al., 1991). However, for valves requiring complex reparative procedures, limited information is available about long-term durability and many surgeons continue to replace the valve, using a mechanical valve or tissue bioprosthesis.

Less commonly, valvuloplasty is performed on the tricuspid valve. Tricuspid regurgitation is often due to annular dilatation secondary to left-sided VHD. If untreated at the time of mitral or aortic valve replacement, it generally persists or progresses and may lead to heart or liver failure (Minale et al., 1990). Tricuspid regurgitation may often be corrected by implantation of a prosthetic ring to support the valve annulus. Because atrioventricular conduction tissue runs through the annulus of the tricuspid valve, complete heart block can result from suturing in close proximity to conduction tissue during the repair.

Reparative procedures for aortic regurgitation are unusual. Repair is occasionally possible in an aortic valve with an isolated perforation of one of the leaflets and no annular dilatation, calcification, or gradient indicative of aortic stenosis. In such an unusual situation, it may be possible to patch the leaflet with glutaraldehyde-treated pericardium to salvage the native valve. Pericardium is very durable and is able to withstand the systemic pressure to which the aortic valve and root are subjected. Repair of an incompetent aortic valve is also possible in some cases of regurgitation secondary to ascending aortic aneu-

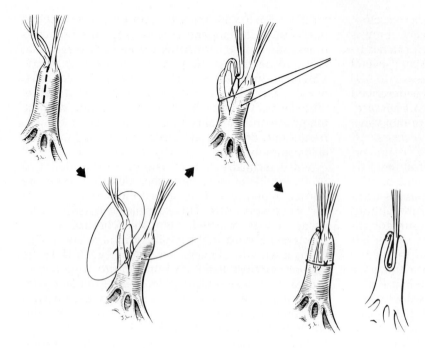

FIGURE 16-1. Diagrammatic representation of chordal shortening to correct mitral regurgitation. After incision of the papillary muscle, the elongated chordae tendinae is drawn into the incised area and sutured in place, thus reducing the length of the chordae by twice the depth of the incision. (Cosgrove DM, 1989: Mitral valve repair in patients with elongated chordae tendineae. J Cardiac Surg 4:250)

rysm or dissection. If the aortic valve itself is normal and regurgitation is caused only by annular distortion from aortic pathology, it may be possible to resuspend the aortic valve and restore competence.

The possibility of delaying or avoiding altogether the need for valve replacement is clearly advantageous. Many patients receive excellent palliation and never require implantation of a valvular prosthesis. Actuarial studies show a lesser risk of thromboembolism and other prosthesis-related complications. Long-term anticoagulation can be avoided. The risk

of reoperation appears to be as low or lower than that for patients with valve replacement.

All of the reparative procedures are associated with potential complications. The primary complication of valvuloplasty is breakdown of the repair, resulting in *acute valvular insufficiency*. The complication is usually detected by acute onset of congestive heart failure and a new murmur. Reoperation and implantation of a valvular prosthesis is required. In a small percentage of patients who undergo mitral valvuloplasty, *systolic anterior motion (SAM)* of the anterior

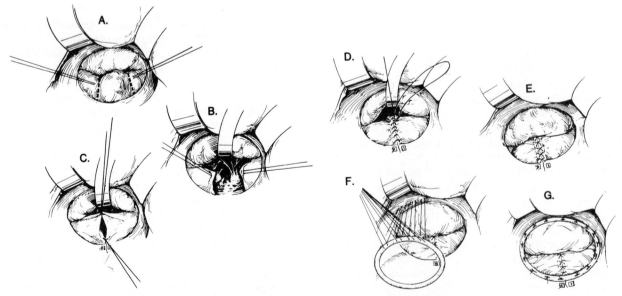

FIGURE 16-2. (**A** through **C**) Initial steps in quadrilateral resection of the mitral valve posterior leaflet to correct mitral regurgitation (**D** through **G**) Completion of mitral valvuloplasty with insertion of prosthetic annuloplasty ring. (Cohn LH, Disesa VJ, Couper GS, et al, 1989: Mitral valve repair for degeneration and prolapse of the mitral valve. J Thorac Cardiovasc Surg 98:988)

leaflet of the mitral valve occurs, causing obstruction of the left ventricular outflow tract. Most often, systolic anterior motion does not produce symptoms but rather is detected by intraoperative or postoperative echocardiography and the presence of a systolic murmur. More severe cases are associated with significant dynamic left ventricular outflow tract obstruction, similar to that occurring in patients with idiopathic subaortic hypertrophic stenosis. Treatment of the two conditions is similar and includes administration of beta-adrenergic blocking agents and avoidance of beta-adrenergic receptor agonists (epinephrine or dobutamine), vasodilatation, diuresis, and cardiac glycosides (Grossi et al., 1992). Systolic anterior motion is usually a self-limiting syndrome.

Valvulectomy (i.e., removal of a valve without implantation of a prosthesis) is a procedure occasionally performed for infective endocarditis of the tricuspid valve (Arbulu et al., 1991). Most tricuspid endocarditis occurs in young adult drug abusers who have no underlying heart disease. Such patients generally tolerate tricuspid regurgitation that is produced by absence of the tricuspid valve. Valvulectomy avoids the necessity for placing prosthetic material in a patient in whom there is significant risk of infecting the new prosthesis.

Some patients who undergo tricuspid valvulectomy experience postoperative symptoms of right-sided heart failure and eventually require implantation of a tricuspid prosthesis. However, if a new prosthesis is implanted electively after the infection has been cured, the risk of prosthetic valve endocarditis is substantially reduced. Alternatively, if the valvular abnormality is limited to the presence of a vegetation, it may be possible to resect the vegetation from the valve leaflet and perform a reconstructive procedure, leaving a competent, native valve.

VALVE REPLACEMENT

Despite advances in reparative techniques, valve replacement is necessary in the majority of patients who require surgical therapy for VHD. The era of cardiac valve replacement began in the early 1950s when Hufnagel implanted a caged ball prosthesis in the descending thoracic aorta to treat aortic regurgitation (Austen, 1989). Successful aortic valve replacement in its native anatomic position and mitral valve replacement were accomplished in 1960 by Harken and Starr, respectively (Hildenberg & Austen, 1989). Since that time, thousands of valve replacement operations have been performed using a variety of mechanical and biologic tissue valves.

Almost all surgical procedures on cardiac valves are performed through a median sternotomy incision. Rarely, reoperative procedures on the mitral valve are performed through a left thoracotomy incision to avoid potential injury of cardiac structures during repeat sternotomy. Using cardiopulmonary bypass, the aorta (aortic valve replacement), left

atrium (mitral valve replacement), right atrium (tricuspid valve replacement), or pulmonary artery (pulmonic valve replacement) is opened and the native valve excised. An appropriately sized valvular prosthesis is selected by measuring the native annulus using a sizing instrument. A series of sutures are placed around the circumference of the native annulus and through the corresponding location on the sewing ring of the prosthesis. The valvular prosthesis is then positioned in the annulus and the sutures tied (Fig. 16-3).

In patients undergoing *mitral valve replacement* for mitral regurgitation, consideration is given to preservation of the native subvalvular apparatus, especially if left ventricular function is significantly impaired. Mitral valve replacement causes deterioration of left ventricular function in the early postoperative period because afterload is acutely increased by restoring mitral valve competence. If a decision is made to preserve subvalvular structures, caution must be taken in prosthesis selection and implantation technique to ensure that native chordae tendineae do not impede proper prosthesis function. Proper sizing of a mitral prosthesis is also imperative to achieving optimal hemodynamic performance. A prosthesis that is excessively large may compromise left ventricular contraction; one that is too small may produce an unacceptably large transvalvular gradient.

An unusual but usually lethal complication of mitral valve replacement is *left ventricular rupture* secondary to disruption of the left atrioventricular groove. The injury is estimated to occur in approximately 1% of patients who undergo mitral valve replacement (Karlson et al., 1988). It is more likely in women and in patients with small left ventricles (Kirklin & Barratt-Boyes, 1993a). The defect generally becomes apparent within minutes after discontinuation of cardiopulmonary bypass or within hours of operation when the patient develops massive bleeding and hypotension. When left ventricular rupture becomes apparent, emergent surgical repair is attempted, using cardiopulmonary bypass to arrest and decompress the heart and to maximize exposure. Occasionally late ventricular rupture occurs, leading to the development of a left ventricular false aneurysm (Karlson et al., 1988).

During *aortic valve replacement*, the conventional antegrade technique of administering cardioplegic solution into the aortic root to enhance myocardial protection is not possible. Alternatively, cardioplegic solution is delivered directly into each of the coronary artery ostia or in a retrograde fashion into a catheter placed through the right atrium into the coronary sinus. Special techniques may be necessary during aortic valve replacement if the aortic root is extremely small or heavily calcified. It is important to select a prosthesis with the greatest effective orifice to sewing ring ratio. In extreme cases, it may be necessary to perform an *aortoplasty*, or enlargement of the aortic root with a synthetic patch, in addition to aortic valve replacement. Aortic valve replacement in combina-

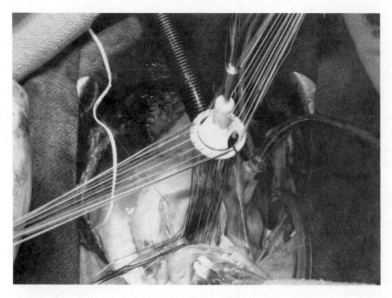

FIGURE 16-3. Implantation of a St. Jude aortic valve prosthesis. Photograph is taken from above the patient's head, looking downward into the aortic root. The native valve has been excised, and sutures have been placed around the circumference of the aortic valve annulus and the sewing ring of the prosthesis.

tion with replacement of the ascending aorta is discussed in Chapter 17, Surgery on the Thoracic Aorta.

Aortic valve replacement may be complicated by (1) inadequate debridement of annular calcium resulting in perivalvular leaks, (2) vigorous debridement resulting in aortic or left ventricular perforation or interruption of conduction pathways, (3) detachment of the mitral valve anterior leaflet during aortic valve excision, (4) heart block from sutures placed in or around the bundle of His, (5) occlusion of the coronary artery ostia by the prosthesis sewing ring, and (6) lodging of detached calcium in the left coronary artery or left ventricle with subsequent embolization (Massimiano & Hammond, 1991). Ensuring removal of all air from the aorta, left ventricle, and coronary arteries is extremely important after opening the left atrium or aorta to replace the mitral or aortic valve, respectively. Air remaining in the systemic circulation can produce catastrophic embolization when cardiopulmonary bypass is discontinued and the heart is allowed to eject.

Multiple valve replacement is sometimes necessary. Rheumatic and, rarely, endocarditic damage of multiple valves can occur. In addition, mitral or tricuspid regurgitation due to annular dilatation may develop secondary to chronic ventricular enlargement caused by the dysfunction of another valve. When multiple prostheses are necessary, selection of the type of prostheses to be used is partially based on technical considerations of implantation. Mechanical valves are more likely to be selected because of their durability and to avoid the significant risk of reoperation in these patients. Multiple valve replacement procedures require a longer duration of cardiopulmonary bypass and more dissection in the area of the conduction system. In addition, patients who require multiple valve replacement usually have more underlying ventricular dysfunction. Accordingly, double or triple valve replacement is associated with a higher operative mortality and a greater risk of postoperative heart

block, bleeding, and low cardiac output. Valve replacement for infective endocarditis necessitates special techniques to debride all infected material. Some surgeons bathe the endocardial surfaces with antibiotic solution before implanting the valvular prosthesis. If the prosthetic material becomes infected, it is almost impossible to sterilize and death due to intramyocardial infection follows. There is some controversy regarding the best type of valvular prosthesis to implant in patients with active endocarditis. Data suggest that allograft valves are more resistant to recurrent infection when used for aortic valve replacement in patients with active infective endocarditis (Haydock et al., 1992).

TYPES OF VALVULAR PROSTHESES

A variety of artificial prostheses are available for replacement of native valves (Table 16-2; Fig. 16-4). Some prostheses, such as the St. Jude Medical, the Starr-Edwards, and the Medtronic-Hall, are mechanical, constructed of synthetic materials. Others, such as the Carpentier-Edwards or Hancock porcine,

---

TABLE 16-2. SELECTED CARDIAC VALVULAR PROSTHESES

Mechanical

St. Jude Medical
Starr-Edwards
Medtronic-Hall

Tissue

Carpentier-Edwards (porcine)
Hancock (porcine)
Allograft (human cadaver)
Edwards-Shiley (bovine pericardial)

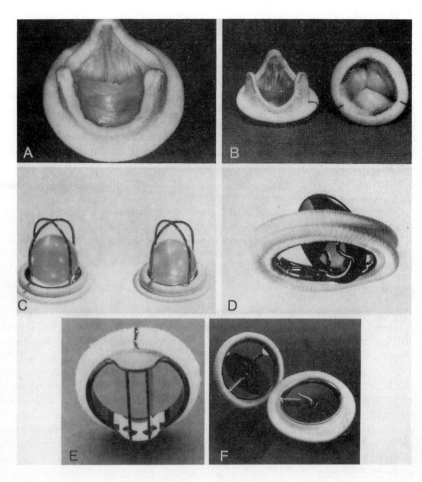

FIGURE 16-4. Types of cardiac valvular prostheses. The two most commonly implanted bioprostheses are the Hancock porcine bioprosthesis **(A)** and the Carpentier-Edwards porcine bioprosthesis **(B)**. Mechanical prostheses include the Starr-Edwards **(C)**, Bjork-Shiley **(D)**, St. Jude **(E)**, and Medtronic-Hall **(F)** prostheses. (Gray RJ, Matloff JM, 1990: Follow-up after valve replacement. In Medical Management of the Cardiac Surgical Patient, p. 339. Baltimore, Williams & Wilkins)

Edwards pericardial, and human cadaver allograft valves, are made of biologic animal or human tissue. The most important characteristics of any of the valvular prostheses are (1) minimal impedance to forward flow when open and no regurgitation when closed, (2) proper opening and closing in response to changes in pressure gradient, (3) nonthrombogenicity, (4) biocompatibility (i.e., lack of rejection and trauma to blood elements), (5) durability, (6) ease of insertion, and (7) inaudibility (Weiland, 1983, Bonchek, 1987; Hildenberg & Austen, 1989).

No currently available prosthesis achieves all of these objectives. Each has features that makes it more or less suited for a given clinical situation. Therefore, the decision about the specific prosthesis to implant in an individual patient is based on a number of factors, including patient age, associated medical problems, underlying cardiac pathology, life-style, and aptitude for compliance. In women who desire a future pregnancy, valve selection is complicated by two factors: (1) a hypercoagulable state accompanies pregnancy, and (2) anticoagulation with warfarin sodium therapy is contraindicated during pregnancy because of fetal wastage, fetal hemorrhage, and fetal malformations caused by the teratogenic effects of warfarin compounds (Badduke et al., 1991).

The most important determination in valve selection is whether to implant a mechanical or biopros-

thetic valve (Table 16-3). The principal differences between mechanical valves and bioprostheses are durability and thrombogenicity characteristics. Mechanical valves are more durable but are more thrombo-

---

TABLE 16-3. RATIONALE FOR PROSTHESIS SELECTION

Patients Likely to Receive Mechanical Prostheses

Children
Young adults (except childbearing women)
Patients with renal failure
Patients with small valvular annulus
Patients with high reoperative risk
Patients with another indication for anticoagulation (e.g., atrial fibrillation)
Patients requiring aortic root replacement

Patients Likely to Receive Tissue Prostheses

Elderly patients in whom long-term durability is less important
Persons in whom chronic anticoagulation is ill advised:
  History of major bleeding episode
  Anticipated future pregnancy
  Demonstrated noncompliance with medical therapy (drug abuser, alcoholic)
  Life-style with high risk for trauma
  Advanced age (potential for dosage error or fall)
Patients at increased risk for thromboembolism

genic and necessitate anticoagulation. Bioprostheses (i.e., biologic valvular prostheses) do not necessitate chronic anticoagulant therapy but are likely to degenerate, necessitating subsequent reoperation. Comparison of mechanical and bioprosthetic valves at 10 years reveals that in the long term, the risk of primary valve failure in bioprostheses is counterbalanced by the risk of anticoagulant-related hemorrhage and perivalvular regurgitation in mechanical valves; survival and overall freedom from valve-related complications at 10 years are similar whether a bioprosthetic or mechanical valve is implanted (Hammermeister et al., 1991a, 1991b). Older patients (>65 years) have a greater risk of valve-related complications with mechanical prostheses, whereas younger patients (<40 years) are at greater risk with bioprostheses (Jamieson, 1993).

MECHANICAL PROSTHESES

Mechanical valves account for approximately 60% of prostheses implanted in patients in the United States and worldwide (Akins, 1991). Mechanical prostheses commonly implanted in patients in the United States include the St. Jude Medical, Starr-Edwards, and Medtronic-Hall. All of these valves have one of three basic design types: (1) bileaflet, (2) caged ball, or (3) tilting disc. The *St. Jude Medical valve* is the most commonly implanted valvular prosthesis. Available since 1977, it has a bileaflet, low-profile design that provides central flow and excellent hemodynamic performance characteristics (Czer et al., 1990). Bileaflet valves are least obstructive to forward flow, especially when a small valve size is required; however, they also have the highest regurgitation fraction (Whittlesey & Geha, 1991).

The *Starr-Edwards valve* has a caged-ball design (i.e., a cage attached to the sewing ring that houses a ball inside). The ball rests on the sewing ring when the valve is in a closed position and moves forward into the cage as a pressure gradient forces the valve open (Whitman, 1987). Various models have been in use since 1961 and have displayed excellent durability. Caged ball valves produce more turbulent flow due to central obstruction by the ball itself; the valve may also partially obstruct the ventricular outflow tract when used in the mitral position due to its high profile (Whittlesey & Geha, 1991). The *Medtronic-Hall valve* has a cageless, tilting-disc design. It also has excellent durability and less obstruction to forward flow than caged-ball valves.

The predominant concern with any of the mechanical prostheses is thromboembolism. Two factors predispose to thrombosis when a large foreign surface is in contact with the bloodstream: (1) turbulence, shearing forces, stagnation, and eddy currents trigger the release of biochemical factors that evoke clotting; and (2) valve materials themselves may precipitate thrombosis (Hildenberg & Austen, 1989). Because of the potential for thromboembolism, long-term anti-

coagulation with warfarin sodium is recommended in patients with all currently available mechanical prostheses (Stein et al., 1992). In the event that oral anticoagulation is discontinued, such as before a planned operation or if the patient is unable to take oral medications, intravenous heparin is necessary. If a patient with a mechanical prosthesis develops gastrointestinal bleeding or another contraindication to chronic anticoagulation, elective replacement of the prosthesis may become necessary. All of the mechanical valves cause some hemolysis, but it is usually not clinically significant (Whittlesey & Geha, 1991).

BIOPROSTHESES

Bioprosthetic heart valves are made from animal or human tissue that has been processed to make it biologically inert. Most common among the bioprostheses is the porcine valve, constructed from the aortic valve of a pig and preserved with glutaraldehyde. Less commonly used are human cadaver aortic valves (i.e., allografts) and bovine pericardial valves. Biologic tissue valves are attractive because of their lower propensity for thromboembolic complications as compared with mechanical prostheses.

Porcine valves have been used extensively since the early 1970s. Except in small sizes, they have hemodynamic characteristics that are comparable to mechanical prostheses (Hartz et al., 1986). In the smallest sizes porcine valves may provide significant obstruction to forward flow due to the large sewing ring. Porcine valves are often implanted in patients in whom it is desirable to avoid chronic anticoagulation (i.e., elderly persons, women in child-bearing years, and those with a medical contraindication to anticoagulation). The low rate of serious thromboembolism and virtual lack of valve thrombosis eliminate the necessity of long-term anticoagulation with its associated risk of related hemorrhagic complications (Jamieson et al., 1990). However, thromboembolism can occur with bioprostheses, particularly during the first postoperative month and in the presence of atrial fibrillation or low cardiac output (Whittlesey & Geha, 1991). The major drawback to porcine valves is the well-documented incidence of valve failure, particularly in young patients. Primary valve degeneration can be expected at 10 years in 73% of patients younger than 30 years of age at time of implantation, in 23% of patients aged 30 to 59 years, and in 17% of patients aged 60 years or older (Jamieson et al., 1988).

Primary valve failure occurs more frequently in mitral bioprostheses (28% at 10 years) than in aortic bioprostheses (21%) (Jamieson et al., 1990). The reasons why bioprostheses in the mitral position are more susceptible to structural dysfunction than those in the aortic position remain undetermined. Structural valve deterioration of mitral bioprostheses also appears to be accelerated in women, although the responsible mechanism has not been identified (Burdon et al., 1992).

In most cases, valve degeneration occurs gradually, owing to leaflet calcification and fibrosis (Fig. 16-5). Occasionally, acute leaflet rupture causes precipitous valve failure. Aside from the durability problem, the valve itself is rarely a cause of mortality, thromboembolism, or permanent morbidity. Bioprostheses are therefore best suited for use in the aortic position in elderly patients because chronic anticoagulation is not necessary and the prosthesis is likely to remain durable for the remainder of the patient's natural life span. Bioprostheses are seldom implanted in persons younger than 60 years of age (except in women who desire pregnancy), those who have experienced degeneration of a previous bioprosthesis, or those who require anticoagulation for another reason. Young persons who do receive tissue prostheses will almost certainly require a subsequent cardiac operation.

An *allograft aortic valve* or *homograft* is harvested from a human cadaver heart. Although most commonly used for valve replacement in children, in some centers they are also considered the prosthesis of choice for replacement of the aortic valve in adults (Kirklin & Barratt-Boyes, 1993c). Allografts are obtained from organ donors in whom the heart is unsuitable for transplantation but the cardiac valves are satisfactory. The aortic valve is harvested with a portion of the surrounding aorta and cryopreserved (i.e., ultrafrozen using liquid nitrogen) for long-term storage. The donor valve is matched to a recipient by size and ABO blood type. The need for ABO typing is controversial because it is unclear whether any living cells remain after cryopreservation. For the same reason, postoperative immunosuppression, as would be administered after organ transplantation, is generally not considered necessary after allograft implantation.

Allografts, like other bioprostheses, have a low incidence of thromboembolism, negating the need for chronic anticoagulant therapy (Massimiano & Hammond, 1991). Although long-term data are limited, durability appears good and failure occurs gradually without precipitous hemodynamic compromise. Allograft aortic valves are not well suited for aortic valve replacement in patients in whom the ascending aorta is diffusely enlarged and thin walled, and in the presence of severe systemic hypertension (Kirklin & Barratt-Boyes, 1993c).

Institutions that use allografts must have a system in place for harvesting and storing donor aortic tissue, which is then transported to the cryopreservation processing center. In return, needed sizes of processed allografts are returned to the institution. Availability of allografts in the United States is limited because most donor hearts are used for heart transplantation.

Bovine pericardial xenografts have been used in some centers as an alternative to porcine valves. Two manufacturers (Ionescu-Shiley and Hancock) have withdrawn pericardial valves from use. Prevalent structural dysfunction due to tears in the valve cusps have caused a high incidence of valve failure (Masters et al., 1991; Walley et al., 1991). The Carpentier-Edwards pericardial valve, which has a different structural design, remains in use. Cusp rupture has not occurred, and the valve has been demonstrated to have good intermediate-term (7-year follow-up) durability and low rates of valve-related morbidity (Frater et al., 1992).

POSTOPERATIVE CONSIDERATIONS

RESULTS OF VALVE REPLACEMENT

Operative mortality with valve replacement ranges from 5% to 15% in most centers. However, the risk to an individual patient is quite variable depending on the specific type of operation, etiology of valvular disease, status of ventricular function, and need for concomitant procedures. Risk of operative death may be as low as 3% for a patient who undergoes elective aortic valve replacement for aortic stenosis or as high as 50% for a patient requiring emergent mitral valve replacement for acute, ischemic mitral regurgitation. Operative mortality does not appear to be influenced by the type of prosthesis that is implanted.

Unless irreversible ventricular dysfunction or pulmonary hypertension has developed before surgical intervention, most patients who undergo valve replacement can expect a significant improvement in functional capacity. Dyspnea caused by a dysfunctional valve is often significantly diminished even during the first postoperative week. However, underlying ventricular dysfunction is frequently present

FIGURE 16-5. Explanted mitral valve bioprosthesis demonstrates leaflet degeneration and calcification (*arrow*). (Courtesy of David J. Mehlman, MD)

and postoperative recovery is generally slower than that seen in cardiac surgical patients with normal ventricular function. Typically, it takes months or even as much as a year to achieve full improvement from valve replacement.

VALVE-RELATED MORBIDITY

The potential for morbidity or mortality from a valvular prosthesis remains as long as the valve is in place. The major types of morbidity associated with the presence of a prosthetic cardiac valve are valve failure, thromboembolism, anticoagulant-related hemorrhage, and endocarditis. *Valve failure* is suggested by auscultation of a change in heart sounds and is documented by transthoracic or transesophageal echocardiography. It may be caused by (1) periprosthetic leak, (2) mechanical dysfunction (mechanical prosthesis), or (3) leaflet degeneration or calcification (bioprosthesis). A *periprosthetic leak* is regurgitation of blood around the sewing ring of the prosthesis. Although its occurrence is unusual, it is twice as common in patients with mechanical as opposed to bioprosthetic valves (Whittlesey & Geha, 1991). A periprosthetic leak in the early postoperative period is almost always due to suture disruption or a technical problem with placement of the prosthesis. It is most likely in those patients in whom annular tissue is friable secondary to endocarditis or myocardial infarction.

Primary valve failure is defined as dysfunction of the prosthesis itself. Primary failure of a mechanical valve can occur due to improper or failed motion of one of the valve components. Although mechanical valve failure is unusual, it usually produces acute hemodynamic instability. An occasional cause of mechanical valve failure is thrombus or pannus formation on the valve. *Valve thrombosis* is more likely if anticoagulation is discontinued or inadequate but occurs rarely even with therapeutic anticoagulation (Fig. 16-6). *Pannus* is a fibrinous coating that occasionally develops on the surfaces of the prosthesis (Fig. 16-7). Depending on the amount and type of thrombus or fibrinous material on the valve, it may be necessary to surgically debride the prosthesis or explant the prosthesis and implant a new one. In bioprosthetic valves, primary valve failure consists of leaflet degeneration or calcification as previously discussed.

The incidence of *thromboembolism* has decreased due to anticoagulant therapy and the fact that currently available mechanical prostheses are less thrombogenic than earlier models (Altman et al., 1991). Nevertheless, thromboembolism remains a major complication of prosthetic cardiac valves. Thromboembolic events can occur with any type of prosthesis but are more often associated with mechanical valves. Consequently, all currently available mechanical prostheses necessitate life-long anticoagulation with the inherent potential for anticoagulant related hemorrhage. Anticoagulant therapy is also recom-

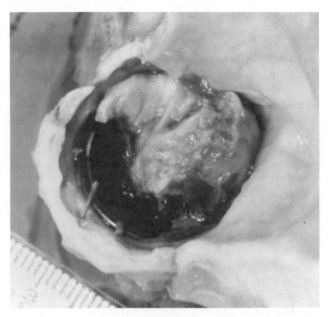

FIGURE 16-6. Autopsy specimen reveals massive thrombus covering aortic surface of mechanical aortic valve prosthesis in patient with inadequate anticoagulation. (Courtesy of David J. Mehlman, MD)

mended for the first 3 months after implantation of bioprosthetic valves in the mitral position (Stein et al., 1992).

Even with systemic anticoagulation, thromboembolic events occur in patients with mechanical prostheses at rates ranging between 0.7% and 3.1% per patient-year (Whittlesey & Geha, 1991). Rates of thromboembolic complications vary among the various mechanical valves, and regimens for anticoagula-

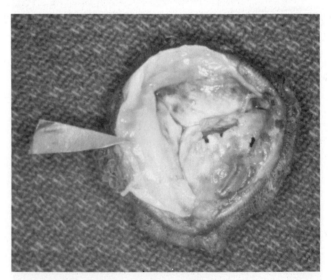

FIGURE 16-7. Porcine aortic bioprosthesis explanted 13 years after implantation; marker illustrates extensive pannus formation along valve sewing ring. (Courtesy of David J. Mehlman, MD)

tion are based on the thrombogenicity of the specific prosthesis. Risk of thromboembolism is lower after aortic valve replacement and greatest after multiple valve replacement (Whittlesey & Geha, 1991). Embolization can occur to the cerebral circulation, resulting in a cerebral vascular accident or transient ischemic attack, or to the peripheral circulation, resulting in ischemia or infarction of tissue distal to the embolus.

Generally, administration of warfarin sodium is begun on the second postoperative day, after mediastinal drainage tubes have been removed. Most surgeons prefer to abstain from initiating anticoagulation earlier because the use of cardiopulmonary bypass impairs coagulation during the early postoperative period (Elefteriades & Geha, 1985). If chronic anticoagulation therapy is necessary, serial prothrombin time measurements are performed and used to adjust the dosage of warfarin.

The lack of standardization of tissue thromboplastin used as the reagent in prothrombin time assays and the resultant variability between laboratories in prothrombin time results has been the focus of recent attention in the United States (Vanscoy & Krause, 1991). The *international normalized ratio* (INR) is being advocated as a more accurate means of reporting results of prothrombin time testing. It is a value calculated from the prothrombin time assay result, taking into account the sensitivity of the reagent used to perform the prothrombin time assay. Recommended international normalized ratio values for various patient groups receiving anticoagulant therapy are still evolving. For the present, both the prothrombin time and international normalized ratio values should be taken into consideration in determining proper dosage of warfarin.

It usually takes several days to establish the dose of warfarin necessary to achieve and maintain therapeutic anticoagulation in a particular patient. Warfarin is a very potent and potentially dangerous medication. *Anticoagulant-related hemorrhage* is a potential risk, particularly in patients who are elderly, are malnourished, or have chronic liver dysfunction secondary to VHD. The most serious form of anticoagulant related bleeding is intracerebral hemorrhage, although gastrointestinal bleeding or profuse bleeding with trauma can also occur. Patient education is of great importance. Both the patient and family are instructed about implications of anticoagulant therapy. A plan for routine prothrombin time testing and for physician monitoring of results is essential. Conditions such as pregnancy, required surgical procedures, trauma, or development of gastric ulcers may occur subsequent to valve implantation and greatly complicate anticoagulant therapy.

Implantation of a valvular prosthesis also imposes a higher risk of infective endocarditis. Prophylaxis against *prosthetic valve endocarditis* is extremely important. Appropriate antibiotic prophylaxis is essential before surgical procedures or instrumentation, particularly dental work (Dajani et al., 1990). If patients who have undergone valve replacement require invasive procedures in the early postoperative period, such as reinsertion of a urinary drainage catheter, antibiotic prophylaxis is especially important and must not be omitted.

In patients with endocarditis related to drug abuse, drug addiction is the primary disease and should be addressed while the patient is hospitalized in a controlled environment (Finkelmeier et al., 1989). As many as 49% of patients with endocarditis due to drug addiction may return to use of drugs after being cured of endocarditis (Arbulu et al., 1991). Aggressive efforts are made to enroll the patient in a drug rehabilitation program directly from the acute hospital setting. If a valvular prosthesis becomes infected through continued intravenous drug use, the prognosis for survival is dismal (Fig. 16-8).

Prosthetic endocarditis, or infection of a valvular prosthesis, is a major complication of valve replacement with an associated mortality of up to 65% (Haydock et al., 1992). The complication occurs when transient bacteremia leads to seeding of the prosthetic material with pathogenic organisms. With mechanical and bioprosthetic valves, prosthetic endocarditis is most common in the first 6 weeks after operation; allograft valves appear to be more resistant to infection during this early period (Haydock et al., 1992). Comparison between mechanical and bioprosthetic valves at 10 years reveals no difference in the incidence of endocarditis (Hammermeister et al., 1991a).

Prosthetic endocarditis is a potentially life-threatening complication, particularly if it occurs during the early postoperative months. At best, it necessitates prolonged hospitalization and treatment with organism-specific intravenous antibiotics for at least 6

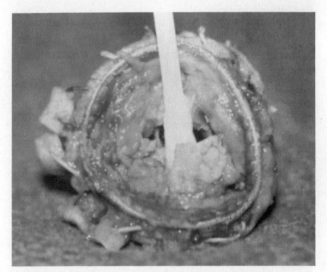

FIGURE 16-8. Porcine aortic bioprosthesis explanted at autopsy from patient who continued intravenous drug abuse after valve replacement for infective endocarditis. Note presence of extensive vegetations covering valve leaflets. (Courtesy of David J. Mehlman, MD)

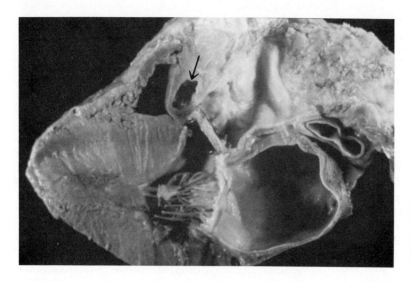

FIGURE 16-9. Autopsy specimen from patient who died of prosthetic valve endocarditis reveals intramyocardial abscess in perivalvular tissue adjacent to prosthetic aortic valve (*arrow*). (Courtesy of David J. Mehlman, MD)

weeks. It may also lead to urgent reoperation for removal of the infected prosthesis and reimplantation of another. The severity of the infection and type of therapy differ depending on the specific pathogenic organism. Streptococcal infections are less virulent than those due to *Staphylococcus*. Fungal infections are extremely difficult to eradicate with antimicrobial therapy and often require emergent valve replacement. Treatment of prosthetic endocarditis is complicated by the presence of artificial material, which is difficult to sterilize. Septic embolization and intramyocardial abscesses are common sequelae of prosthetic endocarditis that is not checked by antibiotic therapy or removal of the infected prosthesis (Fig. 16-9).

REFERENCES

Abe T, Tukamoto M, Yanagiya M, et al., 1989: DeVega's annuloplasty for acquired tricuspid disease: Early and late results in 110 patients. Ann Thorac Surg 48:670

Akins CW, 1991: Mechanical cardiac valvular prostheses. Ann Thorac Surg 52:161

Altman R, Rouvier J, Gurfinkel E, et al., 1991: Comparison of two levels of anticoagulant therapy in patients with substitute heart valves. J Thorac Cardiovasc Surg 101:427

Arbulu A, Holmes RJ, Asfaw I, 1991: Tricuspid valvulectomy without replacement. J Thorac Cardiovasc Surg 102:917

Austen WG, 1989: Choosing a heart valve substitute. In Grillo HC, Austen WG, Wilkins EW, et al. (eds): Current Therapy in Cardiothoracic Surgery. Toronto, BC Decker

Badduke BR, Jamieson WR, Miyagishima RT, et al., 1991: Pregnancy and childbearing in a population with biologic valvular prostheses. J Thorac Cardiac Surg 102:179

Bonchek LI, 1987: The basis for selecting a valve prosthesis. In McGoon DC (ed): Cardiac Surgery, ed. 2. Philadelphia, FA Davis

Burdon TA, Miller DC, Oyer PE, et al., 1992: Durability of porcine valves at fifteen years in a representative North American patient population. J Thorac Cardiovasc Surg 103:238

Czer LS, Chaux A, Matloff J, et al., 1990: Ten-year experience with the St. Jude Medical valve for primary valve replacement. J Thorac Cardiovasc Surg 100:44

David TE, Bos J, Rakowski H, 1991: Mitral valve repair by replacement of chordae tendineae with polytetrafluoroethylene sutures. J Thorac Cardiovasc Surg 101:495

Dajani AS, Bisno AL, Chung KJ, et al., 1990: Prevention of bacterial endocarditis: Recommendations of the American Heart Association. JAMA 264:2919

Deloche A, Jebara VA, Relland JY, et al., 1990: Valve repair with Carpentier techniques. J Thorac Cardiovasc Surg 99:990

Duran CM, 1991: Acquired disease of the mitral valve. In Baue AE, Geha AS, Hammond GL, et al. (eds): Glenn's Thoracic and Cardiovascular Surgery, ed. 5. Norwalk, CT, Appleton & Lange

Elefteriades JA, Geha AS, 1985: Additional topics. In House Officer Guide to ICU Care: The Cardiothoracic Surgical Patient. Rockville, MD, Aspen Publishers

Finkelmeier BA, Hartz RS, Fisher E, Michaelis LL, 1989: Implications of prosthetic valve implantation: An eight year follow-up of patients with porcine bioprostheses. Heart Lung 18:565

Frater RW, Salomon NW, Rainer WG, et al., 1992: The Carpentier-Edwards pericardial aortic valve: Intermediate results. Ann Thorac Surg 53:764

Galloway AC, Colvin SB, Baumann FG, et al., 1988: Current concepts of mitral valve reconstruction for mitral insufficiency. Circulation 78:1087

Grossi EA, Galloway AC, Parish MA, et al., 1992: Experience with twenty-eight cases of systolic anterior motion after mitral valve reconstruction by the Carpentier technique. J Thorac Cardiovasc Surg 103:466

Hammermeister KE, Sethi GK, Oprian C, et al., 1991a: Comparison of occurrence of bleeding, systemic embolism, endocarditis, valve thrombosis and reoperation between patients randomized between a mechanical prosthesis and a bioprosthesis: Results from the VA randomized trial. J Am Coll Cardiol 17:362-A

Hammermeister KE, Sethi GK, Oprian C, et al., 1991b: Comparison of outcome an average of 10 years after valve replacement with a mechanical versus a bioprosthetic valve: Results of the VA randomized trial. J Am Coll Cardiol 17:41-A

Hartz RS, Fisher EB, Finkelmeier BA, et al., 1986: An eight-year experience with porcine bioprosthetic cardiac valves. J Thorac Cardiovasc Surg 91:910

Haydock D, Barratt-Boyes B, Macedo T, et al., 1992: Aortic valve replacement for active endocarditis in 108 patients. J Thorac Cardiovasc Surg 103:130

Hendren WG, Morris AS, Rosenkranz ER, et al., 1992: Mitral valve repair for bacterial endocarditis. J Thorac Cardiovasc Surg 103:124

Hildenberg AD, Austen WG, 1989: Heart valve substitutes. In Eagle KA, Haber E, DeSanctis RW, Austin WG (eds): The Practice of Cardiology, ed. 2. Boston, Little, Brown

Jamieson WR, 1993: Modern cardiac valve devices—bioprostheses and mechnical prostheses: State of the art. J Cardiac Surg 8:89

Jamieson WR, Allen P, Miyagishima RT, et al., 1990: The Carpentier-Edwards standard porcine bioprosthesis. J Thorac Cardiovasc Surg 99:543

Jamieson WR, Rosado LJ, Munro AI, et al., 1988: Carpentier-Edwards standard porcine bioprosthesis: Primary tissue failure (structural valve deterioration) by age groups. Ann Thorac Surg 46:155

Karlson KJ, Ashraf MM, Berger RL, 1988: Rupture of left ventricle following mitral valve replacement. Ann Thorac Surg 6:590

Kirklin JW, Barratt-Boyes BG, 1993a: Mitral valve disease with or without tricuspid valve disease. In Cardiac Surgery, ed. 2. New York, Churchill Livingstone

Kirklin JW, Barratt-Boyes BG, 1993b: Tricuspid valve disease. In Cardiac Surgery, ed. 2. New York, Churchill Livingstone

Kirklin JW, Barratt-Boyes BG, 1993c: Aortic valve disease. In Cardiac Surgery, ed. 2. New York, Churchill Livingstone

Korzeniowski OM, Kaye D, 1992: Infective endocarditis. In Braunwald E (ed): Heart Disease: A Textbook of Cardiovascular Medicine, ed. 4. Philadelphia, WB Saunders

Larbalestier RI, Kinchla NM, Aranki SF, et al., 1992: Acute bacterial endocarditis. Circulation 86 (Suppl II):II-68

Massimiano PS, Hammond GL, 1991: Aortic valve disease and hypertrophic myopathies. In Baue AE, Geha AS, Hammond GL, et al. (eds): Glenn's Thoracic and Cardiovascular Surgery, ed. 5. Norwalk, CT, Appleton & Lange

Masters RG, Pipe AL, Bedard JP, et al., 1991: Long-term clinical results with the Ionescu-Shiley pericardial xenograft. J Thorac Cardiovasc Surg 101:81

McGrath LB, Gonzalez-Lavin L, Bailey BM, et al., 1990: Tricuspid valve operations in 530 patients. J Thorac Cardiovasc Surg 99:124

Minale C, Lambertz H, Nikol S, et al., 1990: Selective annuloplasty of the tricuspid valve. J Thorac Cardiovasc Surg 99:846

Schlant RC, 1991: Mitral stenosis. In Hurst JW (ed): Current Therapy in Cardiovascular Disease, ed. 3. Philadelphia, BC Decker

Spencer FC, 1990: Acquired disease of the mitral valve. In Sabiston DC, Spencer FC (eds): Surgery of the Chest, ed. 5. Philadelphia, WB Saunders

Stein PD, Alpert JS, Copeland J, et al., 1992: Antithrombotic therapy in patients with mechanical and bioprosthetic heart valves. Chest 102 (Suppl):445S

Ting W, Silverman N, Levitsky S, 1991: Valve replacement in patients with endocarditis and cerebral septic emboli. Ann Thorac Surg 51:18

Vanscoy GJ, Krause JR, 1991: Warfarin and the international normalized ratio: Reducing interlaboratory effects. DICP Ann Pharmacother 25:1190

Walley VM, Rubens FD, Campagna M, et al., 1991: Patterns of failure in Hancock pericardial bioprostheses. J Thorac Cardiovasc Surg 102:187

Weiland A, 1983: A review of cardiac valve prostheses and their selection. Heart Lung 12:498

Whitman GR, 1987: Prosthetic cardiac valves. Prog Cardiovasc Nurs 2:116

Whittlesey P, Geha AS, 1991: Selection and complications of cardiac valve prostheses. In Baue AE, Geha AS, Hammond GL, et al. (eds): Glenn's Thoracic and Cardiovascular Surgery, ed. 5. Norwalk, CT, Appleton & Lange

17

SURGERY ON
THE THORACIC AORTA

The most common pathologic processes necessitating surgery on the thoracic aorta are aneurysm and dissection. Although these conditions can coexist, they are distinct entities. A third pathologic process, transection, is much less common and is discussed in Chapter 32, Cardiac and Thoracic Trauma. Repair of congenital aortic abnormalities, such as coarctation and patent ductus arteriosus, is discussed in Chapter 19, Surgical Treatment of Congenital Heart Disease in Adults.

THORACIC AORTIC ANEURYSM

An *aneurysm* is a localized area of transmural thinning and dilatation of the aortic wall. Thoracic aortic aneurysms most commonly are atherosclerotic in origin but can also develop secondary to other conditions, including Marfan's syndrome, cystic medical necrosis, aortitis, trauma, chronic dissection, or infection. A true aneurysm is one in which blood is contained by aortic wall composed of the three normal layers (intima, media, adventitia). A false aneurysm is one in which partial or complete disruption of the aortic wall has occurred but blood is contained by the ad-

ventitial layer or periaortic fibrous tissue (Cohn, 1990).

Aneurysms are described according to shape and location. A fusiform aneurysm widens the aorta circumferentially, and a saccular aneurysm distorts only one side of the aortic wall. Because aneurysmal dilatation is generally localized, thoracic aneurysms are typically categorized as ascending (between the aortic valve and innominate artery origin), transverse arch (between the innominate and left subclavian artery origins), descending (originating distal to the left subclavian artery but above the diaphragm), or thoracoabdominal (involving both descending thoracic and abdominal aortic segments). Less commonly, multiple segments or the entire thoracic aorta is aneurysmal.

The most threatening consequence of an aortic aneurysm is spontaneous aortic rupture with almost certain death. Thoracic aneurysm is fatal in 75% of patients within 5 years of diagnosis, and almost half the deaths are due to rupture (Lindsay et al., 1990). Occurrence of aneurysmal rupture is unpredictable, but risk is known to increase in direct proportion to aneurysm diameter (Eagle & DeSanctis, 1992). Increased stretching of the aortic wall increases wall tension (law of Laplace), making rupture more likely (Cohn, 1990). Natural history data for patients with thoracic aneurysms are somewhat limited, but fusiform aneurysms greater than 7 cm are more likely to rupture than smaller ones (Eagle & DeSanctis, 1992). Normal aortic diameter is 2.5 to 3.0 cm.

In addition to aortic rupture, aneurysm expansion can occur, producing disabling symptoms as the enlarging aortic segment encroaches on surrounding structures. Common symptoms are chest or back pain, hoarseness, cough, and dyspnea. Aneurysms in the ascending aorta often distort the aortic valve annulus, leading to progressive symptoms of aortic regurgitation.

INDICATIONS FOR OPERATION

Thoracic aneurysm is a life-threatening condition for which surgical therapy is the only treatment. As recently as 10 to 15 years ago, resection of a thoracic aortic aneurysm was associated with considerable mortality. Since that time, technical advances have lowered the risk associated with operations on the aorta. As a result, indications for surgical repair of thoracic aortic aneurysms have expanded.

In otherwise healthy patients, some surgeons advocate resection of any fusiform thoracic aneurysm that is 6 cm or greater in diameter, even in the absence of symptoms. Others reserve surgical resection for those patients with symptoms related to the aneurysm, radiographic evidence of aneurysm expansion, or moderate to severe aortic regurgitation (Akins, 1989). In patients with Marfan's syndrome, operative intervention is frequently recommended for aneurysms 5.0 to 5.5 cm in diameter regardless of symptomatology. The extensive cystic medial necrosis frequently present in patients afflicted with Marfan's syndrome predisposes to degenerative changes in the aortic wall and makes aneurysm rupture or expansion more likely.

Aortography is performed before operative therapy to assess the size and extent of the aneurysm and its relation to branch vessels arising from the aorta. If the ascending aorta is involved in the aneurysmal process, cardiac catheterization is essential to define the origin of the coronary arteries as they arise from the ascending aorta. Preoperative knowledge of coronary artery anatomy is key to the surgeon's ability to plan and perform a successful operation. Abnormalities such as coronary artery lesions, anomalous origin of the coronary artery ostia, or obstruction of the ostia by the aneurysm may be revealed. Occasionally, diffuse aneurysmal disease is demonstrated in multiple segments of the aorta. In such cases, operative resection is generally accomplished in staged procedures. The order of repair is based on size and associated symptoms or on cardiac complications of the aneurysms (Crawford, 1989).

Most often, aneurysm repair can be performed electively, unless rapid expansion or rupture is sus-

pected (Akins, 1989). If aortic rupture occurs and is contained, the patient may survive long enough to be considered for emergent operative therapy. A *contained rupture* is one in which the adventitia, or outer layer of aortic wall, is disrupted but periaortic, pericardial, or pleural tissue contains the blood and prevents rapid exsanguination and death. Severe chest pain, and radiographic evidence of mediastinal widening or pleural effusion suggest contained rupture. *Leaking aneurysm* and *impending rupture* are other terms commonly used to describe this condition. Urgent operative therapy is also undertaken for *mycotic*, or *infected, aneurysms* because of their propensity for rupture despite antimicrobial therapy (Crawford, 1989).

OPERATIVE TECHNIQUES

Surgical repair of aortic aneurysm consists of resecting the aneurysmal segment and replacing it with a prosthetic graft. Grafts used for replacement of diseased aortic segments are generally made of low-porosity woven Dacron. Just before implantation, the graft is "preclotted" by saturating it with albumin, nonheparinized blood, or fibrin glue (Rose et al., 1991). Most commonly, preclotting consists of immersing the graft in an albumin solution and then briefly autoclaving the graft. Preclotting renders the graft impervious to blood (i.e., blood-tight) (Kouchoukos, 1991).

Operative technique is planned according to aneurysm location and underlying aortic pathology. Often, the graft is sewn inside the aneurysm. Native aorta is not resected but instead is wrapped around the graft. This so-called *inclusion technique* is thought to assist in hemostasis and may assist in protecting the prosthesis from infection (Fig. 17-1). *Interposition* describes an alternative technique in which the aneurysmal tissue is excised and replaced with a prosthetic tube graft interposed between the two aortic remnants. In selected situations, a *sutureless intraluminal prosthesis* may be used to avoid prolonged aortic occlusion. The intraluminal graft, which has a stiff ring on each end, is placed inside the aortic lumen, and tapes are tied circumferentially around the aorta over the rings. Eliminating sutured anastomoses considerably shortens the time that blood flow through the aorta is interrupted. Occasionally, *local excision* of saccular aneurysms, without aortic occlusion or graft placement, is possible (Akins, 1989).

Ascending Aneurysm

Most *ascending aortic aneurysms* are associated with cystic degeneration of the medial layer; other etiologies include arteriosclerosis, aortitis, post-stenotic dilatation from aortic stenosis, infection, and trauma (Kouchoukos, 1991). For operative repair of the ascending aorta, a median sternotomy incision is used

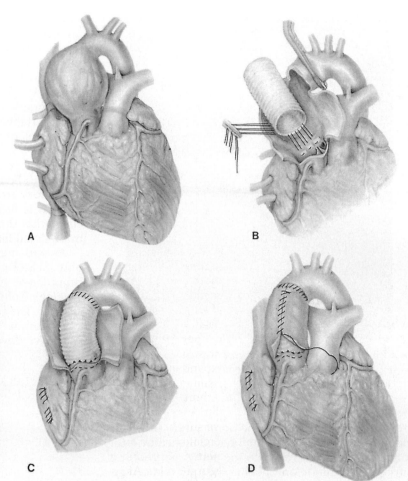

FIGURE 17-1. One technique for surgical management of a fusiform aneurysm of the ascending aorta. **(A)** Aneurysmal dilatation begins above the aortic annulus and does not involve the origin of the coronary arteries. **(B and C).** The aneurysm is opened and replaced with a prosthetic tubular graft. **(D)** The wall of the aneurysm is closed around the graft to minimize blood loss. (Robicsek F, 1984: Aneurysms of the thoracic aorta. In Haimovici H [ed]: Haimovici's Vascular Surgery: Principles and Techniques, ed. 2, p. 650. Norwalk, CT, Appleton & Lange)

and cardiopulmonary bypass (CPB) is necessary. The distal portion of the ascending aorta or the transverse arch may be used for arterial cannulation unless the aneurysm extends to the innominate artery or occurs secondary to chronic dissection. In these cases, the femoral artery is cannulated for CPB.

After the ascending aorta is adequately exposed, CPB is instituted. Cardioplegic solution is injected into the coronary arteries (either directly or using a retrograde technique) to protect the myocardium from ischemic damage during the repair. The diseased aortic segment is resected, and a prosthetic tube graft is sewn in its place. After proximal and distal graft anastomoses are completed, air is evacuated before reestablishing aortic flow. Anastomotic sites are inspected carefully to ensure hemostasis.

In patients with Marfan's syndrome, cystic medial necrosis, or granulomatous or syphilitic aortitis, adjacent but nondiseased areas of aorta are usually resected because of the likelihood of future aneurysmal dilatation secondary to the underlying disease process. If the aneurysm has caused annular dilatation of the aortic valve (annuloaortic ectasia), or if coexisting aortic valve disease is present, the valvular abnormality is concomitantly addressed. Either resuspension

of the valve annulus, valvuloplasty, or valve replacement may be required to restore valvular competence. In patients with Marfan's syndrome who undergo ascending aortic aneurysm resection, prophylactic replacement of the aortic valve is recommended because of the known propensity for myxomatous degeneration of the valve that may lead to aortic regurgitation in the future.

If both the ascending aorta and aortic valve must be replaced, a *composite graft* (i.e., a prosthetic tube graft containing a mechanical aortic valve prosthesis), may be used (Fig. 17-2). A composite graft, also called a valve conduit, avoids possible aneurysmal dilatation of aortic root tissue left in place between a separately implanted tube graft and aortic valve prosthesis. When a composite graft is implanted, the entire aortic root is resected, including tissue from which the coronary arteries originate. Therefore, surgical reconstruction must include reestablishment of blood flow from the aorta into the coronary arterial circulation.

One of three methods is generally used to accomplish this. The first is removal of the right and left coronary ostia from the aortic wall, along with a surrounding cuff of aortic tissue. The two coronary ostia

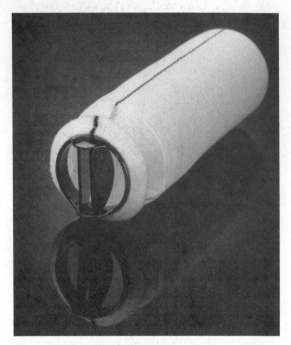

FIGURE 17-2. Composite aortic graft with St. Jude valvular prosthesis. (Courtesy of St. Jude Medical, St. Paul, MN)

clavian arteries). Special intraoperative techniques are needed to protect the brain and heart during the repair and to reconstruct the aorta to restore circulation to the head, neck, and upper and lower extremities (Crawford & Coselli, 1991). Until the past decade, operations on the aortic arch were associated with considerable risk. A major factor in reducing operative mortality was the introduction by Griepp and colleagues of profound hypothermia and circulatory arrest for aortic arch replacement (Griepp et al., 1975; Galloway et al., 1989). This method of protection against ischemia allows cessation of blood flow (i.e., circulatory arrest) for up to 60 minutes while the aortic arch is reconstructed. Techniques for preserving circulation during aortic operations are described in more detail later in the chapter.

As with ascending aortic repair, a median sternotomy incision and CPB are used. The femoral artery is cannulated. After clamping the proximal aorta, cardioplegic solution is administered into the coronary arteries. The aortic repair is performed with profound hypothermia and circulation totally arrested or at very low flows. Reparative techniques are variable

are then reimplanted into the aortic graft. This technique is not well suited for all cases. Sometimes, the coronary ostia lie so close to the aortic root that it is impossible to reimplant them in the graft without applying undue tension to the anastomotic site. In the case of aortic dissection, aortic tissue surrounding the coronary ostia may be friable or disrupted (Kouchoukos, 1991).

A second method of restoring aorta to coronary artery continuity is the *Cabrol procedure* (Fig. 17-3). A prosthetic graft, comparable in size to the diameter of the coronary artery ostia, is sewn in end-to-end fashion: one end to the right and the other end to the left coronary artery ostium. The graft is then laid over the anterior surface of the composite graft. An opening is made in the posterior surface of the small graft and in the anterior surface of the composite graft. A side-to-side anastomosis is then fashioned between the two openings. A third method of reestablishing blood flow to coronary arteries is by attaching saphenous vein grafts from the aortic prosthetic graft to the native coronary arteries in the same manner as would be done during coronary artery bypass grafting.

Arch Aneurysm

Aneurysms of the aortic arch are less common than in other aortic segments. However, they present a formidable challenge for the thoracic surgeon. They are likely to involve the origins of the brachiocephalic vessels (i.e., the innominate, left carotid, and left sub-

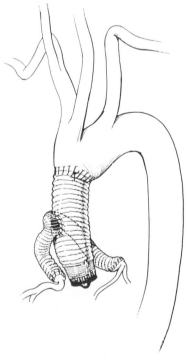

FIGURE 17-3. Composite graft with Cabrol technique of restoring aorta–coronary artery continuity. The two ends of the smaller diameter graft are sewn in end-to-end fashion to the aorta surrounding the right and left coronary artery ostia; a side-to-side anastomosis is created between the smaller graft and the composite graft. (Coselli JS, Crawford ES, 1993: Composite aortic valve replacement and graft replacement of the ascending aorta plus coronary artery reimplantation: How I do it. Semin Thorac Cardiovasc Surg 5:61)

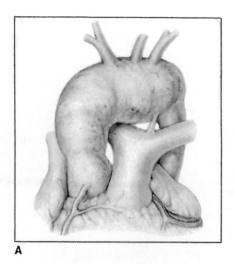

A

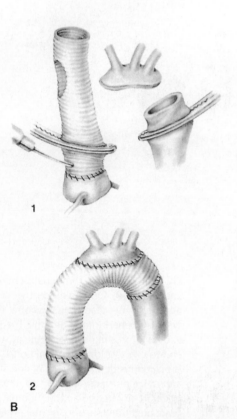

1

2

B

FIGURE 17-4. (A) An aneurysm of the transverse aortic arch. **(B)** One technique for surgical management: *1.* The aneurysm is resected and replaced with a tubular prosthetic graft anastomosed in end-to-end fashion to the ascending and to the descending aorta. The origin of the aortic arch branches is excised with a cuff of aortic wall. *2.* The island of aorta containing the origin of the arch vessels is anastomosed to an opening in the superior surface of the tubular graft. (Robicsek F, 1984: Aneurysms of the thoracic aorta. In Haimovici H [ed]: Haimovici's Vascular Surgery: Principles and Techniques, ed. 2, p. 657. Norwalk, CT, Appleton & Lange)

because aneurysms of the transverse arch vary widely in size and extent (Kirklin & Barratt-Boyes, 1993a). One technique of arch reconstruction includes implanting a prosthetic tubular graft and suturing an island of aortic tissue containing the origins of the arch vessels to an opening in its superior surface (Fig. 17-4). Alternatively, a graft designed with arch branches or an aortic arch cadaver homograft may be used to replace the diseased segment.

Descending Aneurysm

Aneurysms of the descending thoracic aorta account for 30% to 40% of all thoracic and thoracoabdominal aneurysms; the majority occur secondary to degenerative disease or atherosclerosis (Rose et al., 1991). Descending thoracic aneurysms are repaired through a left posterolateral thoracotomy incision (Fig. 17-5). The operation is usually performed without CPB. A double-lumen endotracheal tube is used to provide single lung ventilation. The right lung is ventilated, while the left lung is maintained in a deflated state to provide adequate exposure of the aorta and prevent retraction injury of the lung (Crawford, 1989). Because the descending thoracic aorta must be clamped during the repair, an aortic shunt or a form of CPB may be used to reduce the possibility of ischemic injury to the spinal cord or kidneys. These techniques are described later in the chapter.

Thoracoabdominal Aneurysm

The repair of *thoracoabdominal aneurysms* can be quite complex because aortic branches to abdominal viscera are involved and must be reimplanted into the graft (Fig. 17-6). As with descending thoracic aorta aneurysm repair, prevention of ischemic damage to the spinal cord and kidneys is essential. In addition, the incision required for adequate exposure of a thoracoabdominal aneurysm (lateral chest wall, extending down the middle of the abdomen) is extensive and is likely to compromise patient mobility and pulmonary hygiene in the early postoperative period (Fig. 17-7).

RESULTS OF ANEURYSM RESECTION

Mortality associated with thoracic aneurysm resection varies according to aneurysm location and underlying aortic pathology. Cohn (1990) summarizes operative mortality as follows: ascending, 5% to 15%; arch, 10% to 30%; descending, 5% to 15%; and thoracoabdominal, 10% to 40%. Variance in results between surgical centers remains significant. Common causes of death after thoracic aortic aneurysm resection include bleeding and cardiac dysfunction. Elderly patients, and those with underlying cardiac, renal, or pulmonary disease, are at increased risk for operative death or complications.

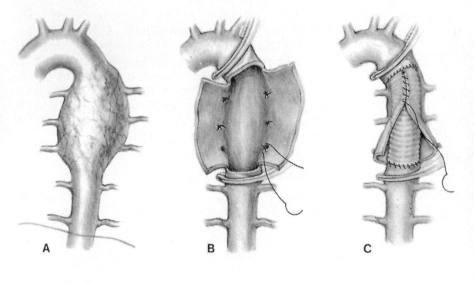

FIGURE 17-5. **(A)** Aneurysm of the mid-descending thoracic aorta. **(B and C)** One technique of surgical management. (Robicsek F, 1984: Aneurysms of the thoracic aorta. In Haimovici H [ed]: Haimovici's Vascular Surgery: Principles and Techniques, ed. 2, p. 662. Norwalk, CT, Appleton & Lange)

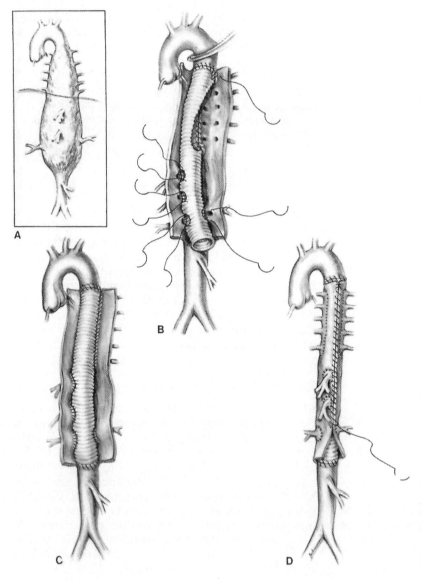

FIGURE 17-6. **(A)** Thoracoabdominal aortic aneurysm. **(B)** One method of surgical management. After clamping the aorta, the aneurysm is opened longitudinally. The proximal end of a prosthetic tube graft is sutured in end-to-end fashion to normal aorta. The graft is placed inside the aneurysm and side-holes are created to correspond to the ostia of visceral, intercostal, and lumbar arteries branching from the aneurysmal portion of the aorta. Graft openings are sutured circumferentially around the corresponding vessel ostia. **(C)** The distal end of the graft is anastomosed in end-to-end fashion to the distal aorta. **(D)** After all anastomoses are completed, the wall of the aneurysm is sutured around the graft. (Robicsek F, 1984: Aneurysms of the thoracic aorta. In Haimovici H [ed]: Haimovici's Vascular Surgery: Principles and Techniques, ed. 2, p. 672. Norwalk, CT, Appleton & Lange)

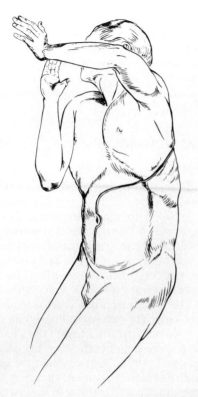

FIGURE 17-7. Thoracoabdominal incision. The patient is in the semidecubitus position. A posterolateral thoracotomy incision is begun between the sixth to eleventh thoracic vertebrae, then is continued downward and anteriorly to the midline where it is extendeddown the middle of the abdomen. (Ernst CB, Reddy DJ, 1989: Thoracoabdominal aortic aneurysm. In Haimovici H [ed]: Haimovici's Vascular Surgery: Principles and Techniques, ed. 3, p. 618. Norwalk, CT, Appleton & Lange)

AORTIC DISSECTION

Aortic dissection is the longitudinal separation of the aortic wall layers. Disruption of the intima, or innermost layer, provides an entry point for blood from the true lumen of the aorta to dissect the medial layer, creating a false lumen or second channel for blood flow. The column of blood entering the false channel is propelled by the force of arterial pressure, stripping the intima from the adventitia for variable distances along the length of the aorta (Cohn, 1990).

Cystic medial necrosis is present in approximately 20% of patients with aortic dissection (Kirklin & Barratt-Boyes, 1993b). It is frequently related to a connective tissue disorder such as Marfan's syndrome or, less commonly, Ehlers-Danlos syndrome. Other etiologic factors include hypertension, pregnancy, congenital bicuspid aortic valve, and coarctation (Wheat, 1987; Wolfe & Moran, 1981). Iatrogenic aortic dissection may occur secondary to catheterization, instrumentation, or surgical procedures involving the aorta.

Aortic dissection is considered acute if it is recognized within 2 weeks of its onset because most of the associated mortality occurs during this interval (Eagle et al., 1989). Dissection detected more than 2 weeks after its presumed occurrence is considered chronic. The Stanford classification system is commonly used to categorize aortic dissection according to location. *Type A dissection* involves the ascending aorta and may involve the descending aorta as well. *Type B dissection* involves only the descending aorta distal to the left subclavian artery. Distinction between type A and type B dissection is important in determining therapy.

Although dissection is the most common catastrophic illness involving the aorta, many patients do not survive long enough to receive treatment. The arterial hypertension usually associated with the condition produces progressive dissection that can occur in both retrograde and antegrade directions from the original point of intimal disruption. Without treatment, more than 25% of patients die within 24 hours, more than 50% within 1 week, and more than 75% within 1 month; fewer than 10% of patients survive 1 year (Eagle & DeSanctis, 1992).

Three major pathologic consequences can result from aortic dissection (Eagle et al., 1989). First, retrograde dissection can disrupt the aortic valve annulus leading to acute aortic valve incompetence, with resultant pulmonary edema or cardiogenic shock. Second, rupture of intraluminal blood through the adventitia can occur anywhere along the length of the aorta. Free rupture produces rapid exsanguination; rupture into the pericardium or mediastinum causes cardiac tamponade.

Third, because all body tissues receive blood from branches of the aorta, perfusion to any of the vital organs can be compromised. Branches of the aorta may be involved in the dissection, may be occluded by the dissection, may stay in communication with the aorta by the false channel, or may be uninvolved (Kirklin & Barratt-Boyes, 1993b). Dissection of a coronary artery, usually the right, may cause acute myocardial infarction. Involvement of the arteries arising from the aortic arch may produce altered mental status or focal neurologic deficits (Fann et al., 1989). Compromised blood flow to the spinal cord, kidneys, intestines, or lower extremities may cause paraplegia, renal dysfunction, bowel infarction, or limb ischemia, respectively.

Patients with aortic dissection usually become acutely symptomatic, either with sudden, severe chest or back pain or with manifestations of occlusion of one of the major organs supplied by the aorta. Other findings may include mediastinal widening on chest roentgenogram, hypertension despite a general appearance of shock, unequal pulses, and a diminishing hematocrit. The diagnosis is confirmed with aortography, computed tomography, or, more recently, transesophageal echocardiography.

INDICATIONS FOR OPERATION

The decision whether to perform surgical repair of a dissection is determined in large part by its location and extent. Type A dissection (involving the ascending aorta or arch) is almost always treated with emergent surgical therapy unless the patient has already suffered irreversible major organ system damage. Replacement of the ascending aorta is performed to prevent death from (1) cardiac tamponade due to intrapericardial rupture, (2) acute myocardial infarction as a result of coronary artery occlusion, or (3) left ventricular failure caused by acute aortic valve regurgitation (Fann et al., 1989).

In contrast, type B dissection (limited to the descending aorta distal to the left subclavian artery) is usually treated primarily with medical (i.e., antihypertensive) therapy. Surgical and medical therapies provide equal long-term survival rates in patients with uncomplicated descending (type B) aortic dissection (Glower et al., 1990). However, surgical treatment may become necessary for type B dissection if pain persists, if blood pressure cannot be controlled, or if there is evidence of dissection progression, aortic regurgitation, or rupture (Eagle et al., 1989). Progression of dissection is manifested by persistent pain or evidence of compromised blood flow to the spinal cord, abdominal viscera, or lower extremities.

Many surgeons advocate surgical therapy for either type A or B dissection in patients with Marfan's syndrome because of the friable nature of aortic tissue in this disease and the propensity for rupture or recurrent dissection (Eagle et al., 1989). The choice of medical or surgical therapy remains somewhat con-troversial for dissection that originates in the aortic arch because arch resection carries a higher operative risk. Whether or not surgical repair is undertaken, an integral component in treatment of both type A and type B dissections is aggressive pharmacologic therapy to control hypertension and prevent extension of the dissection.

OPERATIVE TECHNIQUES

Type A Dissection

Type A dissection is repaired through a median sternotomy incision. CPB, using femoral artery cannulation, is used to maintain circulation while the ascending aorta is clamped and repaired. Repair of type A aortic dissection consists of resecting the most proximal segment of ascending aorta involved in the dissection process, thus preventing further retrograde dissection into the aortic valve annulus or pericardium. The aortic arch is included in the resection in patients with (1) excessive enlargement and impending or actual rupture of the false channel in the arch or (2) a large degenerative aneurysm in the arch (Crawford et al., 1992). A synthetic tube graft is used to replace the resected segment of aorta. The graft is sutured proximally and distally to the aorta, obliterating the false channel between intimal and adventitial layers (Fig. 17-8).

The site of intimal disruption is included in the repair if it is located in the ascending aorta. If the intimal disruption is located in the arch or descending aorta, resective therapy for type A aortic dissection may still be limited to repairing the ascending aorta.

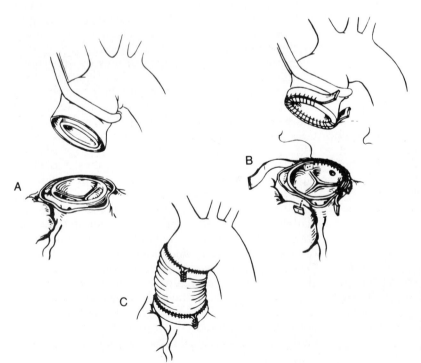

FIGURE 17-8. Surgical repair of type A aortic dissection. **(A)** Resection of the ascending aorta containing the intimal tear. **(B)** Resuspension of the aortic valve at commissures and preparation of the proximal and distal aortic walls for anastomosis of the graft. **(C)** Completed resection and graft replacement of the ascending aorta. (Ergin MA, Galla JD, Lansman S, Griepp RB, 1985: Acute dissections of the aorta: Current surgical treatment. Surg Clin North Am 65:730)

Reconstruction of the aortic arch increases operative risk because of the technical difficulties associated with interrupting blood flow through the brachiocephalic arteries. Also, an intimal tear beyond the arch may not be accessible with a sternotomy exposure. Some surgeons, however, advocate resection of the intimal tear in all cases (Ergin et al., 1991).

In 60% to 70% of cases, type A dissection is associated with aortic valvular regurgitation (Fann et al., 1991). Aortic valve repair or replacement may be necessary if the dissection has damaged the valve or distorted the annulus. Whether it is best to salvage a native aortic valve, using a reparative technique, or replace the valve is controversial; operative and long-term survival are similar (Fann et al., 1991). Valve replacement is usually performed in patients with Marfan's syndrome. As with aortic aneurysm repair, the amount of aortic tissue resected is determined by the nature and extent of underlying pathology. In patients with cystic medial necrosis or other diseases likely to cause recurrent dissection, the entire aortic root and aortic valve are replaced with a composite graft because the underlying disease process makes future aneurysm formation and aortic regurgitation likely.

Type B Dissection

Type B dissection, that involving only the aorta distal to the left subclavian artery, is repaired through a left thoracotomy incision. With proximal and distal control, the aorta is clamped and the aortic segment containing the intimal disruption is resected (Ergin et al., 1991). Aortic continuity is restored with a tubular graft, obliterating the false lumen at the proximal and distal ends. If blood flow into arterial branches of the aorta has been compromised, adequate blood supply to organs supplied by the branches must be restored.

The same considerations about occluding the descending thoracic aorta during aneurysm resection apply to dissection repair. However, the risk of spinal cord damage associated with repair of aortic dissection is higher than that for operative repair of atherosclerotic aortic aneurysms or congenital coarctation in which collateral vessels to the spinal cord are usually well developed. Repair of type B aortic dissection is associated with a 10% to 20% incidence of paraplegia.

Chronic Dissection

Chronic aortic dissection may also be treated surgically if it is associated with aneurysmal dilatation, chronic aortic regurgitation, or progression of the dissection (Eagle et al., 1989). During operative repair of chronic aortic dissection, the false channel is not obliterated because it may be the source of blood supply to aortic branches. Fenestrations are created in the prosthetic graft, and the distal end of the graft is sutured to the outer wall of the dissected aorta to preserve flow into the false lumen (Ergin et al., 1991).

RESULTS OF DISSECTION REPAIR

Operative mortality is 10% to 20% for acute type A and 16% for type B dissections (Ergin et al., 1991). Residual aortic pathology and coexisting cardiovascular disease are significant causes of late death and morbidity (Glower et al., 1991).

PRESERVATION OF CIRCULATION DURING AORTIC OPERATIONS

For most operative procedures on the aorta, it is necessary to occlude blood flow through a segment of the aorta. Because the aorta supplies blood to all vital organs, maintenance of adequate perfusion to vital organs is a particular challenge. The reduction in mortality and morbidity associated with aortic surgery is largely due to better techniques of CPB and organ preservation during the period of aortic cross-clamping. The specific techniques used depend on what segment of the thoracic aorta must be repaired.

Involvement of the aortic root (ascending aorta) in the disease process necessitates use of CPB to maintain circulation while blood flow into the proximal aorta is interrupted. Depending on the type and location of pathology, arterial perfusion is accomplished with cannulation of the femoral artery, distal ascending aorta, or transverse arch. Perfusion of the coronary ostia with cold cardioplegic solution is performed to protect the myocardium from ischemic injury during the repair. Alternatively, a retrograde technique may be used for perfusing the coronary arteries. Techniques of CPB and myocardial protection are described in more detail elsewhere in the text.

Operations on the aortic arch require attention to protection of cerebral circulation because blood flow through the carotid arteries must be interrupted. Instead of the moderate hypothermia and CPB perfusion techniques used in most cardiac operations, profound hypothermia and circulatory arrest are used. This technique has proven successful in protecting the brain against ischemic damage during periods of up to 1 hour of interrupted blood flow. With the patient on CPB, body temperature is lowered to 18°C to 20°C, clamps are applied to the proximal aorta and the three brachiocephalic arteries, and cold cardioplegic solution is administered to establish total circulatory arrest. The profound hypothermia technique and shorter periods of cerebral vessel occlusion have decreased the incidence of neurologic sequelae. However, great care must be taken to evacuate all air and debris from the aortic lumen before reestablishing flow to the brain (Akins, 1989).

Despite these protective measures, neurologic complications remain the predominant type of morbidity associated with operative procedures on the aortic arch. Some surgeons pack the patient's head in ice to provide additional, topical cooling of the brain.

Also, the repair is sometimes performed without applying clamps to the aorta; avoidance of clamping lowers the risk of causing cerebral embolization or aortic dissection secondary to manipulation and clamping of diseased aortic tissue (Galloway et al., 1989).

Operations on the descending thoracic aorta (e.g., type B aortic dissection, descending thoracic and thoracoabdominal aneurysms, or aortic transection) necessitate occluding the descending thoracic aorta. Diminished perfusion to organs and tissue distal to the clamp can cause ischemic damage to the spinal cord, kidneys, liver, or intestines (Laschinger et al., 1987; Qayumi et al., 1992). The spinal cord is most vulnerable to ischemic injury. Although the descending thoracic aorta can generally be clamped for approximately 30 minutes before ischemic damage occurs, paraparesis or paraplegia sometimes occurs unpredictably even with shorter cross-clamp duration. Multiple factors are thought to account for postoperative paraplegia, including variable location of collateral blood supply to the anterior spinal artery (usually between T6 and L2, but sometimes higher), duration of aortic occlusion, hypotension, and hypoxia (Akins, 1989).

Clamping the aorta also elevates proximal aortic pressure. The resulting rise in afterload can cause increased cardiac work and myocardial oxygen consumption (Rose et al., 1991). Therefore, aortic pressure above the clamp must be carefully regulated during the period of cross-clamping to prevent left ventricular failure. Pharmacologic vasodilation may be used to counteract proximal hypertension. However, significant reduction of upper body arterial pressure during cross-clamping or hypotension after the cross-clamp is removed can produce ischemic damage to the kidneys or spinal cord (Kirklin & Barratt-Boyes, 1993a).

One of three techniques may be used for spinal cord protection and to relieve proximal hypertension: (1) a heparin-bonded shunt, (2) left-sided heart (i.e., partial) bypass, or (3) CPB with femoral artery and vein cannulation (femorofemoral bypass). In the first method, a *heparin-bonded shunt* is placed proximal (in the aorta, left subclavian artery, or left ventricular apex) and distal (in the descending thoracic aorta or femoral artery) to the occluded aortic segment (Akins, 1989). In the second method, *partial ("left heart") bypass,* blood is drained from a cannula in the left atrium, circulated through a centrifugal pump, and returned to the systemic circulation through a femoral artery cannula. Because blood still flows through the right side of the heart and pulmonary vasculature normally, an oxygenator in the circuit is not necessary and only low doses of heparin are required.

In the third method, the femoral artery and vein are cannulated and full *CPB* is instituted. Blood is drained through the venous cannula and circulated through the CPB circuit before being returned to the

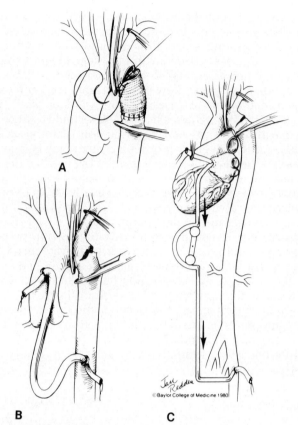

FIGURE 17-9. Several of the techniques described in the text are demonstrated in this drawing depicting repair of a traumatic transection of the descending thoracic aorta, including the "clamp and sew" technique **(A),** a heparinized shunt placed proximal and distal to the clamped segment of aorta **(B),** and partial (left heart) bypass with cannulation of the left atrium and femoral artery **(C).** (Mattox KL, 1991: Thoracic trauma. In Baue AE, Geha AS, Hammond GL, et al [eds]: Glenn's Thoracic and Cardiovascular Surgery, ed. 5, p. 100. Norwalk, CT, Appleton & Lange)

body through the femoral artery cannula. The first two methods have the advantage of requiring little or no anticoagulation, thus reducing the likelihood of hemorrhagic complications (Ergin et al., 1991). Full anticoagulation is required for femorofemoral CPB. Neither use of partial or full CPB during the procedure nor use of a shunt to maintain blood flow from above to below the occluded segment has eradicated the occurrence of postoperative paraplegia. Consequently, some surgeons perform the repair with a *"clamp and sew" technique* in which the aorta is clamped and the repair performed without using a shunt or either form of CPB (Fig. 17-9).

POSTOPERATIVE CONSIDERATIONS

An important feature of early postoperative management in patients who have undergone aortic surgery is blood pressure control. Many patients with aortic aneurysm or dissection have underlying hypertension. After aortic operations, blood pressure is maintained in a low normal range (80 to 90 mm Hg systolic) to protect the multiple anastomotic suture lines. Often, patients have previously been taking a beta-blocking medication, such as propranolol. Antihypertensive therapy is resumed when oral medications are reinstituted. Because hypertension is a predominant risk factor and one that can usually be controlled with pharmacologic therapy, it is imperative that affected patients understand the need for life-long medical supervision with sustained control of hypertension.

The most common complications of aortic surgery are bleeding and ischemic organ injury. Procedures that include extensive replacement of the thoracic aorta may be associated with 2000 to 7000 mL of blood loss; hemorrhage may be more severe in the event of technical problems, prolonged CPB, excessive hemodilution, or coagulation defects (Kouchoukos & Wareing, 1991).

Operations on the ascending aorta or aortic arch may be associated with stroke or generalized cerebral dysfunction secondary to embolization of air or particulate matter (Kouchoukos & Wareing, 1991). Paraplegia occurs unpredictably in a small percentage of patients undergoing descending aortic surgery despite all currently employed techniques to prevent or predict it. Similarly, acute renal failure may occur due to intraoperative ischemic damage to the kidneys.

An unusual but very serious complication of surgical procedures on the thoracic aorta is infection of the vascular prosthesis. In most instances, graft infection is thought to be due to contamination at operation (Kouchoukos & Wareing, 1991). Risk factors associated with development of vascular prosthesis infection include presence of infection elsewhere in the body, diabetes, preoperative use of steroids, and postoperative sepsis. The infection usually produces a false aneurysm at the suture line (Crawford, 1989).

Continued medical evaluation of patients with aortic disease is essential, especially in those with aortic dissection or Marfan's syndrome. Recurrent dissection or fusiform aneurysm formation can develop in weakened areas of dissected aortic wall (Crawford, 1989). Also, the remainder of the patient's aorta is subject to the same pathologic process that affected the resected segment of aorta. In patients afflicted with Marfan's syndrome, multiple segments or even the entire aorta may eventually be affected by aneurysm formation or dissection. Multiple operations for repair of diseased ascending aorta, aortic arch, or descending aorta may be necessary and may considerably extend life expectancy (Crawford, 1989).

REFERENCES

Akins CW, 1989: Nondissecting aneurysms of the thoracic aorta. In Eagle KA, Haber E, DeSanctis RW, Austin WG (eds): The Practice of Cardiology, ed. 2. Boston, Little, Brown

Cohn LH, 1990: Thoracic aortic aneurysms and aortic dissection. In Sabiston DC Jr, Spencer FC (eds): Surgery of the Chest, ed. 5. Philadelphia, WB Saunders

Crawford ES, 1989: Replacement of the thoracic aorta. In Grillo HC, Austen WG, Wilkins EW Jr, et al. (eds): Current Therapy in Cardiothoracic Surgery. Toronto, BC Decker

Crawford ES, Coselli JS, 1991: Aneurysms of the transverse aortic arch. In Baue AE, Geha AS, Hammond GL, et al. (eds): Glenn's Thoracic and Cardiovascular Surgery, ed 5. Norwalk, CT, Appleton & Lange

Crawford ES, Kirklin JW, Naftel DC, et al., 1992: Surgery for acute dissection of ascending aorta. J Thorac Cardiovasc Surg 104:46

Eagle KA, DeSanctis RW, 1992: Diseases of the aorta. In Braunwald E (ed): Heart Disease: A Textbook of Cardiovascular Medicine, ed. 4. Philadelphia, WB Saunders

Eagle KA, Doroghazi RM, DeSanctis RW, Austen WG, 1989: Aortic dissection. In Eagle KA, Haber E, DeSanctis RW, Austin WG (eds): The Practice of Cardiology, ed. 2. Boston, Little, Brown & Co

Ergin MA, Lansman SL, Griepp RB, 1991: Dissections of the aorta. In Baue AE, Geha AS, Hammond GL, et al. (eds): Glenn's Thoracic and Cardiovascular Surgery, ed 5. Norwalk, CT, Appleton & Lange

Fann JI, Glower DD, Miller DC, et al, 1991: Preservation of aortic valve in type A aortic dissection complicated by aortic regurgitation. J Thorac Cardiovasc Surg 102:62

Fann JI, Sarris GE, Miller C, et al, 1989: Surgical management of acute aortic dissection complicated by stroke. Circulation (Suppl I):I-257

Galloway AC, Colvin SB, LaMendola CL, et al., 1989: Ten-year operative experience with 165 aneurysms of the ascending aorta and aortic arch. Circulation (Suppl I):I-249

Glower DD, Fann JI, Speier RH, et al, 1990: Comparison of medical and surgical therapy for uncomplicated descending aortic dissection. Circulation 82 (Suppl IV):IV-39

Griepp RB, Stinson EB, Hollingsworth JF, et al., 1975: Prosthetic replacement of the aortic arch. J Thorac Cardiovasc Surg 70:1051

Kirklin JW, Barratt-Boyes BG, 1993a: Chronic thoracic and thoracoabdominal aortic aneurysm. In Cardiac Surgery, ed. 2. New York, Churchill Livingstone

Kirklin JW, Barratt-Boyes BG, 1993b: Acute aortic dissection. In Cardiac Surgery, ed. 2. New York, Churchill Livingstone

Kouchoukos NT, 1991: Aneurysms of the thoracic aorta. In Baue AE, Geha AS, Hammond GL, et al. (eds): Glenn's Thoracic and Cardiovascular Surgery, ed 5. Norwalk, CT, Appleton & Lange

Kouchoukos NT, Wareing TH, 1991: Management of complications of aortic surgery. In Waldhausen JA, Orringer MB (eds): Complications in Cardiothoracic Surgery. St. Louis, Mosby–Year Book

Laschinger JC, Izumoto H, Kouchoukos NT, 1987: Evolving concepts in prevention of spinal cord injury during operations on the descending thoracic and thoracoabdominal aorta. Ann Thorac Surg 44:667

Lindsay J Jr, DeBakey ME, Beall AC, 1990: Diseases of the aorta. In Hurst JW, Schlant RC, Rackley CE, et al (eds): The Heart, ed. 7. New York, McGraw-Hill

Qayumi AK, Janusz MT, Jamieson WR, Dyster DM, 1992: Pharmacologic interventions for prevention of spinal cord injury caused by aortic cross-clamping. J Thorac Cardiovasc Surg 104:256

Rose DM, Laschinger JC, Cunningham JN Jr, 1991: Descending thoracic aortic aneurysms. In Baue AE, Geha AS, Hammond GL, et al. (eds): Glenn's Thoracic and Cardiovascular Surgery, ed. 5. Norwalk, CT, Appleton & Lange

Wheat MW, 1987: Acute dissection of the aorta. In McGoon DC (ed): Cardiac Surgery, ed. 2. Philadelphia, FA Davis

Wolfe WG, Moran JF, 1981: Dissecting Aneurysms. In Gay WA (ed): Cardiovascular Surgery (Goldsmith Practice of Surgery—revised edition). Philadelphia, Harper & Row

CHAPTER 18

SURGICAL TREATMENT OF CARDIAC RHYTHM DISORDERS

CARDIAC RHYTHM DISORDERS
    Classification of Arrhythmias
    Pathogenesis of Tachyarrhythmias
    Treatment Modalities

SURGICAL THERAPY
    Operations to Eradicate Supraventricular
        Tachyarrhythmias
    Operations to Eradicate Ventricular
        Tachyarrhythmias
    Antitachycardia Devices

CARDIAC RHYTHM DISORDERS

CLASSIFICATION OF ARRHYTHMIAS

Cardiac arrhythmias are generally categorized as bradyarrhythmias or tachyarrhythmias. The primary treatment modality for persistent or recurring symptomatic bradycardia is permanent pacing, discussed in detail in Chapter 20, Permanent Cardiac Pacemakers. Tachyarrhythmias that represent a *chronic cardiac rhythm disorder* are the focus of this chapter. They almost always occur secondary to underlying cardiac pathology or abnormality. Tachyarrhythmias are further categorized as supraventricular or ventricular according to whether the site of origin or perpetuation is above or below the bifurcation of the bundle of His (Guiraudon et al., 1991). Transient cardiac arrhythmias caused by a specific precipitant, such as myocardial ischemia, proarrhythmic agents, or electrolyte imbalance, are discussed in Chapter 25, Cardiac Arrhythmias.

PATHOGENESIS OF TACHYARRHYTHMIAS

Most clinically important tachyarrhythmias are thought to arise due to a reentrant mechanism (Rosenthal & Josephson, 1990). Normally, an impulse originating in the sinus node is transmitted to all car-

diac cells and is extinguished when all cells have been depolarized and are completely refractory (Zipes, 1992a). *Reentry* occurs in an area of unidirectional block and slow conduction through an alternate pathway. Retrograde conduction through the region of unidirectional block can initiate a continuous, circuit-like electrical wavefront. Because the wavefront is always preceded by excitable tissue, reentrant arrhythmias can continue indefinitely (Cox, 1990). Patients who have the substrate for reentrant tachyarrhythmias are likely to experience recurrent arrhythmic episodes, which may be associated with syncope or sudden cardiac death (SCD).

Although many tachyarrhythmias result from reentry, some tachyarrhythmias are presumed to arise from an *automatic mechanism*. In other words, they occur due to enhanced spontaneous depolarization of normally latent automatic cardiac cells. Arrhythmogenesis of most clinically occurring arrhythmias is somewhat presumptive because present diagnostic modalities cannot unequivocally determine the etiologic mechanism (Zipes, 1992a).

TREATMENT MODALITIES

Treatment of supraventricular and ventricular tachyarrhythmias consists of (1) pharmacologic antiarrhythmic agents, (2) catheter ablation therapy, and

Betsy Finkelmeier: CARDIOTHORACIC SURGICAL NURSING.
© 1995 J.B. Lippincott Company.

(3) surgical therapy. Frequently, a combination of therapies is necessary. Chronic therapy with antiarrhythmic medications is limited by several factors. All currently available antiarrhythmic medications have associated adverse effects that make chronic therapy unappealing, particularly in young patients. Many of the agents are proarrhythmic, that is, they can cause arrhythmias. Some significantly depress myocardial contractility. Most importantly, none has proven completely effective in preventing arrhythmia recurrence. Life-threatening arrhythmias can recur despite predicted success based on rigorous testing during hospitalization (Rosenthal & Josephson, 1990).

Catheter ablation is the most rapidly expanding form of therapy. It consists of using radiofrequency delivered through an intracardiac catheter to eradicate arrhythmogenic tissue. The procedure is curative and, in contrast to surgical intervention, does not necessitate general anesthesia, sternotomy, or cardiopulmonary bypass. Catheter ablation techniques are effective in eradicating reentrant forms of supraventricular tachycardia (SVT), particularly those involving posteroseptal bypass tracts and dual atrioventricular (AV) nodal pathways (Rosenthal & Josephson, 1990). Catheter ablation may also be performed for eradication of ventricular tachycardia (VT). Appropriate candidates include patients with frequent episodes of VT that do not produce hemodynamic instability and that are not well controlled with antiarrhythmic medications. Antiarrhythmic medications and catheter ablation are discussed in greater detail in Chapter 4, Cardiac Rhythm Disorders.

SURGICAL THERAPY

The role of surgical therapy in treatment of tachyarrhythmias continues to evolve as more knowledge is gained regarding electrophysiologic mechanisms of arrhythmias and as less invasive forms of therapy are refined. Despite the evolution of sophisticated diagnostic techniques and therapeutic approaches, a paradox exists in surgical treatment of cardiac rhythm disorders. Although the mechanism in most forms of SVT is well understood, the responsible anatomic tissue cannot be distinctly visualized; conversely, electrophysiology of ventricular arrhythmias remains unclear but the responsible anatomic tissue is often visually apparent (Cox, 1990).

A number of surgical techniques have been developed over the past decade for the correction or treatment of tachyarrhythmias, including (1) *intraoperative mapping* (i.e., programmed electrical stimulation of cardiac endocardium and epicardium to localize reentrant pathways or arrhythmogenic foci), (2) *cryoablation* (i.e., direct application of an extremely cold [−60° C] probe to arrhythmogenic tissue to destroy it), (3) surgical excision of arrhythmogenic endocardial or epicardial tissue, and (4) implantation of antitachy-

cardia pacing or defibrillating devices. Often, combinations of these techniques are used.

Cryoablation and surgical excision are techniques used for arrhythmia eradication. The objective of such procedures is to excise, isolate, or interrupt cardiac tissue responsible for the initiation, maintenance, or propagation of the tachycardia while preserving or improving myocardial function (Zipes, 1992b). In patients in whom this is not feasible, implantable devices may be used to treat the tachyarrhythmia each time it occurs.

OPERATIONS TO ERADICATE SUPRAVENTRICULAR TACHYARRHYTHMIAS

Surgical therapy may be performed to eradicate one of the various reentrant forms, or less commonly an automatic form, of SVT. Reentrant SVT is generally categorized according to location of the reentrant pathway. *Atrial-ventricular* reentry signifies the presence of anomalous, electrically active tissue extending between atrium and ventricle and bypassing normal conduction through the AV node. AV nodal reentry occurs due to a reentrant pathway within the AV node or perinodal tissue. Atrial reentry tachycardia is caused by a reentrant pathway within atrial muscle.

Atrial-Ventricular Reentry Tachyarrhythmias

The most common surgically corrected, supraventricular rhythm disorder is atrial-ventricular reentrant tachycardia produced by the anomalous pathway present in *Wolff-Parkinson-White (WPW) syndrome*. Patients with WPW syndrome have accessory atrial-ventricular pathways, also called Kent bundles, that are present from birth and that may become clinically manifested at any time. Kent bundles may be located in one of the four regions of the coronary sulcus: left free wall, right free wall, posterior septum, or anterior septum (Fig. 18-1) (Holman et al., 1992). Most common is a left posterior free wall Kent bundle. In approximately 20% of patients, more than one accessory pathway is present (Hood et al., 1991). Intermittent or continuous conduction through the accessory pathway can occur antegrade only, retrograde only, or, in some patients, in both an antegrade and retrograde fashion. Because the AV node is bypassed, paroxysmal atrial tachycardia or atrial fibrillation with a rapid ventricular response rate can occur and produce significant hemodynamic compromise.

In many patients, tachyarrhythmias associated with WPW syndrome are suppressed with antiarrhythmic medications. Eradication of the reentrant pathway is recommended for patients with WPW who (1) have recurrent, disabling episodes of SVT despite antiarrhythmic medications, (2) become syncopal or experience SCD with arrhythmic episodes,

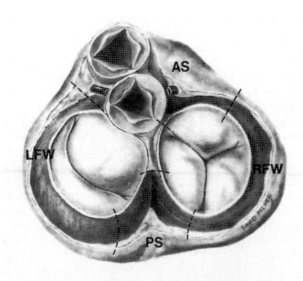

FIGURE 18-1. The heart is sectioned at the AV junction; *dotted lines* indicate the borders of the four anatomic regions of the coronary sulcus in which Kent bundles may be located: *AS*, anteroseptal space; *RFW*, right free wall; *PS*, posteroseptal space; *LFW*, left free wall. (Holman WL, Kirklin JK, Epstein AE, et al, 1992: Wolff-Parkinson-White syndrome. J Thorac Cardiovasc Surg 104:804)

or (3) experience intolerable side effects from antiarrhythmic medications. Either catheter ablation or surgical interruption of the anomalous pathway may be used to eradicate reentrant atrial-ventricular arrhythmias associated with WPW syndrome. With the increasing efficacy of catheter ablative techniques that can be accomplished without an operative procedure, surgical intervention is less often required. It is used primarily for patients in whom catheter ablative therapy fails to eradicate the reentrant pathway, in whom multiple pathways are present, or who require cardiac surgery for a coexisting cardiac problem (Bolling, 1991b).

Surgical division of an anomalous pathway in a patient with WPW syndrome was first performed successfully in 1968 (Cobb et al., 1968). Currently, pathway eradication is performed using one of two techniques depending on location of the accessory pathway as determined by the preoperative electrophysiologic study and preference of the surgeon. The classic *endocardial approach*, developed by Sealy and refined by Cox, is performed through an incision in the atrial endocardium; Guiraudon has described an alternative *epicardial approach* performed through an incision in the atrial epicardium (Page et al., 1990).

The endocardial technique can be used for accessory pathways in all locations. It necessitates use of cardiopulmonary bypass and cardioplegic arrest. Intraoperative mapping, using electrodes positioned around the AV groove, is performed to determine the ventricular and atrial insertion sites of the accessory

pathway (DeMaio, 1991a). By provoking the clinically occurring arrhythmia, abnormal activation sequences are identified and reentrant pathways are localized.

Intraoperative mapping is important because it is more precise than preoperative programmed electrical stimulation. However, the preoperative study is essential because general anesthesia, hypothermia, or trauma to the pathways may preclude arrhythmia induction and thus the ability to map intraoperatively (Zipes, 1992b). After mapping, the appropriate atrium is opened. The atrial and ventricular endocardial surfaces in the area of the pathway are incised to interrupt the reentrant pathway.

The less commonly used epicardial approach consists of interruption of the atrial end of the reentrant pathway by excision or cryoablation of the outer surface of the heart without opening the atrium. The epicardial approach can be performed when the pathway is localized to the right or left free wall or to the posterior septal area (DeMaio, 1991a). An endocardial approach is necessary to divide anterior septal pathways. An advantage of the epicardial technique is that it does not necessitate the inducement of hypothermic, cardioplegic arrest. Because the procedure is performed on a normothermic, beating heart, successful pathway interruption is immediately identified by loss of preexcitation (early ventricular activation representing impulse conduction that bypasses the AV node) on the electrocardiogram. In addition, in patients with right free wall or posterior septal pathways, pathway interruption can sometimes be performed without cardiopulmonary bypass (Mahomed et al., 1988). After either procedure, a postoperative electrophysiologic study is performed to confirm successful arrhythmia eradication. Results of endocardial and epicardial division techniques are comparable. The operation is almost universally successful in eradicating the arrhythmia and the risk of mortality or morbidity is minimal. Some surgeons advocate a combined endocardial and epicardial approach that includes desirable features of each technique (Selle et al., 1991).

Atrioventricular Nodal Reentry Tachyarrhythmias

AV nodal tachycardia arises from a reentrant pathway confined to the AV node or perinodal tissue. The presence of two anatomically or functionally distinct AV nodal pathways is thought to produce the arrhythmia in most patients (Guiraudon et al., 1991). Although catheter ablation is the preferred interventional technique, AV nodal reentry tachycardia may be treated with surgical therapy in patients in whom catheter ablation is unsuccessful. The first surgical therapy for AV nodal reentry was ablation of the His bundle. This technique was unattractive because destruction of AV nodal tissue produced complete heart block and necessitated implantation of a permanent pacemaker. More recent surgical techniques are based on mapping studies demonstrating that a portion of at least one of the pathways resides outside the anatomic AV node in adjacent tissue (Cox et al., 1990; Yagi et al., 1991).

One of two surgical techniques may be used to eradicate AV nodal reentrant pathways. Perinodal cryosurgical ablation is performed by application of a cryoprobe to atrial tissue immediately adjacent to the AV node to ablate arrhythmogenic tissue (Fig. 18-2) (Cox et al., 1990). Alternatively, perinodal tissue in the atrium is sharply dissected (Yagi et al., 1991). Each of these methods eliminates the reentrant pathway while preserving antegrade AV conduction. Surgical techniques for AV nodal reentry tachycardia are successful in approximately 95% of cases (Zipes, 1992b). Heart block is a potential complication.

Atrial Reentry Tachyarrhythmias

Surgical procedures developed for *atrial reentry tachyarrhythmias* (e.g., atrial fibrillation) are being performed in a few centers but are not yet established as conventional alternatives to less invasive forms of therapy. Development of operative procedures for

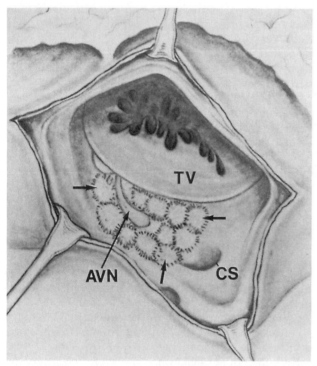

FIGURE 18-2. Cryoablation of AV nodal reentrant tachycardia. Drawing demonstrates surgical exposure through right atriotomy incision with patient's head to left. *TV*, tricuspid valve; *CS*, coronary sinus; *AVN*, region of AV node; *short arrows* point to several of the overlapping 3-mm cryolesions placed in the perinodal region of the atrial septum. (Adapted from Cox JL, Ferguson B, Lindsay BD, Cain ME, 1990: Perinodal cryosurgery for atrioventricular node reentry tachycardia in 23 patients. J Thorac Cardiovasc Surg 99:446)

ablation of atrial reentry arrhythmias has been slow because (1) understanding of the responsible electrophysiologic mechanisms is limited, (2) the anatomic tissue responsible for arrhythmogenesis is not visible, and (3) very few surgeons have acquired experience with the operative techniques (Cox, 1985; Cox et al., 1991a).

Atrial fibrillation is the most common atrial reentry arrhythmia. It is thought to be caused by multiple reentrant circuits that may be simultaneously active, precluding synchronous activation of enough atrial myocardium to generate an identifiable P wave (Cox et al., 1991a). Currently available pharmacologic therapy or electric cardioversion often fails to restore sustained sinus rhythm. Although antiarrhythmic medications may control ventricular rate, many patients continue to experience symptoms from the arrhythmia. In addition, atrial fibrillation is associated with increased risk for cerebral vascular accident due to embolization of thrombus from the left atrium (Repique et al., 1992).

Surgical eradication of atrial fibrillation is feasible because of the anatomically large reentry pathway responsible for the arrhythmia. The *maze procedure*, developed by Cox and associates, may be performed in selected patients with chronic atrial fibrillation and arrhythmia intolerance, drug intolerance, or previous thromboembolism (Ferguson & Cox, 1993). It may also be performed in patients with chronic atrial fibrillation who require cardiac surgery for another reason, such as mitral valve replacement. The Cox/maze procedure consists of multiple atrial incisions to disrupt atrial reentry and allow sinus impulses to activate the entire atrial myocardium (Cox et al., 1991b) (Fig. 18-3).

Automatic Atrial Tachycardia

Ectopic atrial tachycardia is an unusual automatic form of SVT. It occurs most often in children and can lead to cardiomyopathy in untreated patients (Walsh et al., 1992). In selected centers, ectopic atrial tachycardia is treated surgically with an *atrial isolation operation*. After precisely localizing the arrhythmogenic focus, which is usually in the left atrium, that part of the atrium is surgically isolated from the remainder of the heart so that the ectopic impulses cannot be conducted (Hillis et al., 1992).

OPERATIONS TO ERADICATE VENTRICULAR TACHYARRHYTHMIAS

Ventricular Tachyarrhythmias

Ventricular tachyarrhythmias most often occur in patients with coronary artery disease and significant left ventricular dysfunction. Malignant ventricular arrhythmias, that is, VT and ventricular fibrillation (VF), are life threatening. SCD, which is usually related to ventricular tachyarrhythmias, accounts for

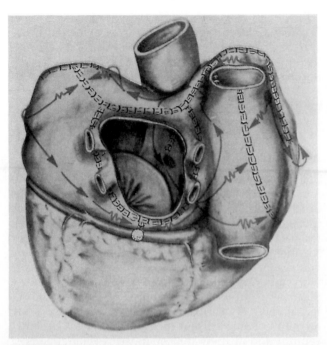

FIGURE 18-3. Posterior view of heart illustrating incisions constituting the Cox/maze operation. (Cox JL, Schuessler RB, D'Agostino HJ, et al, 1991: The surgical treatment of atrial fibrillation: III. Development of a definitive surgical procedure. J Thorac Cardiovasc Surg 101:578)

half of all cardiovascular mortality in North American and Western Europe (Lehmann & Saksena, 1991). Patients who have experienced either cardiac arrest or an episode of VT with syncope have a 22% to 30% risk of significant arrhythmia recurrence within 1 year (Gartman et al., 1990).

In a limited number of patients, ventricular tachyarrhythmias are *ischemia mediated;* that is, they occur secondary to myocardial ischemia. If the arrhythmia is the only consequence of the ischemia, antiarrhythmic drug therapy is usually attempted. However, more often the patient has anginal symptoms as well as the arrhythmia. In this setting, operative therapy may be recommended. Coronary artery revascularization is the primary therapeutic approach for patients who experience VT known to be associated with exercise-induced ischemia (Zipes, 1992b).

More often ventricular arrhythmias are *scar mediated;* that is, they occur due to a reentrant pathway in the subendocardial borders of infarcted myocardium. Currently available pharmacologic therapy for scar-mediated tachyarrhythmias is limited by the ineffectiveness and, in fact, proarrhythmic properties of most conventional antiarrhythmic medications and the frequency of intolerable side effects produced by effective agents. Conventional antiarrhythmic drug therapy successfully controls life-threatening arrhythmias in only 20% to 50% of patients (DeMaio, 1991b). In those patients who cannot be successfully treated with antiarrhythmic medications, surgical treatment may be recommended.

Types of Surgical Procedures

In contrast to ischemia-mediated arrhythmias, coronary artery revascularization does not prevent recurrence of arrhythmias caused by the abnormal electrophysiologic properties of endocardial scar. Left ventricular aneurysmectomy as a means of eradicating arrhythmogenic scar tissue also is ineffective. Current surgical treatment of scar-mediated tachycardia includes (1) eradication of arrhythmogenic scar tissue, (2) implantation of an antitachycardia device (i.e., an implantable cardioverter/defibrillator [ICD]), or (3) a combination of both therapies. The therapies differ in that procedures to eradicate arrhythmogenic tissue are designed to eliminate arrhythmia recurrence while ICDs do not prevent recurrence but rather treat the arrhythmia each time it occurs.

Surgical procedures to eradicate arrhythmogenic tissue in the ventricle began in the late 1970s with introduction of the encircling endocardial ventriculotomy by Guiraudon and associates and endocardial resection by Josephson and associates (Elefteriades et al., 1990). *Encircling endocardial ventriculotomy* is a procedure in which all infarcted and bordering endocardium is excluded from electrical continuity with normal myocardium through a perpendicular ventricular incision that spares only the epicardial surface and coronary vessels (Grusso & Harken, 1991). The procedure is no longer in common use.

Endocardial resection is the surgical excision of arrhythmogenic endocardial scar. Moran and associates (1982) refined endocardial resection, using epicardial and endocardial mapping to direct performance of an *extended endocardial resection,* in which not only the localized area of arrhythmogenesis but all visible fibrotic endocardium is removed. Operative procedures currently used for eradication of ventricular arrhythmias include (1) map-directed limited endocardial resection, (2) extended endocardial resection with or without mapping, (3) cryoablation, and (4) endocardial scar ablation using the neodymium:yttrium-aluminum-garnet (Nd:YAG) laser (Moran, 1990).

Endocardial Resection

Map-directed endocardial resection is the procedure most commonly performed for eradication of ventricular arrhythmias. Before operation, coronary angiography and left ventriculography are usually performed to identify coronary artery lesions and evaluate left ventricular function. In reasonably stable patients, antiarrhythmic drug therapy is discontinued the evening before operation to facilitate intraoperative arrhythmia induction and mapping (Moran, 1990). With the patient on cardiopulmonary bypass, a left ventriculotomy is performed through the aneurysmal segment that is usually present. Intraoperative mapping is performed to identify all potentially arrhythmogenic foci.

Endocardial mapping is performed using a hand-held probe or a multiple electrode array. A technique has also been developed that achieves endocardial mapping using a balloon apparatus that is inserted through an atrial incision, passed across the mitral valve, and inflated in the left ventricle so that electrodes are positioned against the endocardial surface of the ventricle (Mickleborough et al., 1990). A stocking device that fits over the heart allows mapping of epicardial surfaces without significant manipulation of the heart. In 85% to 90% of cases, VT can be induced and mapped (Hargrove & Miller, 1989). With availability of computerized techniques, it is possible to localize the responsible endocardial tissue with one provocation of VT. Guided by the results of mapping, subendocardial tissue identified as responsible for arrhythmogenesis is resected (Fig. 18-4). Programmed electrical stimulation is repeated after resection to confirm ablation of the arrhythmia.

Because VT often cannot be induced in a hypothermic heart, normothermia may be maintained during the procedure (Grusso & Harken, 1991). Advocates of sequential mapping and resection of arrhythmogenic tissue in a normothermic, beating heart believe this method provides more successful arrhythmia eradication while minimizing resection of normal muscle (Hobson et al., 1991). However, a warm, beating heart is more susceptible to myocardial ischemia and many surgeons use cold cardioplegia despite its limiting effect on intraoperative assessment of the success of arrhythmia eradication.

A *visually directed endocardial resection* (without mapping) may be necessary if VT cannot be induced and, therefore, mapped intraoperatively. The resection is extended to include all fibrotic endocardium that is visible to the surgeon. Extended endocardial resection requires a more extensive operative procedure and a longer period of cardiopulmonary bypass (DeMaio, 1991b). It is also less precise than that

which can be achieved with intraoperative mapping because arrhythmogenic tissue is located not in the scar itself but in the border zone between scar and healthy myocardium and because the necessary depth of resection is not visually apparent (Hobson et al., 1991). A postoperative electrophysiologic study is performed after endocardial resection to evaluate success of the operation.

Adjunctive Techniques

Sometimes arrhythmogenic scar is located on the inferior wall of the left ventricle and involves portions of the papillary muscles. If scar tissue extends through the papillary muscles or annulus of the mitral valve, complete resection is not possible without sacrificing the mitral valve. Because of underlying ventricular impairment typically present in patients who undergo endocardial resection, mitral valve replacement imposes a prohibitive operative risk. Alternatively, cryoablation may be used to eradicate arrhythmogenic tissue, especially over the ventricular septum and at the papillary muscles (Elefteriades et al., 1990). *Nd:YAG laser ablation* is also being used investigationally to eradicate arrhythmogenic tissue. Cryoablation and laser ablation are useful adjuncts because they destroy electrically active tissue while leaving structural elements intact (DeMaio, 1991b). Often coronary artery bypass grafting is performed concomitantly with endocardial resection. If a discrete ventricular aneurysm is present, it may be resected.

Results of Endocardial Resection

With the evolution of ICD devices, endocardial resection has become less favored as a treatment modality owing to significant operative mortality and arrhythmia recurrence in some patients. The proce-

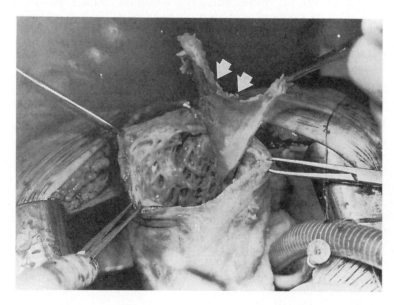

FIGURE 18-4. Intraoperative photograph demonstrating endocardial resection. The aneurysmal segment of the left ventricular wall has been resected; endocardial tissue is being removed from the left ventricular chamber (*arrows*). (Grosso MA, Harken AH, 1991: Ventricular tachyarrhythmias. In Baue AE, Geha AS, Hammond GL, et al [eds]: Glenn's Thoracic and Cardiovascular Surgery, ed. 5, p. 1869. Norwalk, CT, Appleton & Lange)

TABLE 18-1. FACTORS AFFECTING CHOICE OF SURGICAL THERAPY FOR VENTRICULAR TACHYARRHYTHMIAS

Factors Favoring Endocardial Resection

Frequent arrhythmic episodes
Monomorphic ventricular tachycardia
Mild to moderate left ventricular impairment
Discrete anterior aneurysm

Factors Favoring Implantable Cardioverter/Defibrillator Implantation

Infrequent arrhythmic episodes
Polymorphic ventricular tachycardia or fibrillation
Severe left ventricular impairment
Posterior aneurysm

(Adapted from Elefteriades JA, Biblo LA, Batsford WP, et al, 1990: Evolving patterns in the surgical treatment of malignant ventricular arrhythmias. Ann Thorac Surg 49:94)

dure is curative if successful but carries a higher operative risk than implantation of an ICD, particularly in patients with severely impaired left ventricular function. Endocardial resection remains useful in carefully selected situations. It is best suited to patients with a discrete anterior aneurysm, fairly good ventricular function, and frequent VT. In such patients, the risk of operative death is not prohibitive and long-term freedom from arrhythmia recurrence has been achieved. With careful candidate selection, operative mortality of 4% to 9% and arrhythmia suppression in 85% to 89% of patients is currently reported (Kron et al, 1990; Grusso & Harken, 1991; Ferguson & Cox, 1993).

Endocardial resection is unsuited to patients with global left ventricular dysfunction, polymorphic VT, or extensive scar that involves the papillary muscles or mitral valve annulus. In such patients, a combination of pharmacologic antiarrhythmic therapy and ICD implantation is preferable. Cardiac transplantation may be considered in patients with an ejection fraction less than 20%, diffuse hypokinesis, and no discrete aneurysm (Lawrie et al., 1991). Table 18-1 is a list of factors that are considered in determining the best form of surgical therapy for ventricular tachyarrhythmias.

ANTITACHYCARDIA DEVICES

Antitachycardia Pacing

An *antitachycardia pacemaker* is a device capable of sensing tachycardia and delivering four or five pacing stimuli in succession at progressively shorter intervals. Contemporary devices are activated by sensing (1) a rate that exceeds a programmed limit, (2) suddenness of onset of the tachycardia (to differentiate from sinus tachycardia), and (3) rate stability of the tachycardia (to differentiate from atrial fibrillation)

(Barold et al., 1992). Antitachycardia pacing is used almost exclusively to treat refractory, reentrant SVT in patients in whom electrophysiologic testing has demonstrated reproducible tachycardia termination with pacing without proarrhythmic effects (Rosenthal & Josephson, 1990). The effectiveness of catheter ablation and surgical eradication techniques for reentrant SVT have made antitachycardia pacing applicable to only a small number of patients. Antitachycardia pacing of the ventricle for treatment of VT is precluded by the prohibitive risk of inducing VF. However, newer implantable cardioverter/defibrillators incorporate an antitachycardia function that is useful in selected patients.

Implantable Cardioverter/Defibrillator

The *implantable cardioverter/defibrillator* is a battery-operated, prosthetic device capable of detecting tachyarrhythmias and delivering electrical countershocks. ICDs are used to provide rapid restoration of a stable cardiac rhythm in patients with chronic rhythm disorders associated with SCD or sustained VT with hypotension. Without such rapid defibrillation, these arrhythmias are usually fatal.

The first automatic defibrillator was implanted by Mirowski in 1980 (Mirowski et al., 1980). Since then, thousands of ICDs have been implanted and device technology has evolved considerably. Current devices consist of a pulse generator and a lead system with electrodes for sensing of cardiac activity and for countershocking the heart. The ICD discharges when the sensing electrodes detect a cardiac rhythm at a rate that exceeds the programmed upper limit of the device. Alternatively, the device may discharge only when both rate and probability density function (PDF) criteria are met. PDF describes electrogram morphology, specifically the proportion of the electrogram that is isoelectric (i.e., on the baseline). Because less isoelectric time occurs with VT and VF, these arrhythmias produce a PDF that is distinct from sinus rhythm. From a practical standpoint, however, the PDF feature is often not activated because it depletes battery life and because many patients who require ICDs have underlying bundle branch block or a VT morphology that negates its value.

When VT or VF is sensed, a high-energy pulse is delivered through the electrodes (Grusso & Harken, 1991). A series of five shocks may be delivered; the first occurs 10 to 25 seconds after the arrhythmia is detected, and if unsuccessful, four subsequent shocks will be delivered unless the heart rate falls below the programmed rate. After five shocks, the device remains quiescent until it detects 35 seconds of an alternative cardiac rhythm (DeBorde et al., 1991). It then resets and regains its capability of delivering another series of five shocks.

Availability of ICDs has changed the treatment of SCD survivors and patients with malignant ventricular tachyarrhythmias. The devices are best suited to patients in whom arrhythmia suppression or eradication cannot be achieved with conventional therapy. ICD implantation is often preferable to chronic antiarrhythmic drug therapy because of the lack of proven long-term effectiveness and substantial toxic and adverse effects associated with available pharmacologic agents. The most common indication for ICD placement is the occurrence of arrhythmias that are refractory to pharmacologic therapy as assessed by electrophysiologic inducibility or major arrhythmic event despite antiarrhythmic therapy. Although data from randomized trials are not available, patients with ICDs have a 5% probability of SCD within 5 years as compared with a 20% probability for similar drug refractory patients before availability of ICD therapy (Barold & Zipes, 1992).

ICD implantation is a particularly useful therapeutic option in patients who are not candidates for endocardial resection (e.g., those with poor ventricular function and those in whom endocardial fibrosis is extensive and would require sacrifice of the mitral valve to eradicate the arrhythmogenic focus). Another group of patients benefiting from ICD therapy are those with dilated cardiomyopathy who are awaiting heart transplantation. The limited supply of donor hearts often necessitates a waiting period of 1 to 2 years for transplantation. As left ventricular dysfunction associated with the cardiomyopathy progresses, the propensity for malignant ventricular arrhythmias and SCD increases (Wenger et al., 1990). Many patients die during this waiting period, and approximately 80% of the deaths are related to arrhythmias (Bolling et al., 1991a).

In most patients, ICD implantation can be performed transvenously using a single endocardial lead system. The endocardial lead is inserted through the right or left subclavian or jugular vein and positioned with the catheter tip in the apex of the right ventricle. With the catheter in this position, the sensing electrode is in the right ventricular apex; the defibrillating electrodes are in the superior vena cava and right ventricle (Fig. 18-5). A defibrillating patch electrode may be placed in the subcutaneous tissue as well. The proximal portion of the lead or leads is tunneled subfascially into the upper abdomen and connected to the pulse generator, which is implanted through a separate abdominal incision in a subcutaneous pocket. The generator is large, weighing 200 to 250 g.

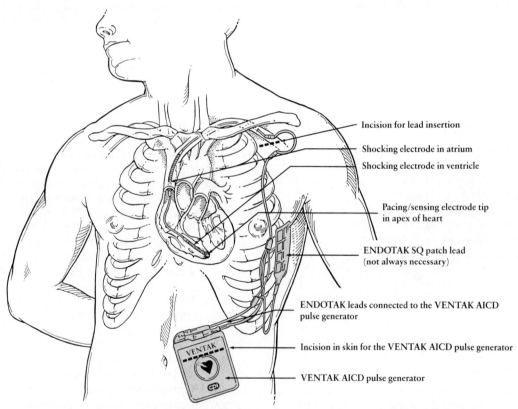

Incision for lead insertion

Shocking electrode in atrium

Shocking electrode in ventricle

Pacing/sensing electrode tip in apex of heart

ENDOTAK SQ patch lead (not always necessary)

ENDOTAK leads connected to the VENTAK AICD pulse generator

Incision in skin for the VENTAK AICD pulse generator

VENTAK AICD pulse generator

FIGURE 18-5. CPI implantable cardioverter/defibrillator (Ventak) with single endocardial lead system (Endotak). Both sensing and defibrillating electrodes are located on a single endocardial lead implanted transvenously in the right side of the heart. An additional defibrillating patch electrode may also be placed in the subcutaneous tissue. The lead system is connected to a pulse generator implanted in the subcutaneous tissue of the upper abdomen. (Courtesy of Cardiac Pacemakers, Inc, St. Paul, MN)

The device is tested at the time of implantation, using rapid pacing, programmed stimulation, or alternating current to induce VT and VF (Bolling et al., 1991a). With each arrhythmia induction, energy output from the ICD is increased or decreased as necessary to determine the *defibrillation threshold,* or lowest pulse amplitude that successfully terminates the induced arrhythmia (Bardy et al., 1993). A low defibrillation threshold is important because (1) it may increase over time due to fibrosis at the electrode–tissue interface, (2) antiarrhythmic drugs that increase the defibrillation threshold may be prescribed, and (3) pulse generators implanted in the future may be programmed at lower energy levels (Gartman et al., 1990). To ensure an adequate margin of safety, defibrillation threshold should be at least 10 joules lower than the maximal output that can be delivered by the pulse generator. If energy values near the maximum output of the device fail to terminate VF, the ICD may not function effectively and another treatment option may be necessary. Typically, the defibrillating threshold is 15 to 18 joules.

If it is not possible to achieve adequate defibrillating thresholds using an endocardial lead system, patch electrodes may be implanted directly on the epicardial surface of the heart (Fig. 18-6). Implantation of an epicardial patch lead system requires a surgical incision to expose the epicardial surface of the heart. Usually, a lateral anterior thoracotomy is performed. A subxiphoid approach can also be used, but it provides limited exposure and is not appropriate for obese patients or those with enlarged hearts. A median sternotomy may be used if a concomitant cardiac surgical procedure, such as coronary artery revascularization or endocardial resection, is to be performed.

When epicardial defibrillating electrodes are used, either endocardial or epicardial leads may be used to provide bipolar rate-sensing electrodes. The defibrillating patches are usually placed on the superolateral and inferobasal surfaces of the ventricles to contain the maximum volume of myocardium between them (Grusso & Harken, 1991). In patients who have had or who are likely to have a cardiac operation (e.g., those awaiting transplantation) the patches may be placed in an extrapericardial position, that is, on the outer surface of the pericardium.

In patients undergoing coronary artery revascularization, the decision about the necessity and timing for ICD implantation is sometimes complex. It may not be possible to confirm before coronary artery revascularization whether an arrhythmia is caused by ischemia or scar. Coronary artery bypass grafting may relieve ischemia and yet not prevent arrhythmia recurrence. If arrhythmia recurrence is likely, ICD electrodes may be placed as part of a primary cardiac surgical operation. An ICD generator can then be implanted if inducibility is demonstrated postoperatively.

Placement of epicardial patches at the time of coro-

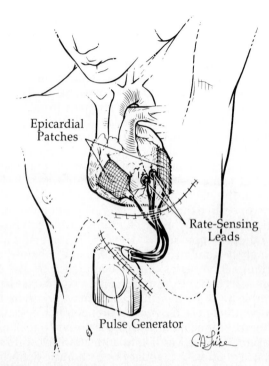

FIGURE 18-6. Implantable cardioverter/defibrillator using an epicardial lead system. If an endocardial lead system cannot be used, rate sensing and defibrillating electrodes may be implanted on the epicardial surface of the heart through a short thoracotomy incision; the pulse generator is placed in a subcostal pocket. (Kron IL, Haines DE, Tribble CG, et al, 1990: Operative risks of the implantable defibrillator versus endocardial resection. Ann Surg 211:601)

nary artery revascularization, however, may cause more pericardial inflammation, increase the risk of infection, cause coronary artery erosion, or affect long-term patency of bypass grafts lying on the surface of the heart. The presence of patches also makes a subsequent cardiac operation more difficult. Reentry through the sternum is complicated by dense adhesions formed because of the presence of the prosthetic material. Finally, epicardial patch electrodes can alter or block current flow through the heart during external defibrillation, thereby significantly elevating defibrillation requirements or even precluding successful transthoracic defibrillation (Lerman & Deale, 1990). With the availability of an endocardial lead system that can be implanted transvenously, the surgeon may determine that it is preferable to avoid the use of epicardial electrodes and, if necessary, implant a transvenous system at a later time.

In a patient who requires both an ICD and a pacemaker, safeguards are important to prevent inappropriate sensing by the ICD of the pacing impulses. The ICD pulse generator detects the spike of highest amplitude as the R wave. If the pacing impulse and R wave are similar in amplitude, the ICD pulse generator may "double count" the heart rate and produce erroneous triggering of a countershock. Conversely, if the patient develops VF, pacing impulses may be substantially taller than the fibrillatory waves and may be sensed by the ICD unit as a normal heart rate. In this case, the ICD would fail to discharge. The two pulse generators are placed as far apart from one another as possible. Also, a bipolar lead system is used for the pacemaker because it produces a pacing impulse of smaller amplitude than that which occurs with a unipolar lead. The ventricular pacing lead is placed at some distance from the rate-sensing electrodes of the ICD unit.

Postoperative care after ICD implantation is similar to that of patients who have undergone other types of cardiothoracic operations. The ICD is generally activated at the time of implantation using a hand-held programmer. A series of tones emitted from the device reveals that the desired change in status has been accomplished. Tachyarrhythmias may occur in the postoperative period owing to preoperative cessation of antiarrhythmic medications, electrolyte imbalance, hypoxemia, or pericardial inflammation. Despite the presence of an ICD, standard transthoracic defibrillation is performed if sustained VT or VF occurs. External paddles are placed in the conventional position on the chest wall. If the first external countershock fails to produce defibrillation, paddle position is adjusted, placing one paddle on the left anterior chest and one posteriorly on the back.

An electrophysiologic study is usually performed during the postoperative period to induce VT or VF and ensure appropriate sensing and reliable termination of the arrhythmia (Stephenson & Combs, 1991). An exercise stress test is also necessary to determine the patient's heart rate with exercise. If the heart rate exceeds the programmed upper rate limit for the ICD, a shock may be delivered inappropriately when sinus tachycardia is mistaken for VT. Pharmacologic therapy may be necessary to prevent sinus tachycardia during exercise. In such cases, a permanent pacemaker may also be necessary.

Patients who receive ICDs require significant education and psychologic support from nursing staff. A protocol for patient education should be designed that includes routine monitoring of the device, implications of the device for daily life, actions to take if the device discharges, and signs and symptoms that should be reported to the physician. Patients are generally encouraged to obtain an identification bracelet or necklace. They may also be instructed to perform "cough CPR" (coughing vigorously every 2 seconds with deep inhalation followed by firm exhalation) at the onset of arrhythmic episodes to avoid loss of consciousness (Brannon & Johnson, 1992).

The ICD is interrogated every 2 months to evaluate battery status and to maintain proper device function by charging and discharging the device (Mason & McPherson, 1992). Current generation ICD pulse generators can be expected to require replacement every 36 months (Moran et al., 1990). Implantation of an ICD device does not necessarily negate the need for antiarrhythmic medications because frequent discharging of the device is not desirable or practical. Therefore, many patients with ICDs continue to require chronic pharmacologic therapy. Because antiarrhythmic medications can alter defibrillation threshold, device function is also tested after changes in the medication regimen. Amiodarone, lidocaine, mexiletine, and flecanide increase defibrillation threshold while bretylium and sotalol decrease threshold (Barold & Zipes, 1992).

Mortality associated with ICD implantation is 1% to 4% (Rosenthal & Josephson, 1990). Although the device is very effective in decreasing death due to arrhythmia, long-term survival is poor, with many patients succumbing to heart failure (Kron et al., 1990). At 5 years there is no significant survival difference between patients receiving ICD therapy and medically treated, matched, high-risk patients (Lehmann & Saksena, 1991). In patients with severe ventricular impairment, cardiac transplantation may be a preferable alternative.

Infection is the major complication of ICD implantation, occurring in 1% to 20% of patients (Rosenthal & Josephson, 1990). Although infection may be localized to the subcutaneous pocket, the presence of prosthetic material connected to the heart may necessitate removal of the entire system. Other complications include generator migration and erosion, lead or generator failure, and inappropriate device discharge (Hobson et al., 1991).

Limitations of ICD therapy include the bulky and somewhat disfiguring device, discomfort and psychologic implications of sudden and unpredictable shocks, and the necessity for frequent follow-up visits (Elefteriades et al., 1990). Patients who have frequent arrhythmic episodes despite pharmacologic therapy are not good candidates for ICD implantation because the resulting frequent discharges quickly deplete battery life and are disturbing to the patient. The device is also generally not used in patients whose survival from noncardiac disease is estimated to be less than 1 year (DeBorde et al., 1991).

Newer defibrillating devices integrate automatic antitachycardia pacing, cardioversion, and defibrillation therapies; antibradycardia (VVI) pacing; memory functions for sensed and therapeutic events; selectable current pathways; and noninvasive programmed electrical stimulation (Fromer et al., 1992). These multiple-option devices are capable of *tiered therapy* (i.e., antitachycardia pacing, low-energy cardioversion, and asynchronous defibrillation) so that electrical therapy can be tailored more specifically to the tachyarrhythmia that occurs. The multiple-option devices are particularly beneficial for patients with frequent episodes of sustained VT who can be spared chronic antiarrhythmic therapy and the discomfort of high-energy shocks (Myerburg & Castellanos, 1992).

REFERENCES

Bardy GH, Johnson G, Poole JE, et al., 1993: A simplified single-lead unipolar transvenous cardioversion-defibrillation system. Circulation 88:543

Barold SS, Zipes DP, 1992: Cardiac pacemakers and antiarrhythmic devices. In Braunwald E (ed): Heart Disease: A Textbook of Cardiovascular Medicine, ed. 4. Philadelphia, WB Saunders

Bolling SF, Deeb GM, Morady F, et al., 1991a: Automatic internal cardioverter defibrillator: A bridge to heart transplantation. J Heart Lunt Transplant 10:562

Bolling SF, Morady F, Calkins H, et al., 1991b: Current treatment for Wolff-Parkinson-White syndrome: Results and surgical implications. Ann Thorac Surg 52:461

Brannon PH, Johnson R, 1992: The internal cardioverter defibrillator: Patient–family teaching. Focus Crit Care AACN 19:41

Cobb FR, Blumenschein SD, Sealy WS, et al., 1968: Successful surgical interruption of the bundle of Kent in a patient with Wolff-Parkinson-White syndrome. Circulation 38:1018

Cox JL, 1985: The status of surgery for cardiac arrhythmias. Circulation 71:413

Cox JL, 1990: The surgical management of cardiac arrhythmias. In Sabiston DC Jr, Spencer FC (eds): Surgery of the Chest, ed. 5. Philadelphia, WB Saunders

Cox JL, Ferguson TB, Lindsay BD, Cain ME, 1990: Perinodal cryosurgery for atrioventricular node reentry tachycardia in 23 patients. J Thorac Cardiovasc Surg 99:440

Cox JL, Schuessler RB, Boineau JP, 1991a: The surgical treatment of atrial fibrillation (I). J Thorac Cardiovasc Surg 101:402

Cox JL, Schuessler RB, D'Agostino HJ, et al., 1991b: The surgical treatment of atrial fibrillation (III). J Thorac Cardiovasc Surg 101:569

DeBorde R, Aarons D, Biggs M, 1991: The automatic implantable cardioverter. AACN Clin Issues Crit Care Nurs 2:170

DeMaio Jr SJ, 1991a: Surgical and catheter ablative therapy of supraventricular arrhythmias. In Hurst JW (ed): Current Therapy in Cardiovascular Disease, ed. 3. Philadelphia, BC Decker

DeMaio Jr SJ, 1991b: Surgical and catheter ablative therapy of ventricular arrhythmias. In Hurst JW (ed): Current Therapy in Cardiovascular Disease, ed. 3. Philadelphia, BC Decker

Elefteriades JA, Biblo LA, Batsford WP, et al., 1990: Evolving patterns in the surgical treatment of malignant ventricular arrhythmias. Ann Thorac Surg 49:94

Ferguson TB, Cox JL, 1993: Surgical treatment of cardiac arrhythmias. Heart Dis Stroke 2:37

Fromer M, Brachmann J, BLock M, et al., 1992: Efficacy of automatic multimodal device therapy for ventricular tachyarrhythmias as delivered by a new implantable pacing cardioverter-defibrillator: Results of a European multicenter study of 102 implants. Circulation 86:363

Gartman DM, Bardy GH, Allen MD, et al., 1990: Short-term morbidity and mortality of implantation of automatic implantable cardioverter defibrillator. J Thorac Cardiovasc Surg 100:353

Grusso MA, Harken AH, 1991: Ventricular tachyarrhythmias. In Baue AE, Geha AS, Hammond GL, et al. (eds): Glenn's Thoracic and Cardiovascular Surgery, ed. 5. Norwalk, CT, Appleton & Lange

Guiraudon GM, Klein GJ, Sharma AD, Yee R, 1991: Surgical treatment of supraventricular tachycardias. In Baue AE, Geha AS, Hammond GL, et al. (eds): Glenn's Thoracic and Cardiovascular Surgery, ed. 5. Norwalk, CT, Appleton & Lange

Hargrove WC, Miller JM, 1989: Risk stratification and management of patients with recurrent ventricular tachycardia and other malignant ventricular arrhythmias. Circulation 79 (Suppl I):I-178

Hillis LD, Lange RA, Wells PJ, Winniford MD, 1992: Surgical treatment of tachyarrhythmias. In Manual of Clinical Problems in Cardiology, ed. 4. Boston, Little, Brown

Hobson CE, DiMarco JP, Haines DE, et al., 1991: The influence of preoperative shock on outcome in sequential endocardial resection for ventricular tachycardia. J Thorac Cardiovasc Surg 102:348

Holman CE, Kirklin JK, Epstein AE, et al., 1992: Wolff-Parkinson-White syndrome. J Thorac Cardiovasc Surg 104:802

Hood MA, Smith WM, Robinson C, et al, 1991: Operations for Wolff-Parkinson-White syndrome. J Thorac Cardiovasc Surg 101:998

Kron IL, Haines DE, Tribble CG, et al., 1990: Operative risks of the implantable defibrillator versus endocardial resection. Ann Surg 211:600

Lawrie GM, Pacifico A, Kaushik R, et al, 1991: Factors predictive of results of direct ablative operations for drug-refractory ventricular tachycardia. J Thorac Cardiovasc Surg 101:44

Lehmann MH, Saksena S, 1991: Implantable cardioverter defibrillators in cardiovascular practice: Report of the policy conference of the North American Society of Pacing and Electrophysiology. Pace 14:969

Lerman BB, Deale OC, 1990: Effect of epicardial patch electrodes on transthoracic defibrillation. Circulation 81:1409

Mahomed Y, King RD, Zipes DP, et al, 1988: Surgical division of Wolff-Parkinson-White pathways utilizing the closed-heart technique: A 2-year experience in 47 patients. Ann Thorac Surg 45:495

Mason P, McPherson C, 1992: Implantable cardioverter defibrillator: A review. Heart Lung 21:141

Mickleborough LL, Usui A, Downar E, et al., 1990: Transatrial balloon technique for activation mapping during operations for recurrent ventricular tachycardia. J Thorac Cardiovasc Surg 99:227

Mirowski M, Reid PR, Mower MM, et al., 1980: Termination of malignant ventricular arrhythmias with an implanted automatic defibrillator in human beings. N Engl J Med 303:22

Moran JM, Kehoe RF, Loeb JM, et al., 1982: Extended endocardial resection for the treatment of ventricular tachycardia and ventricular fibrillation. Ann Thorac Surg 34:538

Moran JM, 1990: Surgical treatment of ventricular arrhythmias. In Karp RB, Kouchoukos NT, Laks H, Wechsler AS (eds): Advances in Cardiac Surgery, Vol. 1. Chicago, Year Book Medical Publishers

Myerburg RJ, Castellanos A, 1992: Evolution, evaluation, and efficacy of implantable cardioverter-defibrillator technology. Circulation 86:691

Page PL, Pelletier LC, Kaltenbrunner W, et al., 1990: Surgical treatment of the Wolff-Parkinson-White syndrome. J Thorac Cardiovasc Surg 100:83

Repique LJ, Shah SM, Marais GE, 1992: Atrial fibrillation 1992: Management strategies in flux. Chest 101:1095

Rosenthal ME, Josephson ME, 1990: Current status of antitachycardia devices. Circulation 82:1890

Selle JG, Gallagher JJ, Colavita PG, et al., 1991: Surgical division of posterior septal accessory pathways in the Wolff-Parkinson-White syndrome: A new modified approach. J Cardiac Surg 6:311

Stephenson NL, Combs W, 1991: Artificial cardiac pacemakers and implantable cardioverter defibrillators. In Kinney MR, Packa DR, Andreoli KG, Zipes DP (eds): Comprehensive Cardiac Care, ed. 7. St. Louis, Mosby—Year Book

Walsh EP, Saul JP, Hulse JE, et al., 1992: Transcatheter ablation of ectopic atrial tachycardia in young patients using radiofrequency current. Circulation 86:1138

Wenger NK, Abelmann WH, Roberts WC, 1990: Cardiomyopathy and specific heart muscle disease. In Hurst JW, Schlant RC, Rackley CE, et al. (eds): The Heart, ed. 7. New York, McGraw-Hill

Yagi Y, Schuessler RB, Boineau JP, Cox JL, 1991: Feasibility of closed heart discrete cryomodification of atrioventricular conduction. J Thorac Cardiovasc Surg 101:1004

Zipes DP, 1992a: Genesis of cardiac arrhythmias: Electrophysiological considerations. In Braunwald E (ed): Heart Disease: A Textbook of Cardiovascular Medicine, ed. 4. Philadelphia, WB Saunders

Zipes DP, 1992b: Management of cardiac arrhythmias: Pharmacological, electrical, and surgical techniques. In Braunwald E (ed): Heart Disease: A Textbook of Cardiovascular Medicine, ed. 4. Philadelphia, WB Saunders

CHAPTER 19

SURGICAL TREATMENT OF CONGENITAL HEART DISEASE IN ADULTS

DEFECTS WITH LEFT TO RIGHT SHUNT
Atrial Septal Defect
Ventricular Septal Defect
Patent Ductus Arteriosus

DEFECTS WITH OUTFLOW OBSTRUCTION
Aortic Stenosis
Coarctation of the Aorta
Pulmonic Stenosis
Tetralogy of Fallot

Surgical treatment of *congenital heart disease* (CHD) began over 50 years ago with the repair of vascular abnormalities such as patent ductus arteriosus and coarctation. With the development of cardiopulmonary bypass in the 1950s, it became possible to repair intracardiac defects as well. Innovative techniques were devised to correct most of the major cardiac deformities. Operative repairs to correct all but the most complex defects have now been available for more than 2 decades. Today, intraoperative techniques to protect organ function and sophisticated perioperative management allow many repairs to be safely performed during infancy.

Congenital heart surgery in adults is relatively uncommon, comprising only a small percentage of adult operative procedures requiring extracorporeal circulation (cardiopulmonary bypass). Untreated CHD in adults is uncommon because of increased awareness and improved noninvasive diagnostic techniques that result in detection of most defects early in life. Nevertheless, a small percentage of congenital defects do remain untreated until adulthood.

In some cases, an asymptomatic lesion is first diagnosed during a physical examination or diagnostic study in an adult. Although the defect may be asymptomatic at the time of diagnosis, natural history data about CHD reveal that many defects are associated with life-threatening complications or a shortened life expectancy. In other cases, pregnancy or aging may precipitate the onset of symptoms that warrant operative correction of the defect.

Adults with unrepaired congenital heart defects almost always have one of the most common and least complex of the many possible types of cardiac deformities. Most are isolated defects that are associated with either (1) a left to right shunt or 2) valvular or vascular obstruction. The discussion in this chapter is limited to surgical treatment of these lesions.

It should be noted, however, that surgical intervention is occasionally required in two other categories of adults with CHD. First, an increasing number of children who underwent repair of a congenital lesion have now survived to adulthood. Surgical therapy is occasionally required in these patients to treat a complication of the operative repair. Second, some individuals with noncorrectable lesions survive to adulthood. Palliative procedures performed during childhood in such patients may require revision. The spectrum of CHD is discussed in greater depth in Chapter 6, Congenital Heart Disease in Adults.

Betsy Finkelmeier: CARDIOTHORACIC SURGICAL NURSING.
© 1995 J.B. Lippincott Company.

DEFECTS WITH LEFT TO RIGHT SHUNT

The most common defects associated with left to right shunting are atrial septal defect (ASD), ventricular septal defect (VSD), and patent ductus arteriosus (PDA). In all of these defects, left to right shunting occurs across the defect because of the differences between systemic (left-sided) vascular resistance and pulmonic (right-sided) vascular resistance. The primary difference between the defects is the level at which shunting occurs: ASD—atria, VSD—ventricles, and PDA—great vessels. The degree of shunting is quantified using a ratio that compares the amount of pulmonary blood flow with the amount of systemic blood flow (Qp:Qs) or cardiac output from the right ventricle as compared with cardiac output from the left ventricle.

The primary consequence of left to right shunting is increased blood flow through the pulmonary vasculature. Congestive heart failure and pulmonary hypertension result and may progress to pulmonary vascular obstruction, a condition characterized by an irreversible increase in pulmonary vascular resistance. In its most severe form, pulmonary arterial pressure may eventually exceed systemic pressure, producing a reversal in direction of shunting. When right to left shunting secondary to increased pulmonary vascular resistance replaces left to right shunting, *Eisenmenger's syndrome* is said to exist. The development of Eisenmenger's syndrome precludes surgical correction of the defect. In the presence of irreversible pulmonary vascular obstructive disease, correcting the intracardiac defect would produce severe right-sided heart failure.

ATRIAL SEPTAL DEFECT

Atrial septal defect accounts for 45% of congenital heart defects found in adults (Henning & Grenvik, 1989). Although ASDs may occur at the junction of the superior vena cava (*sinus venosus ASD*) or at the base of the septum (*ostium primum ASD*), those that remain unrepaired until adulthood are almost always *ostium secundum ASDs* (located in the middle of the septum).

The size of the defect and compliance of the left and right ventricles during diastole determine the amount of shunting across an ASD (Kopf & Laks, 1991). Many adults with ASDs are asymptomatic, although easy fatigability and exertional dyspnea are common (Canobbio, 1989). Because symptoms develop gradually, they may not be recognized as abnormal. In other cases, a previously asymptomatic defect may begin to produce congestive heart failure as the individual ages. Supraventricular arrhythmias are also likely to develop. Common diseases acquired in adulthood (e.g., hypertension or ischemic heart disease) may decrease left ventricular compliance and increase left to right shunting.

Conversely, conditions that decrease right ventricular compliance (e.g., right ventricular myocardial infarction or failure) or that increase pulmonary vascular resistance (e.g., pulmonary embolism or pulmonary vascular obstructive disease) may produce significant right to left shunting with arterial desaturation. In addition, some right to left shunting occurs even when the predominant direction of shunting is left to right. As a result, venous thrombus may migrate across the septal opening and into the systemic circulation. This phenomenon, known as *paradoxical embolism*, is an occasional cause of cerebral vascular accidents in young adults.

Natural history data reveal a shortened life expectancy for persons with ASDs. The average life span for those with uncorrected defects is 50 years, with most patients dying of progressive heart failure (Kopf & Laks, 1991). Although some individuals survive to old age without symptoms, most become increasingly disabled with progressive symptoms (Cowen et al., 1990). Chronic atrial fibrillation may be present in more than 50% of individuals older than 60 years of age (Schaff & Danielson, 1987). Chronic congestive heart failure with fluid retention, hepatomegaly, and severe cardiac cachexia also occur in older adults (Kirklin & Barratt-Boyes, 1993-A).

ASD closure is recommended for defects associated with a greater than 1.5:1 left to right shunt (Spencer, 1990). Some adolescents and young adults may be candidates for nonsurgical closure using an *umbrella clamshell device*. During cardiac catheterization and using fluoroscopy, the device is positioned across the ASD to occlude the defect (Lock, 1991). The umbrella clamshell device remains investigational; at this time the primary method for repairing ASDs is surgical closure.

ASD was the first cardiac lesion successfully repaired using extracorporeal circulation (Kopf & Laks, 1991). The operation is performed through a median sternotomy incision and using cardiopulmonary bypass. After application of a cross-clamp to the aorta and administration of cardioplegic solution, an incision is made in the right atrium to expose the interseptal defect and significant intracardiac structures. ASDs are often closed by direct suturing of the defect in children. In adults, patching the defect with a piece of autogenous pericardium or prosthetic material is recommended (Schaff & Danielson, 1987). Great care is taken during the repair to avoid air entry through the defect into the left atrium and systemic circulation.

A sinus venosus ASD is often associated with *partial anomalous pulmonary venous connection*, that is, one or more of the pulmonary veins empties abnormally into the right instead of the left atrium. Anomalous pulmonary veins allow oxygenated blood to directly enter the right side of the heart and once again circulate through the pulmonary vessels. If anomalous pulmonary veins are present, ASD repair must include baffling the pericardial patch to redirect blood

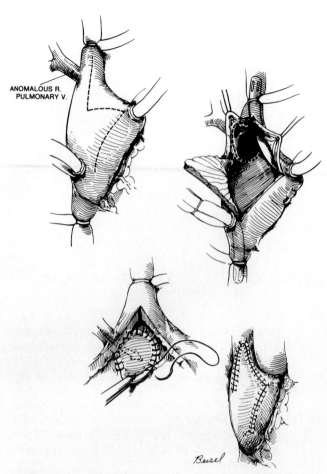

ANOMALOUS R.
PULMONARY V.

Beisel

FIGURE 19-1. Repair of sinus venosus ASD with partial anomalous pulmonary venous connection. After initiating cardiopulmonary bypass, right atrium is opened (**top left**), revealing sinus venous defect and orifice of anomalous right pulmonary vein (**top right**). Pericardial patch is placed to close defect and redirect flow from anomalous vein into the left atrium behind the patch (**lower left**). Incision in right atrial wall and superior vena cava is closed (**lower right**). (Waldhausen JA, Pierce WS, 1985: Congenital heart disease. In Johnson's Surgery of the Chest, ed. 5, p. 331. Chicago, Year Book Medical Publishers)

flow from anomalous veins into the left atrium (Fig. 19-1). Failure to revise anomalous drainage at the time of ASD repair results in a residual left to right shunt and the continued potential for right ventricular failure and pulmonary hypertension. Mitral valve deformities almost always accompany ostium primum ASDs and usually necessitate mitral valve repair or replacement. Closure of an ostium primum ASD is also complicated by the proximity of the defect to AV nodal conduction tissue; postoperative heart block occasionally results (DeAngelis, 1991).

Patients who undergo ASD repair are usually young, otherwise healthy adults. If pulmonary vascular resistance is normal, the operation is associated with less than 1% mortality rate and minimal morbid-

ity (Spencer, 1990). Except for temporary limitations imposed by the sternotomy, the patient can usually return to previous activities within weeks of the operation. Even in the presence of preoperative pulmonary artery hypertension and congestive heart failure, closure of an ASD associated with a significant left to right shunt usually produces symptomatic improvement (Cowen et al., 1990). Warfarin sodium (Coumadin) therapy is often recommended for several months after ASD repair (Backer et al., 1989). Anticoagulation reduces the possibility of thromboembolism from the surface of the repaired defect until it is covered by ingrowth of endothelial tissue.

VENTRICULAR SEPTAL DEFECT

A defect in the ventricular septum may also cause a left to right shunt. *Ventricular septal defects* are described according to their location in one of the four components of the septum; the membranous septum, and three muscular components—the inlet septum, the apical (trabecular) septum, or the outlet (infundibular) septum (Pacifico et al., 1990b). Seventy to 80% of VSDs are located in the membranous septum (Arciniegas, 1991).

Although VSD is one of the most common congenital lesions, large VSDs in adults are infrequent. It is estimated that 40% of VSDs close spontaneously during infancy and 60% close by 5 years of age (Warnes et al., 1991a). Spontaneous closure may even occur during adulthood. Those VSDs that remain open and associated with a significant shunt usually produce symptomatic congestive heart failure that prompts operative repair during childhood. A small VSD in an adult may not require surgical repair. However, surgery is recommended for VSDs associated with greater than 1.5:1 left to right shunting to prevent progressive heart failure and irreversible pulmonary vascular obstructive disease.

Surgical repair of a VSD is performed using a median sternotomy approach and cardiopulmonary bypass. Most defects can be repaired through an incision in the right atrium, thus avoiding the damaging effect of an incision in the ventricle (Fig. 19-2). However, a right ventriculotomy may be necessary for closure of VSDs in certain locations. A prosthetic patch is almost always used to close the defect. Because a small, hemodynamically insignificant residual VSD may persist after operative closure, antibiotic prophylaxis against infective endocarditis is continued after operative repair (Warnes et al., 1991a). The risk of endocarditis continues, despite surgical correction of a congenital heart defect, in patients with residual areas of turbulent flow, valvular or aortic wall abnormalities, and those in whom prosthetic valves have been implanted (McNamara, 1989). Repair of acquired VSDs that occur secondary to myocardial infarction is discussed in Chapter 15, Surgical Treatment of Coronary Artery Disease.

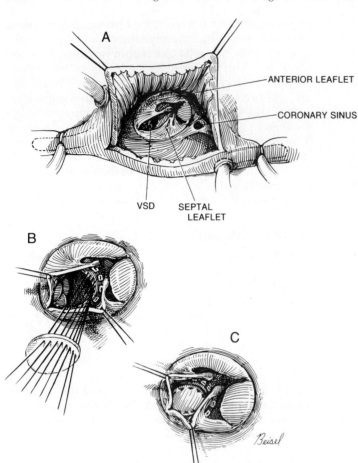

ANTERIOR LEAFLET

CORONARY SINUS

VSD   SEPTAL
       LEAFLET

FIGURE 19-2. Transatrial repair of a perimembranous VSD. **(A)** After establishing cardiopulmonary bypass and inserting a left ventricular vent, cardioplegia is administered and the right atrium is opened widely. The perimembranous VSD is exposed by retracting the septal leaflet of the tricuspid valve. **(B** and **C)** A patch is sutured into place to close the VSD. (Waldhausen JA, 1985: Congenital heart disease. In Johnson's Surgery of the Chest, ed. 5, p. 341. Chicago, Year Book Medical Publishers)

PATENT DUCTUS ARTERIOSUS

Patent ductus arteriosus is a vascular connection between the descending thoracic aorta and the pulmonary artery. Its presence represents a failure of the fetal ductus arteriosus to close at or shortly after birth. A left to right shunt occurs due to the gradient between systemic pressure in the aorta and the much lower pulmonary artery pressure. The degree of shunting is dependent on the size of the ductal lumen and the resistance in the pulmonary vascular bed (Canobbio, 1989). Typically, pulmonary blood flow is increased, producing symptoms of congestive heart failure that prompt surgical repair in infancy or childhood. Even small PDAs without associated symptoms are usually detected during childhood because of the characteristic, continuous murmur produced by left to right shunting throughout the cardiac cycle. The diagnosis can be confirmed by echocardiography; cardiac catheterization is not necessary. Repair is performed whether or not symptoms are present because PDAs are known to be associated with a shortened life expectancy. Potential complications of unrepaired PDA include heart failure, pulmonary hypertension, infective endocarditis, and aortic aneurysm or dissection secondary to degenerative changes in the ductal tissue.

Occasionally, a small or medium-sized PDA remains undetected until adulthood. A third of adults with unrepaired PDAs are asymptomatic; exercise intolerance and dyspnea are the most common presenting symptoms (Fisher et al., 1986). In selected patients, it may be possible to close a PDA by implanting an investigational occluding device into the ductus through a cardiac catheterization technique (Lock, 1991). Most PDAs in adults are surgically repaired. Through a left thoracotomy incision, the ductus is clamped and divided and the two segments are closed by direct suture technique (Fig. 19-3).

Repair of PDA in an adult may be complicated by several features that occur more often than with repair during childhood. These include (1) the frequent presence (21%–81%) of pulmonary hypertension, (2) a tendency for the ductus to be giant in size, (3) the common occurrence of ductal calcification, and (4) the presence of prior or concurrent infective endocarditis (Fuster et al., 1991a). Ductal calcification increases technical difficulty of the repair because the ductus may be easily torn when manipulated (Myers & Waldhausen, 1991). Accordingly, partial cardiopulmonary bypass (i.e., bypass of only the left side of the heart) may be used to increase safety of the procedure. Despite these factors, operative complications

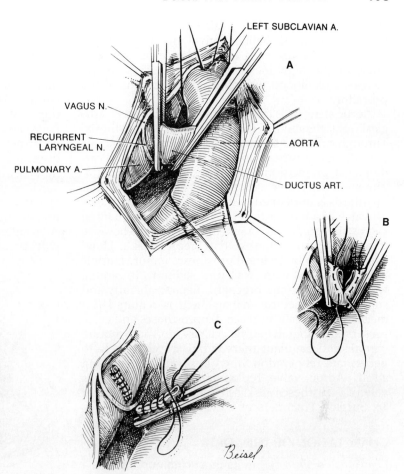

FIGURE 19-3. Surgical division of a patent ductus arteriosus (PDA). **(A)** After exposure of the PDA through a left thoracotomy incision, clamps are applied to the ductus close to the aorta and pulmonary artery. **(B)** The ductus is divided halfway through and partially sutured. **(C)** Each end of the divided ductus is closed with a running mattress suture followed by an over-and-over suture. (Waldhausen JA, 1985: Congenital heart disease. In Johnson's Surgery of the Chest, ed. 5, p. 291. Chicago, Year Book Medical Publishers)

are unusual after PDA repair. The procedure is generally considered curative. However, when the operation is performed in patients with severe, chronic congestive heart failure, death may occur due to the preexisting cardiomyopathy caused by long-standing volume overload of the left ventricle (Kirklin & Barratt-Boyes, 1993b).

DEFECTS WITH OUTFLOW OBSTRUCTION

The following defects are associated with valvular or vascular obstruction: aortic stenosis, coarctation of the aorta, pulmonic stenosis, and tetralogy of Fallot (TOF). TOF differs from the other three in that in addition to the obstructive component, right to left shunting of blood occurs through an associated intracardiac defect (VSD).

AORTIC STENOSIS

Aortic stenosis includes lesions that obstruct left ventricular outflow at the subvalvular, valvular, or supravalvular level. In adults, aortic stenosis is nearly always due to an abnormality at the valvular level. The most common type of congenitally abnormal valve is one that is bicuspid instead of tricuspid (Li-

berthson, 1989a). A nonstenotic, bicuspid valve is estimated to occur in 1% of the population (Fuster et al., 1991b). Although a bicuspid aortic valve may remain functionally normal, more often fibrosis and calcification occur with aging, gradually leading to stenosis (Kaplan, 1991). A bicuspid aortic valve is also more susceptible to infective endocarditis. Congenital aortic valve stenosis is usually progressive. The obstruction to left ventricular outflow causes left ventricular hypertrophy and eventual left-sided heart failure. Few patients survive beyond 60 years of age without serious signs and symptoms (Ungerleider, 1990).

Classic symptoms associated with aortic stenosis include dyspnea, angina, and syncope. Ventricular arrhythmias or sudden cardiac death may also occur. The development of symptoms is ominous, signifying a downward course and the likelihood of death within the next several years. Therefore, the presence of symptoms is an indication for repair or replacement of the stenotic valve. Corrective therapy may also be recommended in asymptomatic patients with a high transvalvular gradient because of an increased incidence of sudden cardiac death.

Balloon valvotomy has been safely and effectively used to dilate stenotic aortic valves in children. It may also play an increasing role in young adults with mobile, noncalcified, bicuspid aortic valves (Lock, 1991).

However, in older adults, calcification of the valve has often occurred. Balloon valvotomy is not recommended in the presence of valvular calcification because of the high incidence of restenosis and the increased likelihood of embolic complications of the procedure.

Aortic stenosis is most commonly corrected by surgical replacement of the valve with a prosthesis. Through a median sternotomy incision and using cardiopulmonary bypass, aortic cross-clamping, and cardioplegia, an incision is made in the ascending aorta. The stenotic, native valve is excised and a valvular prosthesis is implanted in its place. Either a mechanical valve or a bioprosthesis may be used. Mechanical valves are usually preferable in young adults because they are far more durable than bioprostheses. However, all of the mechanical prostheses require chronic anticoagulation with warfarin sodium. In young women who become pregnant, heparin therapy and sophisticated medical management is required if a mechanical valve is in place. Bioprostheses and cryopreserved allograft aortic valves do not require chronic anticoagulant therapy but are very likely to necessitate reoperation when implanted in a young adult. Aortic valve replacement and the various valvular prostheses are discussed in detail in Chapter 16, Surgical Treatment of Valvular Heart Disease.

COARCTATION OF THE AORTA

Coarctation of the aorta, in its most common form, is a segmental narrowing of the aortic lumen that occurs near the origin of the left subclavian artery, opposite the ligamentum arteriosum (Liberthson, 1989b). In some cases, coarctation remains undetected until adulthood. In others, coarctation repaired during childhood recurs in an adult. As many as 5% to 10% of individuals with repaired coarctation may require reoperation for coarctation recurrence (Connery et al., 1991).

Patients with coarctation develop proximal hypertension and a significant gradient in arterial blood pressure between upper and lower extremities. The presence of the coarcted segment causes a series of complex and poorly understood cardiovascular responses designed to maintain needed blood flow to organs below the stricture (Sealy, 1990). Unrepaired coarctation almost always produces symptoms or complications by 40 years of age, and survival beyond 50 years is unlikely (Liberthson, 1989b). Death can occur secondary to left ventricular failure, aortic dissection or rupture, stroke (secondary to hypertension), or infective endocarditis. A bicuspid aortic valve is often associated with coarctation and may become stenotic secondary to calcification or regurgitant due to the association of systemic hypertension with the abnormal valve (Fuster, 1991c).

Because of the potential complications of unrepaired coarctation, surgical correction is undertaken when the condition is diagnosed. In addition to a preoperative aortogram, cardiac catheterization is often performed because of the frequency of associated cardiac defects. Coarctation repair is performed through a left lateral thoracotomy incision. Cardiopulmonary bypass is not generally necessary. The aorta is clamped above and below the site of coarctation while the narrowed segment is removed. In infants, coarctation is often repaired using a flap graft constructed from the subclavian artery. In older children, it is frequently possible to restore aortic continuity with end-to-end anastomosis of the remaining aortic segments. However, the aorta in adults is less elastic and a prosthetic tube graft may be necessary to replace the resected area of coarctation (Fig. 19-4). Alternatively, an aortoplasty, or patching of the aorta with prosthetic material to widen the coarcted seg-

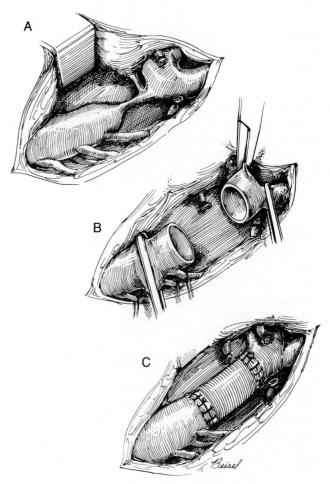

FIGURE 19-4. Surgical repair of coarctation of the aorta using a tubular graft prosthesis. **(A)** The coarctation is exposed through a left lateral thoracotomy incision. **(B)** Clamps are applied to the aorta above and below the area of coarctation and the coarcted segment is excised. **(C)** A tubular prosthetic graft is placed to bridge the defect and sutured to the aorta in end-to-end fashion. (Waldhausen JA, 1985: Congenital heart disease. In Johnson's Surgery of the Chest, ed. 5, p. 313. Chicago, Year Book Medical Publishers)

ment, is performed. However, aneurysm formation has been associated with the patch angioplasty technique and some surgeons recommend avoidance of this method of repair (Myers & Waldhausen, 1991).

Blood pressure control is of primary importance in postoperative management. Hypertension occurs despite complete relief of the gradient, secondary initially to increased epinephrine and then to increased norepinephrine secretion (Myers & Waldhausen, 1991). Intravenous agents may initially be necessary to achieve and maintain blood pressure in a desirable range. Coarctation repair does not necessarily produce normalization of systemic blood pressure (Maron, 1987). Many adults require chronic antihypertensive therapy.

A small percentage of patients undergoing coarctation repair develop postoperative arteritis in arteries arising from the aorta below the coarctation (Sealy, 1990). This acute regional arteritis may produce abdominal pain, ileus, and, in severe cases, small bowel necrosis in the early postoperative period. Accordingly, a nasogastric tube is prophylactically placed at the time of operation and oral feedings are withheld for the first several postoperative days until normal bowel function returns.

Coarctation repair is rarely complicated by postoperative paraplegia. Adults with coarctation generally have well-developed collateral blood vessels that bypass the narrowed segment to augment perfusion to the distal aorta. Even so, ischemic injury to the spinal cord and resultant paraplegia can occur with any operation that necessitates temporary occlusion of blood flow through the descending thoracic aorta. The risk of paraplegia is significantly higher during repair of recurrent coarctation.

Other complications of coarctation repair include restenosis, aneurysm formation, progressive enlargement of the ascending aorta, and infection of the prosthetic graft. Long-term follow-up studies have demonstrated a substantial number of postoperative cardiovascular problems, particularly in individuals who undergo operation at an older age and in those who have had a longer duration of preoperative hypertension (Perloff, 1992). Despite operative repair, patients may suffer premature death due to associated aortic or mitral valve disease, congestive heart failure, infective endocarditis, or aortic or cerebral artery rupture (Maron, 1987). Therefore, adults with repaired coarctation require ongoing medical supervision for potential postoperative sequelae.

PULMONIC STENOSIS

Congenital *pulmonic stenosis* is an unusual lesion in adults. The anomaly most often consists of a dome-shaped valve with a central opening and fused commissures (Warnes et al., 1991b). The functional consequences of pulmonic stenosis depend on the degree of obstruction and the adaptive response of the right ventricle. Over time the right ventricle hypertro-

phies, the pulmonic valve may become increasingly stenotic, and, in severe cases, right ventricular failure and tricuspid regurgitation may ensue (Canobbio, 1989). In patients with significant pulmonic stenosis the lesion may be corrected by balloon or surgical valvotomy or by pulmonic valve replacement.

TETRALOGY OF FALLOT

Tetralogy of Fallot describes a congenital malformation of the heart, classically composed of four elements: (1) VSD, (2) aorta overriding the VSD and communicating with both ventricles, (3) right ventricular outflow tract obstruction, and (4) right ventricular hypertrophy. Right to left shunting with decreased pulmonary blood flow is the primary physiologic consequence of TOF. Depending on the degree of aortic override and right ventricular outflow tract obstruction, shunting may vary from mild to severe (Pinsky & Arciniegas, 1990). If shunting is severe, cyanosis results.

Total correction of TOF is now almost always performed during childhood. However, because the techniques for correction of TOF in infants and children are relatively recent, a small number of adults exist with uncorrected TOF. Often, such patients have had palliative procedures designed to increase blood flow through the pulmonary vasculature and thus decrease the cyanosis associated with TOF. Examples of such palliative procedures include the Blalock-Taussig, Potts, Glenn, and Waterson-Cooley shunts.

Most often, surgery in adults with TOF is performed to revise a previous corrective procedure that has become physiologically dysfunctional. Reoperation becomes necessary in 2% to 13% of patients surviving initial corrective surgery for TOF (Heck et al., 1991). Persistent or recurrent right ventricular outflow tract obstruction, significant pulmonic regurgitation, and residual or recurrent VSD are the most common abnormalities necessitating reoperation (Pacifico et al., 1990a).

Rarely, corrective surgery may be performed initially during adulthood. Operative intervention is generally indicated in adults with uncorrected TOF to avoid troublesome symptoms and a shortened life expectancy. In most adults, uncorrected TOF can be definitively repaired with a low mortality rate (Laks & Pearl, 1991). Corrective repair is performed through a median sternotomy incision and using cardiopulmonary bypass. A right atriotomy or ventriculotomy is performed and the VSD is closed with a prosthetic patch. If the pulmonic valve itself is stenotic, pulmonic valvotomy may be necessary. The right ventricular outflow tract and main pulmonary artery usually require enlargement with patch augmentation. If this does not improve right ventricular outflow, a transannular patch, with sacrifice of the native pulmonic valve, is required. Previously constructed palliative shunts are closed at the time of correction. In most adults who undergo total correction of TOF, cyanosis is relieved and functional status improves (Presbitero et al., 1988).

REFERENCES

Arciniegas E, 1991: Ventricular septal defect. In Baue AE, Geha AS, Hammond GL, et al. (eds): Glenn's Thoracic and Cardiovascular Surgery, ed. 5. Norwalk, CT, Appleton & Lange

Backer CL, Hartz RS, Meyers SN, Davis G, 1989: Coronary embolism following atrial septal defect repair. Ann Thorac Surg 45:561

Canobbio MM, 1989: Congenital heart disease in adults. In Underhill SL, Woods SL, Froelicher ES, Halpenny CJ (eds): Cardiac Nursing, ed. 2. Philadelphia, JB Lippincott

Connery CP, DeWeese JA, Eisenberg BK, Moss AJ, 1991: Treatment of aortic coarctation by axillofemoral bypass grafting in the high-risk patient. Ann Thorac Surg 52:1281

Cowen ME, Jeffrey RR, Drakeley MJ, et al., 1990: The results of surgery for atrial septal defect in patients aged fifty years and over. Eur Heart J 11:29

DeAngelis R, 1991: The cardiovascular system. In Alspach JG (ed): Core Curriculum for Critical Care Nursing, ed. 4. Philadelphia, WB Saunders

Fisher RG, Moodie DS, Sterba R, Gill CC, 1986: Patent ductus arteriosus in adults—long-term follow up: Nonsurgical versus surgical treatment. J Am Coll Cardiol 8:280

Fuster V, Driscoll DJ, McGoon DC, 1991a: Congenital heart disease in adolescents and adults: Patent ductus arteriosus and other aorticopulmonary and coronary abnormal communications. In Giuliani ER, Fuster V, Gersh BJ, et al. (eds): Cardiology: Fundamentals and Practice, ed. 2. St. Louis, Mosby—Year Book

Fuster V, Warnes CA, Driscoll DJ, McGoon DC, 1991b: Congenital heart disease in adolescents and adults: Congenital left-sided outflow obstruction. In Giuliani ER, Fuster V, Gersh BJ, et al. (eds): Cardiology: Fundamentals and Practice, ed. 2. St. Louis, Mosby—Year Book

Fuster V, Warnes CA, McGoon DC, 1991c: Congenital heart disease in adolescents and adults: Coarctation of the aorta. In Giuliani ER, Fuster V, Gersh BJ, et al. (eds): Cardiology: Fundamentals and Practice, ed. 2. St. Louis, Mosby—Year Book

Heck HA, Pacifico AD, McConnell ME, 1991: Management of complications following surgical intervention for tetralogy of Fallot. In Waldhausen JA, Orringer MB (eds): Complications in Cardiothoracic Surgery. St. Louis, Mosby—Year Book

Henning RJ, Grenvik A, 1989: Congenital heart disease in the adult. In Henning RJ, Grenvik A (eds): Critical Care Cardiology. New York, Churchill Livingstone

Kaplan S, 1991: Natural adult survival patterns. J Am Coll Cardiol 18:311

Kirklin JW, Barratt-Boyes BG, 1993a: Atrial septal defect and partial anomalous pulmonary venous connection. In Cardiac Surgery, ed. 2. New York, Churchill Livingstone

Kirklin JW, Barratt-Boyes BG, 1993b: Patent ductus arteriosus. In Cardiac Surgery, ed. 2. New York, Churchill Livingstone

Kopf GS, Laks H, 1991: Atrial septal defects and cor triatriatum. In Baue AE, Geha AS, Hammond GL, et al. (eds): Glenn's Thoracic and Cardiovascular Surgery, ed. 5. Norwalk, CT, Appleton & Lange

Laks H, Pearl JM, 1991: The surgeon's responsibility: Operation and reoperation: The UCLA experience. J Am Coll Cardiol 18:327

Liberthson RR, 1989a: Congenital heart disease. In Congenital Heart Disease. Boston, Little, Brown

Liberthson RR, 1989b: Congenital heart disease in the child, adolescent, and adult. In Eagle KA, Haber E, DeSanctis RW, Austen WG (eds): The Practice of Cardiology, ed. 2. Boston, Little, Brown

Lock JE, 1991: The adult with congenital heart disease: Cardiac catheterization as a therapeutic intervention. J Am Coll Cardiol 18:330

Maron BJ, 1987. Aortic isthmic coarctation. In Roberts WC (ed): Adult Congenital Heart Disease. Philadelphia, FA Davis

McNamara DG, 1989: The adult with congenital heart disease. Curr Probl Cardiol 14:57

Myers JL, Waldhausen JA, 1991: Management of complications following repair of coarctation of the aorta, patent ductus arteriosus, interrupted aortic arch, and vascular rings. In Waldhausen JA, Orringer MB (eds): Complications in Cardiothoracic Surgery. St. Louis, Mosby–Year Book

Pacifico AD, Kirklin JK, Colvin EV, et al., 1990a: Tetralogy of Fallot: Late results and reoperations. Semin Thorac Cardiovasc Surg 2:108

Pacifico AD, Kirklin JW, Kirklin JK, 1990b: Surgical treatment of ventricular septal defect. In Sabiston DC Jr, Spencer FC (eds): Surgery of the Chest, ed. 5. Philadelphia, WB Saunders

Perloff JK, 1992: Congenital heart disease in adults. In Braunwald E (ed): Heart Disease: A Textbook of Cardiovascular Medicine, ed. 4. Philadelphia, WB Saunders

Pinsky WW, Arciniegas E, 1990: Tetralogy of Fallot. Pediatr Clin North Am 37:179

Presbitero P, Demarie D, Aruta E, et al., 1988: Results of total correction of tetralogy of Fallot performed in adults. Ann Thorac Surg 46:297

Schaff HV, Danielson GK, 1987: Advances in the surgical management of congenital heart disease in adults. In McGoon DC (ed): Cardiac Surgery, ed. 2. Philadelphia, FA Davis

Sealy WC, 1990: Paradoxical hypertension after repair of coarctation of the aorta: A review of its causes. Ann Thorac Surg 50:323

Spencer FC, 1990: Atrial septal defect, anomalous pulmonary veins, and atrioventricular septal defects (AV canal). In Spencer FC, Sabiston DC Jr, (eds): Surgery of the Chest, ed. 5. Philadelphia, WB Saunders

Ungerleider RM, 1990: Congenital aortic stenosis. In Sabiston DC Jr, Spencer FC (eds): Surgery of the Chest, ed. 5. Philadelphia, WB Saunders

Warnes CA, Fuster V, Driscoll DJ, McGoon DC, 1991a: Congenital heart disease in adolescents and adults: Ventricular septal defect. In Giuliani ER, Fuster V, Gersh BJ, et al. (eds): Cardiology: Fundamentals and Practice, ed. 2. St. Louis, Mosby–Year Book

Warnes CA, Fuster V, McGoon DC, 1991b: Congenital heart disease in adolescents and adults: Pulmonary stenosis with intact ventricular septum. In Giuliani ER, Fuster V, Gersh BJ, et al. (eds): Cardiology: Fundamentals and Practice, ed. 2. St. Louis, Mosby–Year Book

CHAPTER 20

PERMANENT CARDIAC PACEMAKERS

INDICATIONS FOR PACING	PACING MODES
PACING SYSTEM COMPONENTS	NBG Code
GOALS OF PERMANENT PACING	Single-Chamber Modes
Prevention of Bradycardia	Dual-Chamber Modes
Atrioventricular Synchrony	PACEMAKER IMPLANTATION
Rate Modulation	Implantation Procedure
	Postoperative Follow-Up
	Complications

The development of implantable, permanent pacemakers has significantly increased survival and improved quality of life for many individuals with bradyarrhythmias due to cardiac conduction abnormalities or other disorders. Approximately 2 million persons worldwide have had permanent pacemakers implanted; of those, 500,000 are alive and in the United States (Furman, 1991). Pacemakers were initially developed and remain the primary modality for maintaining an adequate ventricular heart rate in patients with life-threatening bradycardia. However, technologic advances in the past decade have resulted in increasingly complex systems capable of pacing the heart in a more physiologic manner. As a result, pacemaker therapy has become more sophisticated, with new terminology, changing criteria for selection of a pacing system, and increasingly complex electrocardiographic manifestations (Finkelmeier & Salinger, 1986). Major developments responsible for increased capabilities of permanent pacing systems include permanent electrodes that can be reliably positioned in the atrium, pulse generator microcircuitry that can be noninvasively reprogrammed, and sensor systems that detect physiologic indicators of increased metabolic need.

INDICATIONS FOR PACING

Indications for cardiac pacing may be categorized as defects in atrioventricular (AV) conduction, defects in impulse formation, or a combination of both (Furman, 1991). The most common indication for permanent pacing is complete heart block. The most dramatic symptomatic indication is *Stokes-Adams seizure*, characterized by dizziness or fainting with or without associated convulsions (Furman, 1991). Other indications include symptomatic sick sinus syndrome or second-degree heart block, acute myocardial infarction with persistent, advanced second- or third-degree heart block, recurrent syncope associated with hypersensitive carotid sinus syndrome, advanced block with a symptomatic, slow ventricular rate in atrial fibrillation or atrial flutter, and bradycardia secondary to necessary pharmacologic therapy (ACC/AHA Task Force, 1991). In symptomatic patients temporary pacing may be necessary until a permanent pacemaker is implanted.

Although sophisticated electrophysiologic studies are sometimes necessary, diagnosis of the impulse formation or conduction abnormalities can in most instances be established with prolonged ambulatory

(Holter) or inpatient electrocardiographic monitoring. Provocative maneuvers, such as carotid sinus massage, may be necessary to elicit vagally induced arrhythmias.

PACING SYSTEM COMPONENTS

All permanent pacing systems have several basic components: pulse generator, lead, and electrodes (Fig. 20-1). The *pulse generator,* which is quite compact and minimally disfiguring, is implanted under the skin in a subcutaneous pocket. It houses the power source and electronic circuitry, which are encased in a hermetically sealed metal container, rendering it both fluid and air tight (Lowe & German, 1990). A lithium battery is used as the power source in currently implanted generators. Although factors such as frequency of pacing and voltage requirements influence battery life, lithium-powered pulse generators usually perform for 5 to 10 years or more before replacement is required.

Electronic components of a pulse generator include (1) an output circuit that transforms energy from the power source into an electrical pacing impulse, (2) a timing circuit that determines frequency of stimulation, and (3) a sensing circuit that detects intrinsic cardiac depolarization signals (Harthorne, 1989). Pulse generators designed for pacing both the atrium and ventricle have output, timing, and sensing circuits for both chambers as well as a separate timing circuit for the AV delay (Harthorne, 1989). In addition, many currently used pacemakers have circuitry that performs other functions, such as (1) allowing pacing parameters (e.g., pacing rate and shape of the pacemaker pulse) to be noninvasively

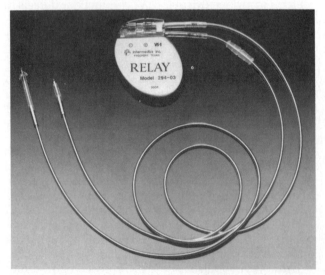

FIGURE 20-1. Dual-chamber pacemaker with bipolar atrial and ventricular leads. (Courtesy of Intermedics, Inc., Angleton, TX)

reprogrammed by an external computer and (2) storing and transmitting data regarding pacemaker function. These features vary among different brands of pacemakers.

The pacemaker *lead* is an insulated length of wire that provides a conduit for electrical energy between the pulse generator and cardiac muscle. Current from the generator travels through the lead to the myocardium (pacing), and cardiac depolarization signals travel from the myocardium to the pulse generator (sensing). Pacing systems are categorized as *single chamber* or *dual chamber,* according to whether sensing or pacing can occur only in the atria or ventricles or in both. In a single-chamber pacing system, a lead is placed only in the chamber to be paced; leads in both the atrium and ventricle are required in a dual-chamber system.

Leads may be placed either on the endocardial surface of a cardiac chamber (transvenous) or on the epicardial surface of the heart (epicardial). Approximately 95% of pacemaker implantations are performed using *transvenous leads* (Hillis et al., 1992). Transvenous leads are further categorized as passive or active. Passive leads are designed with flanges or tines near the tip that catch beneath endocardial trabeculations and hold the lead in position until growth of fibrous tissue around the lead tip permanently fixes its position. Active leads are constructed with a barb, hook, or screw at the tip end and are designed for insertion into a smooth-walled ventricular cavity or placement in the atrial appendage (Lowe & German, 1990) (Fig. 20-2). Because passive leads have better sensing and pacing thresholds, they are most often used. However, active leads are less easily dislodged and may be preferable if lead fixation is difficult.

Epicardial leads are seldom used because they provide less satisfactory chronic pacing thresholds. Also, if the pacing system become infected, a major operation, including sternotomy and dissection of the electrodes from the surface of the heart, may become necessary. Epicardial leads must be used in patients with prosthetic tricuspid valves to avoid positioning the lead across a valvular prosthesis. Epicardial leads may also be preferable in young children and in patients with a right to left shunt, subclavian vein thrombosis, or tricuspid regurgitation.

Electrodes are electrically conductive material that provide the negative (cathode) and positive (anode) terminals of the circuit. Electric current from the pulse generator travels from the cathode to the anode through the patient's tissues, which provide a conductive pathway between the two. The cathode is always located at the distal end of the lead, in contact with viable myocardium. The location of the anode distinguishes a bipolar from a unipolar system (Fig. 20-3). In a bipolar system, both electrodes are located on the lead, spaced several millimeters apart so that they both lie within the heart. A unipolar system has a single electrode (cathode) on the lead's tip; the posi-

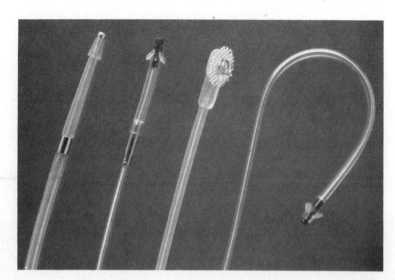

FIGURE 20-2. Examples of pacing leads. From left to right: bipolar flanged, bipolar tined, unipolar screw-in epicardial, and unipolar atrial tined leads. (Courtesy of Intermedics, Inc, Angleton, TX)

tive electrode (anode) required to complete the electrical circuit is located on the casing of pulse generator (Lowe & German, 1990). Current medical opinion favors the use of bipolar leads. They are less likely to sense skeletal muscle myopotentials and environmental electromagnetic interference and are less likely to stimulate the patient's skeletal muscles.

GOALS OF PERMANENT PACING

The primary goals of a permanent pacing system are to compensate for dysfunction of the intrinsic pacemaker (i.e., the sinus node) or the conduction system and to simulate as closely as possible normal physiologic cardiac depolarization and conduction. Recall

that repetitive, spontaneous depolarization of the sinus node and propagation of depolarization throughout atrial and ventricular tissue produce normal sinus rhythm. In this normal pattern of electrical excitation, the impulse propagation wave travels in an orderly fashion from the atria, through the AV node and bundle of His to the ventricles, providing AV synchrony.

When a pacemaker is used to generate a cardiac rhythm, it provides one or more of three basic functions, depending on the type of system: (1) prevention of profound bradycardia, (2) preservation of AV synchrony, and (3) a mechanism for physiologic rate responsiveness or rate modulation. Either a single- (atrial or ventricular) or dual- (atrial and ventricular) chamber system is selected, depending on the type of conduction disorder and which of the three functions is considered most desirable.

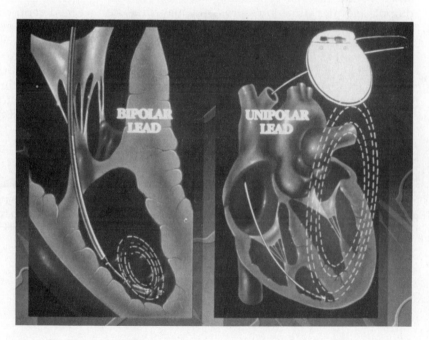

FIGURE 20-3. Bipolar and unipolar pacing systems. With a bipolar system (**left**), electric current flows from the pacemaker through the insulated lead to the negative electrode (cathode) and endocardium; electric current stimulates the heart muscle and flows back to anode, located on a second intracardiac electrode. In a unipolar system (**right**), electric current from the pacemaker flows through the insulated lead and negative electrode (cathode) to the endocardium; electric current stimulates the heart muscle and flows back to the anode, located on the pacemaker itself. (Courtesy of Intermedics, Inc., Angleton, TX)

PREVENTION OF BRADYCARDIA

Prevention of bradycardia is most easily achieved and requires only a single chamber system. If AV nodal function is normal, an electrical stimulus delivered in the atrium (i.e., atrial pacing) is propagated through myocardial cells of both atria and by way of the AV node through both ventricles. However, the AV node is normally the only pathway by which an electrical propagation wave can travel from atrial to ventricular myocardium. In the absence of normal AV nodal function, single-chamber pacing is achieved only with direct electrical stimulation of ventricular myocardium through a ventricular pacing lead. Thus, AV synchrony is present with atrial pacing but absent with ventricular pacing. A dual-chamber system is required to achieve AV synchrony in the presence of AV nodal dysfunction.

ATRIOVENTRICULAR SYNCHRONY

AV synchrony, that is, an appropriately timed atrial contraction preceding each ventricular contraction, provides significant hemodynamic benefit in patients with normal, as well as in those with impaired, ventricular function. First, atrial systole increases ventricular filling, contributing as much as 20% to 30% of cardiac output under certain conditions (Holmes, 1989). Second, the atria empty more completely, which decreases atrial pressure and results in increased venous return to the atria. Third, appropriately timed closing of the mitral and tricuspid valves prevents regurgitation across open valves during ventricular systole and elevated venous pressure resulting from closed valves during atrial systole (Holmes, 1989). Finally, absence of AV synchrony may be associated with retrograde activation of the atria. Ventriculoatrial conduction decreases cardiac output, elevates atrial pressure, and may produce pacemaker-mediated arrhythmias or pacemaker syndrome (Holmes, 1989). Pacemaker syndrome is a phenomenon that sometimes occurs in persons who have single chamber, ventricular pacemakers, and fixed or intermittent normal sinus rhythm. It is discussed later in the chapter.

AV synchrony may also be important in patients with *hypersensitive carotid sinus syndrome*, a disorder characterized by an extreme reflex response to carotid sinus stimulation. In affected persons, lightheadedness or syncope may result from pressure on the carotid artery in the area of the carotid sinus. A collar that is too tight or turning the head suddenly may produce recurring syncope with asystolic periods of three seconds or more. Two components comprise hypersensitive carotid sinus syndrome. The cardioinhibitory component results from increased parasympathetic tone and is manifested by slowing of the sinus rate or prolongation of the PR interval and AV block; the vasodepressor component produces vaso-

dilatation and hypotension secondary to a reduction in sympathetic activity (ACC/AHA Task Force, 1991). In patients with both cardioinhibitory and vasodepressor components of the syndrome, AV sequential pacing is preferable; ventricular pacing may not correct, and may in fact worsen, symptoms related to the vasodepressor component of the syndrome.

RATE MODULATION

A third function incorporated into some current pacemakers is *rate modulation*, which describes a pulse generator's capacity to respond to changing physiologic demands by increasing or decreasing heart rate. Studies examining the contribution of AV synchrony have demonstrated that while it significantly increases cardiac output in patients at rest, its contribution diminishes at higher heart rates, that is, during exercise (Morton, 1991). It has become increasingly evident that a ventricular rate that is responsive to physiologic need is probably the most important factor in increasing cardiac output, particularly in the absence of retrograde atrial activation and in the presence of a fixed atrial arrhythmia (Furman, 1990). Because rate-responsive pacemakers allow increases in heart rate during exercise, they may provide a significant benefit in young and active persons. Rate modulation may also be more important than AV synchrony in patients with chronic congestive heart failure (Fabiszewski & Volosin, 1991).

In patients with normal sinus node function, rate responsiveness is achieved with a dual-chamber pacing system capable of *atrial tracking* or the delivery of a ventricular pacing impulse after each sensed atrial depolarization. Thus, when the patient's sinus rate increases, the ensuing P waves trigger appropriately timed ventricular pacing impulses, resulting in a pacing rate that is controlled by the patient's sinus rate. In patients with sinus node dysfunction, stimuli other than atrial depolarizations must be used to adjust the ventricular pacing rate. A variety of physiologic indicators that reflect changes in metabolic need can be used to modulate changes in pacing rate (Morton, 1991) (Table 20-1).

TABLE 20-1. SELECTED PHYSIOLOGIC INDICATORS USED IN RATE-MODULATED PACING

Mechanical vibration
Minute ventilation
Respiratory rate
Central venous temperature
QT interval

TABLE 20-2. RECOMMENDED PACING MODES

Diagnosis	Optimal Mode
Sinus node dysfunction	AAI-R
Atrioventricular block	DDD
Sinus node dysfunction and atrioventricular block	DDD-R or DDI-R
Chronic atrial fibrillation with atrioventricular block	VVI-R
Hypersensitive carotid sinus syndrome	DDI

(Adapted from British Pacing and Electrophysiology Group, 1991: Recommendations for pacemaker prescription for symptomatic bradycardia. Br Heart J 66:185)

PACING MODES

Several factors are considered in selecting the particular type of pulse generator, including type of conduction abnormality, presence of supraventricular arrhythmias, and age and life-style of the patient. If pacing needs are likely to change over time, a dual-chamber or single-chamber rate-modulated pulse generator with multiprogrammable capability is selected (Finkelmeier, 1991). However, the technology of these devices is complex and the units are more costly. Selection of the proper pacing mode requires careful evaluation of the patient's pacing needs and is sometimes controversial. The choice is based on reliable knowledge of the patient's history and current medications, as well as on the pathophysiology of the underlying cardiac illness. Table 20-2 provides basic guidelines for pacing mode selection according to type of conduction abnormality (BPEG, 1991).

NBG CODE

The various methods by which the pulse generator electrically stimulates the heart (paces) and responds to intrinsic cardiac activity (senses) are called the *modes of pacing*. A standardized coding system for describing pacing modalities was introduced by the Inter-Society Commission for Heart Disease (ICHD) Resources in 1974 (Parsonnet et al., 1974). The coding system has subsequently undergone several revisions as more sophisticated pacing modalities have been developed. The *NBG* (NASPE/BPEG generic) *pacemaker code* is currently used and represents the most recent revision by the North American Society of Pacing and Electrophysiology (NASPE) and British Pacing and Electrophysiology Group (BPEG) (Bernstein et al., 1987).

The NBG Code is a system of classifying pulse generator function using a five-letter code (Table 20-3). The first three letters of the code describe pulse generator functions used to treat bradycardia. The first letter describes the heart chamber in which pacing can occur (e.g., "A" means that the generator is capable of atrial pacing only; "V" means that ventricular pacing only is possible; and "D" signifies that pacing can occur in both chambers. Similarly, the second letter reveals the chamber(s) in which sensing of intrinsic electrical activity occurs. Pulse generator response to sensed cardiac events is designated by the third letter in the sequence. "T" signifies that the pulse generator delivers a ventricular pacing impulse in response to sensed intrinsic atrial activity, "I" means that sensed intrinsic activity inhibits the pulse generator from delivering a pacing impulse, and "D" means that both triggered and inhibited responses are possible under various circumstances.

The fourth letter describes two functions: programmability and rate modulation. The following letters in the fourth position signify a hierarchal progression in function complexity from absence of

TABLE 20-3. THE NASPE/BPEG GENERIC (NBG) PACEMAKER CODE

I Chamber(s) Paced	II Chamber(s) Sensed	III Mode of Response	IV Programmable Functions	V Special Tachyarrhythmia Functions
O—None	O—None	O—None	O—None	O—None
A—Atrium	A—Atrium	T—Triggered	P—Simple programmable	P—Pacing
V—Ventricle	V—Ventricle	I—Inhibited	M—Multiprogrammable	S—Shock
D—Dual	D—Dual	D—Dual	C—Communicating	D—Dual
			R—Rate modulation	

(Adapted from Bernstein AD, Camm AJ, Fletcher RD, et al., 1987: The NASPE/BPEG generic pacemaker code for antibradyarrhythmia and adaptive-rate pacing and antitachyarrhythmia devices. PACE 10:794)

programmability to rate modulation, with each level incorporating features of all levels below it: "O" signifies absence of programmability; "P", simple programmability (one or two programmable parameters); "M", multiple (more than two) programmable parameters; "C", communicating function (telemetry that allows interrogation of the pulse generator); and "R", rate modulation in response to physiologic parameters (Teplitz, 1991). The fifth letter of the code refers to antitachycardia functions. The fourth and fifth letters are often omitted in routine clinical practice. The most commonly selected pacing modes are discussed below.

SINGLE-CHAMBER MODES

AAI

The *AAI pacing mode* provides atrial pacing at a fixed rate with inhibition of pacing by sensed intrinsic atrial activity. The pacing rate is generally programmable. AAI pacing is used in patients who have sinus node dysfunction but intact AV nodal conduction. If rate modulation is desired, AAI-R pacing may be used to additionally provide the rate-responsive feature. Second- or third-degree AV block and atrial flutter or atrial fibrillation are generally contraindications to AAI pacing.

VVI

The *VVI pacing mode* is identical to the AAI pacing mode except that pacing and sensing occur in the ventricle and intrinsic ventricular activity inhibits delivery of pacing impulses. Pacing occurs at a fixed rate. VVI is the operational mode in approximately 70% of currently implanted pacemakers (Furman, 1991). It is most appropriate for patients with (1) no significant atrial contribution to cardiac output (e.g., patients with atrial fibrillation), (2) no evidence of pacemaker syndrome, or (3) special circumstances in which pacing simplicity is a prime concern (e.g., senility) (ACC/AHA Task Force, 1991). VVI-R signifies that the pulse generator also has a rate-responsive feature, that is, the pacing rate increases in response to a selected parameter indicative of increased physiologic demand, usually due to exercise. The VVI-R pacing mode provides rate modulation in patients with an atrial arrhythmia that precludes dual-chamber pacing.

DUAL-CHAMBER MODES

DVI

DVI pacing provides sequential atrial and ventricular pacing at a predetermined rate separated by a programmed AV interval. Intrinsic ventricular events inhibit the pulse generator from delivering pacing impulses. DVI pacing can be either committed or noncommitted. In *committed DVI pacing* the pulse generator always delivers a ventricular pacing impulse one AV interval after delivery of an atrial stimulus (Stephenson & Combs, 1991). *Noncommitted DVI pacing* signifies that the ventricular pacing impulse is delivered only if no intrinsic ventricular activity occurs within the programmed AV interval. Because there is no triggering response with DVI pacing, atrial tracking does not occur. Also, DVI pacing does not provide atrial sensing. Atrial pacing impulses are delivered even during periods when the intrinsic atrial rate exceeds the pacing rate. Therefore, an atrial pacing impulse may be delivered during the vulnerable portion of atrial repolarization, which may result in atrial fibrillation (Ludmer & Goldschlager, 1984). The DVI mode is primarily used in patients with a DDD pacemaker in whom the atrial sensing, but not pacing, capability has failed.

DDI

DDI pacing is similar to DVI pacing except that atrial sensing also occurs. Therefore, intrinsic atrial activity inhibits discharge of an atrial pacing impulse, thereby avoiding competition between the pacemaker and an underlying atrial rhythm (Stephenson & Combs, 1991). Because atrial tracking is not possible with a DDI pacing mode, AV synchronous pacing occurs only at the programmed pacing rate.

DDD

The *DDD pacing mode* is the most sophisticated form of dual-chamber pacing. It provides pacing and sensing in both chambers, as well as the dual responses of triggering and inhibition (Fig. 20-4). With the DDD mode, an intrinsic atrial rate less than the programmed pacing rate results in atrial pacing followed by appropriately timed ventricular pacing or inhibition (like DVI pacing). An intrinsic atrial rate greater than the pacing rate is sensed (atrial tracking), inhibits the atrial output, and triggers ventricular pacing. Spontaneous ventricular events inhibit the ventricular output (like VVI pacing) preventing interference between paced and spontaneous ventricular activity. DDD pacemakers can be programmed to most other pacing modes if the patient's needs change or if malfunction of one of the leads occurs. Because of its versatility, DDD pacing has gained widespread use.

Pacemakers capable of pacing in a DDD-R mode have recently become available. DDD-R pacing provides AV synchrony and rate modulation for patients with fixed sinus bradycardia and complete heart block. It is beneficial for patients who require consistent AV synchrony at rates that vary according to metabolic demands and whose sinus node has lost the ability to respond appropriately to such demands.

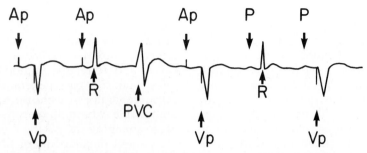

FIGURE 20-4. Simulated drawing demonstrating the possible responses with a DDD pacing mode. From left to right the tracing displays: AV sequential pacing (Ap-Vp); atrial pacing with intrinsic AV conduction resulting in inhibition of ventricular output (Ap-R); premature ventricular complex (PVC) with resetting of escape interval; AV sequential pacing (Ap-Vp); normal sinus complex (P-R), resulting in inhibition of both atrial and ventricular outputs; and sinus depolarization that fails to conduct intrinsically to ventricles, producing a triggered ventricular response (P-Vp). (Finkelmeier BA, Salinger MH, 1986: Dual-chamber cardiac pacing: An overview. Crit Care Nurs 6:19)

PACEMAKER IMPLANTATION

IMPLANTATION PROCEDURE

Implantation of a pacemaker using transvenous leads is performed in an operating room or catheterization laboratory. With the use of local anesthesia, the pacing lead is inserted through the right or left subclavian or jugular vein and positioned in the cardiac chamber to be paced (right atrium or ventricle). Often, the right subclavian vein is used because of the straight vascular pathway it provides into the right side of the heart. Transvenous ventricular leads are positioned in the apex of the right ventricle. Atrial leads are most commonly positioned in the right atrial appendage or on the atrial wall (Holmes et al., 1989). Leads designed for atrial appendage placement have a characteristic "J" shape to allow secure positioning. Fluoroscopy is used to guide lead placement in the heart. For a dual-chamber system, both leads can often be inserted in the same vein, using the same or different puncture sites. Satisfactory lead placement is confirmed by fluoroscopy and measurement of stimulation threshold, lead impedance, and cardiac signal amplitudes of the endocardial electrogram (Furman, 1991; Stephenson & Combs, 1991).

The pulse generator is situated in a pocket below the clavicle, created by separating pectoral muscle fascia from the overlying subcutaneous tissue (Moses et al., 1987). Consideration is given to the patient's life-style when selecting the site for pulse generator placement. For example, placing a pulse generator on the right side is not desirable in a right-handed patient who hunts regularly and uses the right shoulder to brace a shotgun. The pocket should be of adequate size to house the pulse generator without undue tension on overlying skin. Before closing the incision,

hemostasis is achieved to prevent accumulation of blood within the pocket and resultant increased potential for infection.

Epicardial leads will sometimes have been placed prophylactically during a prior cardiac operation in patients considered at high risk for postoperative heart block. Permanent leads are easily secured through the epicardium into the atrial or ventricular myocardium while the chest is open. Alternatively, a small subxiphoid or thoracotomy incision is used for epicardial lead placement. When epicardial leads are used, the pulse generator is placed in a subcutaneous pocket in the abdominal wall.

At the time of pacemaker implantation or shortly thereafter, the pulse generator is programmed to the desired mode. Before discharge from the hospital, verbal instructions and written descriptive information about the pacemaker are given to the patient. Intermittent evaluation of patients with implanted pacemakers is essential, particularly those with more complex dual-chamber systems. Most commonly, this can be accomplished with transtelephonic monitoring, supplemented with periodic visits to a physician's office or pacemaker clinic for pacemaker interrogation and reprogramming.

POSTOPERATIVE FOLLOW-UP

Although pacemakers are highly reliable, they require periodic evaluation by physicians with specialized training. Most often, patients receive this type of specialized surveillance through a pacemaker clinic. Continued evaluation of patients with implanted pacemakers achieves a number of important objectives: (1) assessment of pulse generator battery function and determination of the correct time for replacement, (2) optimal programming of the pacemaker as the patient's physiologic needs change, (3) detection of possible pacing system problems, and, when possible, correction of identified problems via noninvasive reprogramming methods, and (4) maintenance of a data registry of patients with pacemakers so that they can be notified promptly in the event of a device recall. Follow-up of patients with pacemakers is performed through a combination of transtelephonic monitoring and visits to a pacemaker clinic with proper equipment (including pacemaker programming devices) and trained personnel.

Transtelephonic monitoring is a technique that allows transmission of electrocardiographic tracings from the patient's home. Using electrodes placed on the patient's chest or fingertips, the cardiac rhythm tracing is converted into sound waves through a telephone mouthpiece, transmitted to a receiver at the pacemaker clinic, and converted into a printed ECG rhythm tracing (Moses et al., 1987) (Fig. 20-5). The ability to interrogate the pacemaker is called telemetry. With telemetry, diagnostic data can be obtained, including pulse generator model, serial number, date of implant, number of paced and sensed beats, battery and lead impedance, and an intracardiac electrogram (Finkelmeier, 1991). This diagnostic data allows assessment of intrinsic cardiac rhythm, sensing and pacing thresholds, status of AV conduction, presence of ventricular-atrial (retrograde) conduction, and status of battery life (Kleinschmidt & Stafford, 1991). Programmable parameters can be adjusted to accommodate changes in pacing needs. Programmable pulse generators contain predetermined circuits from which one of several features or functions can be se-

lected for variation within a specified range (Hayes, 1989). Parameters that are presently programmable include upper and lower rate limits for pacing, AV interval, pulse generator output, pacing mode, sensitivity, and refractory periods (McErlean, 1991). In rate-responsive pacemakers, settings that control the pulse generator's response to activity are also programmable. Common reasons for reprogramming include changing the pacing mode from DDD to VVI if the patient develops atrial fibrillation, increasing or decreasing the pacing rate, and adjusting sensitivity. Prudent programming of the battery output settings (amplitude and pulse width) can substantially prolong battery life.

COMPLICATIONS

Complications associated with permanent pacemakers are unusual but do occur. The implantation is associated with minimal morbidity. Perforation of the subclavian vein or right ventricle occurs rarely. It is generally detected by fluoroscopy during implantation or by the chest roentgenogram that is routinely obtained after implantation. *Venous perforation* may result in hemothorax, which can usually be treated by tube thoracostomy. *Right ventricular perforation* can produce hemopericardium, which may require pericardiocentesis or, rarely, repair of the ventricle. *Pneumothorax* can occur due to lung puncture.

Pacemaker failure can occur due to battery depletion, pulse generator malfunction, lead dislodgement, or lead fracture. Replacement of a pulse generator is a minor surgical procedure performed using local anesthesia. The incision overlying the generator

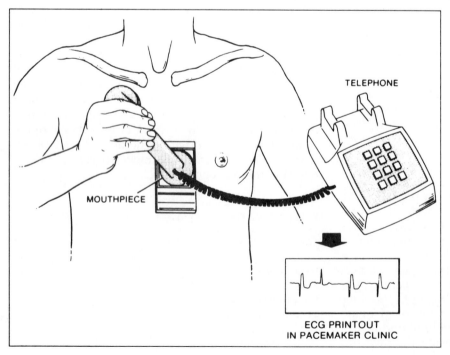

MOUTHPIECE

TELEPHONE

ECG PRINTOUT
IN PACEMAKER CLINIC

FIGURE 20-5. Transmission of rhythm tracing by means of telephone. The patient is shown holding a battery-operated transmitter against the chest. On the back of the transmitter are two electrodes that are pressed firmly against the skin. These electrodes transmit an ECG that is converted into sound waves through the telephone mouthpiece. A receiver at the pacemaker clinic prints the transmitted rhythm tracing. (Moses HW, Schneider JA, Miller BD, Taylor GJ, 1991: Pacemaker technology. In A Practical Guide to Cardiac Pacing, ed. 3, p. 147. Boston, Little, Brown) is reopened, the indwelling generator is detached from the leads and the new generator is inserted in its place in the subcutaneous pocket and attached to the existing leads. Lead problems can sometimes be corrected by repositioning or repairing the lead. Occasionally a new lead must be placed.

Electromagnetic or myopotential interference are both phenomena that can produce inappropriate pacing. *Electromagnetic interference* from common household electrical appliances is unusual with current pulse generators. For example, microwave ovens may be used freely by patients with implanted pacemakers. However, sources of major electrical or magnetic interference, such as arc welding equipment, may cause a problem with pacemaker function. *Myopotential interference* occasionally occurs with a unipolar system because the anodal electrode is located on the casing of the pulse generator and senses regional muscle activity. Pectoral muscle myopotentials can produce inappropriate triggering or inhibition of ventricular pacing because the pulse generator cannot completely discriminate the skeletal muscle electrogram from that of cardiac muscle (Furman, 1991). Myopotential interference, though rare, may cause disabling symptoms in some patients. It is corrected by decreasing pulse generator sensitivity or converting to a bipolar system.

Pacemaker syndrome can occur with VVI pacing systems due to intermittent loss of AV synchrony and retrograde activation of the atrium. It is characterized by sudden decreases in cardiac output and blood pressure that occur during periods of AV asynchrony. The hemodynamic changes are thought to result from loss of the atrial contribution (i.e., "atrial kick") to ventricular filling and from ventriculoatrial conduction that activates atrial stretch reflexes and leads to vagal stimulation and peripheral vasodilatation.

It is estimated that some degree of pacemaker syndrome occurs in 5% to 20% of patients with ventricular pacemakers (Hillis et al., 1992). The syndrome is manifested by episodes of weakness and dizziness during ventricular pacing. When the normal AV sequence of depolarization and contraction is restored by return of sinus rhythm, symptoms are relieved. Pacemaker syndrome is corrected by reprogramming or replacing the pulse generator to provide AV synchronous pacing.

Crosstalk and pacemaker-mediated tachycardia (PMT) are complications unique to dual-chamber pacing systems. *Crosstalk* is inappropriate inhibition of ventricular pacing because the atrial pacing impulse is incorrectly sensed by the pulse generator as an R wave. Crosstalk is corrected by reprogramming the ventricular refractory or blanking interval immediately after delivery of the atrial pacing impulse.

Pacemaker-mediated tachycardia, a rapid ventricular paced rhythm that is sustained by retrograde conduction to the atria, is possible in systems programmed in a VDD or DDD mode. It is generally initiated by an ectopic ventricular impulse that is conducted in retrograde fashion through intrinsic conductive tissue to the atria. The resulting P wave is sensed by the pulse generator, which responds with a triggered ventricular pacing impulse that is again conducted, in retrograde fashion, to the atria. A circular reentrant tachycardia is thus induced. Pacemaker-related tachycardia is terminated by application of a magnet over the pulse generator to produce asynchronous (DOO or VOO) pacing and terminate atrial tracking. The pulse generator is then reprogrammed by increasing the postventricular atrial refractory period or eliminating atrial sensing altogether to prevent recurrence (Ludmer & Goldschlager, 1984).

Pulse generator erosion through the skin occasionally occurs, particularly in elderly, cachectic individuals. The skin over an edge of the generator becomes reddened, and palpation reveals little or no overlying subcutaneous tissue. A new subcutaneous pocket must be created in a different location and the generator moved. If not, skin breakdown eventually occurs, allowing contamination of the device. Rarely, the suture securing the pulse generator in a fixed position becomes disrupted. If this occurs, an unknowing or disoriented patient may manipulate and rotate the pulse generator in the pocket. This so-called *Twiddler's syndrome* can produce lead dislodgment or fracture (Goldberger, 1990). Occasionally, the pulse generator migrates from the original pocket (e.g., into the subcutaneous tissue of the breast in a woman). Repositioning of the generator may be necessary for comfort or cosmetic reasons.

An unusual late complication of pacemaker implantation is *infection* of the pacing system. Infection of the prosthetic material is likely to produce fistula formation and a chronic, indolent infection that continues until all prosthetic material is removed. Typically, an infected subcutaneous pocket containing the pulse generator begins to drain purulent material. The simplest corrective measure is removal of the pulse generator and as much of the leads as is possible. Although this corrects the problem for the moment, infection usually remains along the residual length of the pacing lead and after a quiescent period a sinus tract redevelops and begins to drain again. For this reason, many surgeons recommend removal of the entire pacing system as soon as diagnosis of infection is established.

Infection is a particularly difficult problem when epicardial leads have been secured to the ventricle and is one reason that permanent epicardial pacing systems are not commonly used. Removal of epicardial leads is a formidable task. It usually necessitates a sternotomy incision. Often the heart is densely adherent to the posterior table of the sternum because of the infection. In addition, tissue ingrowth surrounds the area where the leads are attached to the epicardium, making lead removal difficult.

REFERENCES

American College of Cardiology/American Heart Association Task Force on Assessment of Diagnostic and Therapeutic Cardiovascular Procedures, 1991: Guidelines for implantation of cardiac pacemakers and antiarrhythmia devices. J Am Coll Cardiol 18:1

Bernstein AD, Camm AJ, Fletcher RD, et al., 1987: The NASPE/BPEG generic pacemaker code for antibradyarrhythmia and adaptive-rate pacing and antitachyarrhythmia devices. PACE 10:794

British Pacing and Electrophysiology Group, 1991: Recommendations for pacemaker prescription for symptomatic bradycardia. Br Heart J 66:185

Fabiszewski R, Volosin KJ, 1991: Rate-modulated pacemakers. J Cardiovasc Nurs 5:21

Finkelmeier BA, Salinger MH, 1986: Dual-chamber cardiac pacing: An overview. Crit Care Nurs 6:12

Finkelmeier NE, 1991: Pacemaker technology: An overview. AACN Clin Issues Crit Care Nurs 2:99

Furman S, 1990: Rate-modulated pacing. Circulation 82:1081

Furman S, 1991: Cardiac pacing and pacemakers. In Baue AE, Geha AS, Hammond GL, et al. (eds): Glenn's Thoracic and Cardiovascular Surgery, ed. 5. Norwalk, CT, Appleton & Lange

Goldberger E, 1990: Modes of cardiac pacing. In Treatment of Cardiac Emergencies, ed. 5. St. Louis, CV Mosby

Harthorne JW, 1989: Cardiac pacing. In Grillo HC, Austen WG, Wilkins EW, et al. (eds): Current Therapy in Cardiothoracic Surgery. Toronto, BC Decker

Hayes DL, 1989: Programmability. In Furman S, Hayes DL, Holmes DR (eds): A Practice of Cardiac Pacing, ed. 2. Mount Kisco, NY, Futura Publishing

Hillis LD, Lange RA, Wells PJ, Winniford MD, 1992: Temporary and permanent pacing. In Manual of Clinical Problems in Cardiology, ed. 4. Boston, Little, Brown

Holmes DR, 1989: Hemodynamics of cardiac pacing. In Furman S, Hayes DL, Holmes DR (eds): A Practice of Cardiac Pacing, ed. 2. Mount Kisco, NY, Futura Publishing

Holmes DR, Hayes DL, Furman S, 1989: Permanent pacemaker implantation. In Furman S. Hayes DL, Holmes DR (eds): A Practice of Cardiac Pacing, ed. 2. Mount Kisco, NY, Futura Publishing

Kleinschmidt KM, Stafford MJ, 1991: Dual-chamber cardiac pacemakers. J Cardiovasc Nurs 5:1

Lowe JE, German LD, 1990: Cardiac pacemakers and cardiac conduction system abnormalities. In Sabiston DC Jr, Spencer FC (eds): Surgery of the Chest, ed. 5. Philadelphia, WB Saunders

Ludmer PL, Goldschlager N, 1984: Cardiac pacing in the 1980's. N Engl J Med 311:1671

McErlean ES, 1991: Dual-chamber pacing. AACN Clin Issues Crit Care Nurs 2:126

Morton PG, 1991: Rate-responsive cardiac pacemakers. AACN Clin Issues Crit Care Nurs 2:140

Moses HW, Taylor GJ, Schneider JA, Dove JT, 1987: Pacemaker implantation. In: A Practical Guide to Cardiac Pacing, ed. 2. Boston, Little, Brown

Parsonnet V, Furman S, Smyth NP, 1974: Implantable cardiac pacemaker status report and resource guideline. Circulation 50:A21

Stephenson NL, Combs W, 1991: Artificial cardiac pacemakers and implantable cardioverter defibrillators. In Kinney MR, Packa DR, Andreoli KG, Zipes DP (eds): Comprehensive Cardiac Care, ed. 7. St. Louis, Mosby–Year Book

Teplitz L, 1991: Classification of cardiac pacemakers: The pacemaker code. J Cardiovasc Nurs 5:1

CHAPTER 21

SURGICAL TREATMENT OF OTHER CARDIOVASCULAR DISORDERS

CARDIAC TUMORS

TYPES OF TUMORS

Tumors of the heart and pericardium most often represent metastatic spread of lung or breast cancer, melanoma, or leukemia. Such *secondary cardiac tumors* can metastasize to the heart through hematogenous or lymphocytic routes or extend directly from surrounding intrathoracic structures (Schaff et al., 1991). Of the *primary cardiac tumors*, approximately 70% are benign and half of these are myxomas (Van Trigt & Sabiston, 1990; Kirklin & Barratt-Boyes, 1993a). Other benign tumors that occur infrequently are lipomas and papillary fibroelastomas. The most common malignant primary cardiac tumor in adults is angiosarcoma, a tumor that originates in the myocardium and invades both the cardiac chambers and the pericardial space.

INDICATIONS FOR SURGICAL RESECTION

Surgical treatment of intracardiac tumors became possible only after development of cardiopulmonary bypass provided a means of extracorporeal circulation (Novick & Dobell, 1991). It is the recommended treatment for all cardiac tumors, even those that are benign or asymptomatic. The heart has a limited tolerance for any space-occupying lesion, and intracardiac tumors can cause lethal complications, including arrhythmias, cardiac tamponade, pericardial constriction, valvular obstruction, and embolism (Fallon & Dec, 1989; Schaff et al., 1991).

By far the most common cardiac tumor treated with surgical therapy is myxoma. Unfortunately, surgical resection is only occasionally possible for malignant (primary or secondary) cardiac tumors. Because of their rapid growth potential, tumor removal is often precluded by extensive myocardial infiltration, local invasion of adjacent structures, or distant metastases. Since cardiac malignancies are universally fatal if not resected, prognosis for survival is generally poor.

Survival after surgical resection varies depending on the type of tumor and its location. Survival is 90% after surgical resection for myxoma, 50% for other benign tumors, and less than 10% for primary cardiac malignancies (Van Trigt & Sabiston, 1990).

Betsy Finkelmeier: CARDIOTHORACIC SURGICAL NURSING.
© 1995 J.B. Lippincott Company.

207

SURGICAL RESECTION OF MYXOMA

Myxomas are composed of gelatinous, mucoid material and arise from the endocardial surface of one or more of the cardiac chambers. Most myxomas originate in the upper chambers; 75% arise in the left atrium, and 18% occur in the right atrium (Schaff et al., 1991). Typically, atrial myxomas are attached to the interatrial septum by a pedunculated stalk in the area of the fossa ovalis.

Three types of clinical manifestations are associated with myxoma: (1) symptoms related to obstruction of blood flow through the heart, (2) symptoms of systemic embolization of tumor fragments, and (3) constitutional symptoms, such as weight loss, fatigue, and fever. Symptoms are often sudden in onset, intermittent, and related to the patient's body position (Hillis et al., 1992a). Most common is congestive heart failure due to obstruction, valvular regurgitation, or impingement of the cardiac chamber (Sellke et al., 1990).

Despite histologic benignancy, surgical removal of a myxoma is always indicated. Death or catastrophic complications may result from tumor embolization or the hemodynamic abnormalities produced by the presence of an intracardiac foreign body. Because these events can occur precipitously, operative therapy is performed promptly after diagnosis (Schaff et al., 1991). Surgical excision is usually possible because the tumors are primarily intracavitary, rarely extending deeper than the endocardial layer of the heart (Novick & Dobell, 1991).

A median sternotomy approach is used. After instituting cardiopulmonary bypass, aortic cross-clamping, and cardioplegic arrest of the heart, the appropriate cardiac chamber is opened with an incision that allows good visualization of the tumor and makes possible its removal with minimal manipulation (Fig. 21-1). For resection of atrial myxomas one or both atria may be opened. Ventricular myxomas are approached through an incision in the aorta or left atrium (for left ventricular tumors) or right atrium (for right ventricular tumors). These approaches avoid ventricular muscle damage that would result from a ventriculotomy, that is, an incision in the ventricle.

Because myxomatous tissue is gelatinous and very friable, extreme caution is necessary to avoid embolization before and during tumor removal. The heart is handled gently and the chamber containing the myxoma is not manipulated until the aortic cross-clamp is applied and cardioplegic arrest is achieved (Novick & Dobell, 1991). Manipulation of the tumor itself is avoided. Atrial myxomas are handled only by the stalk that anchors the tumor to the interatrial septum.

All myxomatous tissue must be removed because the tumor can recur despite its benignancy. Atrial septal tissue surrounding the tumor pedicle is excised en bloc, creating a small atrial septal defect that is repaired by direct suture technique or with a prosthetic patch (Van Trigt & Sabiston, 1990). After the tumor is evacuated, the chamber is thoroughly irri-

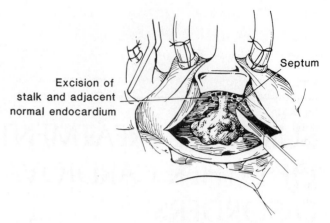

FIGURE 21-1. Left atriotomy performed after initiation of cardiopulmonary bypass reveals myxoma attached to atrial septum; myxoma stalk is excised with adjacent normal endocardium. (DiSesa VJ, Collins JJ Jr, Cohn LH, 1988: Considerations in the surgical management of left atrial myxoma. J Cardiac Surg 3:19)

gated to remove any residual tumor fragments or thrombus that might embolize when the heart is again allowed to eject blood into the systemic circulation. The cardiac valves that contacted the tumor are also carefully inspected for damage (Schaff et al., 1991).

Surgical resection of myxoma is generally curative. Hemodynamic improvement occurs immediately, the risk of embolism is eliminated, and most constitutional symptoms resolve completely (Schaff et al., 1991). Tumor recurrence is unusual, except in individuals with a familial form of myxoma (Novick & Dobell, 1991). Recurring myxomatous tissue may be histologically benign or may become more malignant with each recurrence and may appear in unusual locations, such as the pulmonary artery or aorta (Novick & Dobell, 1991). Because of the possibility of tumor recurrence, serial postoperative echocardiograms are recommended in all patients who have undergone resection of cardiac myxomas (Van Trigt & Sabiston, 1990).

CARDIOMYOPATHIES

HYPERTROPHIC CARDIOMYOPATHY

Hypertrophic cardiomyopathy (HCM), formerly known as idiopathic hypertrophic subaortic stenosis (IHSS), is a primary disease of the heart muscle. Although its etiology is unclear, it is genetically transmitted in most patients. HCM is characterized by inappropriate myocardial hypertrophy, usually involving primarily the interventricular septum of a nondilated left ventricle, and impaired diastolic function (Wynne & Braunwald, 1992). Deformity of the mitral valve apparatus and mitral insufficiency are often present as well (Krajcer et al., 1989).

Clinical Manifestations

The primary abnormality of HCM is dynamic obstruction of the left ventricular outflow tract during systole. Two factors contribute to the obstruction: (1) the septal hypertrophy and (2) abnormal anterior displacement of the mitral valve apparatus and systolic anterior motion of the anterior mitral valve leaflet (Jacobs & Austen, 1990). Left ventricular outflow tract obstruction produces clinical manifestations similar to aortic stenosis (Massimiano & Hammond, 1991). Symptoms, including dyspnea, angina, syncope, and fatigue, most often occur in young adults. Sudden cardiac death can also occur and is a leading cause of death in patients with HCM. The severity of symptoms generally correlates with the extent of ventricular disease and outflow obstruction (Stone et al., 1990).

Symptoms associated with HCM can usually be effectively treated with pharmacologic therapy. Calcium-channel antagonist and beta-blocking medications are used to reduce left ventricular outflow obstruction by decreasing contractility of the hypertrophied muscle. Antiarrhythmic medications may be necessary for control of frequently associated ventricular arrhythmias. Antibiotic prophylaxis against infective endocarditis is also advised.

Surgical Therapy

Surgical treatment is indicated in those patients with significant left ventricular outflow tract gradients who (1) remain symptomatic despite medical therapy or (2) are unable to tolerate pharmacologic therapy. Some surgeons also consider surgical therapy for asymptomatic children and young adults with large left ventricular outflow gradients (Mohr et al., 1989).

The operative procedure most commonly performed for HCM is *myectomy* (i.e., excision of a portion of muscle) (Fig. 21-2). The procedure consists of removing a wedge of the hypertrophied ventricular septum to reduce the dynamic left ventricular outflow tract obstruction. In addition, the operation generally diminishes the degree of mitral regurgitation.

Myectomy is performed through a median sternotomy incision and with cardiopulmonary bypass, aortic cross-clamping, and cardioplegic arrest. Intraoperative echocardiography is used to define septal dimensions, to guide the surgeon in planning the operative approach, and to provide an assessment of operative results. Through an incision in the ascending aorta, the right coronary leaflet of the aortic valve is retracted and a wedge of ventricular septal myocardium is excised. Some surgeons concomitantly plicate

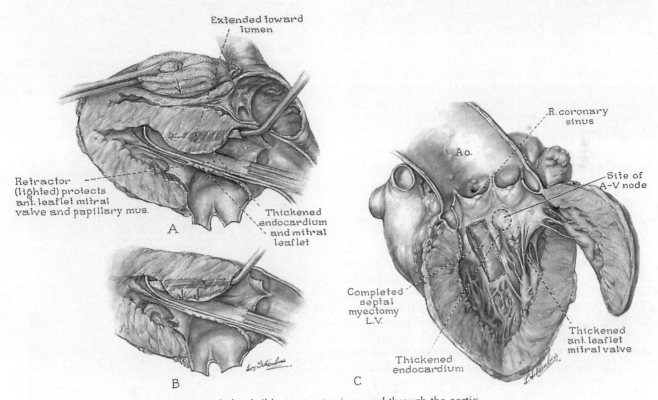

FIGURE 21-2. Myectomy. (**A** and **B**) A lighted ribbon retractor is passed through the aortic valve annulus to the apex; it protects the mitral valve and papillary muscles. An angled knife is used to excise a rectangular piece of the hypertrophied septum. (**C**) View of the left ventricular septum after completion of the septal myectomy. (Morrow AG, 1978: Hypertrophic subaortic stenosis: Operative methods utilized to relieve left ventricular outflow obstruction. J Thorac Cardiovasc Surg 76:425, 429)

the anterior leaflet of the mitral valve to limit its encroachment on the outflow tract (i.e., to eliminate systolic anterior motion) (Cooley, 1991). Replacement of the mitral valve may be necessary if a significant left ventricular outflow gradient or severe mitral regurgitation remains after myectomy.

The largest clinical experience with surgical treatment of HCM has occurred at the National Institutes of Health, where a 3% operative mortality for myectomy is reported (Brown et al., 1991). Surgical correction of the dynamic outflow obstruction relieves symptoms and improves quality of life in the majority of patients. However, the major abnormality of HCM is a myopathic process causing abnormal diastolic compliance (Nishimura et al., 1991). Neither medical nor surgical therapy has been shown to alter the natural history of the disease.

Complications associated with myectomy include left bundle branch block, complete heart block (usually due to left bundle branch block in a patient with preexisting right bundle branch block), and iatrogenic ventricular septal defect (Kirklin & Barratt-Boyes, 1993b). Mild to moderate aortic regurgitation may also occur, although it is rarely severe enough to necessitate aortic valve replacement (Brown et al., 1991). Myectomy is of limited value in patients with a thin septum. Relief of outflow tract obstruction is usually incomplete, and there is increased risk of creating a ventricular septal defect. Mitral valve replacement is sometimes alternatively performed as a primary surgical therapy for relief of symptoms caused by HCM. However, because of potential complications inherent to valvular prostheses, it is generally reserved for patients who have (1) a thin ventricular septum, (2) significant left ventricular outflow tract obstruction after myectomy, or (3) severe mitral regurgitation.

DILATED CARDIOMYOPATHY

Dilated cardiomyopathy (DCM) is a primary heart muscle disease characterized by ventricular dilatation and congestive heart failure. The condition is generally progressive and sometimes leads to death within 1 to 2 years. Approximately 80% of patients die within 10 years (Kirklin & Barratt-Boyes, 1993c). The treatment of choice for end-stage DCM is *cardiac transplantation,* which is discussed in Chapter 31, Heart, Lung, and Heart-Lung Transplantation. However, transplantation is limited by the scarcity of donor organs.

Dynamic cardiomyoplasty is an evolving surgical therapy for those patients with end-stage heart failure who are not acceptable transplant candidates or for whom a donor heart is not available. Because it is still an investigational procedure, it is reserved for patients who have a limited life expectancy with medical therapy alone. However, candidates must be stable enough to withstand a waiting period of 6 weeks while conditioning of the skeletal muscle graft is accomplished (Orie, 1991).

Cardiomyoplasty consists of wrapping the ventricles with a skeletal muscle pedicle graft that is then chronically electrostimulated to contract in synchrony with ventricular systole (Fig. 21-3). Development of dynamic cardiomyoplasty is based on two scientific advances: (1) the concept that skeletal muscle fibers after chronic electrostimulation can be transformed to a fatigue-resistant state and (2) development of a burst pulse generator that synchronizes stimulation of skeletal muscle with ventricular systole (Chachques et al., 1991).

The procedure is performed through a single lateral thoracic incision or two separate incisions: a lateral incision for harvesting the muscle graft and a median sternotomy incision for cardiac access (Moreira et al., 1991). The latissimus dorsi muscle is selected for grafting because of its location, length, blood and nerve supply, and relative ease of surgical transplantation to the heart (Sola et al., 1991). It is harvested with its neurovascular pedicle intact, then transferred as a pedicle graft into the chest and wrapped around the ventricles. Specific operative techniques vary, and the functional importance of wrap orientation, fiber direction, and extent of ven-

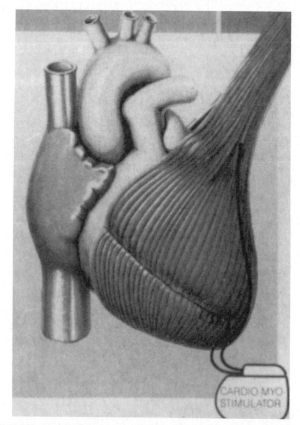

FIGURE 21-3. Dynamic cardiomyoplasty. Latissimus dorsi muscle is wrapped around ventricles and attached to cardiomyostimulator. (Carpentier A, Chachques JC, 1991: Clinical dynamic cardiomyoplasty: Method and outcome. Semin Thorac Cardiovasc Surg 3:137)

tricular coverage remains controversial (Furnary et al., 1991).

Pacing electrodes are implanted in the proximal portion of the muscle and sensing electrodes in the ventricular myocardium. The muscle pacing and heart sensing electrodes are connected to a cardiomyostimulator device, which is implanted in a pocket beneath the rectus abdominus muscle (Carpentier & Chachques, 1991). Stimulation of the muscle graft is not initiated for the first 2 postoperative weeks. This delay allows time for adhesion formation between the graft and the heart, healing of the flap, and development of collateral circulation (Carpentier & Chachques, 1991). Electrical stimulation is then initiated using a progressive muscle-conditioning protocol (Moreira et al., 1990). Eventually, the muscle flap is paced to produce a skeletal muscle contraction synchronously with each cardiac contraction.

Clinical experience with cardiomyoplasty remains limited, and definitive conclusions about its value are not yet established (Moreira et al., 1990). Those patients with left ventricular failure but preserved right ventricular function appear to achieve the most significant improvement (Magovern et al., 1991). Cardiomyoplasty has also been reported as a reconstructive technique when a large portion of ventricle must be resected, such as in the case of a large ventricular aneurysm or tumor (Carpentier & Chachques, 1991).

PERICARDIAL DISEASE

The pericardium is a fibroserous sac that encloses the heart. It is composed of an outer (parietal) layer and an inner (visceral) layer (Shabetai, 1990). The space between the parietal and visceral layers contains a small amount of clear, plasma-like fluid and accommodates physiologic expansion of the heart that occurs with changes in blood volume and posture, respiration, and straining (Shabetai, 1985). Other functions of the pericardium include (1) limiting distention and valvular incompetence at high filling pressures, (2) tethering the heart to adjacent structures, and (3) protecting the heart from inflammation in nearby tissues (Brandenburg et al., 1991).

PERICARDIAL PATHOLOGY

A wide variety of conditions can affect the pericardium, including infection, myocardial infarction, trauma, autoimmune disorders, radiation, uremia, and malignancy. These various etiologies can produce three forms of pericardial pathology: (1) inflammatory pericarditis, (2) pericardial effusion, or (3) constrictive pericarditis. Often a combination of these processes occurs. *Inflammatory pericarditis*, in the absence of pericardial effusion or constriction, is managed with medical therapy, primarily anti-inflammatory agents or corticosteroids. Pericardial effusion and constrictive pericarditis, on the other hand, may

require surgical intervention and are the focus of this discussion.

Pericardial effusion, or abnormal fluid accumulation in the pericardial space, can result from malignancy, infectious processes, postpericardiotomy syndrome, or pericarditis. The degree of symptoms associated with pericardial effusion varies with the volume of the effusion, the rapidity of accumulation, and the physical characteristics of the pericardium (Lorell & Braunwald, 1992). Rapid fluid accumulation, such as occurs with hemorrhage after cardiac surgery, causes cardiac tamponade and acute hemodynamic compromise. Gradual fluid accumulation, such as might occur secondary to malignancy, is more likely to produce progressive shortness of breath.

Constrictive pericarditis is characterized by marked thickening, scarring, or calcification of the pericardium (Franco et al., 1991). It is the end result of chronic pericardial inflammation that may be idiopathic or may be caused by one of a number of disease processes, such as infection (e.g., viral, tuberculous, fungal), uremia, or myocardial infarction.

Large effusions or constrictive pericardial thickening compromise cardiac function by impeding diastolic ventricular filling. Clinical manifestations include ascites, peripheral edema, dyspnea, fatigue, and hepatic congestion (Hillis et al., 1992b). It is often difficult to distinguish clinically between pericardial effusion and pericardial constriction. Echocardiography is generally used to distinguish the two conditions.

SURGICAL PROCEDURES

Symptomatic pericardial effusion is usually treated initially with *pericardiocentesis*. Surgical treatment may be required for recurrent effusions or those inadequately drained by a catheter technique. *Surgical drainage of the pericardium* is achieved by placement of a chest tube under direct exposure. With a subxiphoid approach and a small incision in the pericardium, a chest tube is placed and connected to gravity drainage for several days. Removal of the tube can be performed at the bedside.

In some cases, chest tube drainage is ineffective because the fluid is too viscous or because areas of parietal and visceral pericardium have become adherent to one another, producing loculation (i.e., compartmentalization) of fluid. In such cases, or for chronic recurring pericardial effusions, it may be necessary to remove a portion of the pericardium. *Pericardiectomy* can vary in extent from a small fenestration to almost total excision of the pericardium (Brandenburg et al., 1991).

A *pericardial window* describes a surgical procedure that includes removal of a portion of parietal pericardium and disruption of adhesions to allow free drainage of fluid (Fig. 21-4). It may be performed through a left thoracotomy or subxiphoid incision. Chest tube drainage is required for several postoperative days

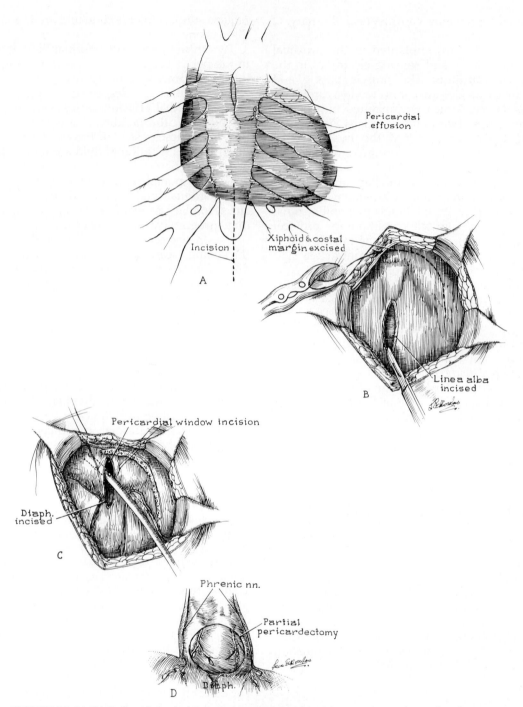

FIGURE 21-4. **(A)** Pericardial window using a subxiphoid incision can be performed under local anesthesia and sedation. **(B)** The incision is carried down to the distal sternum and xiphoid. The upper third of the linea alba is incised; the peritoneum is not opened. The xiphoid process and lower left costal arch are excised. **(C)** The diaphragm is incised in the midline down to the pericardial surface. Stay sutures are placed on either side of the projected pericardiotomy, and the pericardium is incised and drained. A specimen of pericadium is excised. Generally a catheter is placed to allow continued drainage; alternatively, the pericardial window may be opened into the pleural cavity. **(D)** For a partial pericardectomy, the resection of bone and cartilage is extended laterally and most of the pericardium between both phrenic nerves is excised. The edges of the pericardium are sutured to the subcutaneous tissue and the open upper linea alba. (Ravitch MM, Steichen FM, 1988: Diagnostic and therapeutic procedures. In Atlas of General Thoracic Surgery, p. 175. Philadelphia, WB Saunders)

until the amount of drainage is minimal. After the chest tube is removed, fluid that would otherwise accumulate in the closed pericardial space instead seeps into the left pleural space and is reabsorbed.

Constrictive pericarditis may necessitate performance of a *radical pericardiectomy* (i.e., removal of most of the pericardium) to restore adequate cardiac function. Generally, all of the anterior pericardium between the right and left phrenic nerves and, sometimes pericardium beneath the left phrenic nerve, is removed. It is desirable to decorticate (remove the surface layer of pericardium) both atria, both ventricles, and both vena cavae (Franco et al., 1991). Pericardiectomy is usually performed through a median sternotomy incision. A median sternotomy approach better exposes the anterior surface of the heart, especially the right atrium and vena cavae; a left thoracotomy approach better exposes the entirety of the left ventricle, particularly its posterior surface (Brandenburg et al., 1991).

Cardiopulmonary bypass is occasionally used to make pericardiectomy technically easier. Use of extracorporeal circulation allows decompression of the heart, thereby facilitating removal of parietal pericardium from the epicardial surface. Cardiopulmonary bypass may also become necessary if manipulation of the heart induces ventricular fibrillation. Blood loss is often significant during pericardiectomy because of inflammation and adhesions, especially if the procedure is performed with cardiopulmonary bypass and systemic anticoagulation. Transfusion may be necessary. Sometimes, a restrictive cardiomyopathy is present in association with constrictive pericarditis. In such cases, symptomatic improvement after the operation may occur gradually over several months. Most patients, however, eventually experience significant clinical improvement if pericardiectomy is performed early after onset of the condition. Long-standing pericardial restriction, on the other hand, is known to cause irreversible atrophic changes in the myocardium (Brandenburg et al., 1991).

CHRONIC PULMONARY EMBOLISM

Pulmonary emboli usually resolve spontaneously due to intrinsic methods of fibrinolysis. Occasionally, however, *chronic pulmonary embolism* develops as a result of recurring emboli, inadequate lysis, or lack of adequate anticoagulant therapy. Patients with chronic pulmonary embolism may eventually develop incapacitating pulmonary hypertension from accumulation of thrombus in major branches of the pulmonary arteries. Symptoms of progressive respiratory insufficiency and right ventricular failure typically develop.

Pulmonary thromboendarterectomy is a procedure that is performed in selected centers to evacuate thrombotic material and lessen the degree of pulmonary hypertension. Candidates for surgical therapy are patients with (1) severe respiratory insufficiency and hypoxemia from pulmonary hypertension, (2) proximal pulmonary arterial occlusion and adequate bronchial collateral circulation, and (3) minimal impairment of right ventricular function (Lyerly & Sabiston, 1990). Pulmonary thromboendarterectomy is performed through a median sternotomy incision with cardiopulmonary bypass and cardioplegic arrest. Through incisions in the pulmonary arteries, endarterectomy of each of the bronchopulmonary segmental arteries and their subsegmental branches is performed (Daily et al., 1990) (Fig. 21-5). The procedure is associated with significant operative risk but provides considerably improved quality of life in patients with severe symptoms of chronic pulmonary embolism (Daily et al., 1990). Complications of pulmonary thromboendarterectomy include right ventricular failure in patients with long-standing pulmonary hypertension and a hemorrhagic lung syndrome (Lyerly & Sabiston, 1990). Irreversible pulmonary hypertension is alternatively treated with lung or heart-lung transplantation, discussed in Chapter 31, Heart, Lung, and Heart-Lung Transplantation.

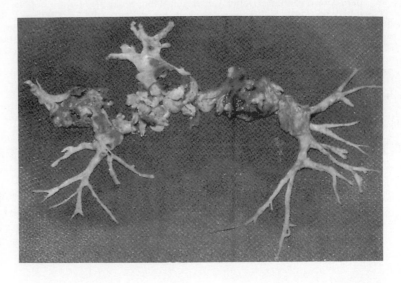

FIGURE 21-5. Endarterectomy specimen; thrombotic material has been removed from the upper, middle, and lower lobe pulmonary artery branches bilaterally. (Jamieson SW, Auger WB, Fedullo PF, et al, 1993: Experience and results with 150 pulmonary thromboendarterectomy operations over a 29-month period. J Thorac Cardiovasc Surg 106:120)

REFERENCES

Brandenburg RO, Click RL, McGoon DC, 1991: The pericardium. In Giuliani ER, Fuster V, Gersh BJ, et al. (eds): Cardiology Fundamentals and Practice, ed. 2. St. Louis, Mosby–Year Book

Brown PS, Roberts CS, McIntosh CL, Clark RE, 1991: Aortic regurgitation after left ventricular myotomy and myectomy. Ann Thorac Surg 51:585

Carpentier A, Chachques JC, 1991: Clinical dynamic cardiomyoplasty: Method and outcome. Semin Thorac Cardiovasc Surg 3:136

Chachques JC, Grandjean PA, Carpentier A, 1991: Patient management and clinical follow-up after cardiomyoplasty. J Cardiac Surg 6 (Suppl):89

Cooley DA, 1991: Surgical techniques for hypertrophic left ventricular obstructive myopathy including mitral valve plication. J Cardiac Surg 6:29

Daily PO, Dembitsky WP, Iverson S, et al., 1990: Risk factors for pulmonary thromboendarterectomy. J Thorac Cardiovasc Surg 99:670

Fallon JT, Dec GW, 1989: Cardiac tumors. In Eagle KA, Haber E, DeSanctis RW, Austin WG (eds): The Practice of Cardiology, ed. 2. Boston, Little, Brown

Franco KL, Breckenridge I, Hammond GL, 1991: The pericardium. In Baue AE, Geha AS, Hammond GL, et al. (eds): Glenn's Thoracic and Cardiovascular Surgery, ed. 5. Norwalk, CT, Appleton & Lange

Furnary AP, Christlieb IY, Magovern JA, et al., 1991: Wrap nomenclature for latissimus dorsi cardiomyoplasty. Semin Thorac Cardiovasc Surg 3:132

Hillis LD, Lange RA, Wells PJ, Winniford MD, 1992a: Primary cardiac tumors. In Manual of Clinical Problems in Cardiology, ed. 4. Boston, Little, Brown

Hillis LD, Lange RA, Wells PJ, Winniford MD, 1992b: Constrictive pericarditis. In Manual of Clinical Problems in Cardiology, ed. 4. Boston, Little, Brown

Jacobs ML, Austen WG, 1990: Acquired aortic valve disease. In Sabiston DC Jr, Spencer FC (eds): Surgery of the Chest, ed. 5. Philadelphia, WB Saunders

Kirklin JW, Barratt-Boyes BG, 1993a: Cardiac tumor. In Cardiac Surgery, ed. 2. New York, Churchill Livingstone

Kirklin JW, Barratt-Boyes BG, 1993b: Hypertrophic obstructive cardiomyopathy. In Cardiac Surgery, ed. 2. New York, Churchill Livingstone

Kirklin JW, Barratt-Boyes BG, 1993c: Primary cardiomyopathy and cardiac transplantation. In Cardiac Surgery, ed. 2. New York, Churchill Livingstone

Krajcer Z, Leachman RD, Cooley DA, Coronado R, 1989: Septal myotomy-myectomy versus mitral valve replacement in hypertrophied cardiomyopathy. Circulation 80(Suppl I):I-57

Lorell BH, Braunwald E, 1992: Pericardial disease. In Braunwald E (ed): Heart Disease: A Textbook of Cardiovascular Medicine, ed. 4. Philadelphia, WB Saunders

Lyerly HK, Sabiston DC Jr, 1990: Chronic pulmonary embolism. In Sabiston DC Jr, Spencer FC (eds): Surgery of the Chest, ed. 5. Philadelphia, WB Saunders

Magovern JA, Furnary AP, Christlieb IY, et al., 1991: Indications and risk analysis for clinical cardiomyoplasty. Semin Thorac Cardiovasc Surg 3:145

Massimiano PS, Hammond GL, 1991: Aortic valve disease and hypertrophic myopathies. In Baue AE, Geha AS, Hammond GL, et al. (eds): Glenn's Thoracic and Cardiovascular Surgery, ed. 5. Norwalk, CT, Appleton & Lange

Mohr R, Schaff HV, Puga FJ, Danielson GK, 1989: Results of operation for hypertrophic obstructive cardiomyopathy in children and adults less than 40 years of age. Circulation 80 (Suppl I):I-191

Moreira LF, Stolf NA, Bocchi EA, et al., 1990: Latissimus dorsi cardiomyoplasty in the treatment of patients with dilated cardiomyopathy. Circulation 82 (Suppl IV):IV-257

Moreira LF, Stolf NA, Jatene AD, 1991. Benefits of cardiomyoplasty for dilated cardiomyopathy. Semin Thorac Cardiovasc Surg 3:140

Nishimura RA, Giuliani R, Tajik AJ, Brandenburg RO, 1991: Hypertrophic cardiomyopathy. In Giuliani ER, Fuster V, Gersh BJ, et al. (eds): Cardiology Fundamentals and Practice, ed. 2. St. Louis, Mosby–Year Book

Novick RJ, Dobell ARC, 1991: Tumors of the heart. In Baue AE, Geha AS, Hammond GL, et al. (eds): Glenn's Thoracic and Cardiovascular Surgery, ed. 5. Norwalk, CT, Appleton & Lange.

Orie JE, 1991: Dynamic cardiomyoplasty: A possible alternative treatment of congestive heart failure. Semin Thorac Cardiovasc Surg 3:98

Schaff HV, Piehler JM, Lie JT, Giuliani ER, 1991: Tumors of the heart. In Giuliani ER, Fuster V, Gersh BJ, et al. (eds): Cardiology Fundametals and Practice, ed. 2. St. Louis, Mosby–Year Book

Sellke FW, Lemmer JH, Vandenberg BF, Ehrenhaft JL, 1990: Surgical treatment of cardiac myxomas: Long-term results. Ann Thorac Surg 50:557

Shabetai R, 1985: The pericardium as a source of cardiac dysfunction. In Utley JR (ed): Perioperative Cardiac Dysfunction, vol. III. Baltimore, Williams & Wilkins

Shabetai R, 1990: Diseases of the pericardium. In Hurst JW, Schlant RC, Rackley CE, et al. (eds): The Heart, ed. 7. New York, McGraw-Hill

Sola OM, Kakulas BA, Haines LC, et al., 1991: Morphology and histology of the latissimus dorsi muscle. Semin Thorac Cardiovasc Surg 3:124

Stone CD, Hennein HA, McIntosh CL, et al., 1990: The results of operation in patients with hypertrophic cardiomyopathy and pulmonary hypertension. J Thorac Cardiovasc Surg 100:343

Van Trigt P, Sabiston DC Jr, 1990: Tumors of the heart. In Sabiston DC Jr, Spencer FC (eds): Surgery of the Chest, ed. 5. Philadelphia, WB Saunders

Wynne J, Braunwald E, 1992: The cardiomyopathies and myocarditides: Toxic, chemical and physical damage to the heart. In Braunwald E (ed): Heart Disease: A Textbook of Cardiovascular Medicine, ed. 4. Philadelphia, WB Saunders

5

P A R T

POSTOPERATIVE MANAGEMENT

CHAPTER 22

POSTOPERATIVE PATIENT MANAGEMENT

INTENSIVE CARE	CARE ON THE POSTOPERATIVE UNIT
Admission and Assessment	Progression of Activity
Early Postoperative Care	Pulmonary Hygiene
Common Problems	Incision Care
	Medications
	Common Problems
	Preparation for Discharge

Patient recovery from cardiac surgery usually follows a routine and predictable course. Intensive care is generally necessary for the first 24 to 48 hours. An intermediate or step-down unit, if available, may be used for postoperative care on the second day. Discharge from the hospital within 6 to 7 days of operation is common.

INTENSIVE CARE

Ideally, the postoperative intensive care unit (ICU) is located adjacent to the cardiac surgical operating rooms. In facilities where the two are geographically separated, it is desirable to keep patients in a recovery room near the operating suite for several hours. This minimizes transfer time during which monitoring and the ability to treat problems are compromised. Also, the patient can be rapidly transferred back to the operating room should excessive bleeding or other urgent reason for operative reexploration develop.

Transfer from the operating room to the ICU is performed after the operation is concluded and when the patient is hemodynamically stable. A self-inflating bag with 100% oxygen is used to ventilate the intubated patient during transport. Portable units

with the capacity for electrocardiographic and pressure monitoring are also used. Continued visibility of the heart rhythm and arterial pressure adds a dimension of safety to the transfer process. First, attachment of monitoring equipment in the ICU can be performed in a less urgent fashion. Second, it allows prompt detection of arrhythmias, hypertension, or hypotension during transfer. Common problems that can occur during patient transport include sudden hypotension due to fluid shifts that occur as the patient is moved, acute hypertension due to sympathetic stimulation, extubation or reflex responses caused by traction on the endotracheal tube, and alteration in dosage or disconnection of intravenous medication infusions (Hendren & Higgins, 1991).

ADMISSION AND ASSESSMENT

Patient admission to the ICU is performed in a systematic manner. Priorities on patient arrival are (1) reestablishing mechanical ventilation, monitoring capabilities, and chest tube suction; (2) confirming hemodynamic stability; and (3) identifying all catheters and pacing equipment (Fig. 22-1). Generally, two nurses participate in the admission process so that necessary tasks can be performed quickly and any sudden problems are treated promptly. The anesthe-

Betsy Finkelmeier: CARDIOTHORACIC SURGICAL NURSING.
© 1995 J.B. Lippincott Company.

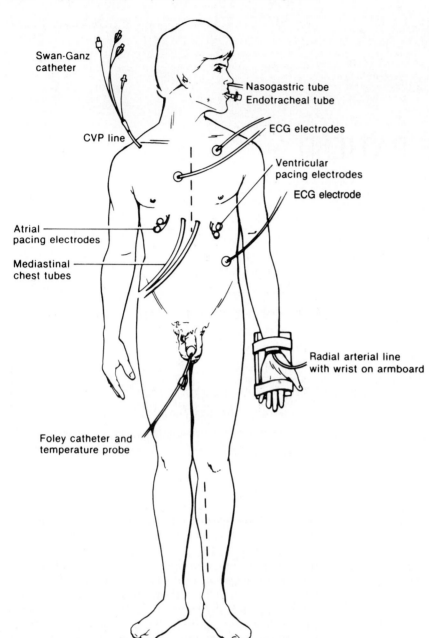

Swan-Ganz catheter

Nasogastric tube

Endotracheal tube

CVP line

ECG electrodes

Ventricular pacing electrodes

ECG electrode

Atrial pacing electrodes

Mediastinal chest tubes

Radial arterial line with wrist on armboard

Foley catheter and temperature probe

FIGURE 22-1. Drawing demonstrates typical appearance of postoperative patient; *dotted lines* represent median sternotomy incision and leg incision for harvesting of saphenous vein. (Adapted from Hudak CM, Gallo BM, Benz JJ, 1990: Intra-aortic balloon pump counterpulsation. In Critical Care Nursing: A Holistic Approach, ed. 5, p. 270. Philadelphia, JB Lippincott)

siologist or surgeon who accompanies the patient communicates the following information to the ICU nurse: the procedure performed, the type of anesthesia used, any significant intraoperative findings or complications, whether the patient has received blood transfusions, current medication and fluid infusions, and desirable hemodynamic parameters.

A respirator with appropriately set parameters should be in place at the bedside when the patient arrives so that mechanical ventilation can be promptly instituted. Electrocardiographic leads are connected to the bedside monitor, and arterial and pulmonary artery catheter transducers are transferred. Chest tube suction is reestablished. The arterial catheter and all intravenous catheters are as-

sessed for patency and proper infusion rates. Catheters typically present include a subclavian or jugular pulmonary artery catheter, a multiple-lumen central venous catheter for administration of medications and fluid, one or two peripheral intravenous catheters, and a radial arterial catheter. If volumetric pumps used in the operating room for infusion of intravenous medications can also be used in the ICU, no exchange of equipment is necessary. If a separate set of pumps is used, a consistent system of exchanging equipment is important so that drug infusion rates are not altered while medication solutions or infusion pumps are changed.

Temporary atrial and ventricular epicardial pacing wires are inspected and properly secured with an insulating cover. An external pulse generator, set in a synchronous mode, may be attached to the ventricular epicardial wire. Drainage tubes and catheters, including mediastinal, and sometimes pleural, chest drainage tubes, a urethral drainage catheter, and a nasogastric tube, are examined for proper functioning. If saphenous veins have been harvested, a drain may be present in the leg and is usually connected to low continuous suction.

As soon as all necessary equipment attachments are made and the admission process is completed, a thorough patient assessment is performed. The purpose of the assessment is to provide a summarized description of all significant findings at a particular point in time (Table 22-1). Information included should complement and expand on that which is recorded on flow sheets used for vital signs and other parameters. Baseline information observed at the time of admission to the ICU is invaluable in evaluating the patient's clinical course over time. The assessment is repeated by each new nurse assuming care of the patient (usually every 8 to 12 hours). A standardized unit protocol for documentation of the patient assessment ensures that information is consistently recorded and easily available to all nurses and physicians caring for the patient.

Often, experienced nurses can integrate performance of the assessment with nursing interventions required during the admission process. The order of patient assessment is less important than its performance in a consistent and thorough fashion so that all relevant data is included. However, certain observations are priorities and should be performed as soon as the patient arrives. These include observation of symmetric chest movement; auscultation of bilateral breath sounds; and documentation of heart rate and rhythm, blood pressure, hemodynamic parameters, chest tube output, and infusion rates of intravenous fluids. Intravenous medication infusions are reviewed for proper concentration, rate of infusion, and location and integrity of infusion site (Lee & Ramos, 1990). Because neurologic complications most often become apparent in the early postoperative hours, the patient's ability to move all extremities and follow simple commands is documented as soon as it is noted.

EARLY POSTOPERATIVE CARE

In the great majority of cases, the admission and early postoperative hours are routine and nursing care can be performed in an organized fashion. However, the first few hours are critical in that potentially life-threatening problems are most likely during this period. The patient, the cardiac rhythm, and the hemodynamic parameters are observed continuously, and vital signs are documented every 15 to 20 minutes to ensure prompt detection of developing complications, particularly hemorrhage, low cardiac output, or arrhythmias. Ongoing monitoring of temperature

TABLE 22-1. ASSESSMENT OF THE POSTOPERATIVE PATIENT

Neurologic Status

Level of consciousness
Reactivity of pupils
Ability to move extremities
Level of orientation
Presence of any neurologic deficits or abnormal reflex responses

Cardiovascular Status

Heart rate, cardiac rhythm
Arterial blood pressure (systolic, diastolic, and mean)
Pulmonary artery pressure (systolic, diastolic, and mean)
Pulmonary capillary wedge pressure, left atrial pressure*
Central venous pressure
Cardiac output/cardiac index
Systemic vascular resistance
Heart sounds
Pacing wires, pulse generator settings
Peripheral perfusion (pulses, capillary refill, color, temperature)
Chest tube output

Respiratory Status

Respiratory rate (ventilator and patient)
Breath sounds
Symmetry of chest movement
Current ventilator settings
Arterial blood gas or oxygen saturation measurement
Respiratory effort

Gastrointestinal Status

Bowel sounds
Presence and function of nasogastric tube
Presence of abdominal distention or tenderness

Renal Status

Urine output
Urine color

Other

Adequacy of pain control and sedation
Intravenous fluids and medications
Chest x-ray and electrocardiogram
Laboratory measurements
Incisional drainage

* Measured in selected patients only.

is performed using a pulmonary artery or urethral catheter equipped with a thermistor. If neither of these is used, rectal temperature is checked every hour.

Standard hemodynamic monitoring of the postoperative patient includes arterial blood pressure, central venous pressure, pulmonary artery pressure, cardiac output, cardiac index, and systemic vascular resistance. Mixed venous oxygen saturation, using blood sampled from the distal port of the pulmonary artery catheter, may also be measured to assess systemic perfusion. Patients undergoing valvular heart surgery occasionally have a left atrial catheter for direct measurement of left atrial pressure. Management of these catheters and principles of hemodynamic monitoring are discussed in detail in Chapter 23, Hemodynamic Monitoring.

The most important hemodynamic indicator in the early postoperative period is cardiac output (Karp & Kouchoukas, 1991). No one parameter, however, should be considered or treated in isolation. Rather, all are evaluated in combination to determine appropriate therapeutic interventions. A thorough understanding of the interplay between the hemodynamic variables is essential. The goal is to maintain adequate systemic perfusion to protect cerebral, myocardial, and visceral function.

Measurement of *arterial blood pressure,* particularly mean arterial pressure, provides essential information about perfusion of the heart, brain, kidneys, and other vital organs. In addition to invasive pressure monitoring, quality of peripheral pulses, color and temperature of the extremities, level of mentation, and adequacy of urine output are important indicators of peripheral perfusion.

Cardiac output is measured using the pulmonary artery catheter and a thermodilution technique. To correct for differences in patient size, the measured cardiac output is divided by body surface area to obtain cardiac index. Cardiac index is affected by preload, afterload, cardiac rhythm, and myocardial contractility. It is often necessary to manipulate these individual parameters in the early postoperative hours to achieve and maintain a normal cardiac index (i.e., one that is greater than 2 L/min/m^2). However, altering preload, afterload, cardiac rhythm, and contractility affects the work done by the heart. When the heart works harder, oxygen consumption is greater. In patients with cardiac pathology, clinical methods for measuring oxygen consumption and determining the optimal relationship between work and energy consumption remain unclear.

Preload is the end-diastolic volume in the ventricle and serves as an estimation of average diastolic fiber length (Smith, 1990). *Starling's law* describes the relationship between end-diastolic fiber length and cardiac output (Hudak et al., 1990a). As filling pressure (as measured indirectly by pulmonary artery diastolic, left atrial, or right atrial pressure) increases, cardiac output also increases until a point is reached at which further filling produces a decrease in cardiac output and congestive heart failure. The preload that provides optimal cardiac output varies from patient to patient. Normal pulmonary artery diastolic pressure is 8 to 15 mm Hg, but in a diseased heart cardiac function is often better when it is 15 to 20 mm Hg.

The cardiac surgeon has an excellent opportunity to assess cardiac function in relation to various levels of preload while the patient is being weaned from cardiopulmonary bypass (CPB). During weaning, venous return to the extracorporeal circuit is partially occluded, allowing some volume to enter and be ejected by the heart. As a result, the surgeon in effect controls the patient's preload by manipulating the proportion of venous blood that is diverted through the venous cannula and that which is returned to the heart. Contractility of the ventricles can be directly observed and cardiac output measured to determine the optimal preload level. When the patient is transferred to the ICU, the surgeon communicates preload values associated with most effective cardiac function. If the patient recovers normally, cardiac function should steadily improve from the time the heart was weaned from CPB. Therefore, one would expect the required preload level not to exceed and to gradually decrease from that required by the heart at the time of weaning from CPB.

Afterload, or the impedance to left ventricular contraction, is assessed by measuring *systemic vascular resistance.* Typically, systemic vascular resistance is elevated in the early postoperative hours secondary to hypothermia and peripheral vasoconstriction. It gradually decreases as the patient's body temperature returns to normal. Pharmacologic vasodilating agents may also be used to decrease afterload. Less commonly, pharmacologic agents are needed to increase afterload that has been abnormally decreased by anesthetic agents or an allergic reaction to protamine sulfate. The clinical indicator for right ventricular afterload is *pulmonary vascular resistance.* Elevated pulmonary vascular resistance is unusual except in patients with cardiac pathology associated with pulmonary artery hypertension.

A third variable affecting cardiac output is *cardiac rate* and *rhythm.* Because of the importance of this factor and the prevalence of cardiac arrhythmias in the early postoperative period, continuous ECG monitoring is essential and is usually performed through the fourth or fifth postoperative day. An optimal cardiac rhythm provides atrioventricular (AV) contractions at an acceptable rate. Epicardial pacing wires are routinely placed on the right atrium and ventricle so that temporary pacing can be performed to manipulate the cardiac rhythm. The epicardial pacing wires are often left in place until the day before discharge. The wires are quite useful therapeutically, are associated with almost no morbidity, and can be easily detached before the patient's discharge from the hospital. In addition, the atrial wire can be used for diagnostic purposes.

A heart rate that is too slow decreases cardiac output, which is a product of heart rate times stroke volume. Atrial or ventricular pacing is used to increase heart rate to 90 to 100 beats per minute, the range that usually provides the best cardiac output during the early postoperative period (Bojar, 1989; Geha & Whittlesey, 1991). Atrial pacing is preferable because it maintains the added ventricular filling that results from an appropriately timed atrial systole (i.e., the "atrial kick"). AV synchrony is maintained with atrial (if AV nodal function is normal) or AV sequential pacing. Because it preserves AV synchrony, AV sequential pacing increases cardiac output as compared with ventricular pacing in postoperative cardiac surgical patients (Finkelmeier & Salinger, 1986). If atrial fibrillation or other supraventricular arrhythmia is present, ventricular pacing must be used to increase heart rate.

Tachycardia may develop in the early postoperative hours as a manifestation of hypovolemia or sympathetic overstimulation. A rapid heart rate lowers stroke volume because ventricular filling time is reduced. Tachyarrhythmias require correction of the precipitating cause or suppression with antiarrhythmic medication.

Myocardial contractility or the inotropic state of the heart describes the ability of heart muscle to shorten, develop tension, or both, independent of variations induced by altering preload or afterload (Bond, 1989). Myocardial contractility is enhanced if necessary by using inotropic pharmacologic agents. Most commonly used are dopamine and dobutamine, although another inotrope may be preferable depending on the specific situation. Each agent has a varying degree of inotropic and other types of effects. Therefore, choice of agent is individualized to the specific clinical situation. These drugs are discussed in detail in Chapter 27, Cardiovascular Medications.

Sedatives are generally administered until the patient is fully rewarmed and hemodynamically stable and chest tube drainage is acceptable (Coyle, 1991). Morphine or diazepam is commonly used to prevent premature wakefulness, which may lead to undesirable hypertension, tachycardia, and resistance to mechanical ventilation. Occasionally, a patient awakens before neuromuscular blocking agents are eliminated or metabolized, resulting in an awake but paralyzed patient. Aggressive pharmacologic therapy with nitrates, alpha- and beta-blocking agents, and calcium-channel blocking medications may be necessary to suppress the autonomic instability resulting from the patient's distress (Hendren & Higgins, 1991). Intravenous bolus doses of morphine are administered intermittently as necessary during the first 24 hours to provide adequate analgesia.

An oral or nasal endotracheal tube remains in place during the early postoperative hours. Intubation and mechanical ventilation with a volume-cycled ventilator are necessary until the patient has awakened from anesthesia and is able to do the work of breathing independently. Most patients awaken by 4 to 8 hours after operation (Karp & Kouchoukas, 1991).

Mechanical ventilation is usually performed using an intermittent mandatory ventilation (IMV) mode to give the patient early control and to allow easy tapering of assisted ventilation (Karp & Kouchoukas, 1991). Specific ventilator settings are individualized for each patient. Typical parameters are as follows: respiratory rate = 8 to 10 breaths per minute; tidal volume = 10 to 15 mL/kg; Fio_2 = 50% to 60%; positive end-expiratory pressure = 5 cm H_2O;, and dead space = 50 mL. *Pulse oximetry* is used for continuous

monitoring of oxygen saturation. Arterial blood gases are measured each time changes are made in ventilatory parameters and as indicated by changes in the patient's condition. A nasogastric tube to keep the stomach decompressed usually remains until the patient is extubated.

During the period of intubation, the patient is turned side to side every 2 hours and endotracheal suctioning is performed every 1 to 2 hours. Atelectasis, particularly of the left lower lobe, is a common occurrence after cardiac operations due to reduced lung volume and small airway closure (Valta et al., 1992). Weaning from mechanical ventilation is accomplished by limiting sedation and decreasing the IMV rate. Depending on the type of anesthetic agents that have been used, the patient is generally extubated either the evening of the operation or early the following morning (Table 22-2). Other factors that influence timing of extubation include efficacy of rewarming, hemodynamic status of the patient, and the expected likelihood of reexploration for bleeding (Hendren & Higgins, 1991).

Humidified oxygen by means of face mask is provided for 24 hours after extubation. A nasal cannula may be used alternatively for oxygen delivery. It is generally more comfortable for the patient, although the inspired oxygen is not as well humidified. Providing supplemental humidity is helpful in loosening pulmonary secretions so that they are more easily expectorated. Unless there is a specific respiratory problem, supplemental oxygen is generally not necessary after the first 48 hours.

Two mediastinal chest tubes are generally placed in cardiac surgical patients for evacuation of blood. One is positioned within the pericardium and one is in the posterior mediastinum. If the pleural space has been opened, a pleural chest tube will be present as well. Protocols for routine "stripping" or "milking" of chest tubes vary from institution to institution. Some surgeons believe stripping tubes is important to maintain patency; others believe the excessive negativity created in the mediastinum by routine stripping

---

TABLE 22-2. CRITERIA FOR EXTUBATION

Pao_2 > 60 mm Hg on 40% Fio_2
$Paco_2$ < 45 mm Hg
Respiratory rate < 35/min
Negative inspiratory force > -20
Tidal volume > 4–5 mL/kg
Vital capacity > 10 mL/kg
Continuous positive airway pressure ≤ 5 cm
Able to protect airway
Hemodynamically stable
Chest tube drainage < 100 mL/h
Temperature > 36°C (96.8°F)

(Adapted from Housestaff Manual for Cardiothoracic Surgery, 1994. Chicago, Northwestern University Medical School)

causes more bleeding and might disrupt vein graft anastomoses. Regardless of whether chest tubes are routinely stripped, they are closely monitored during the early postoperative hours to ensure patency and to record hourly the amount of blood loss. Hematocrit levels are measured on admission to the unit and the following day or sooner if bleeding is excessive.

In most institutions, *autotransfusion* is performed (Fig. 22-2). Autotransfusion is reinfusion of shed mediastinal blood that is defibrinated by contact with the pleura and pericardium (Mahfood et al., 1991) Because average blood loss after cardiac operations is approximately 1 L, autotransfusion represents a significant method of blood conservation (Scott et al., 1990). Standardized protocols are used to guide the nurse in performing autotransfusion. Typically, blood is transfused hourly as it accumulates or every 2 to 4 hours, using a closed chest drainage system, filter, and intravenous infusion pump. Autotransfusion is usually discontinued after approximately 6 hours when active bleeding has subsided. In patients who have a postoperative coagulopathy or who have received large amounts of banked blood, autotransfusion may be discontinued because the shed blood is depleted of clotting factors. However, many surgeons elect to continue autotransfusion in these circumstances to conserve red blood cells.

A portable chest roentgenogram is obtained within the first postoperative hour. The film demonstrates the position of intrathoracic tubes and catheters and provides baseline information for radiographic detection of postoperative problems. The critical care nurse is often the first to review the film and to identify problems that require correction, such as improper positioning of endotracheal, chest, or nasogastric tubes or pulmonary artery or central venous catheters; evidence of blood accumulation within the chest (hemothorax or mediastinal widening); pneumothorax; or gastric distention. Chest roentgenograms are discussed in further detail in Chapter 44, Postoperative Chest Roentgenogram Interpretation.

A 12-lead electrocardiogram (ECG) is obtained within several hours of the patient's arrival in the ICU. Because hypothermia can produce ECG changes that confuse interpretation, the ECG is generally deferred until the patient is normothermic and not shivering. If a temporary pacemaker is being used but the patient has an adequate underlying cardiac rhythm, pacing is discontinued while the ECG is recorded. In patients who are pacemaker dependent, the ECG is generally omitted.

Monitoring fluid status is an important component of early postoperative care. Intake and output are recorded hourly during the first 24 hours and every 2 hours during the next 24 hours to document the amount of fluid administered in comparison with that lost as urine and chest tube drainage. Patients commonly gain 2 to 5 kg of fluid weight during cardiac surgical operations owing to the effects of CPB and hormonal changes associated with a major operation. Both antidiuretic hormone and aldosterone levels are elevated by surgical stress and increase sodium and water retention (Behrendt & Austen, 1985).

Despite increased body weight, intravascular volume may actually be depleted. Large amounts of fluid move from the intravascular to the interstitial space during and up to 6 hours after surgery as a result of (1) the increased fluid volume, (2) the increased capillary permeability secondary to vasoactive substances released during CPB, and (3) the decreased plasma colloid osmotic pressure caused by hemodilution (Hudak et al., 1990b). Thus the extra fluid is primarily in the interstitial tissue (i.e., the "third space"). In addition, most patients experience an osmotic diuresis in the early postoperative hours because of hemodilution and the high glucose concentration of the circulating blood volume while on CPB (Karp & Kouchoukas, 1991). Therefore, volume repletion may be necessary to maintain an adequate preload in the early postoperative hours despite increased body weight. If preload is adequate, total fluid administration is limited to 50 mL/h for the first several days. With the exception of the arterial line, intravenous fluids that contain sodium are not used so that fluid retention is not exacerbated. Furosemide or another diuretic agent is sometimes administered if the patient is oliguric despite an adequate preload level.

After removal of the pulmonary artery and central venous catheter, weights provide the most accurate parameter for assessing fluid status. They are ob-

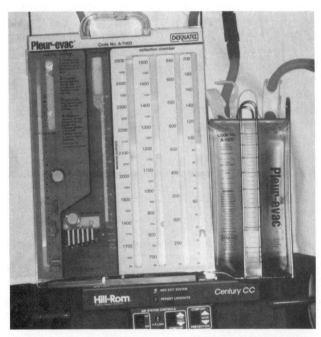

FIGURE 22-2. Example of chest drainage system with autotransfusion bag attached. Blood shed into the autotransfusion bag may be filtered and reinfused through an intravenous catheter.

tained at a consistent time each morning. The preoperative weight provides a baseline value for comparison unless the patient had some degree of heart failure before surgery or the operation was performed emergently and the patient was not weighed. Oral liquids are generally administered beginning on the first postoperative day, after the endotracheal tube has been discontinued and the patient is alert enough to protect the airway. Oral fluids are restricted until the patient returns to preoperative weight. Most patients experience a spontaneous diuresis on the third or fourth postoperative day as fluid is mobilized into the vascular space.

COMMON PROBLEMS

Problems that arise in the early postoperative hours are often of a precipitous nature, requiring immediate interventions by the nurse at the bedside. Consequently, cardiothoracic surgical nurses require a thorough understanding of principles of cardiac physiology, the meaning and relationship of the various hemodynamic parameters, the characteristics of anesthetic agents, the consequences of CPB and rewarming, and the actions of commonly used pharmacologic agents. In most cardiac surgical ICUs, standardized protocols provide nurses with the flexibility to respond to typical problems. Only commonly occurring transient postoperative problems are included in this discussion. The various postoperative complications are discussed in Chapter 28, Complications of Cardiac Operations.

Postoperative bleeding may be caused by a surgically correctable problem, such as a disrupted surgical clip or sutured anastomosis, or by a coagulopathy related to intraoperative anticoagulation, hemodilution, and the extracorporeal circulation of blood during CPB. The most important hemostatic derangement in cardiac surgical patients and a primary cause of postoperative coagulopathy is the reduction in quantity and quality of platelets after CPB (Halfman-Franey & Berg, 1991).

Adequate hemostasis is achieved before transferring a patient out of the operating room. However, bleeding that was not apparent or that was minimal during closure of the chest may increase as the patient's body temperature and blood pressure rise. Bleeding is exacerbated by postoperative hypertension that can occur secondary to elevated systemic vascular resistance or increasing wakefulness and agitation. Factors that increase circulating catecholamines, such as hypoxia, hypercarbia, hypothermia with shivering, and visceral distention, may also contribute to development of hypertension (Hendren & Higgins, 1991). In most situations, mean arterial pressure is maintained below 75 to 80 mm Hg during the early postoperative hours to avoid excessive bleeding. Vasodilating agents, such as nitroprusside or nitroglycerin, are commonly used to accomplish this goal. Sedation of the patient may also be necessary.

Chest tube output is monitored closely to detect sudden increases in the amount of drainage. Patients with more than ordinary amounts of bleeding are observed carefully so that reexploration and hemostasis can be achieved before hemodynamic instability develops. The decision to take a patient back to the operating room for mediastinal reexploration is influenced by the rate and amount of bleeding, the nature of the operation, and the surgeon's assessment of the likelihood of a surgically correctable etiology. In general, reexploration is indicated for greater than 500 mL drainage in any 1 hour, greater than 100 mL/h for 4 to 6 hours, or acute hemodynamic instability despite adequate volume replacement. A dramatic increase in the rate of bleeding is usually indicative of disruption of a clip or suture. In such cases, surgical reexploration is performed at once. A mechanical (surgically correctable) cause of bleeding is found in approximately half the patients who undergo surgical reexploration (Anderson et al., 1991).

If postoperative bleeding is excessive or if chest tubes become clotted, *cardiac tamponade* may occur. As more and more blood accumulates in the pericardial space or mediastinum, the heart is unable to fill adequately, causing cardiac output and blood pressure to fall. Emergent reopening of a portion of the sternal incision may be necessary to prevent cardiac arrest. In some instances, this is performed by the surgeon in the ICU. For this reason, wire cutters and staple removers as well as a chest opening tray should be readily accessible. The patient is returned to the operating room for exploration of the mediastinum and reclosure of the incision under sterile conditions.

A second common problem in the early postoperative period is *low cardiac output*. A low cardiac output state is said to exist when the cardiac index is less than 2.0 L/min/m². The most common causes of postoperative low cardiac output are hypovolemia, myocardial dysfunction, and cardiac tamponade (Hendren & Higgins, 1991). Clinical manifestations include cold, clammy extremities, hypotension, tachycardia, diminished peripheral pulses and capillary refill, decreased urine output, and persistent obtundation (Moreno-Cabral et al., 1988). However, classic signs of shock do not always accompany low cardiac output in the early postoperative hours because of the patient's thermal instability, residual effects of anesthesia, and the osmotic diuresis that usually follows CPB (DiSesa, 1991).

Hypovolemia or inadequate preload is a common etiology of low cardiac output because of the vasodilatation, urinary diuresis, and mediastinal bleeding that occur after cardiac operations. Accordingly, the first method of treatment is to provide sufficient preload to maximize cardiac output without overfilling the heart. Sustained low filling pressures despite volume replacement suggest hemorrhage. Low cardiac output in association with elevated filling pressures indicates a problem with cardiac function. Impaired cardiac function may result from a number of etiologies, including perioperative myocardial infarction, reperfusion of ischemic or infarcted myocardium, inadequate intraoperative myocardial protection, preexisting ventricular damage, or cardiac tamponade. The primary therapy for low cardiac output due to myocardial dysfunction (except that due to tamponade) is continuous intravenous infusion of one or more inotropic pharmacologic agents. Commonly used drugs include dopamine, dobutamine, epinephrine, isoproterenol, and amrinone. Dopamine is often selected as the initial agent of choice because, in low doses, it also stimulates renal dopaminergic receptors, thereby increasing renal perfusion. Often, a low cardiac output state is accompanied by increased afterload, as measured by systemic vascular resistance. Afterload reduction is usually achieved by infusing sodium nitroprusside, a vasodilating agent that directly relaxes smooth muscle in both arteriolar and venous beds, thus lowering systemic vascular resistance, pulmonary vascular resistance, and preload (Greco, 1990). Adequate preload levels must exist before infusing nitroprusside to avoid precipitous hypotension. Nitroglycerin may be used alternatively. Because it vasodilates coronary and pulmonary as well as systemic vessels, it may be preferable for low cardiac output associated with increased pulmonary vascular resistance, coronary artery spasm, or incomplete coronary artery revascularization. In severe cases of low cardiac output secondary to left ventricular failure, intra-aortic balloon counterpulsation may also be used to provide mechanical afterload reduction. Prostaglandin E_1 infusion may be used to produce pulmonary arterial vasodilatation in patients with postoperative right ventricular dysfunction associated with pulmonary hypertension (Kelleher et al., 1991).

Temporary pacing and antiarrhythmic agents are used as necessary to optimize cardiac rate and rhythm. Sedatives are administered to minimize sympathetic overstimulation and its deleterious effects on heart rate and systemic vascular resistance (Moran & Singh, 1989). Mechanical ventilation is continued so that the patient is not subjected to the work of respiration.

Occasionally, *profound hypotension* occurs precipitously in the early postoperative hours. Hypotension detected by arterial pressure monitoring should be verified by cuff measurement or palpation of the femoral artery. All medication infusions are inspected to detect possible interruption of inotropic infusion or bolus of vasodilator infusion. The chest tube drainage system is examined for a sudden increase in blood loss and chest tubes are stripped to ensure patency. In addition to bleeding, diuretic therapy or vasodilatation secondary to rewarming may cause hypovolemia (Hendren & Higgins, 1991). If filling pressures are low, a fluid bolus is administered. Infusion of dopamine, or other inotropic agent, is instituted or increased.

The patient with profound hypotension that is not easily corrected will be almost certainly be taken to the operating room for reexploration of the mediastinum. If an operating room and personnel are not immediately available, part of the sternal incision may be opened by the surgeon in the ICU to detect and relieve possible tamponade. If hemodynamic compromise is due to cardiac tamponade, evacuating blood from the mediastinum will allow the heart to once again fill adequately. Reopening the chest incision increases the risk of subsequent sternal wound infection, particularly if performed in the ICU and if the patient also requires sternal compressions (during closed-chest massage).

If *cardiac arrest* occurs, the endotracheal tube is disconnected from the ventilator and hand ventilation, using a self-inflating bag and 100% oxygen, is begun. The heart rhythm is assessed, and ventricular pacing is instituted for bradycardia or asystole. Defibrillation is performed for ventricular tachycardia or ventricular fibrillation. Although defibrillation is ineffective in converting asystole, what appears to be asystole on the oscilloscope may in fact be a fine ventricular fibrillation that can be converted. Chest compressions (or open cardiac massage if the sternal incision has been opened) is performed, and advanced life support measures are instituted.

Hypertension commonly develops in the early postoperative hours as a consequence of patient emergence from anesthesia, endotracheal suctioning, resistance to mechanical ventilation, or pain (Whitman, 1991). It can also occur as a paroxysmal event in the absence of any of these factors. Certain types of heart disease, such as coarctation of the aorta or aortic valve disease, are particularly likely to be associated with postoperative hypertension.

Although individual patients may require somewhat higher systemic arterial pressures, a mean arterial pressure of 65 to 75 mm Hg is appropriate in most patients in the early postoperative period. Higher arterial pressure increases myocardial work and oxygen consumption. Postoperative hypertension also exacerbates bleeding and may precipitate suture line disruption or loosening of a surgical clip. Careful monitoring of blood pressure and prompt intervention is an important component of postoperative nursing management. Vasodilating agents, such as sodium nitroprusside or nitroglycerin, are commonly used to treat postoperative hypertension. In patients with acceptable cardiac output, beta-blocking agents, such as labetalol or esmolol, may be used (Hendren & Higgins, 1991). Sedation, with morphine or diazepam, may be administered if patient agitation is contributing to hypertension.

Patients are usually mildly hypothermic during the first few postoperative hours. *Hypothermia* is actively induced during cardiac operations to reduce oxygen consumption and thereby diminish the harmful effects of myocardial ischemia. Intraoperative hypothermia is achieved by three techniques: (1) systemic cooling of the blood as it is circulated through the

CPB tubing, (2) topical bathing of the heart with a chilled saline solution, and (3) perfusion of the coronary arteries with chilled cardioplegic solution. In addition, anesthetic agents inhibit the body's normal temperature regulating mechanisms, allowing the temperature to be environmentally controlled (Phillips & Skov, 1988). Thus, a cool room, administration of room temperature intravenous solutions, unwarmed anesthetic gases, exposure of the mediastinal viscera to room air while the incision is open, and application of cold antimicrobial solutions to the skin all play a passive role in cooling the patient (Whitman, 1991).

Rewarming is performed before terminating CPB by increasing the temperature of the circulating blood volume. However, the presence of excessive peripheral vasoconstriction allows retention of cooled blood in peripheral vessels. As these vessels gradually dilate over the next 45 to 90 minutes, they release cold blood to mix with the warmed central blood, producing a 2°C to 5°C decrease in body temperature, referred to as *afterdrop* (Whitman, 1991). The patient's body temperature gradually returns to normal with vasodilatation and restoration of patient thermoregulation (Fig. 22-3).

During the time that the patient is hypothermic, cardiac arrhythmias are common. Hypothermia decreases myocardial conductivity and predisposes the patient to bradyarrhythmias, which may in turn lead to premature ventricular contractions or ventricular tachycardia (Strong, 1991).

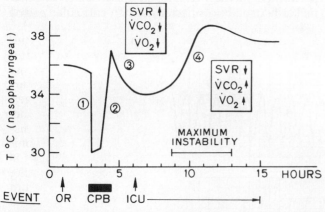

FIGURE 22-3. Nasopharyngeal temperature changes during and after cardiac surgery. *1.* Hypothermia on cardiopulmonary bypass (CPB). *2.* Rewarming on bypass. *3.* Redistribution of heat to the periphery after bypass. *4.* Rewarming after surgery. Systemic vascular resistance (SVR), CO_2 production ($\dot{V}co_2$), and oxygen consumption ($\dot{V}o_2$) vary markedly with temperature changes. A lesser degree of fluctuation is observed in body temperature as measured by thermistors in the bladder or pulmonary artery. (Sladen RN, 1982: Management of the adult cardiac patient in the intensive care unit. In Ream AK, Fogdall RP [eds]: Acute Cardiovascular Management: Anesthesia and Intensive Care, p. 495. Philadelphia, JB Lippincott)

Many patients also experience shivering in response to postoperative hypothermia. Although it is a normal compensatory mechanism to produce heat, it increases the metabolic rate, heart rate, blood pressure, carbon dioxide production, myocardial oxygen demand, and peripheral vasoconstriction (Whitman, 1991). Vasodilating or neuromuscular blocking agents may be administered to eliminate shivering. External measures such as warm blankets or warming devices may be used to facilitate the return to normothermia.

As rewarming and vasodilatation occur in the early postoperative hours, the vascular space increases, with a resultant decrease in preload. Occasionally, rapid fluid infusion may be necessary to restore adequate intravascular volume and correct precipitous hypotension. Volume replacement may be accomplished with crystalloid, colloid, or, in actively bleeding patients, blood component therapy.

Generalized ST segment and T wave changes are common on the postoperative ECG due to operative manipulation of the heart. However, new, localized ST segment elevation, peaked T waves, or Q waves may indicate acute myocardial ischemia or a perioperative myocardial infarction. ECG findings are likely to precede clinical manifestations of ischemia in the sedated patient and should be communicated to the surgeon immediately. In patients who have undergone coronary artery revascularization, ischemia may represent acute graft occlusion or spasm of an internal thoracic artery (also called the internal mammary artery) graft or native coronary artery. Vasodilating agents may be indicated to relieve spasm. Emergent reexploration for examination of graft patency and revision or replacement of jeopardized grafts may be necessary for acute graft closure.

The prevalence of postoperative arrhythmias necessitates familiarity with antiarrhythmic agents, competence in performing the various forms of temporary pacing and defibrillation, and easy access to emergency drugs and equipment. Regardless of the type of arrhythmia, initial nursing interventions consist of prompt assessment of the patient's hemodynamic status, ventricular rate response, and associated signs and symptoms. Possible precipitating factors should be identified with particular attention to hypoxemia, hypokalemia, or proarrhythmic medications, such as digoxin.

Premature ventricular contractions are fairly common. Because the two most likely causes are hypokalemia and hypoxemia, the appearance of ventricular ectopy should prompt measurement of serum potassium and arterial oxygen saturation. Some patients have chronic ventricular ectopy that was well controlled preoperatively with antiarrhythmic medication. Such ectopy can be expected to persist postoperatively, and resumption of the antiarrhythmic agent is usually initiated in the postoperative period. A number of factors are considered in determining the seriousness of new ventricular ectopy. Premature ventricular contractions are of concern if (1) they occur in succession, (2) they have different morphologies (polymorphic), (3) they fall on the T wave of the previous complex, and (4) their frequency is more than six to ten per minute.

Ventricular tachycardia (VT) usually occurs at a rate of 140-220/minute and may be nonsustained or sustained (Moore & Wilkoff, 1991) (Fig. 22-4). Lidocaine is the drug of choice for suppression of VT. An initial intravenous bolus is usually followed by a continuous intravenous infusion. Intravenous procainamide, bretylium, or amiodarone may be used to control VT that is refractory to lidocaine therapy. Temporary pacing is occasionally beneficial if the arrhythmia is precipitated by bradycardia. Defibrillation should be performed at once if hemodynamic compromise or *ventricular fibrillation* (VF) ensues. VF causes immediate cessation of peripheral perfusion and irreversible neurologic injury within minutes (Hillis et al., 1992).

Sustained VT with hemodynamic compromise or VF necessitates initiation of cardiopulmonary resuscitation (CPR) and advanced cardiac life support protocols (Strong, 1991). Defibrillation is the most effective method of treating VF. The likelihood of successful arrhythmia conversion is related to the duration of the arrhythmia (Sanders et al., 1985). Consequently, cardiothoracic surgical nurses are generally trained to promptly defibrillate a patient who develops VF or VT with profound hypotension. CPR is continued until a stable rhythm ensues.

Malignant ventricular arrhythmias are more likely in patients who have a major ventricular wall motion abnormality, severe aortic valve disease, cardiomyopathy, or previous myocardial infarction. Although there are many transient causes of ventricular ectopy

in the early period after cardiac surgery, VT or VF that occurs in high risk patients or without a detectable precipitant warrants further electrophysiologic evaluation to determine if an underlying cardiac rhythm disturbance that requires treatment is present.

In cardiac surgical patients, *wide QRS tachycardias* are most often of ventricular origin. However, aberrantly conducted supraventricular tachycardia (SVT) can also occur. Aberrant complexes are the result of supraventricular impulses that are conducted abnormally through intraventricular pathways, resulting in a wide QRS complex tachycardia that may be difficult to distinguish from VT. Differentiation of the two types of arrhythmias is important. Untreated VT can produce profound hypotension or progress to VF. Conversely, intravenous verapamil, sometimes used to treat supraventricular tachyarrhythmias, may produce hypotension or VF when given to patients with VT (Drew, 1987). Unless aberrancy is confirmed, it is safer to treat the patient as if the arrhythmia is ventricular.

Impaired AV nodal conduction occurs occasionally in patients undergoing valvular surgery and rarely in those undergoing coronary artery revascularization. Usually transient, it may be caused by ischemia, manipulation of cardiac tissue with resultant edema, digoxin toxicity, perioperative myocardial infarction, or mechanical injury to conduction tissue. Temporary pacing is instituted, and medications that slow AV conduction are discontinued. Because of the ease of using pacing wires and the fact that pacing can be performed in the demand mode, an external pacemaker is usually connected to the ventricular pacing

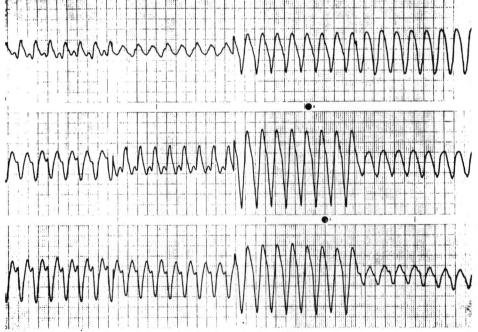

FIGURE 22-4. Ventricular tachycardia in a postoperative patient at a rate of 197 beats per minute. The ventricular origin of this tachyarrhythmia is suggested by concordance of the precordial leads, left axis deviation, and a QRS interval greater than 0.14 second. (Courtesy of Linda Hellstedt, RN, MS)

wire if there is any reason to believe that a patient may develop complete heart block. Pacing thresholds are assessed daily to ensure dependable pacing (Finkelmeier & O'Mara, 1984).

Complete heart block is best treated with AV (dual chamber) sequential pacing, which preserves the atrial contribution to cardiac output. Ventricular pacing is used in patients with atrial fibrillation since atrial capture is not possible. If pacing wires are not present, atropine or isuproterenol should be readily accessible, as well as the necessary equipment to provide for emergency pacing by means of a transvenous or transthoracic pacing system. If a patient is totally reliant on some form of pacing system, an extra pulse generator and cable are placed at the bedside or attached to another set of epicardial wires, if present, to provide backup pacing should the operational pacing system malfunction. If the underlying cardiac rhythm is asystole or profound bradycardia or if external pacing wires are not present, patients remain in an ICU or intermediate care unit for close monitoring until bradycardia is adequately treated.

Supraventricular tachycardia includes atrial tachycardia, atrial flutter, atrial fibrillation, and junctional tachycardia. All are rapid heart rhythms in which the site of impulse formation is above the bifurcation of the bundle of His. These tachyarrhythmias decrease stroke volume by compromising diastolic filling time and thus the effective preload, as well as by decreasing myocardial contractility as a result of altered myocardial oxygen supply and demand (Geha & Whittlesey, 1991).

Atrial flutter and *atrial fibrillation* are particularly common after cardiac surgical procedures, occurring in 20% to 30% of patients. The etiology is not well understood. In some settings, prophylactic digoxin or propranolol is administered during the postoperative period, although their effectiveness in preventing the occurrence of SVT is controversial. Diagnosis of SVT is sometimes difficult because ectopic P waves may be indistinguishable in standard ECG leads used for monitoring. An *atrial electrogram*, obtained using the atrial epicardial wire, can be extremely useful. Atrial electrograms increase the amplitude of atrial activity and diminish that of other electrical components and extracardiac artifact (Finkelmeier & Salinger, 1984).

Treatment of postoperative SVT may consist of oral or intravenous medications, rapid atrial pacing, or cardioversion. In most postoperative patients, SVT produces unpleasant palpitations or sensations but does not significantly affect blood pressure. However, in those with low cardiac output or underlying ventricular impairment, hemodynamic compromise can occur due to loss of effective atrial contraction and the rapid ventricular rate.

The standard therapy for SVT at rates greater than 120 beats per minute is intravenous digitalization, followed by a maintenance regimen of oral digoxin. In most cases, digoxin successfully controls the ventricular rate response and eventually facilitates conversion to normal sinus rhythm. If the patient has already been receiving digoxin, digitalization is not necessary, but rather the drug is administered in doses of 0.125 mg every 1 to 2 hours until the ventricular rate is less than or equal to 100 beats per minute or a total of 1.0 to 1.5 mg has been administered.

Propranolol and verapamil are alternative medications that can be used for treatment of SVT. It is important to note that both of these drugs can produce severe hypotension when administered intravenously, and thus caution must be exercised. If the rhythm is atrial flutter, quinidine may be used to slow the atrial flutter rate. Digoxin is given concomitantly to slow conduction through the AV node and prevent 1:1 AV conduction as the atrial rate slows.

Type I atrial flutter (i.e., with an atrial rate between 240 and 340 beats per minute) can be treated with rapid atrial pacing using the temporary atrial epicardial pacing wires (Waldo, 1989). The procedure, which is relatively painless and easy to perform, is often combined with pharmacologic therapy to prevent recurrence. SVT that produces significant hypotension is treated with prompt cardioversion. Electrical cardioversion may also be considered if SVT persists in a patient who was in normal sinus rhythm preoperatively. The spectrum of cardiac arrhythmias is discussed in depth in Chapter 25, Cardiac Arrhythmias. Temporary pacing techniques and defibrillation are discussed in Chapter 26, Temporary Pacing and Defibrillation.

Electrolyte imbalances may occur during the early postoperative period because of fluid shifts between the vascular space and interstitial tissues and because of manipulation of intravascular volume with intravenous fluids and diuretics. *Hypokalemia* is most common due to the urinary diuresis that commonly follows operations in which CPB is used. Potassium levels are measured every 4 to 8 hours and after the administration of intravenous potassium supplements. Ideally, the serum potassium level is kept between 4.0 and 5.0 mEq/L to avoid ventricular arrhythmias associated with hypokalemia.

Potassium supplementation is generally given concomitantly with diuretic therapy, unless there is a contraindication, such as renal failure. A sliding scale protocol is often developed to guide potassium replacement during the early postoperative period. A central venous catheter must be used for administration of intravenous potassium because of its caustic effect on peripheral veins. A rate-regulating pump is also necessary because rapid infusion of intravenous potassium can produce cardiac asystole.

Maintaining a normal acid–base balance is essential. Fluctuations may occur in arterial pH during the early postoperative hours as a result of any of a number of physiologic factors. Most common is *metabolic alkalosis* that results from extracellular volume and potassium depletion (Smith, 1990). It is corrected with volume and potassium repletion. *Metabolic acidosis* may occur as a result of low cardiac output. The diminished metabolic rate and carbon dioxide production associated with hypothermia may compensate for a moderate degree of metabolic acidosis during the first few postoperative hours (Moreno-Cabral et al., 1988). However, as rewarming occurs, metabolic acidosis may be unmasked.

Serum glucose is almost always elevated owing to the intraoperative administration of large volumes of intravenous solutions that contain glucose and the surgically induced increases in serum catecholamine and cortisol levels (Gray, 1990). Except in patients with diabetes, blood glucose gradually returns to normal levels without treatment. In diabetic patients,

fluctuations in postoperative insulin requirements are common owing to hormonal responses to surgery, immobility, and anorexia. Serial measurements of blood glucose are performed to guide titration of insulin doses until the dosage requirement stabilizes.

CARE ON THE POSTOPERATIVE UNIT

PROGRESSION OF ACTIVITY

Patients who recover in routine fashion are transferred to a general cardiothoracic surgical unit with telemetry monitoring after 24 to 48 hours (Fig. 22-5).

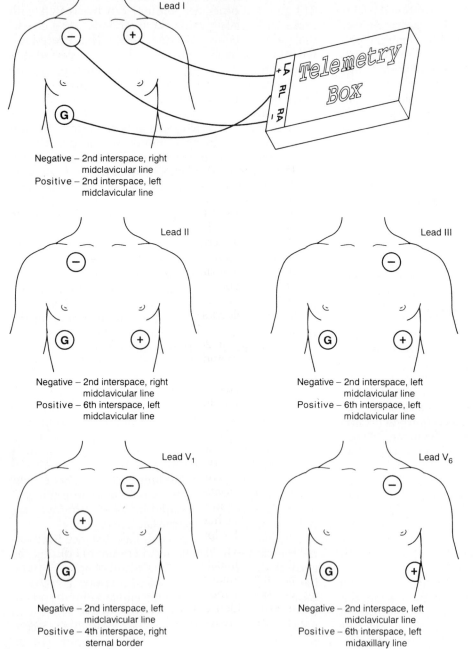

FIGURE 22-5. Telemetry monitoring; various leads may be monitored depending on electrode positions. (Huff J, Doernbach DP, White RD, 1993: Cardiac monitors. In ECG Workout, ed. 2, p 23. Philadelphia, JB Lippincott)

If recovery is routine, almost all invasive catheters will have been removed by this point and the patient can ambulate freely. The plan for progression of activity is based on the patient's age, baseline functional status, degree of ventricular impairment, associated medical problems, type of surgical procedure, and perioperative course. Most patients will be able to walk to the bathroom on the second postoperative day and ambulate in the hallway on the following day. By the time of discharge from the hospital, most patients will be ambulating independently and taking four or five walks in the corridors each day.

Certain groups of patients are much slower in recovering and should not be expected to progress according to the routine regimen. Specifically, the following types of patients require more recovery time and assistance with ambulation: (1) those who undergo a procedure that includes ventriculotomy, such as ventricular aneurysmectomy or endocardial resection; (2) those with end-stage valvular heart disease, (3) those with perioperative myocardial infarction, (4) those with severe ventricular impairment, and (5) those with prolonged preoperative immobility. Elderly patients also progress more slowly and may require more assistance with daily activities.

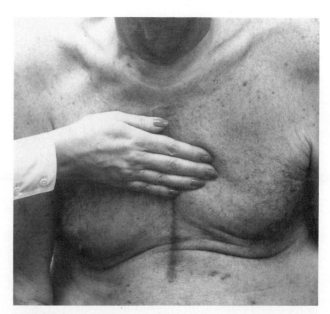

FIGURE 22-6. Sternal stability is assessed by applying firm pressure over the sternal incision while the patient turns his head from side to side or coughs.

PULMONARY HYGIENE

The provision of adequate pulmonary hygiene is one of the most important components of nursing care on the postoperative unit. Postoperative lung function and respiratory mechanics may be substantially impaired by the adverse effects of anesthetic agents, the thoracic incision and surgical manipulation, and CPB (Sivak, 1991). Routine pulmonary hygiene measures include encouraging deep breathing and coughing every hour. Diminished breath sounds, rhonchi, fever, and hypoxemia are signs of atelectasis or retained secretions and indicate the need for more aggressive interventions. Intermittent ultrasonic nebulization administered by face mask helps loosen secretions so that they may be more easily expectorated. Nasotracheal suctioning is occasionally necessary to remove secretions and allow airway expansion if the patient cannot cough effectively. Wheezing is indicative of bronchospasm and may be treated with a bronchodilating agent, such as aminophylline. Bilateral rales suggest pulmonary edema and the need for diuresis.

INCISION CARE

The sternum is palpated daily for stability (Fig. 22-6). Failure of the sternal halves to heal (i.e., *sternal nonunion*) or separation of the sternal halves (i.e., *sternal dehiscence*) is most likely in patients who are obese, diabetic, or receiving corticosteroids or who have had previous sternotomy, postoperative reexploration of the incision, or closed-chest massage. Female patients with large, pendulous breasts are instructed to wear a brassiere except when bathing during the first several weeks to help support the breasts and reduce tension on the sternal incision. Patients who are paraplegic, who have had lower extremity amputations, or who must use crutches will require special nursing and physical therapy assistance to avoid injuring the sternal closure during the early postoperative period. Use of the upper extremities in transferring in and out of bed or for manipulating crutches or an overbed trapeze is avoided since it may lead to sternal dehiscence.

After the first 24 hours, the incision is cleaned daily with soap and water and left uncovered. Close attention is given to the appearance of the sternal incision to detect evidence of infection. Any incisional redness or drainage is reported to the surgeon. Small amounts of serous drainage may occur, usually representing necrosis of subcutaneous fat. Purulent or copious drainage is more ominous.

Leg incisions are cared for in the same manner. As ambulation is increased, patients almost always develop *lower extremity edema* due to disruption of lymphatic channels in the leg or legs from which saphenous veins were harvested. Supportive stockings and elevation of the lower extremities when sitting are prescribed. Leg swelling may persist for several months but almost always resolves. Occasionally, a *seroma*, or cyst-like collection of serous fluid, develops under the skin and drains through the leg incision. If there is no evidence of incisional infection, dry dressings are the only necessary treatment until the drainage abates.

MEDICATIONS

Unless contraindicated by another medical problem, aspirin therapy is initiated in all patients who undergo coronary artery revascularization. Aspirin is generally regarded as the most effective antiplatelet agent for augmenting long-term patency of vein grafts (Goldman et al., 1990). Often aspirin therapy is initiated on the operative day with administration of a rectal suppository. When an oral diet is resumed, one aspirin tablet a day is usually prescribed and continued indefinitely.

Postoperative anticoagulation with warfarin sodium (Coumadin) may be necessary in patients with prosthetic heart valves, chronic atrial fibrillation, or a history of pulmonary embolism. If so, it is generally initiated on the second postoperative day, after chest drainage tubes have been removed. In most patients, anticoagulation is begun with an initial dose of 5 to 10 mg of warfarin. Subsequent doses are determined by daily measurement of prothrombin time (PT). Usually, the PT measurement is obtained in the morning and warfarin is given in the evening because the peak effect of a dose of warfarin is reached 36 to 72 hours after its administration. Serial PT levels and daily warfarin doses are documented and monitored by both physicians and nurses (Table 22-3). Vigilant attention is given to determining the proper dose of warfarin. Before administering warfarin, the most recent PT value is considered. If it is more than 20 seconds, the physician may elect to give no warfarin or only a small dose. Anticoagulant-related hemorrhage can produce catastrophic complications or death.

The international normalized ratio (INR) is gaining recognition in the United States as a more accurate measure of anticoagulation (Vanscoy & Krause, 1991). The INR, a value calculated from the PT assay result, corrects for lack of standardization in the reagent (tissue thromboplastin) used to perform the PT assay. Recommended INR values for the various patient groups receiving warfarin are still being refined. For the present, both PT and INR values are generally taken into consideration.

Certain groups of patients require more cautious anticoagulation. These include small, elderly, or frail individuals; those with long-standing mitral or tricus-

pid valve or liver disease; and those receiving the antiarrhythmic medication amiodarone. A single dose of 10 mg in these patients may produce a PT of 30 seconds or more. If the PT does become dangerously elevated, ambulation is permitted only with direct supervision to prevent potential life-threatening bleeding that could occur with a fall.

Selected patients, particularly those in whom prolonged immobilization is anticipated, may require short-term anticoagulation with intravenous heparin as prophylaxis against *deep venous thrombosis* and *pulmonary embolism*. Patients at greatest risk for postoperative deep venous thrombosis and pulmonary embolism include those requiring prolonged ventilatory or circulatory support; obese, elderly, or debilitated patients; and those who lack lower extremity muscle tone to augment venous return (paraplegic or hemiplegic persons and those with lower extremity amputations).

Specific regimens for postoperative antibiotic prophylaxis vary. Typical is a daily dose of a broad-spectrum cephalosporin (vancomycin for penicillin allergic patients) through the second postoperative day after coronary artery revascularization. If a prosthetic cardiac valve has been implanted, some surgeons continue antibiotic prophylaxis several days longer. However, antibiotic use longer than 48 hours has not been demonstrated to be beneficial and may lead to development of resistant organisms and increased toxicity (Doebbeling et al., 1990).

COMMON PROBLEMS

Low grade fevers are common during the first few postoperative days. The most common etiology is atelectasis. However, sputum, urine, and blood cultures are obtained when a temperature greater than 38.5°C (101.3°F) occurs after the first 48 hours. Wounds are carefully examined for any evidence of infection. Particularly if prosthetic material has been placed in or around the heart, the source of the fever must be promptly identified and treated.

Avoidance of postoperative infection is particularly important in patients who have undergone implantation of prosthetic material, such as a prosthetic cardiac valve, an implantable cardioverter/defibrillator, pacemaker, or vascular graft. In this group of patients, invasive catheters are discontinued as early as possible. If instrumentation such as reinsertion of a urethral catheter is performed in patients with prosthetic heart valves, prophylactic antibiotics are given according to the American Heart Association recommendations (Dajani et al., 1990).

Pain control is rarely a significant problem after cardiac operations performed through a median sternotomy. In contrast to thoracic and abdominal incisions, no muscles need be divided during sternotomy and the divided sternum is secured tightly at the completion of the operation. Although some postoperative chest discomfort is usually present, it is easily con-

TABLE 22-3. EXAMPLE OF REGULATING ANTICOAGULANT THERAPY

Postoperative Day	Prothrombin Time	International Normalized Ratio	Warfarin (Coumadin) Dose
3	11.3	0.9	5.0 mg
4	11.3	0.9	10.0 mg
5	13.6	1.4	5.0 mg
6	18.0	2.5	2.5 mg
7	16.4	2.1	5.0 mg

trolled with analgesic medications and does not generally interfere with patient mobility. However, because all the muscles throughout the chest wall are stretched when the sternal halves are separated, pain in the back, particularly between the shoulder blades and in the neck, is typical. Also, patients who have undergone harvesting of one or both internal thoracic arteries can be expected to experience more anterior chest wall discomfort.

Oral pain medications are generally administered as necessary. Sneezing and coughing are particularly painful because they provoke forceful movement of the chest wall. A pillow may be used to brace the sternum during these times. Heat is often effective in relieving chest wall discomfort; hot showers or a heating pad may provide relief during the latter portion of the hospitalization and the first weeks at home. A heating pad should not be applied directly over the incision.

Disorientation is a common postoperative phenomenon, particularly in elderly patients. Factors thought to contribute include general anesthesia, narcotic analgesics, sleep deprivation, severe preoperative anxiety, use of CPB, and the ICU environment. Alertness to the development of disorientation during the first few postoperative days is important to prevent patient injury. Most commonly, disoriented patients attempt to disconnect attached invasive catheters or tubes or they attempt to get out of bed. If a patient demonstrates any tendency to pull at necessary tubes or catheters, wrist restraints may be necessary. Patients who attempt to climb out of bed or ambulate without adequate assistance may require a sitter in the room, particularly at night. A restraining vest may also be used but may increase the risk of sternal wound disruption caused by the patient straining against the vest. From a legal perspective, nurses are particularly vulnerable if they fail to adequately protect disoriented patients from injury. Other typical problems that affect patients on the postoperative unit are listed in Table 22-4.

PREPARATION FOR DISCHARGE

Most patients are ready for discharge from the hospital by the sixth or seventh postoperative day. Discharge preparation is initiated on the third or fourth postoperative day or as soon as the patient is able to focus on planning for continued recovery at home. Written and oral instructions are given to the patient and family regarding (1) medications, (2) activity, (3) restrictions, (4) diet, and (5) follow-up appointments. Most of the discharge information can be standardized for all types of cardiac surgery. Special attention should be given to those instructions that are specific to a particular patient.

Discharge medications vary depending on the specific operation performed and the patient's underlying cardiac disease. Most patients who undergo coronary artery revascularization procedures are discharged on antiplatelet therapy (aspirin) to enhance graft patency. A coated or buffered aspirin is often better tolerated during the early postoperative period. However, for long-term use, many patients tolerate a less expensive, generic form of aspirin. If the patient has a history of ulcer disease or gastrointestinal bleeding, aspirin therapy may be contraindicated.

Patients who have undergone valve replacement or who have other indications for chronic anticoagulation will be discharged on warfarin sodium. If so, it is imperative that thorough instructions are given to the patient and family. Dosage errors or lack of appropriate monitoring can lead to lethal hemorrhage. Medications and activities that are contraindicated while taking warfarin are reviewed and patients may be encouraged to obtain an identification bracelet, necklace, or wallet card describing anticoagulant use. Written instructions given to the patient and included in the medical record should contain documentation that clearly states (1) current dosage regimen, (2) name of the physician who will monitor PT, and (3) date and place for the next PT measurement. Although warfarin is available in a variety of doses, it is practical to use either 2 or 5 mg tablets. The tablets are scored, and thus can be easily divided. Therefore, a 2-mg tablet allows 1-mg dose modification increments for patients requiring doses in the range of 1 to 5 mg. Similarly, for those patients requiring doses in the range of 2.5 to 12.5 mg, adjusting the dose in increments of 2.5 mg is possible with the 5-mg tablets.

Iron supplementation is generally prescribed in the first few months. Because infectious hazards of homologous blood transfusions have become more apparent, patients are more commonly discharged with a moderate degree of anemia. Unfortunately, iron preparations are often not well tolerated in patients who are already somewhat anorexic and constipated. If the patient cannot tolerate oral iron supplementation, it may take somewhat longer for postoperative anemia to resolve.

Oral pain medications may be prescribed for the first few weeks at home. Pain tolerance is quite variable, and many patients do not desire pain medications, even while in the hospital. Patients can be advised that chest wall discomfort will vary in intensity with level of activities, weather changes, and positioning during sleep. In patients who have had dissection and use of one or both internal thoracic arteries, pain may be more of a problem. In a small number of these patients, chest wall pain and paresthesia may persist for several months.

Most patients are ambulatory and able to perform self-care activities before discharge. The specific regimen for increasing activity at home depends on a number of factors, including general functional status before the operation, underlying cardiac disease, presence of recent myocardial infarction, and perioperative course. Fatigue is common during the first postoperative month. Because it causes patients to be

TABLE 22-4. MISCELLANEOUS POSTOPERATIVE PROBLEMS

Problem	Possible Causes	Treatment
Anorexia	General anesthesia Iron supplementation Pain medications Decreased activity Digoxin toxicity	Liberalization of dietary restrictions Discontinue digoxin
Constipation	General anesthesia Iron supplementation Pain medications Decreased activity	Laxative therapy
Diarrhea	*Clostridium difficile* Impaction Digoxin toxicity Quinidine	Antibiotic therapy Disimpaction Discontinue digoxin Discontinue quinidine
Emotional lability	Hormonal response to surgical stress Impaired physical stamina	Supportive counseling

Fatigue	Effects of general anesthesia and surgical
	    procedure
	Use of caloric intake for wound healing
	Altered sleep patterns
		Scheduled rest periods interspersed with
		    periods of activity

Fever	Atelectasis Postpericardiotomy syndrome Infection	Identify source and treat
Insomnia	Altered sleep patterns Decreased activity	Progressive activity during day Sleep medications
Pleural effusion	Harvesting internal thoracic artery Local hypothermia Postpericardiotomy syndrome	Thoracentesis (if moderate to large)
Postpericardiotomy syndrome	Surgical opening of pericardial sac	Nonsteroidal antiinflammatory agents Steroids (if severe)
Sore throat	Endotracheal intubation	Lozenges, viscous lidocaine
Ulnar paraesthesia	Nerve compression during operation	None—self-limited
Weight loss	Decreased caloric intake	Ensure adequate calories to meet nutritional needs

(Adapted from Manual of Cardiothoracic Nursing, 1984. Chicago, Northwestern Memorial Hospital)

less active during the day, insomnia is an almost universal complaint. The patient should spend most of the day out of bed and incorporate several periods of walking into the daily schedule. Family members are instructed to limit visitors in the early days at home, since this can be quite tiring for the patient.

Discharge instructions include goals to guide progression of activity. Patients are advised to gradually increase daily activities and take rest periods according to level of fatigue. In general, patients can be expected to increase their activities during the first few days at home just by virtue of being in their own surroundings. Walking is the best form of exercise. After the first week at home, the patient should begin to consciously increase the amount of walking each day. If weather is prohibitive, shopping malls provide an excellent area of level surface for walking.

Patients with good ventricular function who undergo coronary artery revascularization are generally walking 4 to 6 miles per day within 6 weeks of the operation. The pace of walking is less important than the amount. Stair climbing may be done, although this is more tiring than walking on level ground, and most patients with stairs at home choose to limit trips up and down to the minimum necessary during the first few weeks. Sexual activity can usually be resumed within several weeks of discharge when the patient is able to ambulate several blocks or flights of stairs without tiring excessively.

Many patients are eager to resume work. If the job is fairly sedentary and the patient can control the amount of hours worked, working on a limited basis can usually be resumed within several weeks of discharge. The patient is cautioned against taking on responsibilities that require undue physical or emotional stamina. Similarly, the patient should avoid social engagements that might prove too tiring. Heavy physical labor should not be resumed for at least 2 to 3 months. Occasionally, cardiac function is compromised to the point that job modification or change may be necessary. The managing cardiologist usually makes this determination.

There are very few activities that are specifically contraindicated during the early period at home. One of these is lifting items that weigh more than 10 pounds. Because the sternum has been surgically divided and the halves resutured together, it must be treated like a broken bone. Although initial healing produces sternal stability within a few weeks, it is 2 to 3 months before the bone regains its full strength. Thus, the sternum should not be subjected to undue stress by using the arms for heavy lifting. Likewise, any exercise or sport that involves vigorous upper extremity motion should be deferred for the same time period. This includes golf, swimming, tennis, using a rowing machine or exercise bicycle with movable handlebars, push-ups, sit-ups, and chin-ups. Additionally, common household activities that stress the sternum, such as manually raising a garage door or shoveling snow, should be avoided during this period.

Most surgeons instruct patients not to drive for at least 1 month after the operation. This prevents patients from attempting to drive when reaction times may still be somewhat slowed by the surgery and postoperative course or by pain medications. In addition, it avoids injury to the healing sternum should an accident occur and result in a forceful blow of the sternum against the steering wheel. It is acceptable for patients to ride in a car and, in most cases, travel by train or airplane.

Instructions are given about any necessary dietary modifications. Patients with coronary artery disease are instructed in low cholesterol diets. If the patient has hypercholesterolemia, more extensive dietary counseling may be necessary, and this is usually prescribed by the managing cardiologist. Modifications in salt intake are often necessary for those patients with valvular heart disease or hypertension.

The cosmetic appearance of the incisions may be a source of great concern, particularly in younger patients. The use of a subcutaneous closure technique has greatly enhanced the appearance of surgical scars. Nevertheless, all scars are somewhat disfiguring. If the patient is concerned, a strip of paper tape may be worn over the incision, except when showering, for several months. The slight pressure of the tape flattens the scar, making it less prominent. Taping the incision is not instituted until the skin edges are healed, approximately 2 weeks after the operation. If infection or skin irritation develops from the tape, its use should be discontinued. Vitamin E or aloe lotion may also be applied to help soften the scar.

The scar will darken in color over the first few months and then eventually fade to approximately the patient's own skin tone. Cosmetic products designed for covering discolored skin are available in major department stores for those few patients in whom the scar remains prominent after several months and is bothersome. In rare cases, keloid scar formation occurs; corticosteroid injections may be considered if the patient is distressed by the scar's appearance.

REFERENCES

Anderson DR, Stephenson LW, Edmunds LH, 1991: Management of complications of cardiopulmonary bypass: Complications of organ systems. In Waldhausen JA, Orringer MB (eds): Complications in Cardiothoracic Surgery. St. Louis, Mosby–Year Book

Behrendt DM, Austen WG, 1985: Complications of other organ systems. In: Patient Care in Cardiac Surgery, ed. 4. Boston, Little, Brown

Bojar RM, 1989: Cardiovascular management. In Manual of Perioperative Care in Cardiac and Thoracic Surgery. Boston, Blackwell Scientific Publications

Bond EF, 1989: Physiology of the heart. In Underhill SL, Woods SL, Froelicher ES, Halpenny CJ (eds): Cardiac Nursing, ed. 2. Philadelphia, JB Lippincott

Coyle JP, 1991: Sedation, pain relief, and neuromuscular blockade in the postoperative cardiac surgical patient. Semin Thorac Cardiovasc Surg 3:81

Dajani AS, Bisno AL, Chung KJ, et al., 1990: Prevention of bacterial endocarditis: Recommendations of the American Heart Association. JAMA 264:2919

DiSesa VJ, 1991: Pharmacologic support for postoperative low cardiac output. Semin Thorac Cardiovasc Surg 3:13

Doebbeling BN, Pfaller MA, Kuhns KR, et al., 1990: Cardiovascular surgery prophylaxis. J Thorac Cardiovasc Surg 99:981

Drew BJ, 1987: Differentiation of wide QRS complex tachycardias. Prog Cardiovasc Nurs 2:130

Finkelmeier BA, O'Mara SR, 1984: Temporary pacing in the cardiac surgical patient. Crit Care Nurse 4:108

Finkelmeier BA, Salinger MH, 1984: The atrial electrogram: Its diagnostic use following cardiac surgery. Crit Care Nurse 4:42

Finkelmeier BA, Salinger MH, 1986: Dual-chamber cardiac pacing: An overview. Crit Care Nurse 6:12

Geha AS, Whittlesey D, 1991: Postoperative low cardiac output. In Baue AE, Geha AS, Hammond GL, et al. (eds): Glenn's Thoracic and Cardiovascular Surgery, ed 5. Norwalk, CT, Appleton & Lange

Goldman S, Copeland J, Moritz T, et al., 1990: Internal mammary artery and saphenous vein graft patency. Circulation 82 (Suppl IV):IV-237

Gray RJ, 1990: Normal convalescence. In Gray RJ, Matloff JM (eds): Medical Management of the Cardiac Surgical Patient. Baltimore, Williams & Wilkins

Greco SA, 1990: Vasoactive drugs. In Underhill SL, Woods SL, Froelicher ES, Halpenny CJ (eds): Cardiovascular Medications for Cardiac Nursing. Philadelphia, JB Lippincott

Halfman-Franey M, Berg DE, 1991: Recognition and management of bleeding following cardiac surgery. Crit Care Nurs Clin North Am 3:675

Hendren WG, Higgins TL, 1991: Immediate postoperative care of the cardiac surgical patient. Semin Thorac Cardiovasc Surg 3:3

Hillis LD, Lange RA, Wells PJ, Winniford MD, 1992: Ventricular tachycardia and ventricular fibrillation. In Manual of Clinical Problems in Cardiology, ed. 4. Boston, Little, Brown

Hudak CM, Gallo BM, Benz JJ, 1990a: Heart failure. In Critical Care Nursing: A Holistic Approach, ed. 5. Philadelphia, JB Lippincott

Hudak CM, Gallo BM, Benz JJ, 1990b: Cardiac surgery and heart transplantation. In Critical Care Nursing: A Holistic Approach, ed. 5. Philadelphia, JB Lippincott

Karp RB, Kouchoukas NT, 1991: Postoperative care of the cardiovascular surgical patient. In Baue AE, Geha AS, Hammond GL, et al. (eds): Glenn's Thoracic and Cardiovascular Surgery, ed. 5. Norwalk, CT, Appleton & Lange

Kelleher RM, Rose AA, Ordway L, 1991: Prostaglandins for the control of pulmonary hypertension in the postoperative cardiac surgery patient: Nursing implications. Crit Care Nurs Clin North Am 3:741

Lee RE, Ramos R, 1990: Nursing care of the cardiac surgical patient. In Gray RJ, Matloff JM (eds): Medical Management of the Cardiac Surgical Patient. Baltimore, Williams & Wilkins

Mahfood SS, Higgins TL, Loop FD, 1991: Management of complications related to coronary artery bypass surgery. In Waldhausen JA, Orringer MB (eds): Complications in Cardiothoracic Surgery. St. Louis, Mosby–Year Book

Moore SL, Wilkoff BL, 1991: Rhythm disturbances after cardiac surgery. Semin Thorac Cardiovasc Surg 3:24

Moran JM, Singh AK, 1989: Cardiogenic shock. In Grillo HC, Austen WG, Wilkins EW Jr, et al. (eds): Current Therapy in Cardiothoracic Surgery. Toronto, BC Decker

Moreno-Cabral CE, Mitchell RS, Miller DC, 1988: Perioperative care. In Manual of Postoperative Management of Adult Cardiac Surgery. Baltimore, Williams & Wilkins

Phillips R, Skov P, 1988: Rewarming and cardiac surgery: A review. Heart Lung 17:511

Sanders AB, Kern KB Atlas M, et al., 1985: Importance of the duration of inadequate coronary perfusion pressure on resuscitation from cardiac arrest. J Am Coll Cardiol 6:113

Scott WJ, Kessler R, Wernly JA, 1990: Blood conservation in cardiac surgery. Ann Thorac Surg 50:843

Sivak ED, 1991: Management of ventilator dependency following heart surgery. Semin Thorac Cardiovasc Surg 3:53

Smith PK, 1990: Postoperative care in cardiac surgery. In Sabiston DC Jr, Spencer FC (eds): Surgery of the Chest, ed. 5. Philadelphia, WB Saunders

Strong AG, 1991: Nursing management of postoperative dysrhythmias. Crit Care Clin North Am 3:709

Valta P, Takala J, Elissa T, Milic-Emili J, 1992: Effects of PEEP on respiratory mechanics after open heart surgery. Chest 102:227

Vanscoy GJ, Krause JR, 1991: Warfarin and the international normalized ratio: Reducing interlaboratory effects. DICP Ann Pharmacother 25:1190

Waldo AL, 1989: Arrhythmias following open heart surgery: Role of cardiac pacing and recording. In Grillo HC, Austen WG, Wilkins EW Jr, et al. (eds): Current Therapy in Cardiothoracic Surgery. Toronto, BC Decker

Whitman GR, 1991: Hypertension and hypothermia in the acute postoperative period. Crit Care Nurs Clin North Am 3:661

CHAPTER 23

HEMODYNAMIC MONITORING

ARTERIAL PRESSURE	PRINCIPLES OF MONITORING
INTRACARDIAC PRESSURES AND INDICES	ASSOCIATED COMPLICATIONS
Pulmonary Artery Pressures	
Left Atrial Pressure	
Right Atrial Pressure	
Calculated Indices	

Hemodynamic monitoring is an essential component of caring for postoperative or critically ill cardiac surgical patients. Cardiac function in these patients is often abnormal because of underlying ventricular impairment, acute dysfunction secondary to the operative procedure and use of cardiopulmonary bypass, or a combination of the two. The word "hemodynamic" literally means "blood power." Hemodynamic monitoring describes the observation and recording of the forces generated within the vasculature that are associated with the movement of blood. By using invasive vascular catheters and sophisticated electronic equipment, quantitative data are obtained that can be used to detect correctable abnormalities and guide therapeutic interventions.

Hemodynamic monitoring is almost always performed using intravascular catheters, pressure transducers, and an amplifier/monitoring system. Fluid pressure at the catheter tip is transmitted by the fluid column inside the catheter to an external transducer (Grossman, 1992). The pressure is exerted on a diaphragm within the transducer causing the diaphragm to be displaced a small amount depending on the size of the force. Most commonly used medical transducers are "strain gauge" transducers. When the diaphragm is displaced, it causes corresponding changes in the resistance of an electronic circuit within the transducer. These resistance changes cause an electric current to vary in exactly the same pattern as the patient's pressure. The varying electric current is used as the input signal to the monitoring system that amplifies it to a readable level. Both a digital numeric value and a graphic representation of the pressure waveform are usually displayed.

Pressures commonly measured in cardiac surgical patients include arterial pressure, central venous pressure, and pulmonary artery pressure. Cardiac output is also routinely measured, and a cardiac index (CI) may be derived by adjusting cardiac output for an individual patient's body surface area. Cardiac output is used to calculate systemic vascular resistance (SVR) using a simple formula known as Ohm's law (i.e., flow = pressure/resistance). In selected patients with complex cardiac pathology, other parameters may also be useful, such as monitoring of left atrial pressure or mixed venous oxygen saturation (Svo_2) and calculation of pulmonary vascular resistance (PVR), stroke volume index (SVI), or stroke work index (SWI).

ARTERIAL PRESSURE

Arterial pressure monitoring is essential in postoperative cardiac surgical patients. It allows continuous display of systolic, diastolic, and mean arterial pressures as well as vascular access for obtaining arterial blood samples for frequent blood gas analysis. Arterial pressure is an important indicator of systemic perfusion, particularly that to the heart, brain, kid-

Betsy Finkelmeier: CARDIOTHORACIC SURGICAL NURSING.
© 1995 J.B. Lippincott Company.

TABLE 23-1. CALCULATED HEMODYNAMIC INDICES

Index	Formula	Normal Values
MAP	DP + [(SP − DP) ÷ 3]	70–105 mm Hg
CI	CO ÷ BSA	2.5–3.5 L/min/m²
SVR	[(MAP − RAP) ÷ CO] × 80	800–1200 dynes · sec · cm⁻⁵
PVR	[(PAPm − PCWP) ÷ CO] × 80	100–250 dynes · sec · cm⁻⁵
SVI	[CI ÷ Heart rate] × 1000	35–45 mL/beat/m²
LVSWI	SVI × (MAP − PCWP) × 0.136	40–75 g/m²/beat

MAP, mean arterial pressure; DP, diastolic pressure; SP, systolic pressure, CI, cardiac index; CO, cardiac output; BSA, body surface area; SVR, systemic vascular resistance; RAP, right atrial pressure; PVR, pulmonary vascular resistance; PAPm, mean pulmonary artery pressure; PCWP, pulmonary capillary wedge pressure; SVI, stroke volume index; LVSWI, left ventricular stroke work index.

neys, and other vital organs. *Systolic blood pressure* (normal range, 100 to 140 mm Hg) represents the maximal pressure with which blood is ejected from the left ventricle. *Diastolic pressure* (normal range, 60 to 90 mm Hg) reflects the elasticity of arterial walls and the rapidity of blood flow. *Mean blood pressure* (normal range, 70 to 105 mm Hg) is the average of systolic and diastolic pressure with respect to time. Because the factor of time is involved, mean blood pressure is approximately equal to the diastolic pressure plus one third of the difference between systolic and diastolic pressures (Table 23-1).

All three values (systolic, diastolic, mean) are used to assess adequacy of systemic perfusion. The same mean blood pressure can represent a wide (high systolic, low diastolic) or narrow (low systolic, high diastolic) pulse pressure; the latter is more desirable because systolic work is less and diastolic coronary perfusion is enhanced (Daily, 1989). Also, arterial pressure alone does not adequately reflect cardiac function. Because of the relationships expressed by Ohm's law, arterial pressure may remain in a normal range despite a low cardiac output if SVR is elevated. Consequently, arterial pressure must be evaluated in concert with cardiac output and SVR. In addition to monitored arterial pressure, noninvasive indicators of systemic perfusion include quality of peripheral pulses, color and temperature of the extremities, level of mentation, and adequacy of urine output.

The graphic representation of the arterial pressure provides additional information (Fig. 23-1). The highest point is read as systolic pressure, the lowest as diastolic. The waveform changes in morphology as it moves from the aortic root to the periphery; in peripheral arteries, systolic pressure is higher, diastolic and mean pressures are lower, and the waveform has increased amplitude (Lake, 1990). The arterial pressure waveform in a peripheral artery should have a sharp, rapid upstroke with a clear dicrotic notch and a definite end of diastole. An arterial pressure waveform with a slow upstroke and prolonged peak can represent partial occlusion of the catheter, aortic ste-

nosis, or decreased stroke volume. An abrupt upstroke with a brief peak and rapid fall may be caused by anxiety, fever, anemia, vasodilation, or aortic regurgitation. Ventricular bigeminy produces an irregular waveform rate and pulse waves of alternating amplitude.

In the early hours after cardiac operations, a mean arterial pressure in the range of 65 to 75 mm Hg is desirable in most patients (Moreno-Cabral et al., 1988). Mean pressure may be maintained at a somewhat higher level in older patients because cerebral vascular disease is more prevalent (Hendren & Higgins, 1991). A mean arterial pressure less than 60 mm

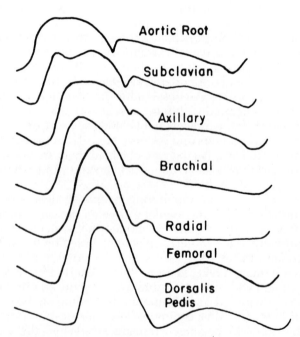

FIGURE 23-1. The arterial pulse waveform changes in morphology as it moves from the central circulation to the periphery. (Bedford RF, 1990: Invasive blood pressure monitoring. In Blitt CD [ed]: Monitoring in Anesthesia and Critical Care Medicine, ed. 2, p. 102. New York, Churchill Livingstone)

Hg indicates inadequate tissue perfusion. It is generally treated with volume replacement if the patient is hypovolemic or with inotropic pharmacologic agents. Conversely, excessive arterial pressure in the postoperative period exacerbates bleeding and increases myocardial oxygen consumption. Pharmacologic vasodilation or sedation is used to maintain mean arterial pressure less than 90 to 100 mm Hg.

The *radial artery* is the first choice for arterial monitoring. It is easy to cannulate and amenable to hemostatic control, and collateral circulation to the hand is generally good. Before insertion of a radial artery catheter, an Allen test is performed to evaluate adequacy of ulnar arterial circulation. The *brachial artery* is used infrequently if radial artery cannulation is not possible. It is a large vessel that is easy to catheterize and amenable to hemostatic control but collateral blood supply to the hand is lacking. A brachial arterial catheter also limits the patient's movement of the elbow. The *femoral artery* is sometimes used for intraoperative monitoring but is not desirable for long-term use because insidious bleeding is more likely (particularly in obese patients), patient mobility is limited, and the catheter's location in the groin makes infection secondary to contamination likely. The *pedal artery* is also used rarely. Although collateral circulation to the foot is adequate, pedal pressure does not as accurately reflect core blood pressure.

INTRACARDIAC PRESSURES AND INDICES

Intracardiac pressures are measured to provide an estimation of preload, which along with afterload, heart rate, and contractility is a major determinant of cardiac output. *Preload* is the end-diastolic volume in the ventricle and provides an estimation of diastolic fiber length (Smith, 1990). As represented by *Starling's law*, as end-diastolic volume increases, cardiac output also increases until a point is reached at which further filling causes a decrease in cardiac output and congestive heart failure. Because there is no method for clinical measurement of intracardiac volumes, fluid pressure is monitored instead. Therefore, preload is clinically defined as the pressure in the ventricle just before systole or *ventricular end-diastolic pressure*.

Insertion of a catheter into the left ventricle for direct measurement of left ventricular end-diastolic pressure is not feasible. Instead, diastolic pressure in the pulmonary artery or, occasionally, left atrial pressure, is measured to provide an indirect method of estimating the *left ventricular end-diastolic pressure* (LVEDP). Similarly, right atrial pressure provides an estimation of *right ventricular end-diastolic pressure* (RVEDP), or right ventricular preload. These indirect measurements are possible because of relationships that exist between intracardiac pressures in the normal heart. Interpretation of measured parameters requires an understanding of these relationships.

Figure 23-2 displays normal intracardiac pressures. Note that pressures in the atria are the same as diastolic pressures in the ventricles. This is because the open position of the atrioventricular (tricuspid and mitral) valves during ventricular diastole allows equilibration of atrial and ventricular pressures. Similarly, when semilunar (pulmonic and aortic) valves are open during ventricular systole, the right and left ventricular systolic pressures in the normal heart are the same as the systolic pressures in the pulmonary artery and aorta, respectively. Finally, because there are no valves in the pulmonary capillaries and veins, pulmonary artery diastolic pressure provides a reasonable measure of left atrial pressure, which in turn approximates LVEDP.

In patients without cardiac pathology, right atrial pressure can also provide an estimate of LVEDP. However, in the presence of dysfunction of one of the ventricles or pulmonary vascular pathology, pressure measurements obtained from the right side of the heart do not accurately reflect left-sided pressures. Patients who undergo cardiac surgery typically have pathology that primarily affects left ventricular function, such as coronary artery disease or valvular heart disease. The left ventricular dysfunction commonly present precludes reliance on right atrial pressure monitoring to promptly detect changes in left ventricular function. Intraoperative and postoperative monitoring of left ventricular preload is essential because of wide fluctuations that can occur and the impact they have on cardiac output.

PULMONARY ARTERY PRESSURE

A pulmonary artery (Swan-Ganz) catheter is almost always used in cardiac surgical patients to continuously monitor left ventricular preload. Most commonly used is a triple-lumen catheter that allows simultaneous recording of right atrial and pulmonary artery pressure (Fig. 23-3A). The catheter also incorporates a thermistor for measuring cardiac output using a thermodilution technique (Becker, 1989a). The proximal lumen of the catheter communicates with a port positioned to lie in the right atrium; the distal lumen communicates with a port in the pulmonary artery and the balloon inflation lumen leads to a balloon positioned just proximal to the distal port. A separate lumen contains wires leading to a thermistor, positioned near the distal end of the catheter so that it lies in the pulmonary artery. Some catheters incorporate an additional proximal lumen, called the venous infusion port, that allows infusion of fluid or medications without interruption of right atrial and pulmonary artery pressure monitoring (Gardner & Woods, 1989) (see Fig. 23-3B). Pulmonary artery catheters may also provide means for temporary cardiac pacing. One model of pulmonary artery catheter has a right ventricular port to allow insertion of a wire for temporary transvenous pacing of the heart. Another model has atrial and ventricular pacing electrodes at-

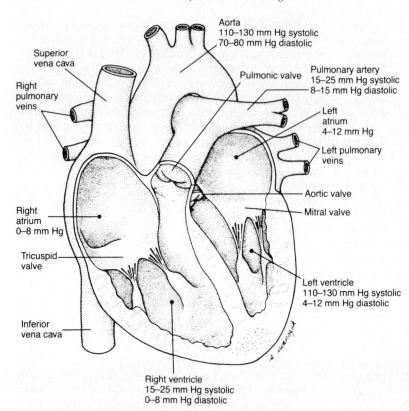

FIGURE 23-2. A schematic representation of the heart displaying normal pressures in the cardiac chambers and great vessels. (Darovic GO, 1987: Cardiovascular anatomy and physiology. In Hemodynamic Monitoring: Invasive and Noninvasive Clinical Application, p. 38. Philadelphia, WB Saunders)

tached to the catheter itself. The newest addition to the arsenal of pulmonary artery catheters is a model that provides continuous cardiac output readings without using thermodilution.

A pulmonary artery catheter is generally inserted percutaneously through the subclavian or jugular vein. Before insertion, the catheter is threaded through a sterile plastic sleeve. The balloon is then inflated to test its integrity and to ensure that it extends beyond the catheter tip when inflated. The proximal and distal ports of the catheter are flushed with heparinized saline solution. A large-bore catheter (8 to 9 F), commonly referred to as an introducer, is usually placed in the vein initially and the balloon-

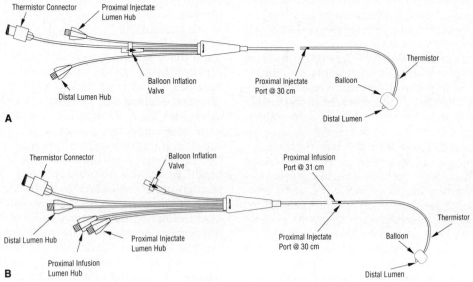

FIGURE 23-3. (A) Standard pulmonary artery catheter. **(B)** Pulmonary artery catheter with proximal venous infusion lumen. (Courtesy of Baxter Healthcare, Edwards Critical-Care Division, Santa Ana, CA)

tipped, flow-directed catheter is passed through the introducer into the vein. The external end of the distal lumen is attached to a transducer so that the pressure waveform can be used to guide catheter advancement.

Waveforms transmitted from the right atrium, right ventricle, pulmonary artery, and pulmonary artery when occluded each have characteristic features that identify location of the catheter tip (Fig. 23-4). When a right atrial pressure waveform demonstrates that the distal lumen has reached the right atrium, the balloon on the distal end of the catheter is inflated. The balloon, typically inflated with 1.5 mL of air, serves two purposes: (1) it acts as a cushion so that the catheter tip is less likely to puncture any vessels and (2) it facilitates advancement of the catheter tip in the proper direction. Acting similarly to a sail on a boat, the inflated balloon is easily caught up in the flow of blood, hence the term *flow-directed* catheter.

The catheter is advanced across the tricuspid valve into the right ventricle and across the pulmonic valve into the pulmonary artery. Passage of the catheter through the heart is monitored by changes in the waveform tracing. As the catheter moves through the right ventricle, transient, clinically insignificant ventricular arrhythmias almost always occur. Right bundle branch block occurs rarely.

When the balloon enters a branch of the left or right pulmonary artery, the vessel diameter narrows enough for the balloon to occlude the artery lumen, or "wedge," represented by a change in the pressure tracing from the characteristic pulmonary artery tracing to a flattened wedge tracing. The balloon is then deflated, and the sterile sleeve is extended distally and attached to the external hub of the introducer. The introducer is secured at the skin with a suture to prevent migration. Proper positioning of the pulmonary artery catheter is assessed by a chest roentgenogram and by the shape of the pressure waveform at the catheter tip. If the catheter tip has been advanced too far, the catheter, with the balloon deflated, is withdrawn a few centimeters at a time until proper positioning is verified. While the catheter is in place, pulmonary artery systolic, diastolic, and mean pressures are continuously displayed and pulmonary capillary wedge pressure may be obtained. Using measured intracardiac and arterial pressures and thermodilution cardiac output determinations, other parameters can be calculated, including SVR, PVR, SVI, and SWI (see Table 23-1).

Pulmonary artery diastolic pressure (PADP), an indirect measurement of LVEDP, is most often used to assess preload and guide clinical therapy. PADP in a normal heart is 8 to 15 mm Hg. However, patients with cardiac disease often require a PADP of 15 to 20 mm Hg to sustain an adequate cardiac output. Optimal preload varies among individual patients. During cardiac operations, the surgeon has the opportunity to assess cardiac function in relation to various levels of preload while the patient is weaned from cardiopulmonary bypass (CPB). Before terminating CPB, venous return to the extracorporeal circuit is partially occluded, allowing some volume to enter and be ejected by the heart. The degree of cannula occlusion therefore controls the patient's preload. Ventricular contractility is directly observed, and the surgeon evaluates the level of preload that provides optimal

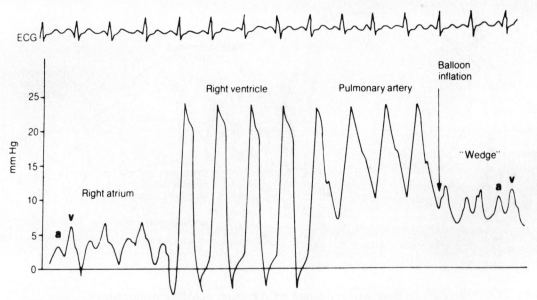

FIGURE 23-4. Characteristic waveforms transmitted from a balloon-tipped pulmonary artery catheter in the right atrium, the right ventricle, the pulmonary artery, and the occluded pulmonary artery, respectively. (Matthay MA, 1983: Invasive hemodynamic monitoring in critically ill patients. Clin Chest Med 4:234)

myocardial contractility. As cardiac function improves, the level of preload necessary for adequate cardiac output and blood pressure can be expected to gradually decrease from that necessary at the termination of CPB.

During the early postoperative hours, a decreased PADP may represent intravascular hypovolemia due to a number of physiologic sequelae of operations that necessitate CPB, including (1) active bleeding, (2) vasodilation, (3) osmotic diuresis, and (4) "third spacing" of fluid. Elevated PADP may represent transient myocardial dysfunction (i.e., low cardiac output syndrome) or overzealous fluid replacement.

In most instances, PADP provides a sufficient indication of LVEDP. However, measurement of *pulmonary capillary wedge pressure* (PCWP) is important in selected situations. PCWP measures pressure beyond the balloon tip, that is, that transmitted from the left atrium into the pulmonary veins and capillaries (Fig. 23-5). It is obtained by inflating the balloon with a small volume (1 to 1.5 mL) of air so that the tip of the catheter is no longer exposed to pressure transmitted from the proximal pulmonary artery. Balloon inflation creates a static column of blood from the catheter tip through the pulmonary veins to the left atrium (Rutledge et al., 1989).

PCWP is therefore a truer representation of mean left atrial pressure and LVEDP than is PADP. Conditions that increase PVR, such as cor pulmonale, pulmonary embolus, and pulmonary fibrosis, alter the correlation between PADP and PCWP, resulting in a PADP that exceeds PCWP (Becker, 1989b). Therefore, it may be preferable to intermittently measure PCWP in the presence of elevated PVR. Because serial balloon inflations can cause pulmonary artery rupture, inflation is maintained only long enough to read the pressure displayed in the mean mode. A characteristic pulmonary artery waveform should reappear as soon as the balloon is deflated.

LEFT ATRIAL PRESSURE

Left atrial pressure (LAP) is the most accurate clinical indicator of LVEDP. Monitoring of LAP is accomplished using a catheter inserted directly into the left atrium during a cardiac operation, passed through the chest wall, and connected to a pressurized fluid administration system (Fig. 23-6). The left atrial pressure waveform comprises three components: (1) the *a wave*, representing atrial contraction, (2) the *c wave*, representing pressure against the closed mitral valve during ventricular systole, and (3) the *v wave*, representing filling of the atrium during late ventricular systole. Because catastrophic consequences can occur if air enters the systemic circulation through the catheter, left atrial catheters are generally placed only when PADP or PCWP is not a reliable indicator of LAP (and indirectly of LVEDP). A left atrial catheter is not used for fluid or medication administration, and precautions are taken to prevent accidental air entry into the systemic circulation.

RIGHT ATRIAL PRESSURE

Right atrial pressure (RAP) or *central venous pressure* (CVP) *monitoring* is used to assess adequacy of venous return, intravascular blood volume, and right ventricular function (Schwenzer, 1990). It is an indi-

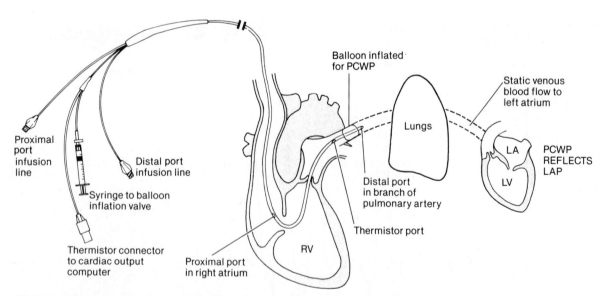

FIGURE 23-5. Pulmonary capillary wedge pressure (PCWP) is measured by momentarily inflating the balloon on the distal end of the pulmonary artery catheter. Balloon inflation creates a static column of blood between the catheter tip and left atrium, thus providing a more accurate representation of left atrial pressure (LAP). (Adapted from Kersten LD, 1989: Hemodynamic monitoring—respiratory applications. In Comprehensive Respiratory Nursing: A Decision Making Approach, p. 758. Philadelphia, WB Saunders)

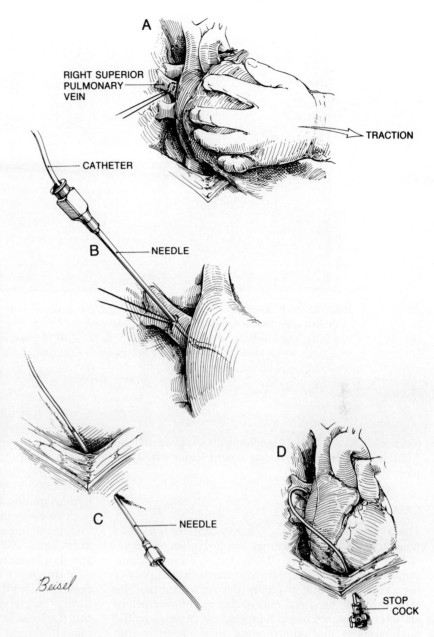

FIGURE 23-6. Intraoperative insertion of a left atrial catheter. **(A)** The right atrium is retracted to the left side by an assistant to expose the right pulmonary vein. **(B)** A pursestring suture is placed at the junction of the vein and the left atrium. A 17-gauge epidural needle with a catheter within is inserted through the pursestring and into the left atrium. The catheter is advanced approximately 5 cm into the left atrium and the needle is carefully withdrawn, leaving the catheter in place. The pursestring suture is tied. **(C)** A separate, longer needle is passed from the skin into the pericardial space. The free end of the left atrial catheter is passed through this needle to the outside of the chest wall. **(D)** The proper length of the catheter is ascertained, and the external end of the catheter is severed and attached to a stopcock. The stopcock is sutured to the skin. (Waldhausen JA, 1985: Pump oxygenators, techniques of cardiopulmonary bypass. In Johnson's Surgery of the Chest, ed. 5, p. 257. Chicago, Year Book Medical Publishers)

rect measure of left ventricular preload in patients in whom right ventricular function, PVR, and the mitral valve are normal (Friedman & Bernstein, 1990). Continuous monitoring of RAP may be performed using the proximal port of the pulmonary artery catheter. If a pulmonary artery catheter is not in place, monitoring is accomplished using a catheter placed through the subclavian or jugular vein. Central venous pressure can be accurately measured if the catheter tip is in the right atrium or any large intrathoracic vein (Varon & Civetta, 1990). In addition to pressure measurements, the catheter can be used for rapid volume infusion or continuous infusion of cardiotonic or vasoactive pharmacologic medications.

RAP monitoring is almost always performed using a transducer rather than the formerly common water

manometer method. In addition to providing a more accurate measurement of mean CVP, pressures obtained with a transducer allow continuous monitoring and analysis of the actual waveform (Daily & Schroeder, 1989a). A normal right atrial waveform is similar in morphology to the left atrial waveform (Fig. 23-7).

Low RAP in conjunction with low PADP usually indicates hypovolemia or dilatation of venous capacitance vessels and the need for volume replacement. High RAP with low PADP suggests right-sided heart failure or elevated PVR. If both RAP and PADP are increased, biventricular failure may be present. Pharmacologic pulmonary artery vasodilation with nitroglycerin, isoproterenol, or prostaglandin E_1 may be instituted to decrease PVR (i.e., right ventricular af-

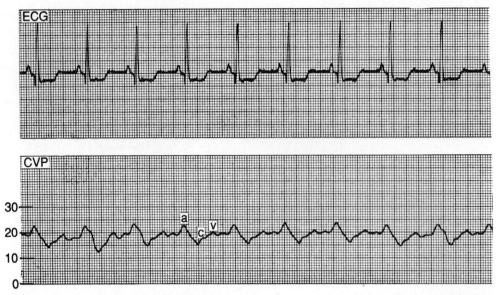

FIGURE 23-7. Right atrial waveform with a, c, and v waves present. The a wave is usually seen just after the P wave of the ECG. The c wave appears at the time of the RST junction on the ECG. The v wave is seen in the TP interval. (Kern LS, 1993: Hemodynamic monitoring. In Boggs RL, Woolridge-King M [eds]: AACN Procedure Manual for Critical Care, ed. 3, p. 304. Philadelphia, WB Saunders)

terload). Occasionally, mechanical support of the right side of the heart, using a ventricular assist device, is necessary.

CALCULATED INDICES

The triple-lumen pulmonary artery catheter is used to measure *cardiac output* using a *thermodilution technique.* A known quantity of cold solution at a known temperature is injected rapidly into the proximal port of the catheter so that it enters the right atrium. The thermistor at the distal end of the pulmonary artery catheter measures blood temperature changes as the cold bolus is ejected from the right ventricle into the pulmonary artery and past the tip of the catheter. The faster the decay of the cold bolus measured by the thermistor, the greater the cardiac output (Elefteriades & Geha, 1985). A computer is used to analyze the temperature changes, known as a thermodilution curve, and calculate cardiac output, expressed as liters per minute. Usually three measurements are obtained in succession and averaged to compensate for sampling error. Measurement of cardiac output using a thermodilution technique is based on the assumption that cardiac output from the right and left sides of the heart are the same. The measured cardiac output divided by the patient's body surface area to correct for body size is termed *cardiac index.*

Cardiac output is the most important hemodynamic parameter in the early period after cardiac operations (Karp & Kouchoukas, 1991). Low cardiac output (<2.0 L/min/m²) may result from hypovolemia or transient myocardial dysfunction. It is corrected by manipulation of those factors that determine cardiac output (i.e., heart rate, preload, afterload [SVR], and contractility). A high cardiac output may represent a hyperdynamic state or sepsis.

Systemic vascular resistance, or *left ventricular afterload,* is the impedance against which the left ventricle must eject. Although SVR cannot be directly measured, it is calculated by a formula in which the pressure difference between the proximal (mean arterial pressure) and distal (right atrial pressure) ends of the cardiovascular system is divided by the cardiac output (Daily & Schroeder, 1989b). The result is multiplied by 80 and expressed in absolute resistance units (dyne · sec · cm⁻⁵). SVR is often elevated in the early postoperative hours secondary to peripheral vasoconstriction and hypothermia. SVR decreases as body temperature returns to normal, sometimes causing precipitous hypotension as it does. SVR may be pharmacologically lowered to reduce left ventricular work. Most commonly, vasodilating agents, such as sodium nitroprusside or nitroglycerin, are used. Intra-aortic balloon counterpulsation is quite effective in providing mechanical afterload reduction. Occasionally, SVR is abnormally low owing to residual effects of anesthetic agents or an allergic reaction to protamine sulfate given to reverse the effects of intraoperative systemic anticoagulation. A low SVR may also occur due to sepsis. Under these circumstances, an alpha-adrenergic agent may be administered to cause vasoconstriction and restore normal SVR.

Because right ventricular dysfunction is relatively uncommon, *PVR*, or *right ventricular afterload*, is not routinely calculated. However, calculation of PVR is important in patients with postoperative right ventricular failure or pulmonary hypertension. It is derived in a similar manner to SVR. The pressure difference between mean pulmonary artery pressure and PCWP is divided by cardiac output, then multiplied by 80.

Mixed venous oxygen saturation (Svo$_2$) may be determined by sampling blood from the distal port of the pulmonary artery catheter while the balloon is deflated. The blood sample must be aspirated slowly and gently to avoid obtaining oxygenated blood from the pulmonary circulation. Pulmonary artery blood is used to measure Svo$_2$ because venous blood returning from various parts of the body has become mixed. In contrast, right atrial blood contains streams of highly desaturated blood entering from the coronary sinus as well as less desaturated blood returning from the superior and inferior vena cavae. Svo$_2$ provides an estimation of systemic perfusion and is helpful in determining the need for inotropic therapy if measurement of cardiac output by thermodilution is unreliable (DiSesa, 1991). Abnormally low Svo$_2$ in the presence of normal arterial Po$_2$ indicates maximal oxygen extraction and a low cardiac output. Pulmonary artery catheters that incorporate a fiberoptic channel for continuous monitoring of mixed venous oxygen saturation are sometimes used.

Stroke volume is the amount of blood ejected by the ventricle with each heartbeat. It is derived by dividing cardiac output by heart rate. When normalized for body surface area, it is termed *stroke volume index*. *Stroke work index* (i.e., stroke work corrected for body surface area) reflects contractility, or the inotropic state of the myocardium, specifically the velocity of fiber shortening during systole (Daily & Schroeder, 1989c). A low stroke work index may indicate the need for inotropic therapy. The formula for calculating left ventricular SWI is displayed in Table 23-1.

PRINCIPLES OF MONITORING

Hemodynamic monitoring is accomplished by attaching an appropriate intravascular catheter to an amplifier/monitor using special connecting tubing, a transducer, and a connecting cable (Fig. 23-8). The connecting tubing, also called *pressure tubing,* is stiff, noncompliant, and relatively short (Lee & Ramos, 1990). These characteristics are necessary to prevent distortion or reduced amplitude of transmitted fluid pressures. The pressure tubing also contains stopcocks for zeroing of the transducer and aspiration of blood samples as well as a device for manually flushing the catheter. Locking connectors are used to prevent tubing disconnection, and lower limit alarms may be adjusted to signal a decrease in pressure if disconnection occurs.

A *pressurized flush solution* is connected to the tubing circuit by means of a continuous, slow flush device that delivers 3 to 5 mL/h of heparinized solution and prevents backflow of blood through the catheter (Fig. 23-9). A dextrose flush solution may be used for pulmonary artery or left atrial catheters, but normal saline is used for arterial catheters because it is less injurious to the artery than dextrose. Heparin is added to the flush solution to prevent thrombus formation around the catheter tip.

The transducer is maintained at the level of the patient's *phlebostatic axis* (i.e., an imaginary point that intersects the fourth intercostal space and the midaxillary line) (Fig. 23-10). Pressure readings obtained with the transducer higher or lower than the phlebostatic reference point will be falsely low or high, respectively. *Zeroing* of the pressure monitoring system consists of confirming that the monitor records a pressure of 0 mm Hg when the transducer is at the phlebostatic axis and is open to the atmosphere. It is performed two to three times daily and whenever there is a question about accuracy of measurements. Most monitoring systems use disposable transducers and provide *internal calibration*. When the calibration control is activated, an electrical signal is introduced to the monitor as if calibration pressure had been applied to the transducer itself (Varon & Civetta, 1990).

Before obtaining pressure measurements, quality of the waveform is assessed and position of the transducer is verified. Accuracy of abnormal pressure measurements should be confirmed before any treatment is initiated. *Damping,* or poor transmission of a pressure waveform, can occur as a result of air bubbles, blood clots, loose fittings, catheter kinking, or positioning of a catheter tip against a vessel wall (Summer & deBoisblanc, 1991). Aspiration and manual flushing may be necessary to evacuate air bubbles or thrombus from the catheter lumen. Catheter kinking may be corrected by splinting the extremity in which the catheter is inserted or by manipulating the catheter position.

Pulmonary artery pressure varies normally with respiration. In spontaneously breathing patients, pressure decreases slightly during inspiration. Conversely, it increases during inspiration in patients receiving positive pressure mechanical ventilation. Therefore, measurements are performed consistently on or off the ventilator and at the same point in the respiratory cycle, typically at end-expiration. High levels of positive end-expiratory pressure (PEEP) artificially elevate pulmonary artery pressure readings because pressure is transmitted to the pulmonary artery catheter. Physiologically, PEEP lowers preload because the increased intrathoracic pressure decreases venous return to the heart. Pulmonary artery pressure is infrequently distorted by *catheter whip artifact,* caused by excessive catheter movement with right ventricular contractions. If this occurs, mean pulmonary artery pressure may provide a more accurate assessment of preload.

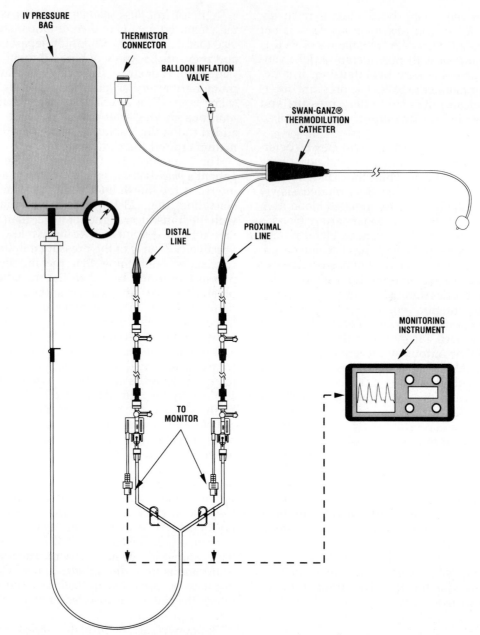

FIGURE 23-8. Diagrammatic representation of monitoring system. In this example two pressure transducers and a pulmonary artery catheter are used to monitor pulmonary artery and right atrial pressures. (Courtesy of Baxter Healthcare, Edwards Critical-Care Division, Santa Ana, CA)

Inflation of the balloon when the pulmonary catheter is incorrectly positioned can cause serious complications. The balloon is always inflated slowly, while monitoring the pulmonary artery waveform for the change from a pulmonary artery pressure to a wedge pressure. If the catheter tip has migrated a short distance distally, only a small amount of air is necessary to cause wedging; inflating the balloon with the usual 1.5 mL increases the risk of pulmonary artery damage or rupture. Consequently, air is injected into the balloon only until a wedge tracing appears. Once the PCWP has been obtained, the balloon is deflated. *Sustained balloon inflation* or *catheter tip migration* that causes pulmonary artery occlusion is detected by the presence of a PCWP waveform. It may be corrected by (1) ensuring full balloon deflation, (2) asking the patient to take deep breaths and cough, (3) repositioning the patient, or (4) withdrawing the catheter a slight distance until a pulmonary artery waveform reappears. *Balloon rupture* may be detected by a loss of

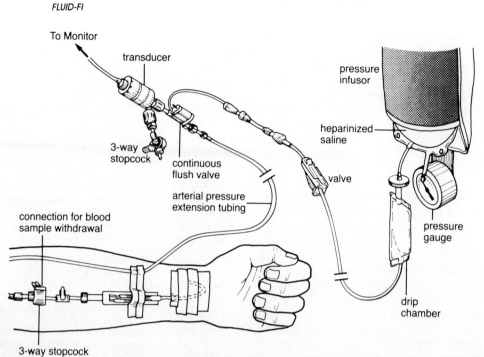

FLUID-FI

To Monitor

transducer

3-way stopcock

continuous flush valve

arterial pressure extension tubing

connection for blood sample withdrawal

3-way stopcock

pressure infusor

heparinized saline

valve

pressure gauge

drip chamber

FIGURE 23-9. A pressurized flush system delivers 3 to 5 mL per hour of heparinized saline through the arterial catheter. The slow infusion prevents backflow of blood into the extension tubing and thrombus formation around the catheter tip. (VanRiper J, VanRiper S, 1987: Fluid-filled monitoring systems. In Darovic GO [ed]: Hemodynamic Monitoring: Invasive and Noninvasive Clinical Application, p. 86. Philadelphia, WB Saunders]

resistance when air is injected in the balloon lumen, by an inability to pull back the syringe plunger when attempting to deflate the balloon, or by an inability to obtain a PCWP waveform. Balloon rupture does not necessitate catheter removal as long as the balloon lumen port is covered and labeled clearly to prevent subsequent attempts to inflate the balloon.

Movement of the tip of a pulmonary artery catheter into the right ventricle is evidenced by a right ventricular pressure waveform. The catheter may be advanced if a sterile sleeve was placed over the catheter before its insertion. Repositioning of an intravascular catheter should be performed only by those experienced in catheter insertion techniques. In the

absence of a protective sheath, the nonsterile catheter is not advanced because it predisposes to catheter-related infection. Instead, if the patient's condition mandates continued pulmonary artery pressure measurements, the catheter is completely removed and replaced with a sterile catheter.

The insertion site of an intravascular catheter is covered with an occlusive, sterile dressing, and aseptic dressing changes are performed daily. Catheter sites should not be covered with large, bulky dressings that might obscure catheter disconnection or insidious bleeding. Flush solutions and tubing are changed according to institutional standards (e.g., flush solution every 24 hours, tubing every 48 hours) to minimize the risk of infection.

Intravascular monitoring catheters are generally removed 24 to 48 hours after cardiac operations. Pulmonary artery and left atrial catheters are usually removed by physicians. Before removing a pulmonary artery catheter, balloon deflation is confirmed. Because removal of left atrial catheters can cause bleeding, a chest tube is often left in place until the catheter has been removed. Removal of any catheter inserted through a central vein is performed with the patient in a supine position in the bed. The head of the bed is lowered and pressure is maintained over the insertion site as the catheter is withdrawn to prevent air embolism. Firm pressure is applied to the skin overlying the vessel puncture site for approximately 5 minutes. Pressure is applied for longer periods in anticoagulated patients, when removing a femoral artery catheter, or if bleeding from the puncture site does not subside.

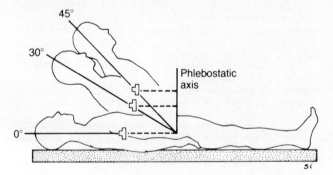

45°

30°

0°

Phlebostatic axis

FIGURE 23-10. When the level of head elevation is changed, the position of the transducer dome is adjusted to maintain the air–fluid interface at the level of the phlebostatic axis. (Darovic GO, 1987: Pulmonary artery pressure monitoring. In Hemodynamic Monitoring: Invasive and Noninvasive Clinical Application, p. 161. Philadelphia, WB Saunders)

ASSOCIATED COMPLICATIONS

Arterial pressure monitoring is almost always performed using the radial artery and complications are rare. While the catheter is in place, the hand distal to the catheter is assessed for evidence of ischemia or emboli. Loss of arterial waveform or an inability to flush the catheter suggests thrombus formation along the catheter and should prompt catheter removal unless the problem is easily corrected (Finkelmeier & Finkelmeier, 1991). Complications associated with insertion of central venous catheters through the subclavian or jugular vein include pneumothorax, hemothorax or hematoma, arterial cannulation, and vessel injury. Disconnection of an indwelling arterial or central venous catheter can result in significant blood loss if not detected promptly. Air embolism can occur with central venous catheter disconnection.

Pulmonary artery catheters are associated with a number of potential complications. The presence of an indwelling catheter in the right ventricle may cause persistent ventricular arrhythmias that necessitate catheter removal. Serial balloon inflation can cause complications, particularly in patients with pulmonary hypertension. Overinflation may cause pulmonary artery rupture, prolonged inflation may cause pulmonary infarction, and injection of air into a ruptured balloon may produce air embolization (Hudak et al., 1990). Occasionally, pulmonary artery rupture occurs even without inflating the balloon, during catheter insertion or migration. Pulmonary artery catheters can also cause tricuspid or pulmonic valve damage and endocarditis (Summer & deBoisblanc, 1991).

Infection is a potential complication with any invasive catheter. Factors that influence the risk of catheter-related infection include insertion technique, length of time the catheter is place, the type of solution infused through the catheter, age of the patient, and the underlying disease process (Yanelli & Gurevich, 1988). Redness or purulent drainage at the catheter insertion site, or unexplained fever and white blood cell count elevation are suggestive of catheter-related infection. If any of these occur, the catheter is removed, its tip is cultured for bacteria, and, if necessary, a new catheter is inserted.

REFERENCES

Becker A, 1989a: Pulmonary artery catheterization: I. Insertion techniques and guidelines for use. In Rippe JM (ed): Manual of Intensive Care Medicine, ed. 2. Boston, Little, Brown

Becker A, 1989b: Pulmonary artery catheterization: II. Interpretation of hemodynamic data. In Rippe JM (ed): Manual of Intensive Care Medicine, ed. 2. Boston, Little, Brown

Daily PO, 1989: Hemodynamic monitoring of the postoperative cardiac surgery patient. In Dailey EK, Schroeder JS (eds): Techniques in Bedside Hemodynamic Monitoring, ed. 4. St. Louis, CV Mosby

Daily EK, Schroeder JS, 1989a: Central venous and pulmonary artery pressure monitoring. In Dailey EK, Schroeder JS (eds): Techniques in Bedside Hemodynamic Monitoring, ed. 4. St. Louis, CV Mosby

Daily EK, Schroeder JS, 1989b: Intra-arterial pressure monitoring. In Dailey EK, Schroeder JS (eds): Techniques in Bedside Hemodynamic Monitoring, ed. 4. St. Louis, CV Mosby

Daily EK, Schroeder JS, 1989c: Clinical management based on hemodynamic parameters. In Dailey EK, Schroeder JS (eds): Techniques in Bedside Hemodynamic Monitoring, ed. 4. St. Louis, CV Mosby

DiSesa VJ, 1991: Pharmacologic support for postoperative low cardiac output. Semin Thorac Cardiovasc Surg 3:13

Elefteriades JA, Geha AS, 1985: Hemodynamic monitoring and the Swan-Ganz catheter. In House Officer Guide to ICU Care: The Cardiothoracic Surgical Patient. Rockville, MD, Aspen Systems

Finkelmeier BA, Finkelmeier WR, 1991: Iatrogenic arterial injuries resulting from invasive procedures. J Vasc Nurs 9:12

Friedman A, Bernstein H, 1990: Hemodynamic monitoring during and after cardiac surgery. In Gray RJ, Matloff JM (eds): Medical Management of the Cardiac Surgical Patient. Baltimore, Williams & Wilkins

Gardner PE, Woods SL, 1989: Hemodynamic monitoring. In Underhill SL, Woods SL, Froelicher ES, Halpenny CJ (eds): Cardiac Nursing, ed. 2. Philadelphia, JB Lippincott

Grossman W, 1992: Cardiac catheterization. In Braunwald E (ed): Heart Disease: A Textbook of Cardiovascular Medicine, ed. 4. Philadelphia, WB Saunders

Hendren WG, Higgins TL, 1991: Immediate postoperative care of the cardiac surgical patient. Semin Thorac Cardiovasc Surg 3:3

Hudak CM, Gallo BM, Benz JJ, 1990: Hemodynamic pressure monitoring. In Critical Care Nursing: A Holistic Approach, ed. 5. Philadelphia, JB Lippincott

Karp RB, Kouchoukas NT, 1991: Postoperative care of the cardiovascular surgical patient. In Baue AE, Geha AS, Hammond GL, et al. (eds): Glenn's Thoracic and Cardiovascular Surgery, ed. 5. Norwalk, CT, Appleton & Lange

Lake CL, 1990: Monitoring of arterial pressure. In Lake CL (ed): Clinical Monitoring. Philadelphia, WB Saunders

Lee RE, Ramos R, 1990: Nursing care of the cardiac surgical patient. In Gray RJ, Matloff JM (eds): Medical Management of the Cardiac Surgical Patient. Baltimore, Williams & Wilkins

Moreno-Cabral CE, Mitchell RS, Miller DC, 1988: Perioperative care. In Manual of Postoperative Management of Adult Cardiac Surgery. Baltimore, Williams & Wilkins

Rutledge FS, Sharpe M, Sibbald WJ, 1989: Cardiovascular monitoring in the critically ill. In Henning RJ, Grenvik A (eds): Critical Care Cardiology. New York, Churchill Livingstone

Schwenzer KJ, 1990: Venous and pulmonary pressures. In Lake CL (ed): Clinical Monitoring. Philadelphia, WB Saunders

Smith PK, 1990: Postoperative care in cardiac surgery. In Sabiston DC Jr, Spencer FC (eds): Surgery of the Chest, ed. 5. Philadelphia, WB Saunders

Summer WR, deBoisblanc BP, 1991: Bedside hemodynamic monitoring. In Parrillo JE (ed): Current Therapy in Critical Care Medicine, ed. 2. Philadelphia, BC Decker

Varon AJ, Civetta JM, 1990: Hemodynamic monitoring. In Berk JL, Sampliner JE (eds): Handbook of Critical Care, ed. 3. Boston, Little, Brown

Yannelli B, Gurevich I, 1988: Infection control in critical care. Heart Lung 17:596

CHAPTER 24

TWELVE-LEAD ELECTROCARDIOGRAPHY AND ATRIAL ELECTROGRAMS

ELECTRICAL COMPONENTS OF THE CARDIAC
    CYCLE
ELECTROCARDIOGRAPHIC LEADS
ELECTRICAL AXIS

ELECTROCARDIOGRAPHIC ABNORMALITIES
    Myocardial Ischemia and Infarction
    Chamber Enlargement
    Bundle Branch Block
ATRIAL ELECTROGRAMS

The *electrocardiogram* (ECG) is a graphic summary of the electrical events that make up each cardiac cycle. The six major deflections (P, Q, R, S, T, U) of the normal ECG represent the movement of charged particles across myocardial cell membranes (i.e., depolarization and repolarization) (Erickson, 1991). Energy created by these electrical events is detected by electrodes on the body surface, transmitted to the electrocardiograph, amplified, and recorded in graphic form.

Electrocardiographs are standardized so that both amplitude and duration of the various deflections making up the cardiac cycle can be measured. Graph paper divided in 1-mm segments is used; every fifth segment, or 5.0 mm, is designated by a darker line. Graph paper is advanced through the machine at a speed of 25 mm per second. Thus, the space between two vertical lines (1.0 mm) represents 0.04 second and that between two darkened vertical lines (5.0 mm) represents 0.2 second. Small vertical lines or dots above the graph are spaced to mark 3-second intervals.

Voltage is similarly standardized so that 1.0 mV of electrical current produces a vertical deflection of 10 mm on the graph paper. If a deflection has both upward and downward components of approximately equal amplitude, it is termed *biphasic*. The isoelectric line between cardiac cycles is termed the *baseline*. Deflections above the baseline are considered positive, and those below the baseline are negative.

The most apparent information revealed on an ECG is cardiac rate and rhythm. Heart rate is described in beats per minute and can be quickly estimated in one of two ways: (1) the number of QRS complexes occurring during 6 seconds (two 3-second intervals measured by the vertical lines or dots above the graph) is multiplied by 10, or (2) the number of seconds in 1 minute (60) is divided by the number of seconds between two consecutive R waves (Table 24-1). Cardiac rhythm is determined using standard criteria for rhythm analysis, described in Chapter 25, Cardiac Arrhythmias.

ELECTRICAL COMPONENTS OF THE CARDIAC CYCLE

Each component of the cardiac cycle can be separately analyzed (Fig. 24-1). The morphology and duration of the various electrical components reveal important diagnostic information about conduction through the heart and cardiac pathology. The first deflection of

TABLE 24-1. ESTIMATION OF HEART RATE*

Number of Boxes† Between R Waves		Heart Rate
One (0.2 second)	= 60/.20 =	300
Two (0.4 second)	= 60/.40 =	150
Three (0.6 second)	= 60/.60 =	100
Four (0.8 second)	= 60/.80 =	75
Five (1.0 second)	= 60/1.0 =	60
Six (1.2 second)	= 60/1.2 =	50

* Obtained by dividing the number of seconds between two consecutive QRS complexes into the number of seconds in 1 minute.

† Large boxes separated by darkened vertical lines on electrocardiograph paper.

the cardiac cycle, the P wave, represents atrial depolarization. A normal P wave has a duration less than 0.12 second (3.0 mm) and voltage less than 0.2 mV (2.0 mm) (Fisch, 1992). Atrial depolarization is followed by an isoelectric line representing a physiologic conduction delay in the atrioventricular (AV) node. Atrial repolarization is not apparent on the ECG because it is masked by other events. The PR interval is measured from the onset of the P wave to the initial (positive or negative) deflection of the QRS complex. It represents intra-atrial, AV nodal, and Purkinje conduction and normally lasts 0.12 to 0.20 second.

The QRS complex represents depolarization of ventricular tissue. It is measured from onset of the first positive or negative deflection of the QRS waveform to termination of the waveform. The normal QRS interval is 0.04 to 0.10 second. Normal voltage of the QRS complex varies depending on the lead. It should be at least 6.0 mm in V_1 and V_6, 8.0 mm in V_2 and V_5, and 10 mm in V_3 and V_4; voltage should not exceed 25 to 30 mm (Conover, 1992a). Morphology of the ventricular depolarization wave varies depending

on the lead in which it is viewed. Although the term *QRS* is commonly used to describe ventricular depolarization on single-lead rhythm tracings, more precise terminology is required when multiple electrocardiographic leads are being analyzed. The standard nomenclature and definitions for the various deflections that make up ventricular depolarization are as follows:

Q wave: First negative deflection, if it is the initial event and is followed by a positive deflection

R wave: First positive deflection

S wave: First negative deflection that follows an R wave

R' wave: Second positive deflection

S' wave: Second negative deflection that follows an R' wave

QS wave: Entirely negative deflection

Thus, Q and S always describe negative deflections and R always describes a positive deflection. The relative size of Q, R, and S deflections is indicated by using a lower case or upper case letter (Fig. 24-2).

Ventricular repolarization is represented by the ST segment and the T wave. The ST segment is the interval between termination of the QRS complex and onset of the T wave. It may be isoelectric or drift slightly (1–2 mm) above the baseline; it does not normally drift more than 0.5 mm below the baseline (Conover, 1992a). The T wave, representing the end of ventricular repolarization, is a gently sloping, asymmetric deflection with usually the same polarity as the QRS complex. In some leads, a low-voltage positive deflection, called the U wave, may be apparent after the T wave. Its cause and clinical significance are not well understood.

The QT interval defines the period from the beginning of ventricular depolarization (onset of QRS complex) to the end of ventricular repolarization (termination of T wave). It coincides with ventricular systole. Normal length of the QT interval varies in-

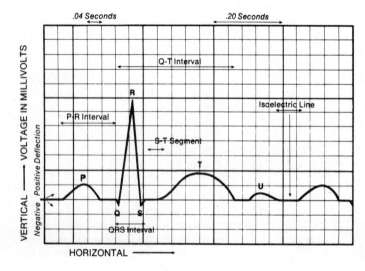

FIGURE 24-1. Electrical components of the cardiac cycle. (Hudak CM, Gallo BM, Benz JJ, 1990: Assessment: Cardiovascular system. In Critical Care Nursing, ed. 5, p. 94. Philadelphia, JB Lippincott)

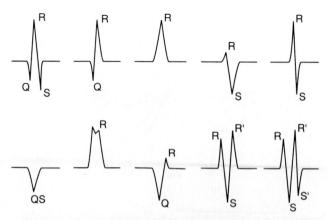

FIGURE 24-2. Diagrammatic representation of QRS variations (see text). (Huff J, Doernbach DP, White RD, 1993: Waveforms, intervals, segments, and complexes. In ECG Workout, ed. 2, p. 13. Philadelphia, JB Lippincott)

versely with heart rate. A general guideline is that at normal heart rates (between 60 and 100 beats per minute) the QT interval should be no longer than one half of the RR interval. When the heart rate is 70 beats per minute, normal QT interval length is 0.40 second (Goldberger, 1990). Measurement of the QT interval is clinically significant because abnormal prolongation is known to provide the substrate for potentially dangerous ventricular arrhythmias.

ELECTROCARDIOGRAPHIC LEADS

An electrocardiographic lead comprises two electrodes of opposite polarity, or one positive electrode and a reference point (Conover, 1992b). Each lead reflects the direction and magnitude of current flow from a particular perspective. Because the heart is three dimensional, electrical current spreads in all directions. The more points from which this electrical energy is measured, the more accurate the depiction of conduction through atrial and ventricular muscle. The standard electrocardiograph examines electrical events of the cardiac cycle from 12 different leads. Surface electrodes are placed on each of the four limbs and on six standard reference points on the chest. The right leg electrode serves only as a ground. The six frontal leads provide information about left, right, superior, and inferior current flow; the six precordial leads assess anterior, posterior, right, and left current flow (Conover, 1992c).

The right arm, left arm, and left leg electrodes are used to obtain the six *limb* or *frontal leads* (I, II, III, aVR, aVL, aVF). The first three limb leads, I, II, and III, are bipolar. That is, each of these leads measures differences in polarity between two skin electrodes, with one acting as the negative and one as the positive pole. Lead I measures electrical polarity between the right (negative pole) and left (positive pole) arms,

lead II between the right arm (negative pole) and left leg (positive pole), and lead III between the left arm (negative pole) and left leg (positive pole).

An imaginary line between the two poles of a particular lead is termed the *axis* of that lead. The axes of the three bipolar limb leads form *Einthoven's triangle. Einthoven's law* describes the relationship between the three bipolar leads: the complex in lead II is always equal to the sum of the complexes in leads I and III (Conover, 1992b). Leads aVR, aVL, and aVF are unipolar leads. They measure polarity differences between the electrical center of the heart and three reference points on the body surface: the right arm, left arm, and left leg, which serve as the positive poles for aVR, aVL, and aVF, respectively. The three unipolar leads are each perpendicular to one of the three bipolar leads.

The *chest,* or *precordial, leads* (V$_1$, V$_2$, V$_3$, V$_4$, V$_5$, and V$_6$) display electrical activity in a horizontal plane. The precordial leads are unipolar, comparing polarity between the electrical center of the heart and six points that act as positive poles on the anterior and left lateral chest wall. Electrodes for V$_1$ and V$_2$ are placed at the fourth intercostal space, just to the right and left sides of the sternum, respectively. The V$_4$, V$_5$, and V$_6$ electrodes are positioned at the fifth intercostal space, on the midclavicular, anterior axillary, and midaxillary lines, respectively. The V$_3$ electrode is positioned equidistant between V$_2$ and V$_4$ (Fig. 24-3). Proper placement of precordial electrodes is essential for accurate interpretation of the ECG. Deviation of as little as 1.5 cm from the standard positions can produce significant variations in measurements of electrocardiographic parameters (Hill & Goodman, 1987).

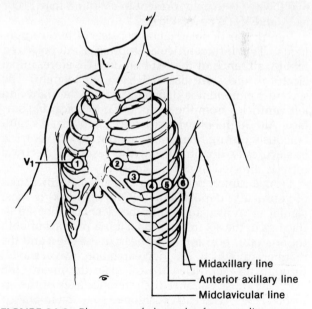

FIGURE 24-3. Placement of electrodes for recording precordial leads. (Hudak CM, Gallo BM, Benz JJ, 1990: Intra-aortic balloon pump counterpulsation. In Critical Care Nursing, ed. 5, p. 106. Philadelphia, JB Lippincott)

ELECTRICAL AXIS

The depolarization of cardiac cells produces electrical currents that flow from depolarized to polarized tissue. These currents can be represented by vectors, which have magnitude and direction. The magnitude is represented by the length of the vector arrow and the direction by the arrowhead. When analyzing a particular lead of the ECG, one must keep in mind the axis and location of the positive pole for that lead. A positive deflection represents a depolarization wave parallel to the axis of the lead and directed toward the positive pole of the lead. Similarly, a negative deflection represents electrical activity parallel to the axis and directed away from the positive pole. Biphasic deflections or an isoelectric line indicates electrical activity directed perpendicular to the axis of the lead. If the mean direction of current flow falls between being parallel and perpendicular to the axis of the lead, the complex will be predominantly positive or negative depending on whether the bulk of electrical energy is directed toward or away from the positive pole of the lead.

Electrical axis describes the mean direction of electrical current or force through the atria (P wave axis) and ventricles (QRS axis). Although electrical current flows in a multitude of directions, cardiac depolarization basically occurs from the base to the apex of the heart and in a leftward direction. Atrial depolarization normally originates in the sinus node, located high in the right atrial myocardium, near the orifice of the superior vena cava. Accordingly, sinus node discharge depolarizes atrial cells in a right to left and inferior direction. Therefore, the P wave is usually upright in leads I, II, aVF, and V_3 through V_6; a negative P wave is usually present in aVR and may occur in V_1 and V_2 (Woods, 1989).

Ventricular depolarization consists of two components. The intraventricular septum is depolarized first by a branch of the left bundle. Therefore, initial electrical forces are directed from left to right. The second component is depolarization of the right and left ventricles from the endocardial to epicardial surface. Although both ventricles are depolarized simultaneously during this phase, the thicker left ventricle is electrically dominant and the resultant electrical force is directed from right to left.

From a clinical perspective, the mean electrical axis of ventricular depolarization (QRS complex) is most significant. Calculated from the electrocardiographic tracings in the six frontal leads, it is a product of both the anatomic position of the heart in the chest and the manner in which the depolarization wave travels through the ventricles. To calculate the mean QRS axis, one must visualize the reference axes of the six frontal leads, with each positioned so that it intersects the electrical center of the heart, as shown in Figure 24-4. Beginning with the positive pole of lead I, each of the negative and positive poles of the six leads is labeled using numerical degrees to represent its posi-

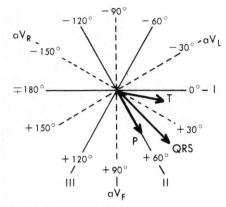

FIGURE 24-4. The hexaxial reference system divides the frontal plane into 30° intervals. All degrees in the upper hemisphere are labeled as negative degrees, and all degrees in the lower hemisphere are labeled as positive degrees. The P vector normally lies along the +60° axis, the mean QRS vector between 0° and +90°, and the mean T vector between −10° and +75°. (Zipes DP, Andreoli KG, 1991: Introduction to electrocardiography. In Kinney MR, Packa DR, Andreoli KG, Zipes DP [eds]: Comprehensive Cardiac Care, ed. 7, p. 83. St. Louis, Mosby–Year Book)

tion. Lead I is used as a starting point and is labeled 0°; positive degrees are assigned to the points moving clockwise and negative degrees to those moving counterclockwise.

Mean QRS axis may be estimated by identifying two factors: (1) the lead with a biphasic QRS complex and (2) the lead with the R wave of tallest amplitude. Mean axis is perpendicular to the lead with the biphasic complex and at the pole with the tallest R wave. The normal adult QRS axis ranges from −30° to +110°. Axes outside this range may represent cardiac pathology. If the axis falls between +110° and +180°, *right axis deviation* is present; an axis of −30° to −90° constitutes *left axis deviation;* an axis of −90° to −180° is considered either extreme right or extreme left axis deviation. An *indeterminate axis* is present when all the QRS complexes in the frontal leads are biphasic.

Right axis deviation may occur normally or as a result of pulmonary disease, right ventricular hypertrophy, lateral wall myocardial infarction, or left posterior hemiblock (Goldberger, 1990). An axis between +90° and +110° is considered borderline right axis deviation and may be due to a vertically positioned heart, particularly in a tall, thin individual. Left axis deviation may represent a normal variant, left anterior hemiblock, an inferior wall myocardial infarction, left ventricular hypertrophy, or left bundle branch block. Borderline left axis deviation (axis between 0° and −30°) may occur secondary to a horizontally positioned heart, as would occur during pregnancy or in the presence of ascites.

The precordial leads are not used to calculate the mean electrical axis of the heart, but they provide important information about ventricular depolariza-

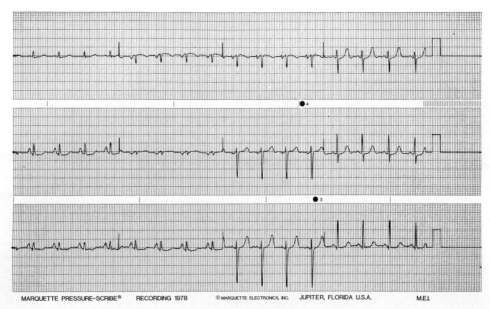

MARQUETTE PRESSURE-SCRIBE®   RECORDING 1978   © MARQUETTE ELECTRONICS, INC.   JUPITER, FLORIDA U.S.A.   M.E.I.

FIGURE 24-5. Precordial leads (V_1–V_6 in this 12-lead ECG demonstrate normal R wave progression. (Courtesy of Richard Davison, M.D.)

tion in the horizontal plane. Normally, the initial septal depolarization, which occurs from left to right, produces a small positive deflection (r wave) in the right leads (V_1, V_2) and a small negative deflection (q wave) in V_6. Septal depolarization is perpendicular to the other precordial leads. The leftward and posterior forces of left ventricular depolarization dominate the remainder of current flow through the ventricles. Thus, negative deflections (S waves) occur in the leads to the right of the left ventricle and positive deflections (R waves) in those to the left. *R wave progression* describes the normal increase in R wave amplitude as the electrocardiographic lead is changed from V_1 through V_5 or V_6 (Fig. 24-5). The R wave is tallest in the lead that is parallel to the mean direction of electrical force.

ELECTROCARDIOGRAPHIC ABNORMALITIES

MYOCARDIAL ISCHEMIA AND INFARCTION

The 12-lead ECG is one of the principal methods used to diagnose myocardial ischemia and infarction. ST segment depression and T wave inversion represent myocardial ischemia. Injured myocardium is evidenced by ST segment and T wave elevation in leads over the affected tissue. Abnormal Q waves appear in leads facing infarcted myocardium because necrotic tissue no longer depolarizes. Although small Q waves representing septal depolarization occur normally in a number of leads, new or large (>0.04 second in duration and >25% of R wave amplitude) Q waves are abnormal and represent transmural myocardial infarction. Q waves do not develop unless a myocardial infarction is transmural (i.e., full thickness). Subendocardial, or nontransmural, myo-

cardial infarction produces only ST segment elevation or depression and T wave inversion.

Changes in specific electrocardiographic leads identify the affected area and, to some extent, the degree of damage to myocardial tissue. Most myocardial infarctions involve the left ventricle. The presence of abnormal Q waves, ST segment elevation, and T wave inversion in leads I, aVL, and V_1 through V_6 represents transmural infarction of the anterior portion of the left ventricle (Fig. 24-6). V_1 through V_3 reveal anteroseptal changes; V_3 through V_4, localized anterior changes; and V_5 through V_6, aVL, and I, anterolateral changes. Inferior wall infarction is revealed by characteristic electrocardiographic changes in leads II, III, and aVF (Hanisch, 1991).

None of the standard surface electrocardiographic leads directly reflect changes in the posterior wall. Instead, posterior infarction is indicated by reciprocal changes in leads opposite the posterior wall (i.e., V_1, V_2, and V_3) (Sweetwood, 1989). In contrast to Q waves, inverted T waves, and ST segment elevation, reciprocal changes include tall R waves; tall, upright T waves; and ST segment depression in these right chest leads. The standard 12-lead ECG is of limited value in diagnosing infarction involving the right ventricle. Right ventricular myocardial infarction, which usually occurs in association with inferior wall myocardial infarction, is best detected by recording the ECG from leads placed on the right side of the chest, in anatomic locations analogous to the conventional left-sided precordial leads (Morton, 1991).

CHAMBER ENLARGEMENT

Atrial enlargement or dilatation produces changes in the normal contour of the P wave. *Right atrial enlargement* causes increased P wave voltage (i.e. >2.5 mm)

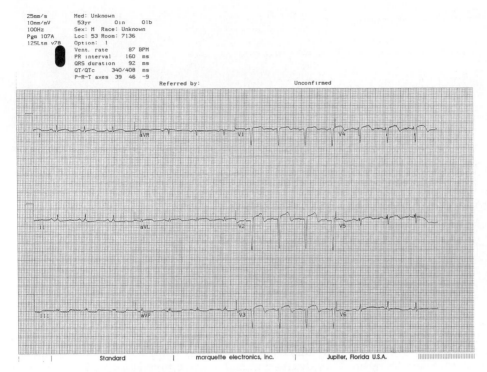

25mm/s   Med: Unknown
10mm/mV   53yr   0in   01b
100Hz   Sex: M Race: Unknown
Pgm 107A   Loc: 53 Room: 7136
12SLtm v78 Option: 1
            Vent. rate   87 BPM
            PR interval   160 ms
            QRS duration   92 ms
            QT/QTc   340/408 ms
            P-R-T axes 39 46 -9
                Referred by: Unconfirmed

Standard   marquette electronics, inc.   Jupiter, Florida U.S.A.

FIGURE 24-6. Twelve-lead ECG demonstrating anterolateral myocardial infarction. Diagnostic findings include Q waves in V$_1$ through V$_2$; slow R wave progression in V$_3$ through V$_5$; ST segment elevation in V$_1$ through V$_5$, I, and aVL; and reciprocal ST segment depression in leads III and aVF. (Courtesy of Richard Davison, M.D.)

but no increase in P wave duration. The characteristic tall, narrow P wave of right atrial enlargement is best visualized in leads II, III, and aVF. *Left atrial enlargement,* on the other hand, causes a widening of the P wave because depolarization of the left atrium occurs slightly later than that of the right atrium. A P wave that is greater than 0.12 second in duration indicates left atrial enlargement. Wide, notched P waves, termed *P mitrale,* occur in the limb leads and in V$_4$ through V$_6$ (DeAngelis, 1991). In addition, the P wave in V$_1$ is often biphasic because lead V$_1$ lies opposite the posteriorly located left atrium. The small, positive deflection that occurs initially represents right atrial depolarization. It is followed by a terminal negative deflection, representing the predominant electrical activity that is directed away from V$_1$ and toward the enlarged left atrium.

Ventricular hypertrophy is demonstrated by increased amplitude of the QRS complex. *Right ventricular hypertrophy* produces large R waves in the right precordial leads (V$_1$, V$_2$) and deep S waves in the left precordial leads (V$_5$, V$_6$). The R wave progression normally apparent from right to left across the precordium is reversed (Morton, 1991). Right precordial T waves are typically inverted. *Left ventricular hypertrophy* produces abnormally deep S waves in V$_1$ or V$_2$ and abnormally large R waves in V$_5$ or V$_6$. ST segment and T wave changes, representing *left ventricular strain* may also be evident in the left chest leads.

BUNDLE BRANCH BLOCK

Normal intraventricular conduction occurs through specialized conduction tissue known as the bundle of His and its branches (Fig. 24-7). The bundle tissue is

trifascicular, composed of a right bundle branch and a left bundle branch that bifurcates into anterior and posterior fascicles. The left bundle also gives rise to a septal branch. Bundle branch block may be fixed or may occur only with a fast (tachycardia-related) or slow (bradycardia-related) heart rate (Hillis et al., 1992). The presence of bundle branch block is revealed by abnormal width and configuration of the QRS complex. Prolongation of the QRS waveform oc-

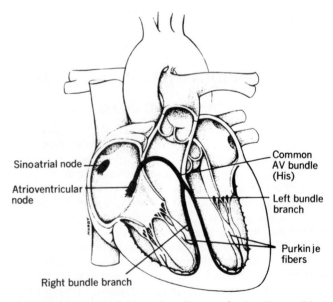

FIGURE 24-7. Distribution of cardiac conduction tissue. (Hudak CM, Gallo BM, Benz JJ, 1990: Physiological anatomy of the cardiovascular system. In Critical Care Nursing: A Holistic Approach, ed. 5, p. 82. Philadelphia, JB Lippincott)

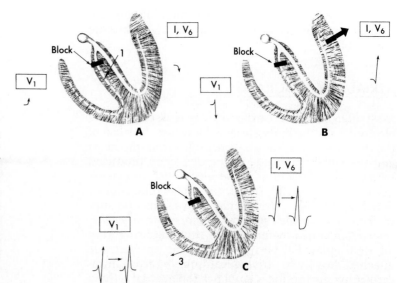

FIGURE 24-8. Schematic representation of ventricular activation in right bundle branch block (RBBB). **(A)** Initial activation of the ventricular septum (*arrow 1*) occurs normally. **(B)** Because of the RBBB, right ventricular activation is delayed and left ventricular activation occurs alone. **(C)** The right ventricle is activated after left ventricular activation, resulting in a terminal R wave in lead V_1 and a terminal S wave in leads I and V_6. (Grauer K, 1992: The QRS interval/bundle branch block. In A Practical Guide to ECG Interpretation, p. 63. St. Louis, Mosby—Year Book)

curs because, instead of simultaneous depolarization, the ventricle supplied by the dysfunctional bundle branch is depolarized slightly after the other ventricle (Drew, 1987). *Complete bundle branch block* produces a QRS complex that is 0.12 second or greater. It does not necessarily imply total absence of conduction through the dysfunctional bundle branch. Rather, if conduction is simply delayed long enough for the ventricles to be depolarized by the other bundle branch, a pattern of complete bundle branch block is present on the ECG (Conover, 1992d).

The configuration of the widened QRS complex in V_1, a right-sided chest lead, and in V_6, a left-sided chest lead, are used to diagnose whether the right or left bundle is dysfunctional. *Right bundle branch block* is most common. In right bundle branch block the initial septal depolarization and left ventricular depo-

larization occur normally. Right ventricular depolarization occurs last, with the impulse wave traveling abnormally from the left ventricular muscle to depolarize the right ventricle. Consequently, the initial portion of the QRS is normal (rS in V_1 and qR in V_6). The terminal portion, representing right ventricular depolarization, consists of an R' wave in V_1 and a deep, wide S wave in V_6. Therefore, right bundle branch block produces an rSR' configuration in V_1 and a qRS configuration in V_6 (Fig. 24-8).

In *left bundle branch block* the depolarization of the septum and ventricles is entirely dependent on the right bundle. Therefore, it occurs entirely in a right to left fashion. The small initial deflection representing septal depolarization is absent. Instead, V_1 displays a QS complex and V_6, a broad RR' wave (Fig. 24-9). If *incomplete bundle branch block* is present, the QRS com-

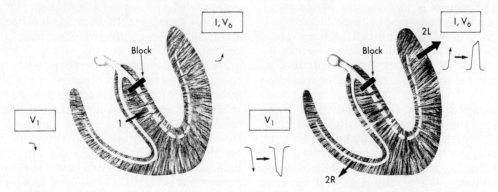

FIGURE 24-9. Schematic representation of ventricular activation in left bundle branch block (LBBB). Initial activation of the ventricular septum (*arrow 1*) occurs abnormally from right to left because of the LBBB. The electrical impulse travels by means of the intact right bundle to activate the right ventricle (*2R*) and spreads across the ventricular septum to activate the left ventricle (*2L*). Ventricular activation thus occurs primarily in a right to left direction, resulting in a QS waveform in lead V_1 and a broad RR' waveform in leads I and V_6. (Grauer K, 1992: The QRS interval/bundle branch block. In A Practical Guide to ECG Interpretation, p. 65. St. Louis, Mosby—Year Book)

plex is typically widened to 0.11 second, although it may be narrower with incomplete right bundle branch block.

ATRIAL ELECTROGRAMS

Most often, electrical cardiac activity is assessed using electrodes on the body surface. However, because of the distance of the sensing electrodes from the heart and the small amplitude of the deflection produced by atrial depolarization, other electrical components or artifacts frequently obscure P waves (Finkelmeier & Salinger, 1984). Arrhythmia analysis may be supplemented in cardiac surgical patients with *atrial electrograms* obtained by recording a rhythm tracing from an atrial epicardial pacing wire. Using an electrode attached directly to atrial epicardium to record intracardiac events produces amplification of atrial activity and diminution of ventricular activity. As a result, atrial activity and its relationship to ventricular activity is elucidated.

One or two pacing wires are routinely attached to the atrial epicardium during cardiac operations. The electrode end of the wire is secured to the epicardium, and the opposite end is brought out through the anterior chest wall. Two types of atrial electrograms may be obtained: (1) a *bipolar electrogram* in which two atrial electrodes are used for recording and (2) a *unipolar electrogram* in which one atrial and one distant electrode are used. Bipolar atrial electrograms provide the best enhancement of atrial activity with minimal visibility of ventricular activity; unipolar atrial electrograms provide some magnification of atrial activity but also clearly demonstrate the relationship between atrial and ventricular activity (Finkelmeier & Salinger, 1984; Moore & Wilkoff, 1991) (Fig. 24-10).

An atrial electrogram is easily obtained at the bedside and should be performed anytime the diagnosis of an arrhythmia is in question. If two atrial epicardial wires have been placed, both bipolar and unipolar tracings may be performed. An appropriately grounded and electrically isolated electrocardiograph is used, preferably one that can produce a simultaneous recording of a surface electrocardiographic lead.

The atrial epicardial wire is attached to the right arm electrode of the electrocardiograph. If a second epicardial wire is present, it is attached to the left arm electrode; if not, the left arm electrode is attached in the usual fashion. The right and left leg electrodes are positioned normally. If both the right and left arm electrodes are attached to atrial epicardial wires, recording a lead I tracing will produce a bipolar atrial electrogram. A lead I tracing with standard electrode placement measures polarity between the right and left arm. Therefore, in this instance it will measure polarity between the two atrial electrodes. When the electrocardiograph is adjusted to obtain a lead II trac-

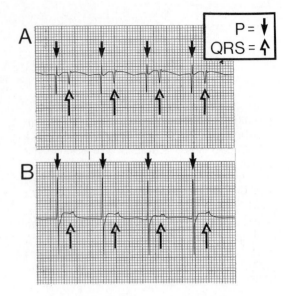

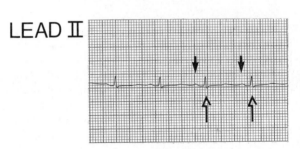

FIGURE 24-10. Normal sinus rhythm: unipolar **(A)** and bipolar **(B)** atrial electrograms are recorded simultaneously with a lead II rhythm tracing. (Finkelmeier BA, Salinger MH, 1984: The atrial electrogram: Its diagnostic use following cardiac surgery. Crit Care Nurs 4:43)

ing (i.e., measuring polarity between right arm and left leg electrodes), it will produce a unipolar electrogram (atrial and left leg electrodes).

If only the right arm electrode has been attached to an atrial wire, recording in either lead I or lead II will produce a unipolar electrogram. A unipolar electrogram may alternatively be obtained by attaching all four limb electrodes in their usual positions and the atrial wire to the V electrode. Recording in the V_1 setting will produce a unipolar atrial electrogram. If a telemetry monitoring system is being used, attaching the right arm electrode to an atrial wire will produce an atrial electrogram. The right arm electrode of a bedside monitoring system may also be used if the equipment is electrically isolated to avoid delivery of current from the monitoring system to the heart through the pacing wire. The electrical safety of the monitoring system must be confirmed before using it to perform an atrial electrogram.

Atrial electrograms are often used when attempting to diagnose supraventricular tachycardias. The atrial electrogram may reveal the presence of P waves

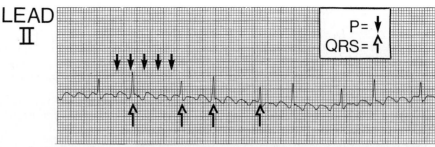

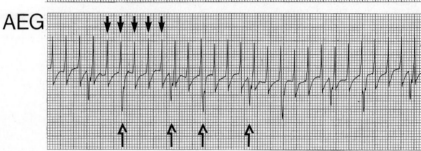

FIGURE 24-11. Atrial electrogram (*AEG*) recorded simultaneously with lead II rhythm tracing clearly reveals atrial flutter waves with a variable block. (Finkelmeier BA, Salinger MH, 1984: The atrial electrogram: Its diagnostic use following cardiac surgery. Crit Care Nurs 4:44)

that are not apparent on the surface ECG (Strong, 1991). During tachyarrhythmias, P wave activity is frequently obscured by the QRS complex or T wave. In addition, it is often difficult to determine if the P wave to QRS complex ratio is more than 1:1. An atrial electrogram of atrial flutter readily reveals flutter waves and allows easy determination of the degree of AV block (Fig. 24-11). In atrial fibrillation, erratic fi-

brillatory waves that may be obscured on the surface ECG are readily detected by an atrial electrogram (Fig. 24-12). An atrial electrogram is also valuable in differentiating ventricular tachycardia and supraventricular tachycardia with aberrancy. Because it more clearly displays the relationship of atrial and ventricular activity, an atrial electrogram may unmask AV dissociation. AV dissociation is present in approximately 50% of cases of ventricular tachycardia (Drew, 1991). As a general rule, AV dissociation during a wide QRS tachycardia is strong presumptive evidence of a ventricular origin of the arrhythmia (Zipes, 1992).

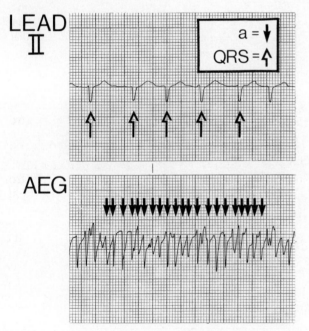

FIGURE 24-12. Atrial electrogram (*AEG*) recorded simultaneously with lead II rhythm tracing during atrial fibrillation reveals erratic atrial activity (a); QRS complexes are obscured in the AEG. (Finkelmeier BA, Salinger MH, 1984: The atrial electrogram: Its diagnostic use following cardiac surgery. Crit Care Nurse 4:45)

REFERENCES

Conover MB, 1992a: Measurement of heart rate and intervals. In Understanding Electrocardiography, ed. 6. St. Louis, Mosby–Year Book

Conover MB, 1992b: Determination of the electrical axis. In Understanding Electrocardiography, ed. 6. St. Louis, Mosby–Year Book

Conover MB, 1992c: The 12-lead electrocardiogram. In Understanding Electrocardiography, ed. 6. St. Louis, Mosby–Year Book

Conover MB, 1992d: Bundle branch block and hemiblock. In Understanding Electrocardiography, ed. 6. St. Louis, Mosby–Year Book

DeAngelis R, 1991: The cardiovascular system. In Alspach JG (ed): Core Curriculum for Critical Care Nursing, ed. 4. Philadelphia, WB Saunders

Drew BJ, 1987: Differentiation of wide QRS tachycardias. Prog Cardiovasc Nurs 2:130

Drew BJ, 1991: Bedside diagnosis of wide QRS tachycardia. Crit Care Nurs Q 14:19

Erickson BA, 1991: Introduction to electrocardiography. In Kinney MR, Packa DR, Andreoli KG, Zipes DP (eds): Comprehensive Cardiac Care, ed. 7. St. Louis, Mosby–Year Book

Finkelmeier BA, Salinger MH, 1984: The atrial electrogram: Its diagnostic use following cardiac surgery. Crit Care Nurse 4:42

Fisch C, 1992: Electrocardiography and vectorcardiography. In

Braunwald E (ed): Heart Disease: A Textbook of Cardiovascular Medicine, ed. 4. Philadelphia, WB Saunders

Goldberger E, 1990: Electrocardiography. In Essentials of Clinical Cardiology. Philadelphia, JB Lippincott

Hanisch PJ, 1991: Identification and treatment of acute myocardial infarction by electrocardiographic site classification. Focus Crit Care 18:480

Hill NE, Goodman JS, 1987: Importance of accurate placement of precordial leads in the 12-lead electrocardiogram. Heart Lung 16:561

Hillis LD, Lange RA, Wells PJ, Winniford MD, 1992: Bundle branch and fascicular blocks. In Manual of Clinical Problems in Cardiology, ed. 4. Boston, Little, Brown

Moore SL, Wilkoff BL, 1991: Rhythm disturbances after cardiac surgery. Semin Thorac Cardiovasc Surg 3:24

Morton PG, 1991: Electrocardiographic assessment of right heart dysfunction. J Cardiovasc Nurs 6:34

Strong AG, 1991: Nursing management of postoperative dysrhythmias. Crit Care Clin North Am 3:709

Sweetwood HM, 1989: Myocardial infarction. In Clinical Electrocardiography for Nurses, ed. 2. Rockville, MD, Aspen Publishers

Woods SL, 1989: Electrocardiography, vectorcardiography, and polarcardiography. In Underhill SL, Woods SL, Froelicher ES, Halpenny J (eds): Cardiac Nursing, ed. 2. Philadelphia, JB Lippincott

Zipes DP, 1992: Specific arrhythmias: Diagnosis and treatment. In Braunwald E (ed): Heart Disease: A Textbook of Cardiovascular Medicine, ed. 4. Philadelphia, WB Saunders

CHAPTER 25

CARDIAC ARRHYTHMIAS

COMMON ARRHYTHMIAS
    Premature Complexes
    Tachyarrhythmias
    Bradyarrhythmias
    Heart Block

DIFFERENTIATION OF WIDE QRS
TACHYCARDIAS

The ability to diagnose cardiac arrhythmias is an essential skill for nurses in cardiothoracic surgical settings. Clinically significant arrhythmias occur quite commonly during the early postoperative period after cardiac operations. Predisposing factors include hypothermia, metabolic derangements associated with cardiopulmonary bypass, alterations in gas exchange and acid–base balance, and underlying cardiac disease (Strong, 1991). Edema of myocardial tissue and pericardial inflammation related to surgical manipulation of the heart are also thought to contribute to postoperative arrhythmias. Patients who undergo pulmonary or esophageal surgery may also develop arrhythmias, particularly in association with extensive pulmonary resection, atelectasis and hypoxemia, or perioperative myocardial infarction.

Arrhythmia identification is performed using a consistent set of criteria applied in systematic fashion. The discussion in this chapter is by no means a complete review of all cardiac arrhythmias and the nuances of diagnosis. Rather, it is confined to summary information regarding diagnosis and management of the most commonly encountered arrhythmias. Each of the selected arrhythmias is defined according to its site of origin, rate, rhythm, waveform appearance, and length of PR and QRS intervals. For the purpose of comparison, the criteria defining *normal sinus rhythm* are included.

Normal Sinus Rhythm (Fig. 25-1)

Origin: sinus node
Rate: 60 to 100 beats per minute
Rhythm: regular
Waveform Appearance: PQRST
PR Interval: 0.12 to 0.20 second
QRS Duration: 0.04 to 0.10 second

A *sinus arrhythmia* is present if the rhythmicity is slightly irregular, with the PP interval varying by more than 0.16 second (Hillis et al., 1992a). The rate variation in sinus arrhythmia is usually related to respiration; the sinus rate increases during inspiration and decreases during expiration.

COMMON ARRHYTHMIAS

PREMATURE COMPLEXES

Premature Atrial Contractions (Fig. 25-2)

Origin: atrial tissue
Rhythm: irregular
Waveform Appearance: P' (ectopic P) QRST
PR Interval: normal or prolonged
QRS Duration: : 0.04 to 0.10 second unless aberrant conduction occurs

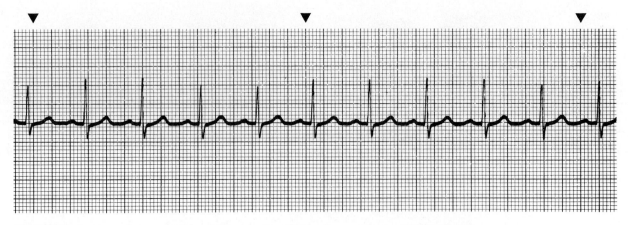

FIGURE 25-1. Normal sinus rhythm with heart rate of 94 beats per minute. (Huff J, Doern-bach DP, White RD, 1993: Atrial rhythms. In ECG Workout, ed. 2, p. 71. Philadelphia, JB Lippincott)

A *premature atrial contraction* (PAC) is the discharge of an ectopic atrial focus that depolarizes the atria and interrupts the dominant rhythm. PACs occur early, vary in frequency, may arise from one or more foci, may be coupled with each normal beat (bigeminy), or may occur in pairs or triads (Waldo & MacLean, 1980). In addition to prematurity, the ectopic P (P') wave may be altered in morphology; that is, it may be taller, shorter, notched, widened, or superimposed on the preceding T wave (Wilkinson, 1991). PACs may be interpolated (i.e., produce no alteration in regularity of the cardiac rhythm), or they may be associated with a noncompensatory or full compensatory pause.

PACs are usually conducted to the ventricles normally, producing a QRS complex identical to that after sinus node discharge. Occasionally, PACs are conducted aberrantly. Aberrancy, defined as a transient abnormality in intraventricular conduction of a complex of supraventricular origin, is discussed in

further detail later in the chapter. If a PAC is very premature, ventricular tissue may still be refractory. If so, the PAC is nonconducted and no QRS complex follows the P' wave. PACs are common after cardiac and pulmonary resection procedures. Although they are usually a precursor of supraventricular tachyar-rhythmias, they otherwise have little clinical significance.

Premature Junctional Contractions

Origin: atrioventricular (AV) nodal tissue

Rhythm: irregular

Waveform Appearance: P' QRST, QRST, or QRST P'

PR Interval: if P' precedes QRS, less than 0.12 second

QRS Duration: 0.04 to 0.10 second unless aberrant conduction occurs

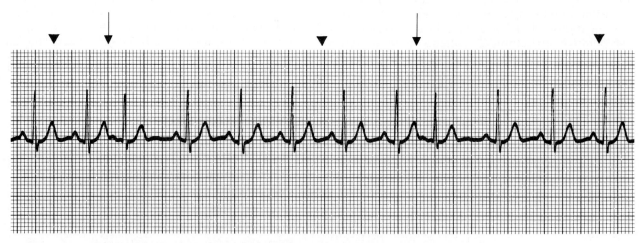

FIGURE 25-2. Normal sinus rhythm with two premature atrial contractions (*arrows*). Note different morphology of ectopic P waves. (Huff J, Doernbach DP, White RD, 1993: Atrial rhythms. In ECG Workout, ed. 2, p. 101. Philadelphia, JB Lippincott)

Premature junctional contractions (PJCs), often a precursor to junctional tachycardia, originate in the AV node. Depolarization of the atria may occur in a retrograde fashion, producing a morphologically abnormal P wave that may appear before, simultaneously with, or after the QRS complex (Hillis et al., 1992b). Alternatively, depolarization of the atria by the sinus node may occur simultaneously with or after AV nodal depolarization. In this case a morphologically normal P wave appears before, during, or after the QRS complex. PJCs that are conducted normally through the bundles produce an appropriately narrow QRS complex. If aberrant conduction occurs, the QRS is widened. PJCs do not require treatment.

Premature Ventricular Contractions (Fig. 25-3)

Origin: ventricular tissue
Rhythm: irregular
PR Interval: none
QRS Duration: more than 0.12 second

Premature ventricular contractions (PVCs) originate from an ectopic focus in the ventricles, usually due to a reentrant mechanism. They are characterized by abnormal width and distorted morphology of the QRS complex as compared with the narrow QRS complex produced by impulses originating in the atria or AV node (Drew, 1987). PVCs may be uniform in morphology or multiformed. Often the T wave after a PVC is opposite the primary deflection of the QRS waveform. PVCs are usually followed by a full compensatory pause; that is, the RR interval surrounding the PVC is exactly twice as long as the RR interval between two complexes of sinus origin. Three or more consecutive PVCs are considered ventricular tachycardia (VT).

In postoperative patients, PVCs may occur transiently due to a precipitant, such as hypoxemia or hypokalemia. However, many patients with organic heart disease have underlying ventricular arrhythmias. It is important to ascertain if the frequency and morphology of PVCs appearing postoperatively differ from the preoperative period. New-onset ventricular ectopy must be promptly evaluated and treated appropriately. Correction of underlying hypoxemia or hypokalemia with oxygen or potassium therapy, respectively, often eradicates ventricular ectopy. Intravenous lidocaine or temporary pacing may also be used to suppress PVCs. In some patients, particularly those with major ventricular wall motion abnormalities, ventricular ectopy represents a chronic arrhythmic disorder and the need for electrophysiologic evaluation and ongoing therapy.

TACHYARRHYTHMIAS

Supraventricular Tachyarrhythmias

Sinus Tachycardia

Origin: sinus node
Rate: 100 to 160 beats per minute
Rhythm: regular
Complex: PQRST
PR Interval: 0.12 to 0.20 second
QRS Duration: 0.04 to 0.10 second

Sinus tachycardia is an acceleration in the rate of normal sinus rhythm. It is generally gradual in onset and termination. P waves have a normal configuration, duration, and axis (Iskandrian, 1991). Both the upper and lower rate limits of sinus tachycardia vary with age. In adults, a sinus rhythm at a rate greater than 100 beats per minute is considered tachycardic; sinus tachycardia rarely occurs at a rate greater than 160 beats per minute.

Sinus tachycardia usually occurs secondary to a hypermetabolic state. Common causes in postoperative patients include fever, pain, anxiety, anemia, hypoxemia, and hypovolemia. The heart works less efficiently during sinus tachycardia because diastolic filling time is reduced. However, the arrhythmia

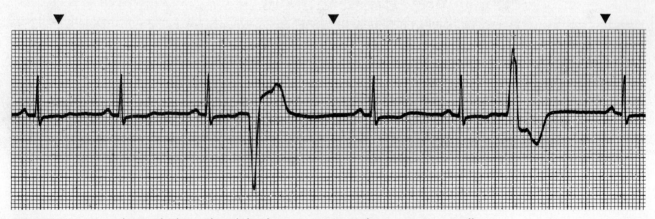

FIGURE 25-3. Normal sinus rhythm with multifocal premature ventricular contractions. (Huff J, Doernbach DP, White RD, 1993: Ventricular rhythms and bundle branch block. In ECG Workout, ed. 2, p. 189. Philadelphia, JB Lippincott)

rarely produces symptoms. Correction of the precipitating factor usually results in return to normal sinus rhythm. Antiarrhythmic medications are generally not necessary.

Supraventricular tachycardia (SVT) includes several arrhythmias, all of which originate above the bifurcation of the bundle of His. Paroxysmal supraventricular tachycardia (PSVT), atrial flutter, and atrial fibrillation are all forms of SVT. The primary distinguishing feature among the various forms is the site of origin (atria or AV node) and rate of atrial depolarization.

Paroxysmal Supraventricular Tachycardia

Origin: atrial or AV nodal tissue
Rate:
Atrial—160 to 250 beats per minute
Ventricular—same, or may be slower if block present
Rhythm: regular
Complex: P'QRST (P' may be superimposed on preceding T wave or inverted), QRST, or QRSTP'
PR Interval: may be shortened
QRS Duration: 0.04 to 0.10 second

Paroxysmal supraventricular tachycardia is the nonspecific term used to describe arrhythmias thought to arise due to reentry and includes tachycardias formerly called *paroxysmal atrial tachycardia* and *paroxysmal junctional tachycardia* (Erickson, 1991). AV conduction usually occurs at a 1:1 ratio, although AV block is sometimes present. Although QRS duration is usually normal, it may be prolonged in the presence of aberrant conduction. PSVT is less common than atrial flutter or atrial fibrillation in postoperative patients. PSVT with block may occur as a manifestation of digoxin toxicity.

Atrial Flutter (Fig. 25-4)

Origin: atrial tissue
Rate:
Atrial—230 to 350 beats per minute (type I); 340 to 430 beats per minute (type II)
Ventricular—rate dependent on degree of block
Rhythm: regularly irregular
Complex: P'P'QRST, P'P'P'QRST, or P'P'P'P'QRST
PR Interval: cannot be determined
QRS Duration: 0.04 to 0.10 second

Atrial flutter is a form of SVT characterized by a rapid, regular atrial rate that may range from 230 to 430 beats per minute (Conover, 1992). In *type I,* or typical, *atrial flutter,* flutter waves occur at a rate of 250 to 350 beats per minute and create a characteristic "sawtooth" baseline (Hillis et al., 1992c). Typically, type I atrial flutter occurs with an atrial rate of 300 beats per minute, 2:1 AV block, and a ventricular rate of 150 beats per minute. Despite the high atrial depolarization rates, mechanically significant contraction of the atria is often preserved (McGuire, 1982).

Type II, or atypical, *atrial flutter* has elements of both atrial flutter and atrial fibrillation. The atrial rate is usually 360 to 380 beats per minute but can range from 340 to 430 beats per minute (Conover, 1992). The flutter waves are less uniform than in type I atrial flutter, varying in morphology and spacing. The term *flutter-fibrillation* is sometimes used to describe type II atrial flutter.

Atrial Fibrillation (Fig. 25-5)

Origin: atrial tissue
Rate:
Atrial—350 to 600 beats per minute
Ventricular—variable

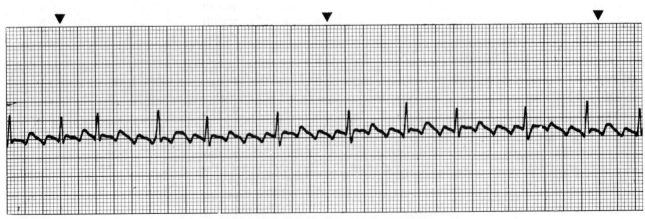

FIGURE 25-4. Atrial flutter with variable degree of block. Note "sawtooth" appearance of flutter waves. (Huff J, Doernbach DP, White RD, 1993: Atrial rhythms. In ECG Workout, ed. 2, p. 105. Philadelphia, JB Lippincott)

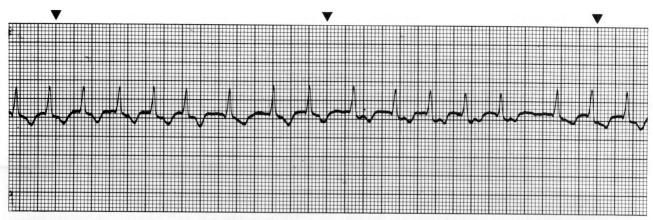

FIGURE 25-5. Atrial fibrillation with ventricular response rate of approximately 140 beats per minute. Note irregular rhythm and fibrillatory baseline without discernible P waves. (Huff J, Doernbach DP, White RD, 1993: Atrial rhythms. In ECG Workout, ed. 2, p. 92. Philadelphia, JB Lippincott)

Rhythm: irregularly irregular
Complex:
Atrial—chaotic fibrillatory waves
Ventricular—QRST
PR Interval: cannot be determined
QRS Duration: 0.04 to 0.10 second

Atrial fibrillation develops when the atrial chambers can no longer sustain a regular, coordinated rhythm and multiple foci in one or both atria begin to discharge hundreds of times per minute (Kastor, 1991). It is probably the most common arrhythmia in postoperative cardiac surgical patients. Its electrocardiographic hallmarks are a fibrillatory baseline in association with an irregularly irregular ventricular rate. Although QRS complexes are usually of normal duration, intermittent aberrant conduction is common due to the rapid and erratic rate of AV nodal depolarization. As a result, occasional widened QRS complexes are typical. It is sometimes difficult to determine if these widened complexes represent aberrancy or PVCs.

The various forms of SVT are common both in postoperative cardiac surgical patients and in patients who have undergone major pulmonary resection, particularly pneumonectomy. Atrial flutter and atrial fibrillation occur most often, usually 3 to 5 days after operation. Although a number of theories have been postulated to explain the frequency of postoperative SVT, the mechanism of arrhythmogenesis remains unclear. In addition, no pharmacologic regimen has proven entirely effective in preventing its occurrence. Atrial electrograms are ideal for magnifying atrial activity and for helping to distinguish among the various forms of SVT and between SVT and ventricular tachycardia (Finkelmeier & Salinger, 1984).

Although SVT is usually not a life-threatening problem, patients with compromised ventricular function or untreated myocardial ischemia may experience clinically significant hypotension. The rapid ventricular rates typically associated with all forms of SVT compromise cardiac output because diastolic ventricular filling time is reduced. Inappropriate timing of mitral and tricuspid valve closure further impairs ventricular filling. In addition, rapid rates increase myocardial oxygen consumption while at the same time shortening diastolic filling time for the coronary arteries (DeAngelis, 1991).

In atrial fibrillation, mechanically effective atrial contractions are absent. Therefore, the proportion of ventricular filling that results from a properly timed atrial systole (i.e., the "atrial kick") is lost and cardiac output may be reduced by 20% to 30% in some patients. Atrial fibrillation is also associated with an increased risk of thromboembolism. Stasis of blood along endocardial surfaces of the quivering or quiescent atria predisposes to thrombus formation. Small fragments of thrombus can embolize from the left atrium into the systemic circulation and from the right atrium into the pulmonary vessels; cerebral, renal, splenic, peripheral, or pulmonary embolism may result (Goldberger, 1990a).

The goals of treating postoperative SVT are twofold: slowing the ventricular rate and conversion to normal sinus rhythm. Treatment may consist of (1) pharmacologic agents, (2) rapid atrial pacing, or (3) cardioversion. Often a combination of therapies is used.

The most common antiarrhythmic agent, used both for prophylaxis and treatment, is digoxin. Digoxin increases the refractory period and decreases conduction velocity in the AV node, thereby slowing the ventricular rate in atrial flutter or atrial fibrillation and prolonging the PR interval in normal sinus rhythm (Smith et al., 1992). Beta-blocking medications, particularly propranolol, are also commonly used to prevent or treat postoperative SVT. In patients with atrial flutter, quinidine is sometimes used to slow the atrial rate. It is always given concomitantly with digoxin because its slowing of the atrial rate and its vagolytic effect on the AV node might otherwise result in a rapid ventricular rate response (Goldberger, 1990b). Verapamil or diltiazem is occasionally used but may not be well tolerated in patients with compromised left ventricular function.

Rapid atrial pacing is sometimes effective in converting PSVT or atrial flutter, particularly when used in combination with pharmacologic therapy. It is not useful in converting atrial fibrillation to normal sinus rhythm because atrial capture cannot be achieved when the atria are fibrillating. Occasionally, postoperative SVT produces acute hemodynamic instability, necessitating emergent cardioversion. Techniques for rapid atrial pacing and cardioversion are described in Chapter 26, Temporary Pacing and Defibrillation.

Ventricular Tachyarrhythmias

Ventricular Tachycardia (Fig. 25-6)

Origin: ventricular tissue
Rate: 100 to 250 beats per minute
Rhythm: regular or slightly irregular
Waveform Appearance:
QRST
P waves (independent of or after QRS)
PR Interval: none
QRS Duration: more than 0.12 second

Ventricular tachycardia is an arrhythmia originating below the bifurcation of the bundle of His. The heart rate is seldom faster than 200 beats per minute and does not exceed 250 beats per minute (Goldberger, 1990b). Atrial activity may occur independent of the ventricular rhythm (AV dissociation), or retrograde ventriculoatrial conduction may be present (Glasser, 1989). If atrial and ventricular activity is dissociated,

fusion or capture beats may occur. *Fusion beats* represent ventricular depolarization partially from a supraventricular focus and partially from a ventricular focus. *Capture beats* are ventricular depolarizations resulting from an impulse originating in the atrium. VT may be monomorphic or polymorphic and may be nonsustained or sustained (Lazarus et al., 1988). *Sustained VT* has a rate greater than 100 beats per minute and lasts more than 30 seconds or requires an intervention to terminate. *Torsades de pointes* is a form of VT characterized by QRS complexes of changing amplitude that appear to twist around the isoelectric line and that occur at rates of 200 to 250 beats per minute (Zipes, 1992).

VT is usually not well tolerated and may produce severe hypotension or deteriorate into ventricular fibrillation (VF). Sustained VT and VF are the most common arrhythmias leading to sudden cardiac death (Drew, 1987). Therefore, VT must be treated promptly, usually with intravenous bolus doses of lidocaine followed by a continuous infusion. Intravenous procainamide or bretylium may also be used if lidocaine fails to suppress VT. Rapid defibrillation is performed if hemodynamic instability is present. Electrophysiologic studies may be necessary to evaluate the likelihood of arrhythmia recurrence and the need for chronic antiarrhythmic therapy.

Ventricular Fibrillation (Fig. 25-7)

Origin: ventricular tissue
Rate: 150 to 300 beats per minute
Rhythm: irregular
Waveform Appearance: chaotic fibrillatory waves
PR Interval: none
QRS Duration: inconsistent

Ventricular fibrillation is characterized by irregular, disorganized, oscillating ventricular complexes. VF rarely terminates spontaneously. If not treated, effec-

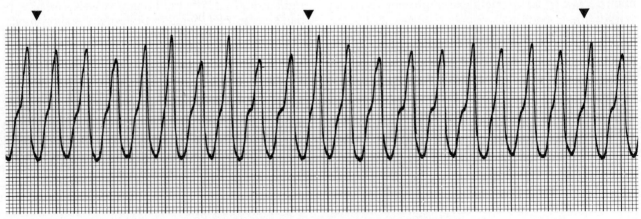

FIGURE 25-6. Ventricular tachycardia at a heart rate of 188 beats per minute; P waves are not identified. (Huff J, Doernbach DP, White RD, 1993: Ventricular rhythms and bundle branch block. In ECG Workout, ed. 2, p. 195. Philadelphia, JB Lippincott)

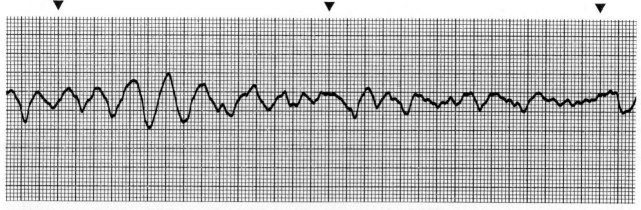

FIGURE 25-7. Ventricular fibrillation. (Huff J, Doernbach DP, White RD, 1993: Ventricular rhythms and bundle branch block. In ECG Workout, ed. 2, p. 190. Philadelphia, JB Lippincott)

tive cardiac output ceases. Death is usually instantaneous since peripheral perfusion ceases immediately and irreversible neurologic injury begins within minutes (Hillis et al., 1992d). For the patient to survive, cardiopulmonary resuscitation and defibrillation must be initiated immediately on detection of VF and continued until organized ventricular activity is restored.

BRADYARRHYTHMIAS

Transient bradyarrhythmias sometimes occur, particularly in the early postoperative period after cardiac surgery. Responsible factors are thought to include perioperative beta-blockade, hyperkalemic or hypermagnesemic damage from cardioplegic solution, and ischemic damage to the conduction system (Smith, 1990).

Sinus Bradycardia

Origin: sinus node
Rate: less than 60 beats per minute
Rhythm: regular
Complex: PQRST
PR Interval: 0.12 to 0.20 second
QRS Duration: 0.04 to 0.10 second

Sinus bradycardia is a rhythm that originates in the sinus node but with a discharge rate less than 60 beats per minute. It may occur (1) as a normal variant, particularly in athletes or during sleep; (2) in response to vagal stimulation, such as with carotid sinus massage or vomiting; (3) as a result of digoxin, beta-adrenergic blocking agents, or calcium-channel antagonists; and (4) secondary to disease processes, such as inferior myocardial infarction or sick sinus syndrome (Jacobson, 1989a).

In most patients, sinus bradycardia is well tolerated. Often, discontinuance of a precipitating medication, such as digoxin, is the only required treatment. In postoperative patients with underlying ventricular dysfunction, it may be beneficial to temporarily increase the heart rate to augment cardiac output. Either atrial or ventricular temporary pacing may be used to increase heart rate during sinus bradycardia. If AV nodal conduction is normal, atrial pacing is preferable because the atrial contribution to ventricular filling is preserved. In patients without epicardial pacing wires, atropine or isoproterenol may be administered. Atropine is given as an intravenous bolus, and isoproterenol is given by continuous intravenous infusion. Both drugs, if effective, increase heart rate within several minutes. Transthoracic or transvenous pacing may also be used.

When sinus node function is depressed, secondary pacemakers, such as the AV node, bundle of His and its branches, or the Purkinje fibers, can form stimuli to initiate the cardiac rhythm (Goldberger, 1990b). Depending on the site of impulse formation, an idiojunctional or idioventricular rhythm results.

Idiojunctional Rhythm (Fig. 25-8)

Origin: AV nodal tissue
Rate: 40 to 60 beats per minute
Rhythm: regular
Waveform Appearance: P'QRST, QRST, or QRST P'
PR Interval: if present, less than 0.12 second
QRS Duration: 0.04 to 0.10 second

Idiojunctional rhythm originates in the AV node and depolarizes the atria and ventricles almost simultaneously. It is usually transient and, in postoperative cardiac surgical patients, is generally treated with temporary atrial or AV sequential pacing to increase heart rate.

Idioventricular Rhythm

Origin: ventricular tissue
Rate: 25 to 40 beats per minute

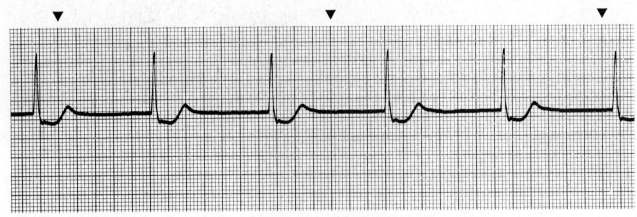

FIGURE 25-8. Junctional rhythm with heart rate of 47 beats per minute; note absence of P waves. (Huff J, Doernbach DP, White RD, 1993: Atrioventricular junctional rhythms and atrioventricular block. In ECG Workout, ed. 2, p. 133. Philadelphia, JB Lippincott)

Rhythm: regular or irregular
Waveform Appearance: QRST
PR Interval: none
QRS Duration: greater than 0.12 second

An *idioventricular* or *ventricular escape rhythm* occurs rarely as a result of complete heart block or suppression of higher pacemakers. The combination of the excessively slow rate and the loss of AV synchrony usually produces symptomatic hypotension. Temporary ventricular or AV sequential pacing is performed until an acceptable heart rhythm resumes or a permanent pacemaker is placed.

HEART BLOCK

Heart block describes arrhythmias in which there is some degree of impairment in transmission of electrical impulses through the conduction system.

First-Degree Heart Block

Origin: sinus node
Rate: 60 to 100 beats per minute
Rhythm: regular
Waveform Appearance: PQRST
PR Interval: greater than 0.20 second
QRS Duration: 0.04 to 0.10 second

In *first-degree heart block* all impulses are conducted through the AV node, bundle of His, and bundle branches, but at a slower than normal rate. The arrhythmia does not produce any abnormality in rate or rhythm. First-degree heart block may result from underlying AV nodal disease, ischemia, pharmacologic agents, or increased vagal tone (DeAngelis, 1991).

Second-Degree Heart Block—Mobitz Type I
(Fig. 25-9)

Origin: sinus node

Rate:
Atrial—60 to 100 beats per minute
Ventricular—slightly less than atrial rate, because some atrial complexes are not conducted
Rhythm:
Atrial—PP interval regular
Ventricular—irregular repetitive cycles of "group beating"
Waveform Appearance: PQRST, intermittent nonconducted P waves
PR Interval: progressively lengthens until P wave is not followed by QRS, then cycle begins again
QRS Duration: 0.04 to 0.10 second

Second-degree heart block describes the condition in which some atrial impulses are conducted to the ventricles and some are not. If the PR interval progressively lengthens from cycle to cycle until an atrial impulse is not conducted, the arrhythmia is termed *Mobitz type I*, or *Wenckebach, second-degree heart block.* After each nonconducted P wave a new cycle begins with a normal or slightly prolonged PR interval (McGuire, 1982).

Second-Degree Heart Block—Mobitz Type II

Origin: sinus node
Rate:
Atrial—60 to 100 beats per minute
Ventricular—slightly less than atrial rate, because some atrial complexes are not conducted
Rhythm:
Atrial—PP interval regular
Ventricular—irregular
Waveform Appearance: PQRST, intermittent nonconducted P waves
PR Interval: normal or prolonged, but not all P waves are conducted
QRS Duration: usually more than 0.10 second

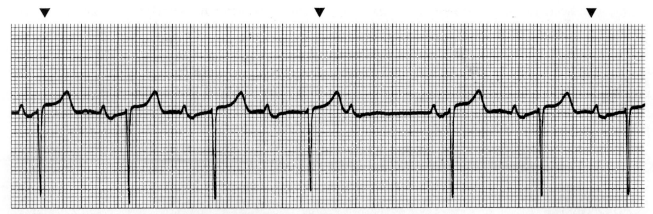

FIGURE 25-9. Mobitz I second-degree heart block. Note that PR interval progressively lengthens (0.2 to 0.48 second) followed by nonconducted P wave and repetition of PR interval lengthening. (Huff J, Doernbach DP, White RD, 1993: Atrioventricular junctional rhythms and atrioventricular block. In ECG Workout, ed. 2, p. 136. Philadelphia, JB Lippincott)

In *Mobitz type II second-degree heart block* some atrial impulses are conducted to the ventricles and some are not, but the PR interval remains constant. The QRS complex is almost always widened because the block occurs in the bundle and one or both branches or in the Purkinje fibers (Goldberger, 1990b). Mobitz type II heart block is more likely than Mobitz type I to progress to complete heart block.

Third-Degree Heart Block (Complete Heart Block) (Fig. 25-10)

Rate:

Atrial—60 to 100 beats per minute

Ventricular—25 to 60 beats per minute, depending on whether escape rhythm originates in AV nodal or ventricular tissue

Rhythm:

Atrial—PP interval regular

Ventricular—RR interval regular

Atrial and ventricular activity unrelated

Waveform Appearance: QRST, P waves independent of QRS waves

PR Interval: none

QRS Duration: normal or wide

In *third-degree* or *complete heart block* no atrial impulses are successfully conducted to the ventricles. Instead, atrial and ventricular activity occur independent of one another; that is, *AV dissociation* is present. Third-degree heart block is recognized by an atrial rate that is faster than the ventricular rate and the absence of a predictable relationship between the two (Gray & Mandel, 1990).

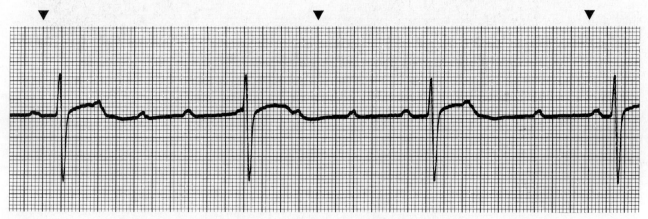

FIGURE 25-10. Complete heart block. Note presence of AV dissociation with ventricular rate of 30 beats per minute and irregular atrial rate of 90 beats per minute. (Huff J, Doernbach DP, White RD, 1993: Atrioventricular junctional rhythms and atrioventricular block. In ECG Workout, ed. 2, p. 144. Philadelphia, JB Lippincott)

Transient heart block occasionally occurs in postoperative cardiac surgical patients, particularly those who have undergone valvular procedures. In all forms of heart block, the electrocardiogram (ECG) is monitored. Possible pharmacologic precipitants, such as digoxin, are discontinued. Second- or third-degree heart block associated with significant bradycardia is treated with temporary ventricular or AV sequential pacing. Postoperative heart block usually resolves within 1 to 2 weeks. If not, implantation of a permanent, transvenous pacemaker may be necessary.

DIFFERENTIATION OF WIDE QRS TACHYCARDIAS

Aberrancy is the abnormal intraventricular conduction of supraventricular impulses. A fixed intraventricular conduction disturbance, such as right or left bundle branch block, results in aberrant conduction of all supraventricular impulses (Nelson, 1989). In other cases, conduction of supraventricular impulses may be normal during sinus rhythm but become aberrant when the heart rate increases or an impulse occurs prematurely. The degree of aberrancy depends on the refractory state of the bundles at the time that the impulse is conducted. If a premature complex is only slightly early, the complex will be slightly abnormal; if it occurs earlier after the preceding complex, it may be extremely widened and bizarre. A premature complex that is very early will find all the fascicles refractory, and the impulse will not be conducted.

SVT with aberrant conduction produces a widened QRS complex and altered T wave that often causes it to be mistaken for VT. Differentiation between VT and SVT with aberrancy is quite important, and yet it is often difficult for both experienced physicians and nurses (Cooper & Marriott, 1989). Sometimes, the arrhythmias may be distinguished by the presence or absence of associated symptoms. VT usually produces hemodynamic deterioration and SVT does not. However, VT without symptoms or SVT with symptoms can also occur.

The therapeutic implications of misdiagnosis are significant. VT that remains untreated can lead to hemodynamic compromise or cardiac arrest due to ventricular fibrillation. Intravenous verapamil, sometimes used to treat SVT, may cause profound hypotension or ventricular fibrillation when given to patients with VT (Drew, 1991). In postoperative patients, and in patients with a history of myocardial infarction or congestive heart failure, the great majority of wide QRS tachycardias are ventricular.

The first response to occurrence of a wide QRS tachycardia is assessment of the patient's hemodynamic status and, if necessary, initiation of resuscitative measures. It is generally safer to err in the direction of treating aberrancy as if it were VT rather than in failing to treat ventricular arrhythmias appropriately. If there is a question about whether a rhythm represents VT or SVT with aberrancy, a 12-lead ECG and a long rhythm tracing are obtained. The patient is monitored closely for hemodynamic sequelae of the arrhythmia, which are treated as necessary.

A number of electrocardiographic criteria have been identified that can assist in diagnosing wide QRS tachycardias. Morphology of the QRS complex in the precordial leads is one distinguishing feature. Although an aberrantly conducted impulse can produce any form of widened QRS, a right bundle branch block (RBBB) morphology of the ectopic complexes (rSR' in lead V_1 and qRS in V_6) is most typical (Fig. 25-11). The right bundle is the longest, thinnest

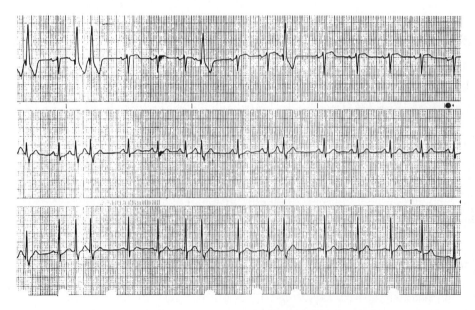

FIGURE 25-11. Simultaneous rhythm tracings of leads V_1 (*top*), II (*middle*), and V_5 (*bottom*) demonstrate sinus rhythm with aberrantly conducted premature atrial contractions. Note right bundle branch block configuration (rSR' in V_1, qRs in V_5) of aberrant beats. Supraventricular origin is also revealed by ectopic p wave preceding wide QRS complexes. (Courtesy of Linda Hellstedt, R.N., M.S.)

TABLE 25-1. ELECTROCARDIOGRAPHIC FEATURES FAVORING SUPRAVENTRICULAR ORIGIN OF ARRHYTHMIA

Isolated Complexes

rSR' morphology in V_1
qRs morphology in V_6
Ashman's phenomenon (long RR, short RR, ectopic complex)
Ectopic P wave preceding QRS
Less than full compensatory pause
Varying coupling interval in atrial fibrillation
Initial deflection identical to sinus complex
QRS ≤ 0.14 second

Tachycardia

Slowing of heart rate with vagal stimulation
Right bundle branch block pattern

(Adapted from Housestaff Manual for Cardiothoracic Surgery. Northwestern University Medical School, 1994)

---

fascicle of the bundle branch system and has the longest refractory period. If a supraventricular impulse is conducted through the AV node before the right bundle is totally repolarized from the previous depolarization, the impulse cannot travel through the right bundle normally and the ventricular portion of the complex is widened with a RBBB configuration.

A second electrocardiographic feature suggesting SVT with aberrancy is ectopic beats that occur after a short RR interval preceded by a long RR interval. Refractory time of the bundles varies directly with the interval between ventricular depolarizations. That is, the longer the R-R interval, the longer the refractory period that follows it (Karnes, 1987). The R wave after

the short interval is likely to be conducted aberrantly, displaying a RBBB morphology. Aberrancy caused by R-R interval variation is termed *Ashman's phenomenon*. It is often seen in association with atrial fibrillation because of the irregularity of the rhythm with long RR intervals frequently followed by short RR intervals. The Ashman phenomenon may also occur during sinus arrhythmias with pronounced RR interval variation or with PACs that have a short coupling interval.

Aberrancy may also be suggested by recognition of a P wave superimposed on the T wave preceding the QRS complex (Petrie, 1988). SVT with aberrancy is likely if P wave and QRS rate and rhythm are linked to suggest that ventricular activation depends on atrial discharge (Zipes, 1992). In postoperative cardiac surgical patients, an atrial electrogram may unmask the presence of P waves preceding and linked to each QRS complex. Other electrocardiographic manifestations suggesting SVT with aberrancy are listed in Table 25-1.

Table 25-2 lists those features that favor a diagnosis of VT. A ventricular origin is more likely if QRS duration is more than 0.14 second, unless the patient has preexisting bundle branch block (Drew, 1987) (Fig. 25-12). Other characteristic electrocardiographic manifestations of isolated ventricular complexes include a left bundle branch morphology, full compensatory pauses, a fixed coupling interval, and multiform complexes. VT is most easily confirmed by identification of AV dissociation. Although AV dissociation does not always occur with VT, its presence strongly suggests a ventricular origin (Zipes, 1992). An atrial electrogram may reveal an independent atrial rhythm that is obscured on the surface ECG. The presence of capture or fusion beats also provides evidence of AV dissociation and a ventricular origin of the tachycardia (Jacobson, 1989b).

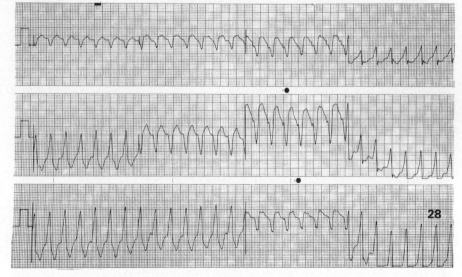

FIGURE 25-12. Twelve-lead ECG demonstrating ventricular tachycardia. Findings suggestive of the diagnosis include a QRS complex duration greater than 0.14 second and a left bundle branch block configuration. (Courtesy of Richard Davison, M.D.)

TABLE 25-2. ELECTROCARDIOGRAPHIC FEATURES FAVORING VENTRICULAR ORIGIN OF ARRHYTHMIA

Isolated Complexes

Rr morphology in V_1
QS or rS morphology in V_6
Initial deflection opposite that of sinus complex
Multiformed complexes
Full compensatory pause after widened complex
Fixed coupling interval in atrial fibrillation
Identical ectopic complexes in sinus rhythm and atrial fibrillation
Short cycle preceding ectopic coupling interval
QRS > 0.14 second

Tachycardia

AV dissociation
Extreme axis deviation ($+180°$ to $-90°$)
Presence of fusion or capture beats
Left bundle branch block pattern
All precordial leads either negative or positive

(Adapted from Housestaff Manual for Cardiothoracic Surgery. Northwestern University Medical School, 1994)

REFERENCES

Conover MB, 1992: Atrial beats and rhythms. In Understanding Electrocardiography, ed. 6. St. Louis, Mosby–Year Book

Cooper J, Marriott HJ, 1989: Why are so many critical care nurses unable to recognize ventricular tachycardia in the 12-lead electrocardiogram? Heart Lung 18:243

DeAngelis R, 1991: The cardiovascular system. In Alspach JG (ed): Core Curriculum for Critical Care Nursing, ed. 4. Philadelphia, WB Saunders

Drew BJ, 1987: Differentiation of wide QRS complex tachycardias. Prog Cardiovasc Nurs 2:130

Drew BJ, 1991: Bedside diagnosis of wide QRS tachycardia. Crit Care Nurs Q 14:19

Erickson BA, 1991: Dysrhythmias. In Kinney MR, Packa DR, Andreoli KG, Zipes DP (eds): Comprehensive Cardiac Care, ed. 7. St. Louis, Mosby–Year Book

Finkelmeier BA, Salinger MH, 1984: The atrial electrogram: Its diagnostic use following cardiac surgery. Crit Care Nurse 4:42

Glasser SP, 1989: Ventricular dysrhythmias. In Henning RJ, Grenvik A (eds): Critical Care Cardiology. New York, Churchill Livingstone

Goldberger E, 1990a: Disorders of cardiac rhythm. In Essentials of Clinical Cardiology. Philadelphia, JB Lippincott

Goldberger E, 1990b: The cardiac arrhythmias. In Treatment of Cardiac Emergencies, ed. 5. St. Louis, CV Mosby

Gray RJ, Mandel WJ, 1990: Management of common postoperative arrhythmias. In Gray RJ, Matloff JM (eds): Medical Management of the Cardiac Surgical Patient. Baltimore, Williams & Wilkins

Hillis LD, Lange RA, Wells PJ, Winniford MD, 1992a: Sinus tachycardia, sinus bradycardia, and sinus arrhythmia. In Manual of Clinical Problems in Cardiology, ed. 4. Boston, Little, Brown

Hillis LD, Lange RA, Wells PJ, Winniford MD, 1992b: Premature beats. In Manual of Clinical Problems in Cardiology, ed. 4. Boston, Little, Brown

Hillis LD, Lange RA, Wells PJ, Winniford MD, 1992c: Atrial flutter. In Manual of Clinical Problems in Cardiology, ed. 4. Boston, Little, Brown

Hillis LD, Lange RA, Wells PJ, Winniford MD, 1992d: Ventricular tachycardia and ventricular fibrillation. In Manual of Clinical Problems in Cardiology, ed. 4. Boston, Little, Brown

Iskandrian AE, 1991: Sinus tachycardia. In Horowitz LN (ed): Current Management of Arrhythmias. Philadelphia, BC Decker

Jacobson C, 1989a: Basic arrhythmias and conduction disturbances. In Underhill SL, Woods SL, Froelicher ES, Halpenny CJ (eds): Cardiac Nursing, ed. 2. Philadelphia, JB Lippincott

Jacobson C, 1989b: Complex arrhythmias and conduction disturbances. In Underhill SL, Woods SL, Froelicher ES, Halpenny CJ (eds): Cardiac Nursing, ed. 2. Philadelphia, JB Lippincott

Karnes N, 1987: Differentiation of aberrant ventricular conduction from ventricular ectopic beats. Crit Care Nurse 7:56

Kastor JA, 1991: Supraventricular tachyarrhythmias. In Horowitz LN (ed): Current Management of Arrhythmias. Philadelphia, BC Decker

Lazarus M, Nolasco V, Luckett C, 1988: Cardiac arrhythmias: Diagnosis and treatment. Crit Care Nurse 8:57

McGuire LB, 1982: Cardiac rhythms. In Beckwith JR: Basic Electrocardiography and Vectorcardiography. New York, Raven Press

Nelson WP, 1989: Supraventricular dysrhythmias. In Henning RJ, Grenvik A (eds): Critical Care Cardiology. New York, Churchill Livingstone

Petrie JR, 1988: Distinguishing supraventricular aberrancies from ventricular ectopy. Focus Crit Care 15:15

Smith PK, 1990: Postoperative care in cardiac surgery. In Sabiston DC, Spencer FC (eds): Surgery of the Chest, ed. 5. Philadelphia, WB Saunders

Smith TW, Braunwald E, Kelly RA, 1992: The management of heart failure. In Braunwald E (ed): Heart Disease: A Textbook of Cardiovascular Medicine, ed. 4. Philadelphia, WB Saunders

Strong AG, 1991: Nursing management of postoperative dysrhythmias. Crit Care Clin North Am 3:709

Waldo AL, MacLean WA, 1980: Diagnosis of cardiac arrhythmias following open heart surgery. In Diagnosis and Treatment of Cardiac Arrhythmias Following Open Heart Surgery. Mount Kisco, NY, Futura Publishing

Wilkinson DV, 1991: Supraventricular premature complexes. In Horowitz LN (ed): Current Management of Arrhythmias. Philadelphia, BC Decker

Zipes DP, 1992: Specific arrhythmias: Diagnosis and treatment. In Braunwald E (ed): Heart Disease: A Textbook of Cardiovascular Medicine, ed. 4. Philadelphia, WB Saunders

CHAPTER 26

TEMPORARY PACING AND DEFIBRILLATION

TEMPORARY PACING

Temporary pacing is an important modality for treating postoperative cardiac arrhythmias. Bradycardia and, in some instances, tachycardia can often be effectively managed with pacing therapy. Goals that can be achieved include one or more of the following: (1) augmentation of cardiac output by increasing heart rate, (2) provision of a safe minimum heart rate, (3) provision of atrioventricular (AV) synchrony, and (4) suppression of arrhythmias. Temporary pacing can be initiated and discontinued rapidly and avoids the adverse effects of antiarrhythmic medications. It may be used alone or in combination with pharmacologic therapy.

COMPONENTS OF THE SYSTEM

The components of temporary pacing systems include pacing leads, a connecting cable, and a pulse generator. The pacing leads and connecting cable provide a pathway between the external pulse generator and the myocardium. Through this pathway, stimulating current travels to the heart and sensed depolarization signals travel to the pulse generator. In patients who undergo cardiac surgical procedures, pacing leads consist of insulated, flexible wires attached to the epicardial surfaces of the right atrium and ventricle (Fig. 26-1). In addition to their therapeutic purpose, atrial pacing wires may also be used diagnostically to obtain atrial electrograms for arrhythmia identification. Atrial electrograms are discussed in Chapter 24, Twelve-Lead Electrocardiography and Atrial Electrograms.

Each pacing wire has an electrode (i.e., electrically conductive material) located at its epicardial end. The electrode is positioned securely in the atrial or ventricular myocardium yet can be easily removed when traction is applied to the external end of the pacing wire. Two electrodes are required to complete the electrical circuit, a pacing and an indifferent electrode. If both electrodes are located in the chamber to be paced, the system is termed *bipolar*. If only the pacing electrode is attached to the chamber being paced, the system is *unipolar*.

By convention, pacing wires attached to the atrial epicardium are brought out through the chest wall to the right of the sternotomy incision (i.e., the patient's right side) and ventricular wires are brought out to the left of the incision (Fig. 26-2). A ground wire is usually placed in the subcutaneous tissue for use as an indifferent electrode. Ground wires are usually of a different color than pacing wires or are identified by a small clip attached to the wire. If emergent pacing becomes necessary in the absence of a second epicardial or a ground wire, a 21-gauge needle inserted tangentially through the subcutaneous tissue may alternatively be used as the indifferent electrode (Moreno-Cabral et al., 1988).

The pulse generator provides the power source. It

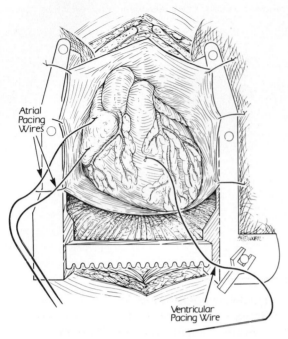

FIGURE 26-1. Placement of atrial and ventricular pacing wires on the epicardial surface of heart. (Finkelmeier BA, O'Mara SR, 1984: Temporary pacing in the cardiac surgical patient. Crit Care Nurs 4:109)

is programmed to discharge electric current of sufficient strength to depolarize myocardial tissue. Pacing is achieved by connecting the epicardial wire from the cardiac chamber to be paced to the negative pole of the connecting cable. A second wire from the same chamber or a ground wire is attached to the positive

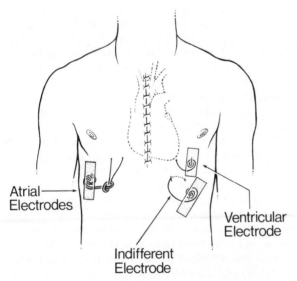

FIGURE 26-2. Position of atrial and ventricular pacing wires and indifferent electrode on chest wall after sternotomy incision has been closed. (Finkelmeier BA, O'Mara SR, 1984: Temporary pacing in the cardiac surgical patient. Crit Care Nurse 4:109)

terminal. The connecting cable is in turn attached to the pulse generator, with negative and positive terminals correctly matched with those of the pulse generator. Three types of external pulse generators are used for temporary pacing in cardiac surgical patients: (1) single chamber, (2) dual chamber, and (3) rapid atrial pulse generators.

PACING MODES

A coding system devised by the North American Society of Pacing and Electrophysiology (NASPE) and British Pacing and Electrophysiology Group (BPEG) provides standard nomenclature for describing pulse generator functions (Bernstein et al., 1987). The NBG (NASPE/BPEG generic) pacemaker code comprises five categories that define *pacing mode* or type of pulse generator function (Table 26-1). The letter in the first position signifies the chamber in which pacing can occur. "A" signifies atrial pacing only; "V", ventricular pacing only; and "D", pacing in both atrial and ventricular chambers. Similarly, the letter "A," "V," or "D" in the second position denotes chambers in which sensing of intrinsic cardiac activity occurs. The letter "O" signifies that sensing is not possible in either chamber. Pulse generator response to sensed cardiac activity is designated by the letter in the third position. "I" signifies that sensed activity inhibits the pulse generator from firing; "T", that intrinsic atrial activity produces a triggered ventricular pacing impulse; and "D", that both inhibited and triggered responses can occur. The fourth and fifth categories describe programmability and antitachycardia functions and are often omitted in routine clinical practice (Teplitz, 1991).

SINGLE-CHAMBER PACING

Indications

Single-chamber pacing is used to provide a consistent minimum heart rate while avoiding undesirable effects of chronotropic medications. Either atrial or ventricular pacing may be performed, using a pulse generator designed for single-chamber pacing (Fig. 26-3). If AV nodal function is normal, atrial pacing is preferable to ventricular pacing because AV synchrony and the atrial contribution to ventricular filling are preserved.

Temporary *atrial pacing* is performed in patients with sinus bradycardia and normal AV nodal function. It may also be used to augment cardiac output by increasing heart rate in patients with normal sinus rhythm and impaired left ventricular function. A heart rate of 90 beats per minute is generally considered optimal during the early postoperative period (Bojar, 1989). In addition, atrial pacing is occasionally used to suppress premature atrial or ventricular complexes. Pacing the atrium is ineffective in the presence of atrial flutter, atrial fibrillation, or AV nodal dysfunction (Lynn-McHale et al., 1991).

TABLE 26-1. THE NASPE/BPEG GENERIC (NBG) PACEMAKER CODE

I Chamber(s) Paced	II Chamber(s) Sensed	III Mode of Response	IV Programmable Functions	V Special Tachyarrhythmia Functions
O—None	O—None	O—None	O—None	O—None
A—Atrium	A—Atrium	T—Triggered	P—Simple programmable	P—Pacing
V—Ventricle	V—Ventricle	I—Inhibited	M—Multiprogrammable	S—Shock
D—Dual	D—Dual	D—Dual	C—Communicating	D—Dual
			R—Rate modulation	

(Adapted from Bernstein AD, Camm AJ, Fletcher RD, et al, 1987: The NASPE/BPEG generic pacemaker code for antibradyarrhythmia and adaptive-rate pacing and antitachyarrhythmia devices. PACE 10:794)

Single-chamber *ventricular pacing* is probably the most common form of temporary pacing in cardiac surgical patients. It is typically used to ensure an adequate heart rate in the presence of AV nodal dysfunction or intermittent sinus bradycardia. Other indications for ventricular pacing include suppression of ventricular ectopy and prophylaxis against profound bradycardia during the early hours after cardiac surgery or when administering medications that slow heart rate or AV conduction. Ventricular pacing is also used when atrial or AV sequential pacing is precluded by chronic atrial fibrillation, intermittent supraventricular tachycardia (SVT), or the absence of atrial epicardial wires.

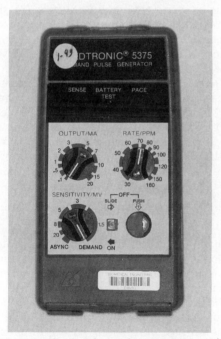

FIGURE 26-3. Single-chamber pulse generator used for temporary atrial or ventricular pacing.

Technique of Pacing

Atrial pacing is performed by attaching an atrial epicardial wire to the negative terminal of the connecting cable and another atrial wire, or a ground wire, to the positive terminal. Atrial pacing is most reliable when a bipolar system is used. Ventricular pacing can be achieved with either a bipolar (two ventricular wires) or unipolar (one ventricular wire and one ground wire) system.

Three settings are programmed when using a single-chamber pulse generator: heart rate, output, and sensitivity. Generally, the pacing rate is ordered by the physician depending on the patient's individual needs. The nurse usually determines the correct output and sensitivity settings for a particular patient. The *output setting* controls the amount of current, measured in milliamperes (mA), that is delivered to the heart with each pacemaker discharge. The correct setting for pulse generator output is established by determining the patient's *stimulation threshold*, defined as the minimum intensity of current needed to produce consistent depolarization of myocardial cells (Finkelmeier & O'Mara, 1984).

To ascertain threshold, the output dial is set between 5 and 10 mA and the pacing rate is temporarily adjusted to exceed the patient's intrinsic heart rate. When this has been accomplished, the monitor should display a 100% paced cardiac rhythm with each pacing artifact immediately followed by an appropriate depolarization (i.e., *1:1 capture*). While the monitor is being observed, pulse generator output is gradually decreased until a loss of capture occurs, evidenced by the appearance of a pacing artifact that is not followed by a cardiac depolarization. The setting at which loss of capture occurs is the patient's stimulation threshold.

Threshold varies depending on the site of electrode placement and the state of the myocardium. Because threshold can be expected to increase over time due to fibrosis at the electrode–myocardium interface, output is set two to three times higher than the patient's threshold and is remeasured daily. However, if the patient's intrinsic heart rate is rapid or the underlying rhythm is unstable, it may be preferable to defer daily measurements after establishing a safe milliamperage setting. Epicardial wires are generally very reliable, and an arbitrary setting of 10 to 15 mA is likely to produce consistent capture for 1 to 2 weeks. If high milliamperage settings are required, pacing discharges may cause an unpleasant twinge of pain or diaphragmatic pacing, evidenced by epigastric twitching or hiccoughs at a rate equal to the pacing rate (Finkelmeier & O'Mara, 1984).

The *sensitivity setting* controls the pulse generator's ability to recognize intracardiac electrical activity (Finkelmeier & Salinger, 1986). Voltage of a specified level is detected and evokes a pulse generator response. Single-chamber pulse generators are capable only of *inhibition* in response to a sensed cardiac event. That is, a sensed depolarization in the atrium or ventricle inhibits delivery of a pacing discharge to that chamber. Pacing modes that provide an inhibition response to sensed depolarizations are referred to as *demand* or *synchronous modes.*

Sensing threshold is the level at which intrinsic cardiac activity is recognized by the sensing electrode (Haskin, 1989). The less sensitive the pulse generator, the higher the voltage of cardiac depolarization necessary for sensing by the pulse generator. Sensing threshold can be determined in a manner similar to determination of stimulation threshold. After the output setting is established, sensitivity is adjusted to a medium setting and the pacing rate is decreased to a level below the patient's intrinsic heart rate. Pulse generator sensitivity is then gradually decreased (by increasing the millivoltage level required for sensing) until an inappropriately premature pacing artifact appears on the monitor, indicating failure of the pulse generator to sense an intrinsic cardiac depolarization.

The setting at which this occurs is the patient's sensing threshold. Once this level is determined, pulse generator sensitivity is increased beyond this point (i.e., by decreasing the millivoltage of intrinsic depolarizations that will inhibit pulse generator firing). It is usually not necessary to individualize the sensitivity setting for each patient. Often, a setting of 1 to 2 millivolts (mV) is chosen unless there is evidence that improper sensing occurs at this level. Adjustment of sensitivity threshold is also omitted if the patient's heart rate is less than 60 beats per minute.

Because atrial depolarizations (P waves) are of low amplitude, they are not accurately sensed for appropriate pulse generator inhibition. Therefore, synchronous temporary pacing of the atrium (AAI) is usually not successful. Instead, an AOO (atrial pacing, nonsensing) pacing mode is used; that is, the sensitivity setting is set in the off position. Since atrial sensing is absent, competition will occur between intrinsic and paced rhythms if rates are nearly the same. In such cases, atrial pacing is terminated or the pacing rate is increased until the intrinsic heart rhythm is suppressed. Delivery of an atrial pacing impulse during atrial repolarization is not dangerous but can induce atrial fibrillation.

When pacing the ventricle, the pulse generator is almost always set in a synchronous, or demand (VVI), mode to avoid pacemaker discharge during ventricular repolarization (R on T phenomenon). The pulse generator is inhibited unless the patient's intrinsic heart rate falls below the pacing rate. Thus, pacing occurs only when the pulse generator senses absence of intrinsic ventricular activity. If the patient has an inadequate underlying ventricular rhythm (heart rate < 50 beats per minute), an asynchronous setting may be desirable to avoid profound bradycardia that might occur in the event of failure of the sensing function.

DUAL-CHAMBER PACING

Indications

Dual-chamber pacing (i.e., sequential pacing of the atrium and ventricle) provides significant hemodynamic benefits in certain clinical situations. As compared with ventricular pacing, dual-chamber pacing has been shown to improve cardiac output in patients with normal ventricular function, as well as in those with valvular heart disease, impaired ventricular function, recent cardiac surgery, and myocardial infarction (Finkelmeier & Salinger, 1986). An appropriately timed atrial contraction preceding each ventricular contraction improves cardiac output through several mechanisms: (1) atrial systole increases ventricular filling, (2) the atria empty more completely, resulting in increased venous return, (3) appropriately timed closing of the mitral and tricuspid valves prevents regurgitation across open valves during ventricular systole, and (4) retrograde activation of the atria is avoided.

AV sequential pacing is most commonly performed in patients with AV nodal dysfunction in whom it is important to preserve the atrial contribution to cardiac output. It may also restore AV synchrony in patients with junctional tachycardia. AV sequential pacing is not suitable for patients with atrial flutter or atrial fibrillation because successful capture of the atria by the pulse generator is not possible.

Two external pulse generators are available for temporary dual-chamber pacing (Fig. 26-4). The two pulse generators differ in the degree of programmable options. Both devices contain atrial pacing circuits, a programmable AV interval, and ventricular pacing circuitry that is inhibited by intrinsic R waves; the more complex of the two dual-chamber pulse generators also contains circuitry for atrial sensing and triggering of ventricular pacing impulses in response to sensed atrial events (Ferguson & Cox,

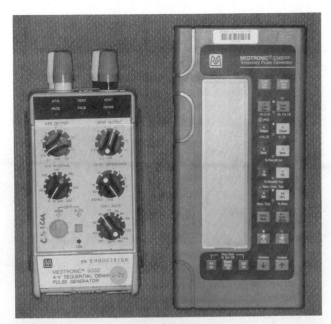

FIGURE 26-4. Two pulse generator models used for temporary dual-chamber pacing.

1991). Dual-chamber pulse generators have two sets of terminals so that pacing and indifferent electrodes for both the atria and ventricles can be attached.

DVI Pacing

The more commonly used of the two pulse generators (Medtronic model 5330) is designed to provide AV sequential pacing in a DVI mode. With DVI pacing the atrium can be paced but atrial activity is not sensed. The ventricular electrode paces the ventricle, and intrinsic ventricular activity is sensed (Goldberger, 1990a). When the intrinsic ventricular rate is less than the pacing rate, the atrium and ventricle are stimulated sequentially (Fig. 26-5). If a paced atrial depolarization is conducted, producing an intrinsic ventricular depolarization, the ventricular pacing dis-

charge is inhibited. Sensing of intrinsic ventricular activity inhibits and resets timing circuits of both atrial and ventricular channels. Because atrial sensing is absent, intrinsic P waves not associated with the atrial pacing impulse may occur (Haskin, 1989).

As with single-chamber pacing, adjustable parameters include heart rate, ventricular output, and ventricular sensitivity. However, two additional settings are programmed to provide AV sequential pacing: atrial output and AV interval. The *atrial output* controls the amount of current delivered to the atrium. Atrial stimulation threshold can be determined in the same manner as is ventricular threshold. The *AV interval setting* allows adjustment of the time interval between delivery of atrial and ventricular pacing discharges. The programmed AV interval simulates the PR interval of an intrinsic cardiac depolarization. The optimal AV interval is thought to be 150 to 175 milliseconds (ms) but may differ from patient to patient and may depend on the selected heart rate (Smith, 1990). Often, the AV interval setting is arbitrarily set at approximately 150 ms (0.15 second). This setting falls within the limits of the normal PR interval (120–200 ms or 0.12–0.20 second).

DDD Pacing

A second, and more complex, temporary dual-chamber pulse generator (Medtronic model 5345) is also available. It is capable of a triggered response to sensed cardiac events. Consequently, it can be used not only for DVI pacing but also for pacing in a DDD mode. This newer, and less commonly used, dual-chamber pulse generator provides *rate modulation,* or the capacity to respond to changing physiologic demands by increasing or decreasing heart rate. It may be preferable in patients with AV nodal dysfunction but normal sinus node function. Rate modulation is achieved by *atrial tracking,* which is the triggering of a ventricular pacing impulse in response to sensed atrial depolarizations. Rate modulation may provide an important contribution to cardiac output in selected patients. Whereas AV synchrony plays a sig-

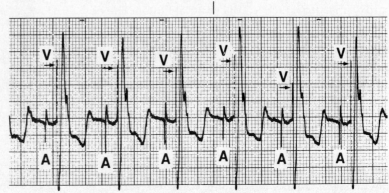

FIGURE 26-5. Electrocardiogram demonstrates AV sequential pacing when the intrinsic pacing rate is less than the programmed pacing rate; *A,* atrial pacing artifact; *V,* ventricular pacing artifact. (Finkelmeier BA, O'Mara SR, 1984: Temporary pacing in the cardiac surgical patient. Crit Care Nurs 4:111)

nificant role in augmenting cardiac output in patients at rest, heart rate becomes the major contributor to cardiac output at higher levels of activity (Fabiszewski & Volosin, 1991)

DDD is the most physiologic of the pacing modes, providing a composite of sensing and pacing in both the atrium and ventricle as required by the patient's underlying rhythm (Kleinschmidt & Stafford, 1991). Either intrinsic or paced atrial depolarizations can occur and are followed by either intrinsically conducted ventricular activity or, in the absence of this, a triggered ventricular pacing discharge. DDD pacing is best suited for use in patients with normal sinus node function, AV nodal dysfunction, and the need for AV synchrony and rate variation according to physiologic needs.

Dual-chamber pacing in a mode that allows atrial tracking requires programming of two additional settings: *upper rate limit* and *total atrial refractory period (TARP)*. The upper rate limit determines the maximum rate of triggered ventricular responses to sensed atrial depolarizations. Establishing an upper rate limit prevents tracking of SVT by activating Wenckebach or 2:1 AV block mechanisms when the intrinsic atrial rate reaches the programmed upper rate limit (Medtronic Technical Manual, 1991).

The TARP is an interval during which the pulse generator is unable to respond to sensed atrial activity. It prevents *pacemaker-mediated tachycardia*, a rapid ventricular paced rhythm that may occur when retrograde ventriculoatrial conduction is sensed and in turn triggers subsequent ventricular pacing discharges. Two settings are adjusted to program the TARP: (1) the AV interval and (2) the *postventricular atrial refractory period* (period after a sensed or paced ventricular event during which sensed atrial activity does not trigger a ventricular response). The programmed TARP should be less than one half of the upper rate limit to prevent development of 2:1 AV block caused by the pulse generator being able to respond to only every other atrial event (Hickey & Baas, 1991).

RAPID ATRIAL PACING

Rapid atrial pacing is used specifically for treatment of paroxysmal atrial tachycardia or atrial flutter. The objectives of rapid atrial pacing are twofold: (1) conversion of the arrhythmia to normal sinus rhythm by overdrive atrial pacing or (2) conversion to atrial fibrillation by stimulating the atrium during the vulnerable phase of atrial repolarization. Atrial fibrillation is more desirable than atrial flutter because the more rapid atrial depolarization rate increases the degree of AV block, thus slowing the ventricular rate. Also, digoxin is more effective in controlling ventricular response rate in atrial fibrillation. In addition, atrial fibrillation induced by rapid atrial pacing is usually transient, lasting only briefly before converting to normal sinus rhythm (Waldo et al., 1984).

Rapid atrial pacing is performed using a pulse generator designed specifically for this purpose (Fig. 26-6). The rapid atrial pulse generator is capable of delivering pacing discharges at rates of up to 800 beats per minute. Because the generator has the capacity for such rapid pacing rates, *it is essential that it is used only with atrial pacing wires*. A ventricular wire is never used, even as the indifferent electrode. Ventricular pacing at such rapid rates would produce ventricular fibrillation and cardiac arrest. Rapid atrial pacing is performed only by physicians who are thoroughly familiar with the procedure.

Two atrial wires or an atrial wire and ground wire are used for rapid atrial pacing. A bedside monitor is always used to allow observation of the electrocardiogram (ECG) during the procedure. An output setting of 15 to 20 mA is generally necessary to achieve atrial capture. The high threshold for atrial capture is presumably due to the relative refractoriness associated with a fast atrial rate (Zoble, 1989).

The rapid atrial pulse generator functions only in an asynchronous mode. With the pulse generator appropriately attached to atrial pacing wires, pacing is initiated at a rate of 80 to 100 beats per minute to ensure that ventricular pacing does not occur. The pulse generator rate is then increased to a rate that is 10% to 15% higher than the intrinsic atrial rate. Atrial capture is evidenced by a change in P wave morphology. However, atrial capture may not be discernible on the ECG. Pacing is usually performed for 15 to 20 seconds and then abruptly terminated; or, alternatively, the rate is gradually reduced (Fig. 26-7). The sequence may be repeated several times if not initially successful in producing sinus rhythm or atrial fibrilla-

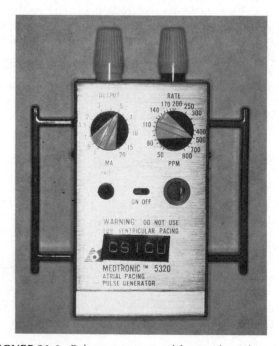

FIGURE 26-6. Pulse generator used for rapid atrial pacing.

FIGURE 26-7. Electrocardiogram demonstrating successful conversion of atrial flutter with rapid atrial pacing: *A*, initiation of pacing at a rate of 450 beats per minute; *B*, termination of pacing is followed by restoration of normal sinus rhythm. (Finkelmeier BA, O'Mara SR, 1984: Temporary pacing in the cardiac surgical patient. Crit Care Nurs 4:110)

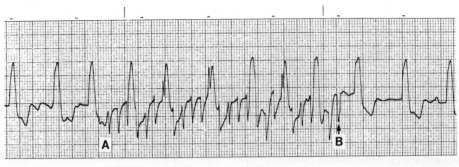

PRINTED IN U.S.A.

tion. Despite conversion with rapid atrial pacing, supraventricular arrhythmias can be expected to persist or recur as long as the responsible stimulus continues (Gray & Mandel, 1990). Therefore, rapid atrial pacing is accompanied by concomitant pharmacologic therapy and is most effective in patients in whom therapeutic serum digoxin levels are present.

PRECAUTIONS AND COMMON PROBLEMS

Although epicardial pacing wires almost never cause morbidity, certain precautions are important to ensure the patient's safety while the wires are in place. Most importantly, epicardial wires provide a pathway by which stray electrical signals can be conducted directly to the myocardium. Therefore, the wires must be electrically isolated to prevent potential ventricular fibrillation caused by stimulation of the myocardium during the vulnerable portion of repolarization. The noninsulated external portion of the pacing wire is covered with a finger cot or nonconductive tape and secured to the chest when not in use. All electric equipment in the patient's environment must be properly grounded and the entire pacing system must be protected from moisture.

Any patient who requires temporary pacing also requires continuous cardiac monitoring, with either a bedside or a telemetry system. Lower alarm rates are set just below the programmed pacing rate so that pacing failure is detected promptly. When temporary pacing is initiated and during any adjustments, bedside monitoring is used so that the cardiac rhythm can be observed while settings on the pulse generator are manipulated. Patients who require temporary pacing for an unstable heart rhythm or profound bradycardia generally remain in a closely monitored unit until the problem resolves or a permanent pacemaker is implanted (Finkelmeier & O'Mara, 1984). An extra pulse generator should be readily available for immediate attachment in the event of pacing failure.

With any type of pacemaker malfunction, the first step is to assess the effect of the malfunction on the patient's hemodynamic status. If the patient is pacemaker dependent, malfunction of the pacing system can lead to cardiac arrest. Cardiopulmonary resuscitation may be necessary if the problem is not immediately corrected or the pulse generator replaced with a

properly functioning unit. More often, problems with temporary pacing systems do not pose an immediate threat to the patient's hemodynamic status. Still, it is important that any dysfunction be promptly corrected to ensure patient safety and obtain maximum benefit from the pacing system.

Two categories of pacemaker malfunction can occur: failure to pace and failure to sense. *Pacing failure* may be categorized as failure to discharge, evidenced on the ECG by the absence of a pacing artifact, or failure to capture, evidenced by a pacing artifact with no resultant depolarization (DeAngelis, 1991) (Fig. 26-8). Pacing failure can result from a variety of factors, such as (1) one of the connections in the system becoming loose, (2) the patient's pacing threshold increasing to a level greater than the current milliamperage setting, (3) pulse generator battery depletion, or (4) disconnection of the pacing wire from the epicardium of the heart.

When pacing failure occurs, all connections from the skin exit site of the pacing wire to the pulse generator itself are examined. The milliamperage setting is increased, and the pacing threshold is remeasured. If these steps fail to correct the problem, the battery and then the cable and pulse generator are replaced. If a DDD pacing mode is being used, adjustment of the pulse width of the pacing impulse may enhance the atrial or ventricular response to the pacing stimulus (Hickey & Baas, 1991).

It is unusual for a previously working system to fail to produce cardiac depolarizations when the milliamperage is adjusted to its maximal setting (20 mA). Inability to correct pacing failure with the above steps probably signifies that the pacing wire is no longer attached to the epicardium, even if it remains secured at the skin surface. If a second epicardial wire attached to the same cardiac chamber is in place, it may be used to replace the failed one. If no other wire is available and the patient requires pacing, *transthoracic* or *transvenous pacing* may be necessary.

In patients with severe cardiogenic shock or cardiac arrest, the electrocardiographic appearance of pacing impulses and resultant depolarizations may occur in the absence of hemodynamic evidence of myocardial contraction or cardiac output (Feeney, 1991). This inability of the myocardium to respond to electrical stimulation is not pacing failure but rather

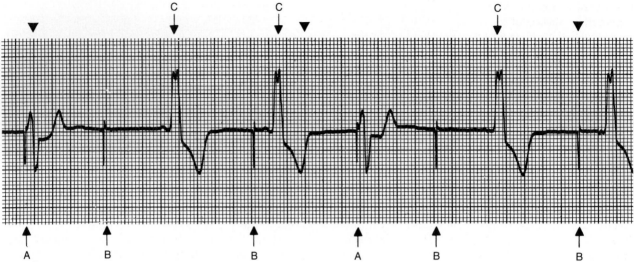

FIGURE 26-8. Only the first and fourth pacing impulses in this rhythm tracing produce appropriate ventricular depolarizations (*A*); failure to pace is demonstrated by pacing impulses that are not followed by ventricular depolarizations (i.e., failure to capture (*B*)); the remaining complexes (*C*) represent intrinsic conduction. (Huff J, Doernbach DP, White RD, 1993: Pacemakers. In ECG Workout, ed. 2, p. 228. Philadelphia, JB Lippincott)

electromechanical dissociation. It is invariably a terminal event.

Two types of sensing failure can occur. *Undersensing* occurs when the pulse generator delivers a pacing impulse before the pacing escape interval. It signifies failure to detect an intrinsic cardiac event (Fig. 26-9). Undersensing is one of the more common types of temporary pacemaker malfunction. If it occurs when the sensitivity dial is adjusted to its most sensitive setting (fully clockwise), the battery, and if necessary the entire pacing system, is changed. Loss of the sensing function is often an early sign of battery depletion (Hickey & Baas, 1991). If battery replacement does not solve the problem, one can replace the wire

currently used as the indifferent lead with another ground wire or, if possible, a pacing wire attached to the same chamber that is being paced. Changing the system from unipolar to bipolar, or vice versa, may correct the problem by providing a different, and larger, electrogram signal for sensing.

Oversensing, on the other hand, occurs when the pulse generator does not deliver a pacing impulse within the escape interval. In this case, pacing has been inappropriately inhibited. The sensitivity dial can be adjusted to decrease pulse generator sensitivity so that sensing of P or T waves, or of noncardiac activity, such as muscle myopotentials or electromagnetic interference, does not inappropriately inhibit

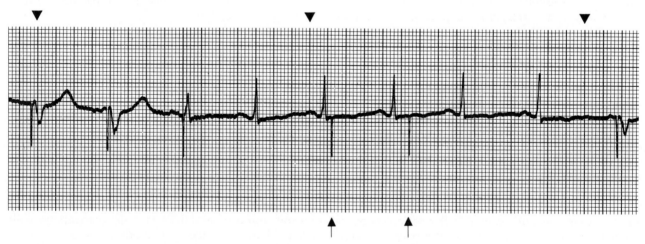

FIGURE 26-9. *Arrows* demonstrate failure to sense intrinsic depolarizations, resulting in inappropriately timed pacing impulses. (Huff J, Doernbach DP, White RD, 1993: Pacemakers. In ECG Workout, ed. 2, p. 222. Philadelphia, JB Lippincott)

delivery of a pacing impulse. If this maneuver fails to correct the problem, all connections are inspected. The battery, and if necessary, the pulse generator and connecting cable, are changed.

A phenomenon known as *pacemaker syndrome* sometimes occurs with VVI pacing in patients who have alternating periods of sinus rhythm and ventricular pacing. It results from intermittent loss of AV synchrony with resultant valvular incompetence and retrograde activation of the atria (Hillis et al., 1992a). Pacemaker syndrome is characterized by a sudden decrease in blood pressure and cardiac output each time the atrial contribution to ventricular filling is lost (Finkelmeier & Salinger, 1986).

Potential problems with temporary, external DDD pacing include (1) obtaining atrial electrode placement that provides effective sensing of P waves and adequate pacing of atrial tissue, (2) the possibility of crosstalk between atrial and ventricular circuits, and (3) the potential for pacemaker-mediated tachycardia (Ferguson & Cox, 1991). *Crosstalk* is inappropriate sensing in one chamber of a pacing discharge or its afterpotential that was intended for the other chamber (Kleinschmidt & Stafford, 1991). The most common form of crosstalk is inappropriate inhibition of ventricular pacing due to sensing of the atrial pacing impulse. It occasionally occurs with AV sequential modes of pacing (DVI, DDD). Crosstalk can often be corrected by decreasing ventricular sensitivity (making the pulse generator less sensitive) or by decreasing amplitude of the atrial pacing impulse (decreasing the atrial output milliamperage setting) (Moungey, 1989).

Pacemaker-mediated tachycardia can occur when AV sequential pacing is performed in patients with intact ventriculoatrial, or retrograde, conduction pathways. It is typically initiated by a paced or spontaneous ectopic ventricular depolarization that is conducted in retrograde fashion, producing atrial depolarization. If the atrial depolarization is sensed by the pulse generator, it triggers a paced ventricular depolarization that is again conducted to the atria, establishing an endless loop tachycardia. Pacemaker-mediated tachycardia is prevented or corrected by lengthening the TARP so that atrial depolarizations produced by retrograde conduction do not trigger ventricular pacing (Finkelmeier & Salinger, 1986).

DEFIBRILLATION

Defibrillation of the heart is the purposeful delivery of an electrical discharge to the heart to simultaneously depolarize the myocardial cells. If defibrillation is successful, the sinus node resumes its role as the dominant pacemaker and normal sinus rhythm ensues. Defibrillation is performed when emergent conversion of an arrhythmia is essential because of profound hypotension or cardiac arrest. Usually, the offending arrhythmia is ventricular tachycardia (VT) or

ventricular fibrillation (VF). Occasionally, SVT with a rapid ventricular response produces hemodynamic compromise. Defibrillation is ineffective in converting asystole. However, a rhythm that appears to be asystole may in fact be a fine VF that may respond to defibrillation.

All nurses caring for cardiac surgical patients should be trained in use of a defibrillator, so that response to a life-threatening arrhythmia is not delayed. Successful conversion of VT or VF is more effective therapy than cardiopulmonary resuscitation. Also, defibrillation is most likely to be successful if performed within 1 to 2 minutes of the onset of VF (Goldberger, 1990b). Paddles are placed on the chest, one just to the right of the sternum and the other on the left midaxillary line at about the fifth interspace (Fig. 26-10). This positioning places most of the heart between the two paddles. All personnel must avoid contact with the patient or bed during defibrillation to avoid accidental shock.

Usually 200 joules of current are used for defibrillation, followed by 300 to 360 joules if the first attempt is unsuccessful (Myerburg & Castellanos, 1992). Cardiopulmonary resuscitation is performed throughout the cardiac arrest, except during defibrillation, until a stable cardiac rhythm is achieved. Repeated electric shocks are delivered, as necessary, in conjunction with other modalities of advanced life support, until a stable cardiac rhythm is restored or a physician pronounces the patient dead.

Defibrillation synchronized to occur during ventricular depolarization, represented by the R wave of the ECG, is termed *cardioversion* or R wave synchronous defibrillation. Synchronized defibrillation reduces the likelihood of inducing VF by stimulating ventricular myocardial cells during the vulnerable

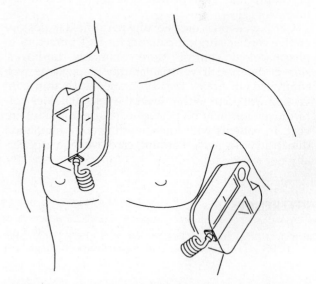

FIGURE 26-10. Standard anterolateral paddle electrode placement for transthoracic defibrillation. (Courtesy of Physio-Control Co., Redmond, WA)

portion of repolarization. Cardioversion is used only for arrhythmias with distinct R waves, such as VT, atrial flutter, or atrial fibrillation. While traditional teaching has been that synchronous cardioversion should always be used for an arrhythmia in which detectable R waves are present, emergent defibrillation may be performed in an unsynchronized mode regardless of the type of arrhythmia. The most important goal in a hemodynamically unstable patient is prompt defibrillation, and using a synchronous setting may delay response time.

Cardioversion is most commonly used for the elective conversion of SVT, most often atrial flutter or atrial fibrillation, or VT in a patient who is hemodynamically stable. If possible, oral intake is withheld for 6 to 8 hours before the procedure. Intravenous access is established, and the patient is placed in a monitored unit. Although the procedure is generally well tolerated, emergency drugs and intubation equipment should be readily accessible. Intravenous diazepam is generally administered to provide amnesia and reduce anxiety.

The cardioverter/defibrillator is placed in a synchronous setting. Electrocardiographic leads are attached to the cardioverter oscilloscope and a lead displaying a tall R wave is selected. It is desirable to use the minimal amount of discharge energy to achieve arrhythmia conversion (Hillis et al., 1992b). Energy requirements vary with the type of arrhythmia. Organized rhythms (e.g., VT or atrial flutter) tend to require less energy than disorganized rhythms (e.g., atrial fibrillation) (Underhill, 1989). As little as 5 joules may be used in the case of atrial flutter; 100 or more joules may be necessary for atrial fibrillation (Goldberger, 1990c). The charge is delivered on the first R wave after depression of the button. If the first electric shock does not convert the arrhythmia, the procedure may be repeated at a higher current setting.

Cardioversion is occasionally performed in postoperative cardiac surgical patients for SVT refractory to pharmacologic control. More commonly, cardioversion is deferred if ventricular rate response is well controlled, in hopes that spontaneous rhythm conversion will occur within several weeks. If it does not, cardioversion may be performed during a follow-up visit. In patients with long-standing atrial fibrillation due to an enlarged left atrium, cardioversion is generally not successful.

REFERENCES

Bernstein AD, Camm AJ, Fletcher RD, et al., 1987: The NASPE/BPEG generic pacemaker code for antibradyarrhythmia and adaptive-rate pacing and antitachyarrhythmia devices. PACE 10:794

Bojar RM, 1989: Cardiovascular management. In Bojar RM (ed): Manual of Perioperative Care in Cardiac and Thoracic Surgery. Boston, Blackwell Scientific Publications

DeAngelis R, 1991: The cardiovascular system. In Alspach JG (ed): Core Curriculum for Critical Care Nursing, ed. 4. Philadelphia, WB Saunders

Fabiszewski R, Volosin KJ, 1991: Rate-modulated pacemakers. J Cardiovasc Nurs 5:21

Feeney MK, 1991: Electrocardiographic interpretation of pacemaker rhythms. AACN Clin Issues Crit Care Nurs 2:159

Ferguson TB, Cox JL, 1991: Temporary external DDD pacing after cardiac operations. Ann Thorac Surg 51:723

Finkelmeier BA, O'Mara SR, 1984: Temporary pacing in the cardiac surgical patient. Crit Care Nurse 4:108

Finkelmeier BA, Salinger MH, 1986: Dual-chamber cardiac pacing: An overview. Crit Care Nurse 6:12

Goldberger E, 1990a: Modes of cardiac pacing. In Treatment of Cardiac Emergencies, ed. 5. St. Louis, CV Mosby

Goldberger E, 1990b: Defibrillation and cardioversion. In: Treatment of Cardiac Emergencies, ed. 5. St. Louis, CV Mosby

Goldberger E, 1990c: Cardiac pacing and cardioversion. In Essentials of Clinical Cardiology. Philadelphia, JB Lippincott

Gray RJ, Mandel WJ, 1990: Management of common postoperative arrhythmias. In Gray RJ, Matloff JM (eds): Medical Management of the Cardiac Surgical Patient. Baltimore, Williams & Wilkins

Haskin JB, 1989: Pacemakers. In Underhill SL, Woods SL, Froelicher ES, Halpenny J (eds): Cardiac Nursing, ed. 2. Philadelphia, JB Lippincott

Hickey CS, Baas LS, 1991: Temporary cardiac pacing. AACN Clin Issues Crit Care Nurs 2:107

Hillis LD, Lange RA, Wells PJ, Winniford MD, 1992a: Temporary and permanent pacing. In Manual of Clinical Problems in Cardiology, ed. 4. Boston, Little, Brown

Hillis LD, Lange RA, Wells PJ, Winniford MD, 1992b: Cardioversion. In Manual of Clinical Problems in Cardiology, ed. 4. Boston, Little, Brown

Kleinschmidt KM, Stafford MJ, 1991: Dual-chamber cardiac pacemakers. J Cardiovasc Nurs 5:9

Lynn-McHale DJ, Riggs KL, Thurman L, 1991: Epicardial pacing after cardiac surgery. Crit Care Nurse 11:62

Medtronic Model 5345 Pulse Generator Technical Manual, 1991. Minneapolis, Medtronic

Moreno-Cabral CE, Mitchell RS, Miller DC, 1988: Postoperative problems. In Manual of Postoperative Management in Adult Cardiac Surgery. Baltimore, Williams & Wilkins

Moungey SJ, 1989: Temporary A-V sequential pacemakers. Prog Cardiovasc Nurs 4:49

Myerburg RJ, Castellanos A, 1992: Cardiac arrest and sudden cardiac death. In Braunwald E (ed): Heart Disease: A Textbook of Cardiovascular Medicine, ed. 4. Philadelphia, WB Saunders

Smith PK, 1990: Postoperative care in cardiac surgery. In Sabiston DC Jr, Spencer FC (eds): Surgery of the Chest, ed. 5. Philadelphia, WB Saunders

Teplitz L, 1991: Classification of cardiac pacemakers: The pacemaker code. J Cardiovasc Nurs 5:1

Underhill SL, 1989: Cardiac arrest and life-threatening arrhythmias without cardiac arrest. In Underhill SL, Woods SL, Froelicher ES, Halpenny J (eds): Cardiac Nursing, ed. 2. Philadelphia, JB Lippincott

Waldo AL, Henthorn RW, Plumb VJ, 1984: Temporary epicardial wire electrodes in the diagnosis and treatment of arrhythmias after open heart surgery. Am J Surg 148:275

Zoble RG, 1989: Cardiac pacing. In Henning RJ, Grenvick A (eds): Critical Care Cardiology. New York, Churchill Livingstone

CHAPTER 27

CARDIOVASCULAR MEDICATIONS

INOTROPIC MEDICATIONS	ANTIANGINAL MEDICATIONS
VASODILATING MEDICATIONS	ANTICOAGULANT, THROMBOLYTIC, AND
ANTIARRHYTHMIC MEDICATIONS	ANTIPLATELET MEDICATIONS
Class I Agents	OTHER SELECTED MEDICATIONS
Class II Agents	Diuretic Agents
Class III Agents	Antihypertensive Agents
Class IV Agents	
Unclassified Agents	

A wide variety of medications are used in the treatment of patients with cardiovascular disease. The discussion in this chapter is limited to summary information about those medications most commonly administered to patients in cardiac surgical settings. For more detailed information concerning pharmacologic actions, precise dosing regimens, and adverse or toxic effects, the reader is referred to a textbook of clinical pharmacology.

INOTROPIC MEDICATIONS

Inotropic medications are those agents that affect contractility of the heart. Because they increase the strength of myocardial contraction at a given point on the Starling curve, increased cardiac output occurs at the same filling pressure, or preload level. Inotropic drugs are most often used for treatment of acute ventricular dysfunction in patients with low cardiac output syndrome or cardiogenic shock. They are commonly administered in cardiac surgical patients because of the transient ventricular impairment that may occur after operations that necessitate cardiopulmonary bypass and cardioplegic arrest of the heart.

A number of medications are categorized as inotropic agents (Table 27-1). They differ in intensity of

action as well as in the other cardiac and systemic effects they produce. With knowledge of the types of actions associated with each agent, choice of the most appropriate drug may be individualized to the specific patient and clinical situation. Sometimes more than one inotrope is infused to take advantage of particular actions of each agent. Often, inotropic drugs are used in combination with a pharmacologic vasodilating agent or intra-aortic balloon counterpulsation to provide concomitant afterload reduction. Most inotropic agents are given by continuous intravenous infusion. Central venous catheters and rate-regulating pumps are almost always used to ensure consistent delivery of a precise dosage. Constant hemodynamic monitoring and close nursing observation are necessary during administration of these potent agents.

Most inotropes act by stimulating *sympathetic*, or *adrenergic*, *receptors* of the autonomic nervous system. Although the heart is innervated by both subdivisions (sympathetic and parasympathetic) of the autonomic nervous system, it is predominantly under sympathetic control. Two types of sympathetic receptor sites exist. The first, alpha-adrenergic receptors, are subclassified as alpha-1 or alpha-2; the second, beta-adrenergic receptors, are subclassified as beta-1 or beta-2. These receptors sites are responsive to endogenously released substances called *catecholamines*

Betsy Finkelmeier: CARDIOTHORACIC SURGICAL NURSING.
© 1995 J.B. Lippincott Company.

TABLE 27-1. COMMONLY USED INOTROPIC AND VASODILATING AGENTS

Drug	Concentration*	Infusion Rate
Inotropes		
Amrinone	250 mg	5–10 μg/kg/min
Dobutamine	250–500 mg	2–10 μg/kg/min
Dopamine	200–400 mg	1–2 μg/kg/min (dopaminergic)
		2–5 μg/kg/min (beta)
		5–10 μg/kg/min (alpha/beta)
Epinephrine	1–2 mg	0.01–0.1 μg/kg/min
Isoproterenol	1–2 mg	0.01–0.1 μg/kg/min
Norepinephrine	1–2 mg	0.01–0.1 μg/kg/min
Vasodilators		
Nitroglycerin	50–100 mg	0.3–3.0 μg/kg/min
Nitroprusside	75–150 mg	0.3–3.0 μg/kg/min

* Amount of drug in 250-mL solution.

that function as neurotransmitters and hormones (Abrams, 1991a).

Sympathetic receptors are located throughout the body. Table 27-2 lists those that influence cardiovascular hemodynamic functioning. Agents that are primarily *alpha-adrenergic agonists,* or stimulators, predominantly cause peripheral vasoconstriction without cardiac enhancement; *beta-adrenergic agonists* increase heart rate and myocardial contractility and cause peripheral vasodilatation (Elefteriades & Geha, 1985a). Norepinephrine, epinephrine, and dopamine are naturally occurring catecholamines that may be administered as pharmacologic inotropes to affect adrenergic receptors. Dobutamine and isoproterenol are examples of *sympathomimetic drugs* (i.e., synthetic agents that act on adrenergic receptors in the same manner as catecholamines). Amrinone, a more recently released inotropic agent, has actions not related to adrenergic stimulation.

Dopamine, an endogenous catecholamine, is often the initial drug chosen for inotropic support of the heart. It is usually administered in a dosage range between 1 and 10 μg/kg/min and has alpha-adrenergic, beta-adrenergic, and dopaminergic effects, depending on the dosage. In low doses, such as less than 2 μg/kg/min, *dopaminergic* effects predominate, causing increased renal blood flow and improved renal function. More commonly, dopamine is given in larger doses (2–5 μg/kg/min) for its beta-adrenergic actions, which increase myocardial contractility. When doses of 7 to 10 μg/kg/min are administered, alpha-adrenergic (vasoconstrictive) effects of dopamine dominate, producing increased systemic vascular resistance and blood pressure (DiSesa, 1991). Accordingly, a vasodilating agent is generally administered concomitantly when higher doses of dopamine are used. The major limiting factor in the use of dopamine is the frequently associated tachycardia. If the patient's heart rate is consistently greater than 110 beats per minute, substitution of another inotropic agent may be desirable. Dopamine may also cause ventricular tachyarrhythmias (Bank & Kubo, 1991). Extravasation of the drug causes local tissue necrosis that can lead to digit loss.

Dobutamine, a synthetic catecholamine, is also used commonly to increase contractility. It differs from dopamine in that its physiologic actions do not vary with dosage. Dobutamine acts primarily on beta-1-

TABLE 27-2. SYMPATHETIC RECEPTOR SITES AFFECTING CARDIOVASCULAR FUNCTION

Receptor	Site	Stimulation Response
Alpha-1	Vascular smooth muscle	Vasoconstriction
Alpha-2	Presynaptic nerve terminals	Inhibits norepinephrine release
Beta-1	Myocardium	Positive inotropic action
		Positive chronotropic action
Beta-2	Arterioles	Vasodilation
	Bronchioles	Bronchodilation

(Adapted from Abrams AC, 1991: Physiology of autonomic nervous system. In Clinical Drug Therapy, ed. 3. Philadelphia, JB Lippincott) adrenergic receptors in the myocardium and to a limited degree on beta-2-receptors and alpha-receptors (Phelan & Klein, 1991). It has little effect on systemic vascular resistance and does not increase renal blood flow (Bond & Underhill, 1990; Smith et al., 1992). Dobutamine does not generally produce tachycardia to the same degree as dopamine but, like dopamine, it can cause ventricular arrhythmias.

Isoproterenol is a pure beta-adrenergic agonist medication. It increases heart rate (positive chronotropic action), increases contractility, and decreases systemic vascular resistance. Because of its vasodilating action, the drug may be safely infused in a peripheral catheter and a separate agent to reduce afterload is not necessary. Isoproterenol produces pulmonary as well as systemic vasodilatation. Consequently, it is effective in decreasing pulmonary vascular resistance, making it a particularly useful agent in patients with chronic pulmonary hypertension or acute right-sided heart failure (Elefteriades & Geha, 1985a). Isoproterenol is a good inotropic choice in bradycardic patients who can benefit from its chronotropic effect. Conversely, its use is limited in some situations by the tachycardia and ventricular arrhythmias that may occur. The drug also is thought to increase myocardial oxygen consumption. Therefore, it is generally not used in the presence of acute myocardial ischemia.

Epinephrine is a naturally occurring catecholamine with both alpha- and beta-agonist actions, including (1) increases in contractility, AV nodal and Purkinje fiber conduction, and sinus node firing through stimulation of beta-1 receptors; (2) vasodilatation and bronchodilatation through stimulation of beta-2 receptors; and (3) at higher doses, vasoconstriction through stimulation of alpha-receptors (Stanley, 1991). Epinephrine is likely to be chosen when it is desirable to rapidly increase heart rate, blood pressure, and cardiac output (Greco, 1990). Because of its alpha-adrenergic effects, a vasodilating medication is usually concomitantly administered. Epinephrine may also be given as an intravenous bolus or occasionally through an endotracheal tube, to restore spontaneous cardiac activity in patients who experience cardiac arrest. Use of epinephrine is limited by tachycardia caused by its chronotropic effects and by its proarrhythmic potential.

Norepinephrine has both beta-adrenergic and chronotropic actions, but it is principally an alpha-adrenergic agent (Ferguson, 1991). Consequently, it increases systolic and diastolic arterial pressure secondary to peripheral vasoconstriction. Norepinephrine is not useful purely as a positive inotropic agent (Hillis et al., 1992a). Because its vasoconstrictive effect increases afterload, norepinephrine may in fact cause cardiac output to decrease and myocardial work to increase. Therefore, it is generally reserved for profound cardiogenic shock, when other inotropic agents fail to correct severe hypotension. Norepinephrine is also used as the agent of choice to increase the profoundly low systemic vascular resistance associated with septic shock.

Amrinone is an inotropic agent that improves cardiac contractility by inhibiting myocardial cellular phosphodiesterase and increasing availability of calcium in the myocardium (Stanley, 1991). It also produces vasodilatation. Therefore, cardiac output is improved both by increased contractility and decreased afterload (Bond & Underhill, 1990). Studies suggest that amrinone has a synergistic effect when infused in combination with adrenergic inotropic agents (DiSesa, 1991). It is administered in a loading dose of 0.75 mg/kg over 2 to 3 minutes, followed by a maintenance infusion of 5 to 10 μg/kg/min (Bank & Kubo, 1991; Smith et al., 1992). The major disadvantage of amrinone is a high incidence of reversible thrombocytopenia when infused for lengthy periods (Phelan & Klein, 1991).

Calcium chloride is sometimes administered to provide acute inotropic support of the heart. Calcium plays an important role in excitation contraction coupling in the myocardium by interacting with active proteins in muscle to initiate contraction (DiSesa, 1991). An intravenous bolus dose of calcium is often given in patients who become profoundly hypotensive. The enhancement of contractility and resulting improvement in cardiac output is transient but may sustain the patient to allow time for initiation of other supportive therapies. It is administered as an intravenous bolus at a dose of 10 mg/kg.

Digoxin is not useful as an inotropic agent in the acute setting but is widely used for chronic inotropic support of the heart. Preoperative patients with impaired ventricular function may be receiving chronic digitalis therapy. Except in those with acute heart failure, the drug may be discontinued in the immediate preoperative period. Its low therapeutic index combined with potassium shifts that occur intraoperatively make perioperative digoxin toxicity likely (Wong, 1991).

VASODILATING MEDICATIONS

Intravenous *vasodilating agents* are frequently used in cardiac surgical patients to reduce afterload, or the impedance to ejection of blood from the ventricle. Vasodilator therapy is based on the sensitivity of ventricular performance to changes in afterload; with fixed preload, the velocity of cardiac contraction diminishes as afterload increases (Barron & Parrillo, 1991). Left ventricular afterload, measured clinically as systemic vascular resistance, is typically elevated in the early hours after cardiac operations secondary to hypothermia and peripheral vasoconstriction. Pharmacologic afterload reduction may be necessary to maintain adequate cardiac output and prevent worsening ventricular dysfunction due to increased left ventricular work and myocardial oxygen consumption. Vasodilating agents are also commonly used in the early postoperative period to correct hypertension that develops as a consequence of patient emergence from anesthesia, endotracheal suctioning, resistance to mechanical ventilation, or pain (Whitman, 1991). If not corrected promptly, postoperative hypertension may cause excessive mediastinal bleeding.

Because both coronary artery disease and valvular heart disease more often damage the left ventricle, left ventricular dysfunction is more common. Consequently, it is usually left ventricular afterload, or systemic vascular resistance, that must be pharmacologically lowered. However, in disorders associated with pulmonary hypertension, such as severe mitral stenosis or postoperative right ventricular failure, agents that lower pulmonary vascular resistance are necessary. The most commonly used intravenous vasodilating agents are nitroglycerin and sodium nitroprusside (see Table 27-1).

Nitroglycerin causes direct relaxation of vascular smooth muscle. It primarily produces venous dilatation, although arterial dilatation may occur at higher doses (Stanley, 1991). The increased volume of the venous capacitance vessels redistributes intravascular blood, effectively reducing preload. Although a less effective afterload-reducing agent than nitroprusside, nitroglycerin provides the added benefit of dilating coronary arteries. It thus increases blood flow through arteries affected by spasm and collateral arteries in areas of myocardium not completely revascularized by coronary artery bypass grafting (Elefteriades & Geha, 1985a). The coronary artery dilatation associated with nitroglycerin also makes it an effective agent for controlling acute myocardial ischemia. Sustained high doses of intravenous nitroglycerin have been associated with a loss of hemodynamic efficacy after 24 to 72 hours of administration (Barron & Parrillo, 1991).

Nitroprusside relaxes vascular smooth muscle, producing almost immediate arterial and venous dilatation. The balanced action lowers both pulmonary and systemic vascular resistances while increasing venous capacitance at the same time (Greco, 1990). The resulting reduction in systemic vascular resistance allows the left ventricle to eject blood more easily, thereby increasing cardiac output. Nitroprusside is quite potent and can produce precipitous, severe hypotension. Also, because cyanogen, cyanide, and thiocyanate are potential breakdown products, cyanate toxicity can occur with high doses or prolonged use (Smith, 1990). Thiocyanate levels are measured intermittently in susceptible patients or if metabolic acidosis or signs of central nervous system dysfunction develop.

Prostaglandin E_1 is a potent pulmonary arterial vasodilating agent that also specifically dilates coronary, renal, and cutaneous vessels (Hendren & Higgins, 1991). The pulmonary vasodilating effects make prostaglandin E_1 useful in patients with right-sided heart failure associated with pulmonary hypertension

(Kelleher et al., 1991). Concomitant norepinephrine infusion may be necessary to compensate for associated systemic vasodilatation caused by the drug.

ANTIARRHYTHMIC MEDICATIONS

Because of the propensity for cardiac arrhythmias in patients who undergo cardiac surgery, any of a number of antiarrhythmic agents may be used. Several considerations are particularly relevant when administering antiarrhythmic agents to cardiac surgical patients. First, many agents have *proarrhythmic actions;* that is, they can actually induce arrhythmias. Second, most antiarrhythmic drugs have negative inotropic effects. Although they may be well tolerated in patients with good ventricular function, they may significantly worsen ventricular function in patients with heart disease, especially when given intravenously (Lewis, 1991). Third, many antiarrhythmic agents alter the thresholds for defibrillation. For example, amiodarone and lidocaine increase defibrillation threshold while bretylium and sotalol decrease threshold (Barold & Zipes, 1992). Antiarrhythmic agents are commonly classified in four categories according to their mechanisms of action (Table 27-3).

CLASS I AGENTS

Class I antiarrhythmic medications are membrane-stabilizing agents. They block the movement of sodium into cardiac conducting cells, thereby stabilizing the cell membrane and decreasing the formation and conduction of electrical impulses (Abrams, 1991b). Class I drugs are subclassified to reflect their predominant effect: (1) class IA agents delay repolarization, thus lengthening action potential; (2) class IB drugs accelerate repolarization, thus shortening action potential; and (3) class IC drugs prolong conduction through the His-Purkinje system (Bond, 1990).

Class IA drugs include quinidine, procainamide, and disopyramide. *Quinidine* is used occasionally in cardiac surgical patients for suppression of supraventricular or ventricular arrhythmias. It has two modes of action: (1) its vagolytic effect enhances conduction through the AV node, and (2) its direct myocardial effect prolongs AV conduction, His-Purkinje conduction times, and the duration of repolarization (Hudak et al., 1990). When using quinidine to treat supraventricular tachycardia (SVT), digoxin is always given beforehand to prevent undesirable acceleration of the ventricular rate due to vagolytic enhancement of AV conduction. However, quinidine administration in digitalized patients increases the serum digitalis level, and the maintenance digoxin dose may need to be reduced to avoid digoxin toxicity (Mandel, 1990). Quinidine usually prolongs the QT interval and, in a small number of patients, causes torsades de pointes, which is a distinctive, polymorphic ventricular tachyarrhythmia (Zipes, 1992).

TABLE 27-3. CLASSIFICATION OF ANTIARRHYTHMIC MEDICATIONS

Class I Membrane-Active Drugs

IA Disopyramide (Norpace)
Procainamide (Pronestyl)
Quinidine (Quinaglute)

IB Lidocaine (Xylocaine)
Mexiletine (Mexitil)
Tocainide (Tonocard)

IC Flecainide (Tambocor)
Propafenone (Rhythmol)

Class II Beta-Adrenergic Blocking Drugs

Atenolol (Tenormin)
Esmolol (Brevibloc)
Propranolol (Inderal)
Metoprolol (Lopressor)
Nadolol (Corgard)
Timolol (Timoptic)

Class III Repolarization Prolonging Drugs

Amiodarone (Cordarone)
Bretylium tosylate (Bretylol)
Sotalol (Betapace)

Class IV Calcium Channel Blocking Drugs

Diltiazem (Cardizem)
Nifedipine (Procardia)
Verapamil (Isoptin)

Unclassified Drugs

Adenosine (Adenocard)
Atropine (Atropine)
Digoxin (Lanoxin)

Quinidine sulfate is administered orally in doses of 200 to 400 mg every 6 hours. Alternatively, a long-acting form, such as quinidine gluconate, may be used. Quinidine is rarely given intravenously because hypotension may result from vasodilatation caused by its alpha-adrenergic blocking effects (Buckingham & Parrillo, 1991). Quinidine is contraindicated in the presence of AV or intraventricular conduction disorders because it slows conduction (Bond, 1990).

Procainamide, an agent similar to quinidine, is occasionally administered by intravenous infusion for ventricular arrhythmias refractory to lidocaine therapy. It works by decreasing rates of conduction through the conducting system and ventricular tissue (Slovis & Brody, 1991). Procainamide is given intravenously at a rate of 100 mg every 5 minutes to a total dose of 500 to 750 mg, followed by a continuous infusion of 2 to 4 mg/min (Kessler et al., 1992). Because procainamide prolongs the QT interval, it may cause serious arrhythmias, such as torsades de pointes or advanced AV block (Moreno-Cabral et al., 1988). *Disopyramide*, another class IA medication, is an oral agent that is sometimes used for chronic treatment of ventricular arrhythmias.

Lidocaine is a class IB drug and is the most commonly used class I antiarrhythmic agent. It is generally accepted as the drug of choice for initial treatment of significant ventricular arrhythmias. It decreases myocardial irritability, or automaticity, in the ventricles with little effect on atrial tissue (Abrams, 1991b). Lidocaine must be given parenterally because significant first-pass hepatic metabolism occurs with oral administration, resulting in unpredictable, low plasma levels and excessive metabolites that can cause toxicity (Zipes, 1992). Lidocaine is administered intravenously, first as a bolus or loading dose (1–1.5 mg/kg) and then by continuous infusion at a rate of 1 to 4 mg/min. Lidocaine acts almost immediately and because of its short half-life must be administered by continuous infusion. Lidocaine toxicity can cause electrocardiographic abnormalities (widening of the PR interval and QRS complex) and a variety of neurologic manifestations, including confusion, seizures, and a depressed level of consciousness (Gahart, 1991a).

Mexiletine and *tocainide* are other class IB agents that are used for treatment of ventricular tachycardia. They have mechanisms of action similar to lidocaine. However, because they do not undergo the significant first-pass hepatic degradation that occurs with lidocaine, they can be administered orally.

Class IC agents include *flecanide* and *propafenone*. These drugs are used infrequently for treatment of life-threatening ventricular tachyarrhythmias refractory to other agents. Flecanide has moderate negative inotropic effects and demonstrated proarrhythmic properties. Propafenone appears to have less of a proarrhythmic effect than flecanide but can cause conduction abnormalities and worsening of heart failure (Zipes, 1992).

CLASS II AGENTS

Class II antiarrhythmic agents are beta-adrenergic blocking medications, such as propranolol, esmolol, and metoprolol. Beta-blocking medications prevent beta-receptors from responding to sympathetic nerve impulses, circulating catecholamines, and beta-adrenergic drugs (Abrams, 1991c). Antiarrhythmic actions of beta-blocking drugs include decreasing (1) heart rate, (2) automaticity in the AV node, and (3) conduction velocity in the atria, AV node, His-Purkinje system, and ventricles (Loveys, 1990).

Beta-blocking agents are sometimes used for treatment of SVT. *Propranolol* is most commonly selected. It may be given in low doses (10 mg orally every 6 hours) as a prophylactic agent to decrease the incidence of postoperative SVT (Smith, 1990). Propranolol may also be used to treat SVT. In patients with atrial fibrillation or atrial flutter, it increases the degree of AV block and reduces heart rate (Hudak et al., 1990). Oral propranolol is given in doses of 10 to 80 mg every 6 hours. Intravenous propranolol may be administered to achieve more rapid ventricular rate control. However, the drug must be injected slowly (0.5–1.0 mg every 5 minutes to maximum of 3 mg) with careful monitoring of blood pressure since it may precipitate profound hypotension. Propranolol is contraindicated in patients with underlying pulmonary disease because its inhibition of beta-2-receptors may cause bronchospasm.

Alternatively, *esmolol* may be used to treat SVT. It is an ultra-short-acting beta-blocking agent that is given by intravenous infusion. Esmolol is an attractive choice in the early postoperative period or in critically ill patients because (1) it is more cardioselective and therefore less likely to produce bronchospasm in patients with mild chronic obstructive pulmonary disease or asthma and (2) its rapid action and metabolic inactivation allow easy control of the magnitude and duration of beta blockade (Blanski et al., 1988). A dose of 500 μg/kg/min is infused for 1 minute, followed by an infusion rate in the range of 50 to 200 μg/kg/min (Loveys, 1990). Hypotension is the most common cardiovascular adverse effect of esmolol; it is most likely to occur within the first 30 minutes after initiating administration of the drug (Morton, 1994). *Metoprolol,* another cardioselective beta-blocking agent, can also be given intravenously (5 mg every 5 minutes to a maximum of three doses) for treatment of postoperative SVT (Antman, 1992). Although not as rapid-acting as esmolol, its effects are more sustained and the patient can be converted to an oral form of the drug. Beta-blocking agents are also sometimes used in patients with ventricular tachycardia to decrease sympathetic tone and the rate of impulse conduction (Slovis & Brody, 1991).

CLASS III AGENTS

Class III antiarrhythmic agents (bretylium tosylate, amiodarone, and sotalol) prolong the action potential duration. *Bretylium* may be given intravenously in postoperative patients for ventricular tachycardia or ventricular fibrillation refractory to suppression with lidocaine therapy. It is administered in intermittent doses (5 to 10 mg/kg) every 15 to 30 minutes (not to exceed 40 mg/kg/d) or as a continuous infusion (1 to 2 mg/min) (Gahart, 1991b). The most significant adverse effect is hypotension, which is usually orthostatic. Hypertension, sinus tachycardia, or other arrhythmias may also occur after initial administration of bretylium (Buckingham & Parrillo, 1991).

Amiodarone, an oral class III agent, is generally considered the most effective antiarrhythmic medication for prevention of recurrent ventricular tachycardia or ventricular fibrillation. A unique feature of amiodarone is its elimination half-life of 30 to 110 days (Hillis et al., 1992b). Because of the drug's long serum half-life, oral therapy is initiated with a loading dose (800 to 1600 mg/d) for 1 to 3 weeks (Abrams, 1991b). Dosage is then gradually reduced to a maintenance dose of 400 mg/d or less. Amiodarone is a very potent medication with a number of quite serious and poten-

tially lethal side effects. Six percent of patients receiving amiodarone develop amiodarone-induced pulmonary toxicity, usually manifested by dyspnea, cough, and new radiographic abnormalities (Dusman et al., 1990). The complication, which can be fatal, is more likely in patients receiving higher maintenance doses and is often reversible if detected promptly. Symptomatic bradycardia, hyperthyroidism, hypothyroidism, and hepatotoxicity can occur in patients receiving amiodarone therapy. Other adverse reactions include corneal microdeposits, photosensitivity, skin pigmentation, and neurologic toxicity (Hudak et al., 1990). Because of its significant side effect profile, it is generally reserved for those patients at high risk for sudden cardiac death or with hemodynamically compromising ventricular tachyarrhythmias in whom other agents are ineffective.

Several considerations are relevant when amiodarone is given to cardiac surgical patients. First, amiodarone has been associated with intraoperative atropine-resistant bradycardia and with vasodilatation and decreased contractility that is not responsive to pharmacologic therapy (Moore & Wilkoff, 1991). Second, life-threatening respiratory failure can develop during the early postoperative period. At particular risk are patients who have had preoperative amiodarone pulmonary toxicity (Nalos et al., 1987). Finally, amiodarone interacts with several cardiovascular medications, such as digoxin, quinidine, procainamide, and warfarin sodium (Giebel, 1987). Extreme caution must be used when initiating anticoagulant therapy with warfarin in patients who are receiving amiodarone.

Sotalol is a class III antiarrhythmic agent with beta-adrenergic–blocking properties. Sotalol, like the other class III agents, is used infrequently to suppress life-threatening ventricular tachyarrhythmias. Its adverse effects are similar to other beta-blocking agents and include fatigue, depression, dizziness, edema, hypotension, bradycardia, and AV block (Hillis et al., 1992c).

CLASS IV AGENTS

Class IV antiarrhythmic medications are calcium-channel antagonists, such as *verapamil, diltiazem,* and *nifedipine.* They work by blocking movement of calcium into both conductive and contractile myocardial cells, thereby reducing automaticity of the sinus node and ectopic pacemakers, slowing conduction through the AV node, and prolonging the AV node refractory period (Abrams, 1991b). Calcium-channel blocking agents are sometimes used to treat SVT in postoperative cardiac surgical patients. Because these agents depress myocardial contractility, they may produce heart failure in patients with impaired ventricular function. Also, intravenous verapamil may cause profound hypotension or ventricular fibrillation if given to a patient with ventricular tachycardia who is misdiagnosed as having SVT (Drew, 1991). Consequently, verapamil is not used for treatment of a wide complex tachycardia unless it is proven to be supraventricular in origin.

UNCLASSIFIED AGENTS

Digoxin is one of the most commonly used antiarrhythmic agents in cardiac surgical patients. Because of the prevalence of SVT after cardiac operations, prophylactic digitalization is sometimes performed in the early postoperative period. Digoxin is also generally administered as the agent of choice for treatment of SVT. It effectively lowers ventricular rate response in atrial flutter or atrial fibrillation by increasing AV block and enhances conversion to normal sinus rhythm. The specific dosing regimen depends on the ventricular rate, the urgency of conversion, patient age, body size, and renal function (Gray & Mandel, 1990). Typically, intravenous bolus doses (0.125- to 0.25-mg doses to a total of 1.0 to 1.5 mg over 24 hours) of digoxin are given to achieve a therapeutic serum level. Subsequent doses of 0.125 to 0.25 mg may be given intravenously until ventricular rate is less than 100 beats per minute or a total of 2 mg has been administered. Digoxin has a low therapeutic index; that is, therapeutic and toxic levels are separated by only a small margin. Digoxin toxicity may cause cardiac arrhythmias, gastrointestinal symptoms (e.g., nausea or diarrhea), and visual abnormalities.

Adenosine is an ultra-short-acting, intravenous agent for treatment of paroxysmal SVT originating in the AV node. Its primary actions are depression of sinus node automaticity, slowing of AV nodal conduction, shortening of the action potential in atrial tissue, and dilatation of coronary vessels (Severson & Meyer, 1992). Because adenosine rapidly slows AV nodal conduction, it is also useful in differentiating wide complex tachycardias of uncertain origin. The usual dose is 6 mg, administered by rapid intravenous injection. Transient adverse effects lasting less than 1 minute are common and include dyspnea, flushing, headaches, and chest pressure (Morton, 1994).

Atropine is an anticholinergic, or cholinergic-blocking, medication that blocks the action of acetylcholine on the parasympathetic receptors of the autonomic nervous system (Abrams, 1991d). It is used to increase the sinus rate and enhance AV conduction in patients with symptomatic bradyarrhythmias. Atropine is given as an intravenous bolus dose (0.5–1 mg) and may be repeated every 5 minutes to a total of 2 mg (Lapsley, 1991).

Magnesium sulfate is an intracellular cation that influences cardiac automaticity, excitability, conduction, and contractility (LeClair & Carlson, 1990). Although its role as an antiarrhythmic agent is somewhat controversial, it is sometimes given in intravenous bolus or infusion form to patients with ventricular tachyarrhythmias.

ANTIANGINAL MEDICATIONS

Three types of medications are used for control of angina pectoris: nitrates, beta-blocking agents, and calcium-channel antagonists. Often a combination of the three types of agents is used.

Nitrates exert a therapeutic effect through four mechanisms: (1) venous vasodilatation resulting in preload reduction, (2) arterial vasodilatation resulting in afterload reduction, (3) dilatation of collateral coronary arteries or the epicardial coronary arteries from which collateral vessels arise, and (4) relaxation of smooth muscle in epicardial vessels narrowed by atherosclerotic lesions or spasm (Kadota & Burke, 1990).

Nitroglycerin is primarily effective because of its dilating effects on coronary arteries. Although it does not increase coronary artery flow that is obstructed by fixed anatomic lesions, it decreases superimposed arterial spasm and dilates collateral arteries that supply jeopardized muscle (Elefteriades & Geha, 1985b). In addition, by reducing preload, nitroglycerin reduces myocardial wall tension and oxygen consumption. Nitroglycerin is available in several forms. In patients with chronic stable angina, it may be administered sublingually to dissipate or forestall periodic anginal episodes (Kutcher, 1991). To provide more extended relief from angina, a time-release patch containing nitroglycerin may be applied topically or an oral, long-acting nitrate (e.g., isosorbide dinitrate) may be given.

In patients with unstable angina, nitroglycerin is administered by continuous intravenous infusion. Arterial pressure monitoring is performed, and dosage is titrated by mean arterial pressure and the occurrence of angina. Typically, dosage in the range of 10 to 200 μg/min is administered to achieve a 10- to 15-mm Hg reduction in systolic blood pressure and elimination of all episodes of angina (Pratt & Roberts, 1991). Adverse effects of nitroglycerin therapy include hypotension and tachyphylaxis (i.e., a reduction in drug efficacy despite a constant infusion rate) (Schaer, 1991). The use of intravenous nitroglycerin therapy for afterload reduction has already been described.

Beta-adrenergic blocking medications decrease myocardial ischemia, and thus anginal pain, by reducing oxygen demands of the myocardium. They inhibit increases in heart rate, AV nodal conduction, and myocardial contractility that result from beta-receptor stimulation (Stanley, 1991). Beta-blocking agents used for angina control include metoprolol, propranolol, atenolol, nadolol, and timolol. The agents differ in duration of action (some allow greater time intervals between doses) and cardioselectivity (i.e., the degree to which beta-receptors outside the heart are affected) (Elefteriades & Geha, 1985b). Intravenous beta-blocking agents, such as metoprolol or propranolol, may be given to selected patients with unstable angina who are hypertensive or tachycardic (Pratt & Roberts, 1991). Because of associated negative inotropic effects, beta-blocking agents may be contraindicated in patients with impaired left ventricular function, particularly in the presence of acute low cardiac output.

The third category of antianginal medication is *calcium-channel blocking*, or *antagonist, medications*. These agents decrease angina by dilating coronary arteries and preventing spasm; to differing degrees, the individual calcium-channel blocking agents also decrease myocardial oxygen consumption by reducing blood pressure, afterload, and contractility (Kutcher, 1991). Diltiazem, nifedipine, and verapamil are examples of calcium-channel antagonists used for anginal control.

ANTICOAGULANT, THROMBOLYTIC, AND ANTIPLATELET MEDICATIONS

Anticoagulation is accomplished with intravenous administration of heparin or, for chronic therapy, with oral administration of warfarin sodium. *Heparin* inhibits clotting of blood by interfering with conversion of prothrombin to thrombin and fibrinogen to fibrin (Christopherson & Froelicher, 1990). It does not dissolve existing thrombus but does prevent its extension. Heparin must be administered intravenously or subcutaneously because it is inactivated by hydrochloric acid in the stomach (Christopherson & Froelicher, 1990).

Systemic anticoagulation with heparin is necessary in all patients who undergo operations necessitating cardiopulmonary bypass. Anticoagulation throughout the period of extracorporeal circulation prevents massive thrombosis that would otherwise occur as blood is circulated outside the body and exposed to the nonbiologic surfaces of the cardiopulmonary bypass circuit. An intravenous bolus of heparin (3 mg/kg) is administered just before initiation of cardiopulmonary bypass. Activated clotting time is measured intermittently to ensure an adequate degree of anticoagulation, and additional bolus doses of heparin are repeated as indicated. *Protamine sulfate*, a heparin antagonist, is given after termination of cardiopulmonary bypass to reverse the anticoagulated state.

Anticoagulation may be also be necessary in selected patients during the preoperative or postoperative period. The most common indication for anticoagulation during the preoperative period is retardation of thrombus formation in patients with acute myocardial infarction or unstable angina. Another common indication for preoperative anticoagulation is a known or suspected source of systemic thromboembolism, such as a mechanical valvular prosthesis, deep venous thrombosis, left ventricular thrombus, or atrial fibrillation. Heparin is used instead of warfarin in preoperative patients because of its shorter half-life. An intravenous heparin infusion may be continued until shortly before the patient is transported to the operating room. Heparin therapy

is usually initiated with a bolus dose of 5000 units, followed by a continuous infusion of 1000 units per hour (Schaer, 1991). The anticoagulant effect of heparin is monitored by a baseline measurement, and then serial measurements of partial thromboplastin time. Dosage is adjusted to achieve a partial thromboplastin time one and one-half to two times greater than the control value.

In postoperative cardiac surgical patients, anticoagulation is usually necessary only in those who have a prosthetic heart valve or a preexisting condition, such as chronic atrial fibrillation or a pulmonary embolus, that necessitates an anticoagulated state. Because the use of cardiopulmonary bypass impairs coagulation during the early postoperative period, anticoagulant therapy is generally not initiated until the second postoperative day, after the chest thoracostomy tubes have been removed.

Warfarin is an oral agent used for chronic anticoagulation. It acts by competing with vitamin K and thus inhibiting hepatic synthesis of vitamin K–dependent clotting factors (factors II, VII, IX, and X) (Christopherson & Froelicher, 1990). Warfarin does not affect circulating clotting factors or platelet function (Abrams, 1991e). It is generally initiated 2 to 3 days after surgery to avoid precipitation of bleeding in the immediate postoperative period. In most patients, anticoagulation is begun with an initial dose of 5 to 10 mg and subsequent doses are determined according to the prothrombin time obtained each morning. Depending on the indication for anticoagulation, doses are titrated to maintain prothrombin times one and one-half to two times greater than the control value. Particular care must be exercised in when anticoagulants are administered to patients who are elderly, who are malnourished, who have chronic liver dysfunction, or who are receiving amiodarone. In these patients, prothrombin times may rise rapidly with only small doses of warfarin.

Thrombolytic medications are agents that destroy thrombus by stimulating conversion of plasminogen to plasmin, which in turn degrades fibrin, fibrinogen, and other procoagulant proteins (Stanley, 1991). Thrombolytic agents are used to lyse thrombus in patients with acute myocardial infarction or massive pulmonary embolism. When given to patients within 4 hours of acute myocardial infarction, thrombolytic agents can often restore blood flow through an acutely occluded coronary artery, thereby preventing myocardial necrosis. Similarly, thrombolytic agents rapidly dissolve pulmonary artery thrombus. They are much more effective than heparin in correcting acute hemodynamic abnormalities caused by massive pulmonary embolism (Rubin & Sherry, 1991). The most commonly used thrombolytic agents are *streptokinase* and *recombinant tissue-type plasminogen activator* (rt-PA). Bleeding is the major complication of thrombolytic therapy; the most significant form is cerebral hemorrhage. Streptokinase may also cause hypotension and allergic reactions. Thrombolytic therapy is discussed in more detail in Chapter 1, Coronary Artery Disease.

The most commonly used *antiplatelet medication* is aspirin (acetylsalicylic acid). *Aspirin* irreversibly inactivates platelet cyclooxygenase, thereby impairing platelet aggregation and reducing the release of platelet-derived vasoconstrictors (Passen & Schaer, 1991). Aspirin is commonly administered in patients with coronary artery disease. It is the mainstay of therapy for unstable angina because of its demonstrated effectiveness in reducing the incidence of myocardial infarction and mortality (Pratt & Roberts, 1991). It is also given indefinitely to patients who have undergone coronary artery bypass grafting to promote long-term vein graft patency. The usual dosage is 325 mg/d. Aspirin therapy is contraindicated in the presence of gastrointestinal bleeding or peptic ulcer disease.

OTHER SELECTED MEDICATIONS

DIURETIC AGENTS

Of the many available diuretic agents, *loop diuretics* are used most commonly in cardiac surgical patients. These are agents that primarily work by actions in the ascending loop of Henle in the renal medulla. Loop diuretics, which include *furosemide, bumetanide*, and *ethacrynic acid*, inhibit absorption of sodium, chloride, and potassium (Cunningham, 1990). All three agents can be given intravenously and begin to act within several minutes.

Furosemide is most commonly used and may be given routinely to postoperative cardiac surgical patients to promote diuresis of fluid retained secondary to use of cardiopulmonary bypass. It is also used to acutely reduce preload in patients with pulmonary edema. Bumetanide or ethacrynic acid may be given alternatively if furosemide does not produce the desired response. Because potassium excretion is enhanced, adequate potassium repletion is essential to avoid potentially lethal hypokalemia-induced arrhythmias. All of the loop diuretics can damage the eighth cranial nerve. Ototoxicity with resultant hearing loss is most likely with high doses or rapid intravenous administration (Makoff, 1990).

ANTIHYPERTENSIVE AGENTS

A variety of agents are used for chronic management of hypertension, and a complete discussion of antihypertensive agents is beyond the scope of this chapter. Many patients who undergo cardiac operations have been on long-term therapy for associated hypertension. Generally, these agents are continued until the time of surgery but may not be necessary during the postoperative hospitalization due to hemodynamic changes associated with surgery. However, patients who required antihypertensive therapy before a cardiac operation usually require resumption of therapy, if not in the early postoperative period, then in the first several months after surgery. Many of the previously discussed vasodilators, beta-blocking agents, and calcium-channel antagonists have antihypertensive actions and may be used for postoperative blood pressure control. *Angiotensin-converting enzyme* (ACE) *inhibiting medications* are also occasionally used and merit mention. These agents act by (1) inhibiting the enzyme responsible for conversion of inactive angiotensin I into active angiotensin II, (2) decreasing circulating angiotensin II and aldosterone, and (3) reducing systemic vascular resistance (Grim, 1990). *Captopril* and *enalapril* are examples of ACE inhibitors.

For rapid blood pressure control, an intravenous agent, such as nitroprusside, nitroglycerin, or esmolol is usually administered. Two antihypertensive agents not previously discussed may also be used. *Labetalol* is a unique agent with both alpha- and beta-adrenergic blocking actions (Makoff, 1990). *Hydralazine* is a vasodilating agent that primarily affects arterial smooth muscle. Both drugs can be administered intravenously to produce rapid reduction of blood pressure.

REFERENCES

Abrams AC, 1991a: Physiology of the autonomic nervous system. In Clinical Drug Therapy, ed. 3. Philadelphia, JB Lippincott
Abrams AC, 1991b: Antiarrhythmic drugs. In Clinical Drug Therapy, ed. 3. Philadelphia, JB Lippincott
Abrams AC, 1991c: Antiadrenergic drugs. In Clinical Drug Therapy, ed. 3. Philadelphia, JB Lippincott
Abrams AC, 1991d: Anticholinergic drugs. In Clinical Drug Therapy, ed. 3. Philadelphia, JB Lippincott
Abrams AC, 1991e: Anticoagulant, antiplatelet, and thrombolytic agents. In Clinical Drug Therapy, ed. 3. Philadelphia, JB Lippincott
Antman EM, 1992: Medical management of the patient undergoing cardiac surgery. In Braunwald E (ed): Heart Disease: A Textbook of Cardiovascular Medicine, ed. 4. Philadelphia, WB Saunders
Bank AJ, Kubo SH, 1991: Congestive heart failure: Inotropic agents. In Parrillo JE (ed): Current Therapy in Critical Care Medicine, ed. 2. Philadelphia, BC Decker
Barold SS, Zipes DP, 1992: Cardiac pacemakers and antiarrhythmic devices. In Braunwald E (ed): Heart Disease: A Textbook of Cardiovascular Medicine, ed. 4. Philadelphia, WB Saunders
Barron JT, Parrillo JE, 1991: Congestive heart failure: Vasodilator therapy. In Parrillo JE (ed): Current Therapy in Critical Care Medicine, ed. 2. Philadelphia, BC Decker
Blanski L, Lutz J, Laddu A, 1988: Esmolol, the first ultra-short acting intravenous beta blocker for use in critically ill patients. Heart Lung 17:80
Bond EF, 1990: Antiarrhythmic drugs. In Underhill SL, Woods SL, Froelicher ES, Halpenny CJ (eds): Cardiovascular Medications for Cardiac Nursing. Philadelphia, JB Lippincott
Bond EF, Underhill SL, 1990: Inotropic agents. In Underhill SL, Woods SL, Froelicher ES, Halpenny CJ (eds): Cardiovascular Medications for Cardiac Nursing. Philadelphia, JB Lippincott
Buckingham TA, Parrillo JE, 1991: Ventricular arrhythmia. In Parrillo JE (ed): Current Therapy in Critical Care Medicine, ed. 2. Philadelphia, BC Decker
Christopherson DJ, Froelicher ES, 1990: Anticoagulant, antithrombotic, and platelet-modifying drugs. In Underhill SL, Woods

SL, Froelicher ES, Halpenny CJ (eds): Cardiovascular Medications for Cardiac Nursing. Philadelphia, JB Lippincott

Cunningham SG, 1990: Diuretics. In Underhill SL, Woods SL, Froelicher ES, Halpenny CJ (eds): Cardiovascular Medications for Cardiac Nursing. Philadelphia, JB Lippincott

DiSesa VJ, 1991: Pharmacologic support for postoperative low cardiac output. Semin Thorac Cardiovasc Surg 3:13

Drew BJ, 1991: Bedside diagnosis of wide QRS tachycardia. Crit Care Nurs Q 14:19

Dusman RE, Stanton MS, Miles WM, et al., 1990: Clinical features of amiodarone-induced pulmonary toxicity. Circulation 82:51

Elefteriades JA, Geha AS, 1985a: Continuous infusion agents. In House Officer Guide to ICU Care: The Cardiothoracic Surgical Patient. Gaithersburg, MD, Aspen Publishers

Elefteriades JA, Geha AS, 1985b: Additional topics. In House Officer Guide to ICU Care: The Cardiothoracic Surgical Patient. Gaithersburg, MD, Aspen Publishers

Ferguson DW, 1991: Cardiogenic shock. In Hurst JW (ed): Current Therapy in Cardiovascular Disease, ed. 3. Philadelphia, BC Decker

Gahart BL, 1991a: Lidocaine hydrochloride. In Intravenous Medications, ed. 7. St. Louis, Mosby–Year Book

Gahart BL, 1991b: Bretylium tosylate. In Intravenous Medications, ed. 7. St. Louis, Mosby–Year Book

Giebel RA, 1987: Amiodarone (Cordarone): Implications for nursing intervention. Prog Cardiovasc Nurs 2:125

Gray RJ, Mandel WJ, 1990: Management of common postoperative arrhythmias. In Gray RJ, Matloff JM (eds): Medical Management of the Cardiac Surgical Patient. Baltimore, Williams & Wilkins

Greco SA, 1990: Vasoactive drugs. In Underhill SL, Woods SL, Froelicher ES, Halpenny CJ (eds): Cardiovascular Medications for Cardiac Nursing. Philadelphia, JB Lippincott

Grim C, 1990: Antihypertensives. In Underhill SL, Woods SL, Froelicher ES, Halpenny CJ (eds): Cardiovascular Medications for Cardiac Nursing. Philadelphia, JB Lippincott

Hendren WG, Higgins TL, 1991: Immediate postoperative care of the cardiac surgical patient. Semin Thorac Cardiovasc Surg 3:3

Hillis LD, Lange RA, Wells PJ, Winniford MD, 1992a: Inotropic agents. In Manual of Clinical Problems in Cardiology, ed. 4. Boston, Little, Brown

Hillis LD, Lange RA, Wells PJ, Winniford MD, 1992b: Amiodarone. In Manual of Clinical Problems in Cardiology, ed. 4. Boston, Little, Brown

Hillis LD, Lange RA, Wells PJ, Winniford MD, 1992c: New antiarrhythmic agents. In Manual of Clinical Problems in Cardiology, ed. 4. Boston, Little, Brown

Hudak CM, Gallo BM, Benz JJ, 1990: Commonly used antiarrhythmic agents. In Critical Care Nursing: A Holistic Approach, ed. 5. Philadelphia, JB Lippincott

Kadota LT, Burke LE, 1990: Nitrates. In Underhill SL, Woods SL, Froelicher ES, Halpenny CJ (eds): Cardiovascular Medications for Cardiac Nursing. Philadelphia, JB Lippincott

Kelleher RM, Rose AA, Ordway L, 1991: Prostaglandins for the control of pulmonary hypertension in the postoperative cardiac surgery patient: Nursing implications. Crit Care Nurs Clin North Am 3:741

Kessler KM, Chakko CS, Myerburg RJ, 1992: Management of premature ventricular contractions. Heart Dis Stroke 1:275

Kutcher MA, 1991: Angina pectoris: Stable. In Hurst JW (ed): Current Therapy in Cardiovascular Disease, ed. 3. Philadelphia, BC Decker

Lapsley DP, 1991: Drug therapy for sudden cardiac death. In Owens PM (ed): Sudden Cardiac Death. Gaithersburg, MD, Aspen Publishers

LeClair HH, Carlson KK, 1990: Agents used to restore electrolyte balance. In Underhill SL, Woods SL, Froelicher ES, Halpenny CJ (eds): Cardiovascular Medications for Cardiac Nursing. Philadelphia, JB Lippincott

Lewis RP, 1991: Supraventricular arrhythmia. In Parrillo JE (ed): Current Therapy in Critical Care Medicine, ed. 2. Philadelphia, BC Decker

Loveys BJ, 1990: Beta-blocking agents. In Underhill SL, Woods SL, Froelicher ES, Halpenny CJ (eds): Cardiovascular Medications for Cardiac Nursing. Philadelphia, JB Lippincott

Makoff DL, 1990: Hypertension. In Berk JL, Sampliner JE (eds): Handbook of Critical Care, ed. 3. Boston, Little, Brown

Mandel WJ, 1990: Cardiac arrhythmias. In Berk JL, Sampliner JE (eds): Handbook of Critical Care, ed. 3. Boston, Little, Brown & Co

Moore SL, Wilkoff BL, 1991: Rhythm disturbances after cardiac surgery. Semin Thorac Cardiovasc Surg 3:24

Moreno-Cabral CE, Mitchell RS, Miller DC, 1988. Postoperative problems. In Manual of Postoperative Management in Adult Cardiac Surgery. Baltimore, Williams & Wilkins

Morton PG, 1994: Update on new antiarrhythmic agents. Crit Care Nurs Clin North Am 6:69

Nalos PC, Kass RM, Gang ES, et al., 1987: Life-threatening pulmonary complications in patients with previous amiodarone pulmonary toxicity undergoing cardiothoracic operations. J Thorac Cardiovasc Surg 93:904

Passen EL, Schaer GL, 1991: Acute myocardial infarction. In Parrillo JE (ed): Current Therapy in Critical Care Medicine, ed. 2. Philadelphia, BC Decker

Phelan J, Klein LW, 1991: The postoperative cardiac surgical patient. In Parrillo JE (ed): Current Therapy in Critical Care Medicine, ed. 2. Philadelphia, BC Decker

Pratt CM, Roberts R, 1991: Angina pectoris: Unstable. In Hurst JW (ed): Current Therapy in Cardiovascular Disease, ed. 3. Philadelphia, BC Decker

Rubin RN, Sherry S, 1991: Pulmonary embolism. In Parrillo JE (ed): Current Therapy in Critical Care Medicine, ed. 2. Philadelphia, BC Decker

Schaer GL, 1991: Unstable angina. In Parrillo JE (ed): Current Therapy in Critical Care Medicine, ed. 2. Philadelphia, BC Decker

Severson AL, Meyer LT, 1992: Treatment of paroxysmal supraventricular tachycardia with adenosine: Implications for nursing. Heart Lung 21:350

Slovis CM, Brody SL, 1991: Cardiac arrest and resuscitation from sudden death. In Hurst JW (ed): Current Therapy in Cardiovascular Disease, ed. 3. Philadelphia, BC Decker

Smith PK, 1990: Postoperative care in cardiac surgery. In Sabiston DC Jr, Spencer FC (eds): Surgery of the Chest, ed. 5. Philadelphia, WB Saunders

Smith TW, Braunwald E, Kelly RA, 1992: The management of heart failure. In Braunwald E (ed): Heart Disease: A Textbook of Cardiovascular Medicine, ed. 4. Philadelphia, WB Saunders

Stanley R, 1991: Cardiovascular drugs. In Kinney MR, Packa DR, Andreoli KG, Zipes DP (eds): Comprehensive Cardiac Care, ed. 7. St. Louis, Mosby–Year Book

Whitman GR, 1991: Hypertension and hypothermia in the acute postoperative period. Crit Care Nurs Clin North Am 3:661

Wong CA, 1991: Physiologic responses to anesthesia. In Shekleton ME, Litwack K (eds): Critical Care Nursing of the Surgical Patient. Philadelphia, WB Saunders

Zipes DP, 1992: Management of cardiac arrhythmias: Pharmacological, electrical, and surgical techniques. In Braunwald E (ed): Heart Disease: A Textbook of Cardiovascular Medicine, ed. 4., Philadelphia, WB Saunders

CHAPTER 28

COMPLICATIONS OF CARDIAC OPERATIONS

RISK FACTORS
CARDIOVASCULAR COMPLICATIONS
  Hemorrhage
  Cardiac Tamponade
  Myocardial Infarction
  Ventricular Dysfunction
  Cardiac Arrhythmias
  Sudden Cardiac Death
  Postpericardiotomy Syndrome
  Pericardial Effusion
  Pulmonary Embolism

NONCARDIAC COMPLICATIONS
  Neurologic Deficits
  Respiratory Complications
  Intra-abdominal Complications
  Renal Failure
  Sepsis
  Wound Complications
  Urinary Tract Complications
  Miscellaneous Complications
DEVICE-RELATED COMPLICATIONS

Postoperative complications can occur after any cardiac operation. They not only cause morbidity and prolong hospitalization, but they also have a direct effect on survival probability. Patients who experience one or more complications have a significantly increased operative mortality rate as compared with those without complications (Hammermeister et al., 1990). Although it is not possible to predict with certainty which patients will develop complications in the perioperative period, one can profile certain groups of patients for whom risk is higher than usual. Unfortunately, an increasing number of cardiac surgical patients fall into these high risk categories.

RISK FACTORS

One of the major determinants of operative risk is the nature and degree of underlying cardiac pathology, especially the status of ventricular function. The most common type of cardiac operation performed in the United States is coronary artery bypass grafting. Patient selection for this procedure has changed substantially in recent years owing to more effective nonsurgical therapies. Improvements in antianginal medications and availability of percutaneous transluminal angioplasty have increased the number of higher-risk patients undergoing surgical revascularization (Christakis et al., 1989). The mean age of patients undergoing operation has increased, and reoperations have become more common. Significant increases have been reported among surgical patients in the degree of ventricular impairment, the incidence of associated medical diseases, the average number of vessels bypassed, and the incidence of emergency operations (Naunheim et al., 1988).

As compared with coronary artery bypass grafting, operative risk is increased in patients who require valve replacement or who require coronary revascularization combined with valve replacement or ventricular aneurysmectomy (Higgins & Starr, 1991). A strong relationship also exists between emergency surgery and postoperative morbidity. Contributing factors in patients receiving emergency operations in-

Betsy Finkelmeier: CARDIOTHORACIC SURGICAL NURSING.
© 1995 J.B. Lippincott Company.

TABLE 28-1. CARDIOVASCULAR COMPLICATIONS OF CARDIAC SURGERY

Hemorrhage
Cardiac tamponade
Myocardial infarction
Ventricular dysfunction
Cardiac arrhythmias
Sudden cardiac death
Postpericardiotomy syndrome
Pericardial effusion
Pulmonary embolism

clude the severity of illness; the likely presence of uncontrolled heart failure, cardiogenic shock, or ongoing myocardial infarction (MI); and the limited amount of preoperative preparation, evaluation, and monitoring (Tuman et al., 1992).

Age is another predisposing factor for operative complications. Increased longevity in the United States has produced a large population of elderly individuals, many of whom develop significant coronary artery disease. As a result, the average age of patients undergoing cardiac operations has been slowly increasing over the past decade. Surgical intervention in septuagenarians and octogenarians is now commonplace. Most series report higher operative mortality in elderly patients, especially when surgery is performed urgently or emergently (Edwards et al., 1991). Higher complication rates have also been consistently demonstrated, probably related to generalized deterioration in the function of major organ systems and the presence of associated chronic medical problems. Neurologic complications are particularly prevalent in elderly patients (Edwards et al., 1991).

Prior heart surgery is a powerful predictor of perioperative complications (Hammermeister et al., 1990). Because both coronary artery revascularization and valve replacement procedures are palliative, some patients require more than one cardiac operation. A previous cardiac operation adds to operative risk primarily because of the advanced nature of disease associated with the need for reoperation and the increased potential for technical problems (Tuman et al., 1992). Entry into the chest is more hazardous because the right ventricle or previously constructed bypass grafts are often adherent to the posterior table of the sternum and may be injured. In addition, the presence of adhesions (internal scarring) from a previous surgical procedure and the loss of distinct tissue planes make intraoperative dissection more difficult. Perioperative bleeding and the need for blood transfusion may be greater. Also, patients undergoing repeat operations are more likely to require postoperative mechanical cardiac assistance (Jones et al., 1991).

Associated arterial occlusive disease is yet another factor that predisposes to postoperative morbidity.

Patients undergoing coronary artery revascularization in particular are likely to have significant cerebral or peripheral occlusive lesions because atherosclerosis is a generalized vascular disease. Carotid or cerebral artery atherosclerosis increases risk for a cerebral vascular accident. Perioperative stroke can also result from embolization of atherosclerotic material in the ascending aorta. An abdominal aortic aneurysm may rupture in the perioperative period. Occlusive arterial disease in the abdominal aorta or femoral arteries may preclude insertion of an intra-aortic balloon catheter for counterpulsation and increases the likelihood of balloon-related complications (Finkelmeier & Finkelmeier, 1991).

Complications also occur more often in patients with other associated medical diseases, such as chronic obstructive pulmonary disease, diabetes mellitus, or renal failure. Although most medications do not add to operative risk, preoperative antiplatelet therapy, specifically with aspirin, increases the likelihood of significant perioperative bleeding. Preoperative use of corticosteroids suppresses the inflammatory process and may impair wound healing.

The most common causes of operative morbidity are discussed in this chapter (Tables 28-1 and 28-2). Occurrence of some types of complications, such as bleeding and heart failure, are fairly predictable. Other complications, such as air embolism, iatrogenic

TABLE 28-2. NONCARDIAC COMPLICATIONS OF CARDIAC SURGERY

Neurologic

Transient ischemic attack
Cerebral vascular accident
Peripheral neurologic deficit
Impaired level of consciousness

Respiratory

Atelectasis
Pleural effusion
Pneumonia
Adult respiratory distress syndrome

Intra-abdominal

Gastrointestinal hemorrhage
Ileus
Small bowel obstruction
Acute pancreatitis
Acute cholecystitis
Intestinal infarction

Renal failure

Infection

Sternal dehiscence/mediastinitis
Other wound
Pneumonia
Urinary tract
Sepsis
Gastrointestinal (*Clostridium difficile*)

aortic dissection, or cardiopulmonary bypass (CPB) system malfunction, may occur unexpectedly. Most complications occur either during the operation or in the first 24 postoperative hours. However, by convention, any complication that occurs either within 30 days of operation or before patient discharge from the hospital is considered operative morbidity.

CARDIOVASCULAR COMPLICATIONS

HEMORRHAGE

Bleeding is a common complication of cardiac operations because of intraoperative anticoagulation of the patient and the use of CPB. Systemic anticoagulation with heparin is necessary to prevent massive thrombosis that would otherwise occur as blood is circulated through an extracorporeal circuit. Although protamine sulfate is given to reverse the effects of heparin when CPB is terminated, normal coagulation is not immediately restored. Exposure to the nonphysiologic surfaces of the extracorporeal circuit reduces the number of platelets, decreases platelet survival time, and alters platelet function (Kirklin & Barratt-Boyes, 1993). In addition, blood is hemodiluted by priming of the cardiopulmonary circuit with crystalloid solution. As a result, levels of coagulation factors (fibrinogen, prothrombin, and factors V and VIII) are reduced by approximately 50% (Halfman-Franey & Berg, 1991). The surgeon achieves adequate hemostasis before closing the chest incision and transporting the patient out of the operating room. Areas that are inspected include anastomotic suture lines; cannulation sites; conduit side branches; internal thoracic artery (also called internal mammary artery) pedicle; and thymic, epicardial, sternal wire, and chest tube sites (Mahfood et al., 1991). However, bleeding may increase substantially as the patient's body temperature warms. Postoperative bleeding is also exacerbated by hypertension, a common problem in the early postoperative hours that may be caused by patient arousal from anesthesia, endotracheal suctioning, the patient's resistance to mechanical ventilation, pain, or that occurs as a paroxysmal event (Whitman, 1991). Even brief periods of hypertension can cause bleeding sufficient to necessitate surgical exploration (Mahfood et al., 1991).

Excessive mediastinal bleeding, or *hemorrhage*, is characterized by sustained chest tube output greater than 100 mL/h or greater than 300 mL in any one hour. It usually occurs within the first 24 postoperative hours. Certain categories of patients are more likely to experience excessive bleeding, including those who (1) have undergone one or more previous cardiac operations, (2) have liver dysfunction secondary to valvular heart disease and passive congestion, (3) have an underlying bleeding disorder, (4) have received aspirin therapy within a week before operation, (5) require lengthy operations necessitating a prolonged period

of CPB, or (6) have friable tissue or an underlying pathologic process likely to be associated with hemorrhage, such as a traumatic cardiac wound, aortic dissection, or ruptured aortic aneurysm.

Postoperative bleeding is categorized as (1) *mechanical* (i.e., surgically correctable) or (2) *nonsurgical* (i.e., generalized bleeding related to a coagulopathy). Mechanical bleeding is found in approximately half the patients who require reexploration (Anderson et al., 1991). Platelet functional impairment is the most important hemostatic derangement after CPB and a major cause of postoperative coagulopathy (Halfman-Franey & Berg, 1991). Nonsurgical bleeding may also be caused by inadequate heparin neutralization, fibrinolysis, complement activation, or decreased levels of factors V, VIII, and XIII, fibrinogen, and plasminogen (Hendren & Higgins, 1991). Coagulopathy is more common in patients who have received antiplatelet agents, thrombolytic therapy, or heparin in the preoperative period (Smith, 1990).

Uncommonly, heparin activity recurs after initial adequate reversal. This so-called *heparin rebound phenomenon* occurs because protamine sulfate, given as an antidote to heparin, is eliminated from the blood before heparin (Ellison et al., 1991). Severe postoperative coagulopathies, such as *disseminated intravascular coagulation*, are rare. They usually occur in patients with low cardiac output, intense peripheral vasoconstriction, and poor tissue perfusion.

Autotransfusion of shed mediastinal blood is routinely performed during the first 6 to 12 hours, or longer if active bleeding continues. If necessary, autotransfusion is supplemented with homologous blood component therapy. Packed red blood cells, platelets, or fresh frozen plasma may be administered to replenish hemoglobin, platelets, or clotting factors. Drugs that improve platelet function (e.g., desmopressin) or prevent fibrinolysis (e.g., aminocaproic acid) may also be administered in selected patients to treat postoperative coagulopathy (Halfman-Franey & Berg, 1991). Heparin rebound is treated with protamine sulfate administration.

If bleeding is excessive or sustained, reexploration may be necessary to detect and correct a mechanical bleeding source. Occasionally, disruption of a suture or loosening of a surgical clip occurs, causing precipitous hemorrhage. In such cases, the patient is immediately transferred to the operating room for reexploration. In the case of massive hemorrhage, the surgeon may open a portion of the sternotomy incision in the intensive care unit to obtain digital control of the bleeding source. Hemorrhage that is inadequately treated leads to hypovolemic shock, exsanguination, or cardiac tamponade.

CARDIAC TAMPONADE

Cardiac tamponade describes a condition in which the heart is compressed by blood that has accumulated in the pericardium or anterior mediastinum. It usually represents a combination of excessive bleeding and inadequate pericardial or mediastinal drainage. To reduce the risk of cardiac tamponade, many surgeons leave the pericardium open and place one of the mediastinal chest tubes in the most dependent part of the pericardial sac near the left ventricle (Geha & Whittlesey, 1991). Also, one of the pleural spaces may intentionally be opened to provide adequate egress for blood if excessive bleeding is anticipated.

The hemodynamic changes associated with cardiac tamponade result from biventricular restriction of end-diastolic volume (Smith, 1990). Clinical manifestations include hypotension; decreased cardiac output; elevation and equalization of filling pressures (central venous, pulmonary artery diastolic, and left atrial pressures); roentgenographic evidence of mediastinal widening; diminished or excessive chest tube drainage; and pulsus paradoxus. The diagnosis should also be suspected any time a cardiac surgical patient's condition suddenly deteriorates, particularly in the early postoperative period and in association with sudden diminution in the amount of chest tube drainage.

Temporizing measures to support cardiac function in the presence of tamponade include administration of fluids and inotropic medications. However, relief of the tamponade is essential to correcting hemodynamic compromise. Chest tubes are stripped to evacuate clotted material and restore patency. If the rate of bleeding is so excessive that tamponade occurs despite patent chest tubes, the surgeon reopens the incision emergently to relieve tamponade and control hemorrhage with digital compression. Depending on the degree of hemodynamic instability, the lower end of the sternotomy incision may be opened in the intensive care unit as a lifesaving measure. If time allows, the patient is instead transported emergently to the operating room. Regardless of where the incision is reopened, eventual transfer to the operating room will be necessary for thorough exploration of the mediastinum and reclosure of the incision under sterile conditions.

Although tamponade most often occurs during the first 24 hours after operation, it occasionally occurs late, almost always in patients who initially had excessive postoperative bleeding or in those who are being anticoagulated (Smith, 1990). Late cardiac tamponade can also occur from bleeding associated with removal of a left atrial catheter or, rarely, an epicardial pacing wire. For this reason, a chest tube is usually left in place until the left atrial catheter is removed and patients are observed in the hospital for 6 to 12 hours after removal of pacing wires.

MYOCARDIAL INFARCTION

Myocardial infarction (MI) is the most common major complication of coronary artery bypass grafting. Clinically significant MIs occur in approximately 5% of patients. However, the incidence of perioperative myocardial necrosis ranges from 3% to 31%, depending on the method used for diagnosis, the population of patients studied, and the skill of the operating room team (Tuman, 1991). Although MI can be a major complication, most perioperative MIs are mild and are detected only by elevated isoenzymes or electrocardiographic changes.

Perioperative MI after coronary artery bypass grafting can be caused by one of several factors. Probably most common is inadequate myocardial oxygenation during CPB, particularly in areas of muscle supplied by diseased coronary arteries. *Arterial spasm* may occur in an internal thoracic artery graft or in native coronary arteries whether or not they have received bypass grafts. *Acute graft closure* of saphenous veins is unusual but can occur as a result of technical difficulties with graft construction, poor conduit quality, or inadequate runoff secondary to distal disease. Although less common, perioperative MI sometimes occurs after other types of cardiac operations. Even in the absence of coronary artery disease, profound hypotension, inadequate myocardial protection during CPB, or air or thrombotic emboli to the coronary circulation can cause significant MI.

An electrocardiogram obtained in the immediate postoperative period is particularly important because it is likely to precede other manifestations of myocardial injury in sedated, intubated patients (Fig. 28-1). In the alert postoperative patient, infarction may be manifested as chest discomfort that is similar to preoperative anginal pain. An electrocardiogram is obtained during the pain, and sublingual nitroglycerin may be ordered by the physician to assess its effectiveness in abating pain.

Arterial spasm is usually treated with intravenous nitroglycerin and calcium-channel antagonists. In severe cases, emergency cardiac catheterization may be performed for instillation of nitroglycerin or papaverine directly into the affected artery (Smith, 1990). If a technical problem with one of the grafts is identified in the first 24 hours, emergent reexploration may be performed, particularly if the patient's condition is unstable. Pharmacologic and mechanical support of the heart may occasionally be necessary if cardiac function is significantly impaired. If graft closure is suspected after the first 24 hours, coronary angiography is performed to definitively assess graft patency. Although it is demoralizing for the patient and surgeon to document early graft closure, it is the most effective means of determining graft viability and planning future therapy.

In asymptomatic or minimally symptomatic patients, treatment and the postoperative course of patients with perioperative MIs are usually similar to that of patients without infarction, except that the return to a normal activity level is more gradual. Beta-blocking medications and other drug therapy shown

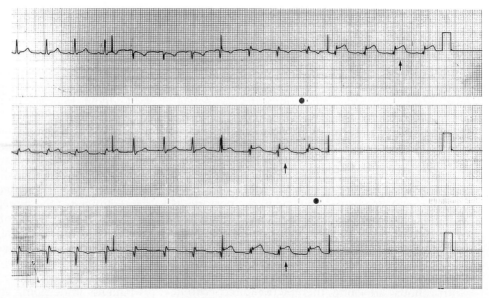

FIGURE 28-1. Twelve-lead electrocardiogram obtained in intubated and sedated patient after uneventful coronary artery bypass grafting (leads V_5 and V_6 not recorded because of presence of bandage). Marked ST segment elevation in leads V_2 through V_4 (*arrows*) represents acute anterior wall injury; subsequent emergent operative exploration revealed severe spasm of the internal thoracic artery (grafted to the left anterior descending coronary artery).

to increase longevity after MI may be initiated (Smith, 1990).

VENTRICULAR DYSFUNCTION

Either left, right, or biventricular dysfunction can complicate cardiac operations. It is probably the most common complication in patients undergoing valvular heart surgery and usually represents an exacerbation of underlying ventricular impairment. In patients with coronary artery disease, ventricular dysfunction is most likely in patients who undergo operation within 1 week of an acute MI, those with compromised ventricular function from previous MIs, and those subjected to long periods of CPB or with inadequate intraoperative myocardial protection. Because both coronary and valvular heart disease most often damage the left ventricle, perioperative left ventricular dysfunction occurs most frequently.

Left ventricular dysfunction is categorized as *low cardiac output syndrome* or *cardiogenic shock*, depending on its severity. Inability of the failing ventricle to sustain adequate tissue perfusion is demonstrated by a cardiac index less than 2.0 L/min/m², systemic vascular resistance greater than 2100 dynes·sec·cm⁻⁵, atrial pressure greater than 20 mm Hg, and urine output less than 20 mL/h (Reedy et al., 1990). Other clinical manifestations include cold, clammy extremities; hypotension; tachycardia; diminished peripheral pulses and capillary refill; and persistent obtundation (Moreno-Cabral et al., 1988). However, residual effects of anesthesia, the patient's thermal instability, and the osmotic diuresis that follows CPB may obscure classic manifestations in the early postoperative hours (DiSesa, 1991).

Low cardiac output or cardiogenic shock is treated by manipulation of those variables that affect cardiac output, that is, heart rate, preload, afterload, and contractility. Temporary pacing may be used to increase heart rate or provide atrioventricular synchrony in the presence of sinus bradycardia or heart block, respectively. Volume replacement with crystalloid or colloid solutions is often necessary to provide an adequate preload, particularly in the presence of postoperative bleeding, diuresis, or vasodilatation.

Afterload reduction and improved myocardial contractility are achieved with a combination of vasodilating and inotropic medications (DiSesa, 1991). Patients are maintained in a sedated state to minimize sympathetic overstimulation and its deleterious effects on heart rate and systemic vascular resistance (Moran & Singh, 1989). Intra-aortic balloon counterpulsation may be necessary if pharmacologic afterload reduction alone is ineffective. In selected patients with cardiogenic shock refractory to pharmacologic therapy or intra-aortic balloon counterpulsation, a ventricular assist device may be used.

Right ventricular dysfunction is less common but may occur in patients with chronic pulmonary hypertension or secondary to left ventricular failure. Pharmacologic pulmonary vascular vasodilatation can be achieved with nitroglycerin or isoproterenol infusion. Prostaglandin E₁ infusion has also proved effective in producing pulmonary arterial vasodilatation in postoperative right-sided heart failure associated with pulmonary hypertension (Kelleher et al., 1991). Norepinephrine may be necessary to counteract the associated significant systemic vasodilatation produced by prostaglandin E₁ (Hendren & Higgins, 1991). Rarely, a right ventricular assist device may be necessary. Cardiac transplantation may be considered in selected patients with irreversible postoperative left ventricular, right ventricular, or biventricular dysfunction.

CARDIAC ARRHYTHMIAS

Arrhythmic complications may be categorized as ventricular tachycardia (VT) or ventricular fibrillation (VF), ventricular ectopy without VT or VF, supraventricular tachycardia (SVT), and conduction disturbances. *Ventricular tachycardia* and *ventricular fibrillation* are the most serious arrhythmic complications. At highest risk for VT or VF are patients with (1) a major ventricular wall motion abnormality secondary to MI, (2) hypertrophic cardiomyopathy, (3) an underlying arrhythmic disorder, or (4) severe aortic valve disease. Life-threatening ventricular tachyarrhythmias may also be precipitated in the postoperative period by perioperative myocardial ischemia from coronary artery or graft occlusion or from transient or sustained low cardiac output (Tam et al., 1991). Rarely, VT or VF occurs in the absence of a detectable precipitant.

Intravenous lidocaine therapy or direct-current cardioversion is used to treat VT that is not associated with hemodynamic instability. VT that causes hemodynamic instability or VF is treated with prompt defibrillation and cardiopulmonary resuscitation as necessary. Except in patients in whom a transient precipitant, such as hypoxemia or hypokalemia, is identified, the occurrence of VT or VF in the postoperative period warrants electrophysiologic evaluation to determine inducibility, likelihood of arrhythmia recurrence, and the most effective form of chronic antiarrhythmic therapy.

Transient, *nonsustained ventricular ectopy* is common in the postoperative period and may result from any of the following factors: hypokalemia, ischemia, hypoxemia, acidosis, digoxin toxicity, edema from surgical manipulation, or mechanical irritation from an intracardiac catheter. Usually such ectopy resolves with elimination of the precipitating cause. An intravenous lidocaine infusion may be necessary temporarily.

Supraventricular tachycardia (i.e., paroxysmal atrial tachycardia, atrial flutter, atrial fibrillation, or junctional tachycardia) occurs in as many as 20% to 30% of patients who undergo cardiac operations. Atrial flutter and atrial fibrillation are most common. Although the arrhythmogenic mechanism is unknown, etiologic factors may include inadequate protection of atrial myocardium against intraoperative ischemia, the high potassium concentration in cardioplegic solutions, and surgical manipulation of the heart. Advanced age also appears to predispose patients to development of postoperative SVT (Leitch et al., 1990; Hashimoto et al., 1991).

In most patients, SVT is tolerated without hemodynamic compromise. It is usually treated with digoxin or propranolol. In fact, these drugs are often given prophylactically during the postoperative period. Type I atrial flutter (atrial rate ranging from 230 to 340 beats per minute) can often be successfully converted with rapid atrial pacing (Waldo, 1989). In patients with compromised cardiac function, SVT may produce significant hypotension necessitating urgent cardioversion.

Atrioventricular block occurs infrequently and is even less often a persistent problem. It is most likely after valve replacement procedures and may represent edema, ischemic damage, or, rarely, mechanical injury of atrioventricular nodal conduction pathways secondary to surgical manipulation. Because significant second- or third-degree heart block is generally transient, it is treated with temporary pacing and usually resolves within 7 to 10 days. If the intrinsic cardiac rhythm is inadequate to support hemodynamic function, the patient remains during this time in a closely monitored intensive or intermediate care unit with easily available back-up pacing and emergency equipment and medications. If atrioventricular block does not resolve, a transvenous permanent pacemaker is implanted.

Patients undergoing coronary artery bypass grafting may develop new *bundle branch blocks* postoperatively; however, complete resolution occurs in most within 2 months (Moore & Wilkoff, 1991). Cardiac arrhythmias and their management are discussed further in Chapter 22, Postoperative Patient Management, and Chapter 25, Cardiac Arrhythmias.

SUDDEN CARDIAC DEATH

Infrequently, cardiac surgical patients experience *sudden cardiac death* in the postoperative period. Precipitous cardiac arrest in a previously stable patient is usually due to an arrhythmia and is most likely to occur during the first 48 hours when electrolyte disturbances, hypoxemia, or myocardial ischemia may be present. Rarely, cardiac arrest occurs late in the postoperative period, presumably caused by an undetected cardiac rhythm disorder. Other less common causes of sudden cardiac death in cardiac surgical patients include undetected cardiac tamponade or pulmonary embolism.

Sudden cardiac death is treated with immediate institution of cardiopulmonary resuscitation and advanced life support measures. In a cardiac surgical patient who does not respond to initial life-saving therapeutic measures, the surgeon will often reopen the sternal incision to detect and relieve possible tamponade. In selected cases, portable CPB using percutaneous cannulation of the femoral artery and vein may be instituted to provide temporary hemodynamic support until definitive therapy to correct the precipitating factor is performed.

POSTPERICARDIOTOMY SYNDROME

Postpericardiotomy syndrome is an inflammatory process that can complicate operations in which the pericardial sac is opened. It occurs in 10% to 50% of patients who undergo cardiac operations (Miller et al., 1988). Although it may be evident as early as the third postoperative day, it more often develops 7 days or more after a cardiac operation (Franco et al., 1991). Postpericardiotomy syndrome has a variable clinical presentation (Horneffer et al., 1990). It usually produces a mild illness. The diagnosis is based on clinical findings, including malaise, fever, a pericardial friction rub, chest pain, and pericardial or pleural effusion. The associated fever is low grade and persists over several days without evidence of local infection.

Treatment with aspirin, indomethacin, or other nonsteroidal anti-inflammatory medication usually results in resolution of symptoms. Antacids are administered concomitantly to reduce gastric irritation, especially in patients who are also receiving warfarin. A single dose of intravenous decadron may also be given. Oral corticosteroids may be necessary in more severe cases. Infrequently, postpericardiotomy syndrome has serious consequences. It is thought to be associated with a higher incidence of saphenous vein graft closure (Horneffer et al, 1990; Smith, 1990). It can also lead to development of significant pericardial or pleural effusions.

PERICARDIAL EFFUSION

Pericardial effusion may represent hemorrhage as described earlier or an increased volume of pericardial fluid secondary to postpericardiotomy syndrome. Clinical manifestations of pericardial effusion include dyspnea, fatigue, pulsus paradoxus, and unexplained hypotension. The degree of symptoms varies with the volume of the effusion, the rapidity of its accumulation, and physical characteristics of the pericardium itself (Lorell & Braunwald, 1992). Large effusions can impede diastolic ventricular filling enough to produce cardiac tamponade.

If tamponade develops or if the effusion does not diminish with medical treatment of postpericardiotomy syndrome, it may be necessary to evacuate the pericardial fluid by means of a pericardiocentesis or a pericardiotomy performed through a left anterior thoracotomy incision. These procedures must be performed with particular care in patients who have had recent coronary artery revascularization to avoid damaging grafts that lie on the anterior surface of the heart. Also, in anticoagulated patients, the procedure may need to be delayed until the prothrombin time is lowered, either by withholding warfarin or with the administration of fresh frozen plasma.

PULMONARY EMBOLISM

Major *pulmonary embolism* is an unusual complication after cardiac operations. However, small pulmonary emboli without associated symptoms may occur more commonly than is clinically detected. At greatest risk are patients with a prior history of deep venous thrombosis or pulmonary embolism, those with coagulation abnormalities, or obese patients with prolonged immobility. Pulmonary emboli originate from the iliofemoral venous system in two thirds of patients and from calf veins in the remaining one third (Van Trigt & Wolfe, 1989). However, clinical evidence of deep venous thrombosis is often absent. Preventive measures against pulmonary embolism include early ambulation and, in high-risk patients, prophylactic anticoagulation.

Clinical manifestations of pulmonary embolism vary. Findings may include shortness of breath, chest pain, new-onset atrial fibrillation, signs and symptoms of deep venous thrombosis, hypotension, and tachycardia. The typical blood gas abnormality associated with pulmonary embolus is a low Pao_2 with respiratory alkalosis (Pratter & Irwin, 1989). Because symptoms vary and noninvasive studies are not definitive, diagnosis may be difficult. Ventilation–perfusion scanning is generally not specific in postoperative cardiac surgical patients because of ventilation–perfusion shunting caused by postoperative atelectasis and increased levels of interstitial fluid in the lungs resulting from CPB. Definitive diagnosis necessitates pulmonary angiography.

On definitive or presumptive diagnosis of a pulmonary embolus, anticoagulation is instituted, initially with heparin and then with warfarin. Supplemental oxygen or intubation and mechanical ventilation may be necessary, depending on the degree of respiratory compromise. Rarely, massive pulmonary embolism occurs, causing severe hypoxemia and right ventricular failure. Such patients are treated with mechanical ventilation, high Fio_2 and positive end-expiratory pressure levels, and inotropic support of the heart. Thrombolytic therapy, using streptokinase or urokinase, may provide dramatic clinical improvement. However, the risk of bleeding precludes its use in patients who develop pulmonary embolism within 10 days after operation (Van Trigt & Wolfe, 1989).

In the hemodynamically compromised patient who is unresponsive to medical therapy, emergent pulmonary embolectomy may be performed. Percutaneous CPB may be necessary as a life-saving measure until the patient can be transported to the operating room and placed on standard CPB. A patient who has recurrent pulmonary emboli despite therapeutic anticoagulation may require placement of a vena caval filter.

NONCARDIAC COMPLICATIONS

NEUROLOGIC DEFICITS

Central neurologic deficits comprise a spectrum of clinical events ranging from isolated *transient ischemic attack* to fatal cerebral injury. *Cerebral vascular accident* is the major cause of neurologic disability after cardiac surgery (Mills & Prough, 1991). Unfortunately, the etiology of perioperative strokes is poorly understood. The most important preoperative risk factor appears to be a history of symptoms suggestive of underlying cerebral vascular disease. In patients with neurologic symptoms or carotid bruits, preoperative ultrasound scanning of carotid arteries is usually performed. Consequently, strokes related to undetected carotid artery disease are fairly uncommon.

More often, perioperative stroke is presumed to be related to cerebral thrombosis or an embolic event. Stroke can also occur due to prolonged hypotension associated with left ventricular failure or due to arterial dissection that occludes cerebral blood flow. A principal source of embolic stroke is atheroma in the ascending aorta and aortic arch that can embolize as a result of manipulation, clamping, or cannulation of the aorta (Wareing et al., 1992). Other potential sources of emboli are (1) thrombus from the left atrium (due to stasis of blood in patients with atrial fibrillation) or ventricle (after MI), (2) air from the arterial perfusion line of the CPB circuit or a chamber of the heart that has been opened or vented, or (3) calcium from the aortic valve area.

Approximately 70% of strokes occur intraoperatively; the remaining 30% occur in the early postoperative period (Mills & Prough, 1991). Neurologic complications most often become apparent as the patient is allowed to awaken from general anesthesia. Less commonly, a patient who is neurologically intact in the immediate postoperative hours develops a new deficit in the ensuing postoperative days. Stroke is diagnosed by physical examination and computed tomography of the brain. Therapy is primarily supportive; if a severe neurologic deficit is present, extensive rehabilitation may be necessary. *Seizures* occasionally occur in postoperative cardiac surgical patients. Although emboli are the probable cause of most postoperative seizures, other factors, such as fluid overload, electrolyte imbalance, and hypoxemia may also precipitate seizures (Anderson et al., 1991).

Peripheral neurologic damage can also result from cardiac operations. Occasionally, *phrenic nerve paralysis* occurs. The phrenic nerves, imbedded in the parietal pleura, can be injured as a result of local hypothermia or surgical trauma during pericardiotomy. Paralysis and elevation of the ipsilateral diaphragm results. Unilateral phrenic nerve paralysis usually does not produce significant problems, except in persons with marginal pulmonary function who may require prolonged ventilatory support. Bilateral injury to the phrenic nerves is manifested by difficulty in weaning from mechanical ventilation. Prolonged ventilatory support may be required.

Compression of the lower trunk of the brachial plexus during retraction of the sternum may produce a *brachial plexus injury* (McLaughlin, 1991). To reduce the risk of this complication, sternal retractors are often placed in a more caudad (toward the lower end of the body) position, thereby avoiding overstretching of the cephalad (toward the head) located nerves. Brachial plexus injury is most commonly manifested

as paresthesia involving the fourth and fifth fingers on the affected side, but it may cause weakness or pain in more severe cases. Although symptoms may persist for several months, they almost always resolve. *Meralgia paresthetica,* or *lateral cutaneous femoral nerve syndrome,* is an unusual neurologic complication characterized by paresthesia and numbness on the anterolateral aspect of the thigh (Parsonnet et al., 1991). Although the precise cause is unknown, it is presumed to occur secondary to intraoperative immobility and positioning of the legs. There is no specific treatment, and symptoms usually resolve within several months.

RESPIRATORY COMPLICATIONS

Atelectasis and pleural effusion are the most common minor respiratory abnormalities. In fact, some degree of atelectasis, particularly of the left lower lobe, is an expected postoperative finding that is usually easily treated with aggressive pulmonary hygiene measures. Factors promoting atelectasis in cardiac surgical patients include reduced lung volume and small airway closure (Valta et al., 1992).

Pleural effusions occur particularly on the left side and in those patients in whom one or both internal thoracic arteries have been harvested for coronary artery bypass grafting. Although pleural effusions generally resolve with time, large or persistent effusions are treated with thoracentesis or chest tube drainage. A persistent effusion that is not drained may eventually cause lung entrapment, necessitating surgical decortication. *Bacterial pneumonia* occasionally occurs, usually due to colonization of the upper respiratory tract in patients who require prolonged intubation. Organism-specific antimicrobial therapy and aggressive pulmonary hygiene measures are instituted.

Acute respiratory failure is uncommon. Patients with severely impaired pulmonary function are at most risk (Bevelaqua et al., 1990). Other patients at risk include those with marginal cardiac function and those who are in a generally debilitated state. Precipitating etiologic factors include atelectasis caused by hypoventilation and retention of secretions, pneumonia (more likely in critically ill patients who are intubated for prolonged periods or who have other infections), and pulmonary edema (usually related to poor ventricular function).

The most severe form of respiratory failure is *adult respiratory distress syndrome (ARDS)*. It is an evolving, severe, diffuse injury of the pulmonary parenchyma that occurs as a response to direct or indirect injury to the lung (Neagley, 1991). In postoperative patients, it is almost always precipitated by sepsis or shock that causes direct injury to pulmonary parenchyma, changes in capillary membrane permeability, and release of bronchoconstrictive mediators. ARDS is characterized by diffuse, bilateral pulmonary infiltrates and severe hypoxemia (Zapol, 1989). Therapy is directed at supporting respiratory function and includes mechanical ventilation, maintaining adequate oxygenation with high FIO_2 and positive end-expiratory pressure levels, and diuresis. Mortality associated with ARDS ranges from 50% to 76%; death is most likely in patients with advanced age, multisystem organ failure, or sepsis (Suchyta et al., 1992).

INTRA-ABDOMINAL COMPLICATIONS

Intra-abdominal complications develop in less than 2% of cardiac surgical patients (Ohri et al., 1991). They are relatively uncommon because the abdomen is not entered and patients are generally immobilized for less than 24 to 36 hours. Although infrequent, abdominal complications can be quite serious. Mortality rates of 12% to 67% are reported and often attributed to delayed diagnosis of abdominal sepsis with resultant multisystem organ failure (Krasna et al., 1988). Types of intra-abdominal complications that may occur include gastrointestinal bleeding, ileus, pancreatitis, cholecystitis, and intestinal ischemia or infarction.

Gastrointestinal bleeding is the most common intra-abdominal complication (Ohri et al., 1991). It may be detected by gradually decreasing hemoglobin levels or when the patient experiences hematemesis or bloody or black stools. Esophagoscopy or colonoscopy is performed to identify the bleeding source. Acute gastritis is the most common etiology of gastrointestinal bleeding. It is treated with antacid therapy and dietary restriction. Bleeding may also arise from gastroduodenal ulcers. Surgical intervention may be required for persistent bleeding or visceral perforation.

Postoperative ileus can develop secondary to excessive analgesia and immobility. It is characterized by abdominal distention; absence of bowel sounds, flatus, or bowel movements; and radiographic evidence of dilated loops of bowel. Nasogastric suction is necessary until bowel motility is restored. An ileus must be differentiated from *small bowel obstruction*, which occurs rarely. The reason for its development during the postoperative period is unclear, but the obstruction is usually related to adhesions from a previous abdominal operation.

Acute pancreatitis is an inflammatory disorder of the pancreas in which pancreatic proteolytic enzymes (i.e., trypsin, chymotrypsin, and elastase) are abnormally activated and destroy tissue in and around the pancreas (Briones, 1991). It produces upper abdominal pain, nausea and vomiting, low-grade fevers, and elevated serum amylase levels. Diagnosis may be delayed by the subtle nature of clinical findings and nonspecific laboratory findings (Krasna et al., 1988). Most cases of pancreatitis in postoperative cardiac surgical patients are self-limited and respond to fluid therapy and nasogastric suction (Shapiro & Gordon, 1990). *Acute cholecystitis* occasionally occurs, manifested by fever, elevated bilirubin level and white blood cell count, and right upper quadrant pain. Cholecystectomy or tube cholecystostomy may be necessary.

Intestinal ischemia is caused by compromised blood flow to the mesenteric arteries. It is most often due to a prolonged low flow state, particularly in association with infusion of alpha-adrenergic agents. Patients at greatest risk are those whose postoperative course is complicated by hemorrhage, low cardiac output, or other major organ system failure. Intestinal ischemia due to embolism is most likely in patients with intracardiac thrombi and arrhythmias.

Intestinal ischemia produces severe abdominal pain, but because patients are typically intubated the pain may remain unrecognized. An important sign heralding development of intestinal ischemia in moribund patients is moderate to severe acidosis. Other signs include elevated white blood cell count, gastrointestinal bleeding, abdominal tenderness, and evidence of sepsis. If bowel ischemia or infarction is suspected, an angiogram of the abdominal aorta may be performed or the patient may be taken directly to the operating room for an exploratory laparotomy. If only a small portion of bowel is necrotic, the involved segment is resected and the patient may survive. However, if a large portion or the entire bowel is infarcted, the condition is fatal and surgical intervention is abandoned.

RENAL FAILURE

Acute renal failure occurs in approximately 1.5% of patients who undergo cardiac operations (Geha & Whittlesey, 1991). In the postoperative setting, it is usually due to acute tubular necrosis precipitated by prolonged hypotension or hypovolemia. The reduced renal blood flow becomes inadequate for normal glomerular filtration. A number of factors associated with CPB can adversely affect renal blood flow, including periods of low perfusion, hypotension, vasoconstrictors (e.g., norepinephrine), and microemboli (Anderson et al., 1991). Other risk factors for development of renal failure include multiple transfusions, low cardiac output, preoperative contrast agents, nephrotoxic drugs, advanced age, prolonged CPB, and preexisting renal dysfunction.

Impending renal failure is manifested by oliguria that is unresponsive to fluid and diuretic therapy and by rising blood urea nitrogen and serum creatinine levels. Therapy includes provision of adequate preload and systemic blood pressure, administration of diuretic agents, and low-dose dopamine infusion (Smith, 1990). Dialysis may become necessary to remove toxic substances, correct metabolic acidosis, and maintain normokalemia and fluid balance (Smith, 1990). Hemodialysis is usually the preferred method in hemodynamically stable patients. In unstable patients, continuous arteriovenous ultrafiltration may be used alternatively to remove excess fluid.

SEPSIS

Sepsis is the presence of microorganisms or their toxins in the bloodstream; *septic shock* describes the systemic response to sepsis, manifested by hypotension, hyperthermia or hypothermia, impaired organ perfusion, metabolic abnormalities, and, if unchecked, progression to multiple organ failure (Luce, 1987). Characteristic hemodynamic indicators of septic shock include high cardiac output, low systemic vascular resistance, and tachycardia. Patients who require prolonged mechanical ventilation and invasive instrumentation for hemodynamic monitoring and support are at greatest risk for systemic infections. Other risk factors include premorbid infection, poor nutritional status, and a debilitated state. The most frequent causative organisms are gram-negative bacteria, notably *Escherichia coli, Klebsiella, Aerobacter, Pseudomonas, proteus,* and *Bacteroides;* common gram-positive organisms are *Staphylococcus, Streptococcus,* and pneumococcus (Anderson & Visner, 1990).

In postoperative patients who develop high or persistent fevers or who deteriorate clinically for unexplained reasons, serious infection should be suspected. Cultures of blood, sputum, urine, and any draining wounds are obtained. Sometimes a septic syndrome occurs without an obvious source of infection. If an overt source cannot be identified, evaluation of the nasal sinuses and abdomen may reveal sinusitis caused by nasotracheal intubation or a covert intra-abdominal infection (e.g., abscess or acalculous cholecystitis) (Zapol, 1989). Therapy for sepsis includes organism-specific antimicrobial therapy and supportive therapy to sustain adequate tissue perfusion and organ function.

WOUND COMPLICATIONS

Sternal wound complications include sternal dehiscence and superficial or deep wound infection. Factors that have been implicated as placing patients at greater risk for sternal wound complications include operative reexploration through the same incision; closed chest massage; prolonged CPB; factors that adversely affect wound healing, such as obesity, diabetes, nutritional depletion, or corticosteroids; diminished tissue perfusion secondary to low cardiac output syndrome; infection elsewhere in the body; deliberate nonclosure of the sternal incision secondary to hemodynamic instability; and the presence of a tracheostomy, which allows colonization of bacteria in close proximity to the sternal incision.

Mobilization of one or both internal thoracic arteries for bypass grafting may also contribute to sternal wound problems, particularly in patients with other risk factors. The internal thoracic arteries provide the major source of blood supply to the sternum, and mobilization of an internal thoracic artery significantly devascularizes the sternal half from which it is harvested (Ulicny & Hiratzka, 1991). Risk is greatest in patients who undergo harvesting of both internal thoracic arteries, especially in the presence of diabetes (Grossi et al., 1991). Because of the prevalence of osteoporosis in elderly women, internal thoracic artery harvesting may contribute to greater risk in this population.

Sternal dehiscence is the postoperative separation of the sutured sternal halves. At the completion of operations that necessitate median sternotomy, the surgically divided sternum is securely reapproximated using heavy suture material or thin wire. Normally the sternal halves fuse together and the sternum regains its full strength over a course of 8 to 12 weeks. If the edges of the sternal halves fail to heal properly or if the suture or wire becomes disrupted before this can occur, sternal dehiscence results. Although usually associated with deep infection of the sternal wound, it may also occur in the absence of wound infection. At particular risk are patients with chronic obstructive pulmonary disease and excessive postoperative coughing who exert greater force on the healing sternum.

A sterile, or noninfected, sternal dehiscence is termed a *mechanical dehiscence.* A division of the sternum that is off center (paramedian) contributes to the likelihood of dehiscence by leaving small segments of bone that can fracture or separate from the tension of the closure. Other factors contributing to mechanical dehiscence are a technically inadequate closure, erosion of wire or suture through the bone, sutures that are not tight, the type of suture material used, patient noncompliance with limitations on activities involving the upper extremities, and a failure of the bone to heal.

Mechanical dehiscence is likely to occur earlier in the postoperative course than does dehiscence associated with infection. Sterile dehiscence occurs most often within several days after operation, whereas infective dehiscence is more likely to become evident 1 to 2 weeks after operation. Mechanical dehiscence is corrected by reoperation to resecure the sternal halves. Heavy bands may be applied to help maintain sternal approximation. A major concern associated with sternal dehiscence is damage to bypass grafts lying on the anterior surface of the heart from movement of the unstable sternum during respiration or at the time of operative restabilization.

Occasionally, mechanical dehiscence occurs late, usually as a result of vigorous upper extremity activity initiated before the bone is fully healed. If only a small portion of the sternum is separated and the patient has a fairly sedentary life-style, the surgeon may elect to follow the patient over several months to determine if sternal healing will occur. In most cases, operative reclosure is required.

Sternal wound infection may result from intraoperative contamination of the operative field, hematogenous spread of pathogens from elsewhere in the body, or postoperative wound contamination. *Staphylococcus aureus* and *S. epidermidis* are the most common pathogenic organisms causing clean wound infections; enteric gram-negative rods are less frequent causes (Doebbeling et al., 1990). Superficial infection involving only the subcutaneous tissue is manifested by small amounts of purulent drainage and localized areas of erythema surrounding the incision. It is treated with local drainage, wound care, and organism-specific antimicrobial therapy.

Signs of deep sternal infection are copious purulent drainage from or extensive cellulitis surrounding the sternal incision, localized tenderness, fever, sternal instability, and malaise. Deep infection of a sternal wound produces significant morbidity and prolongation of hospitalization. It frequently causes sternal dehiscence, *osteomyelitis* of the sternum, and *mediastinitis*.

Treatment of deep sternal wound infection associated with dehiscence includes operative exploration for the purpose of sternal debridement and antibiotic irrigation of the mediastinal cavity. Early exploration improves the patient's outcome by reducing the damage caused by a prolonged and contained infection. An indwelling catheter is usually placed in the mediastinum through which an antibiotic solution, dilute povidone-iodine, or saline is continuously infused over 3 to 5 days (Loop et al., 1990). Chest tubes are placed to evacuate the solution. If possible, primary closure is performed by reapproximating the sternal halves. The skin is often left open for secondary healing.

In the case of severe osteomyelitis, radical operative debridement of all necrotic, avascular tissue may be necessary (Ulicny & Hiratzka, 1991). The bone and cartilage are poorly vascularized structures and, once infected, are very difficult to sterilize. Much or all of the sternum and a significant amount of costal cartilage may need to be removed. The procedure is performed with ready availability of CPB because of the danger of injury to bypass grafts or entry into a cardiac chamber. Unless chronic obstructive pulmonary disease is present, most patients do not suffer impairment of respiratory effort with only fibrous union or even with complete absence of the sternum. However, protection against trauma to the anterior chest is no longer present.

If a significant amount of sternum is excised, reconstruction with *muscle flaps* may be necessary to primarily close the wound (Fig. 28-2). Use of muscle flaps has been a major advance, markedly reducing morbidity and mortality. Applying muscle flaps brings a rich network of blood supply to the poorly vascularized bone (Jeevanandam et al., 1990). The improved blood supply is thought to increase oxygen tension and intravascular delivery of antibiotics to jeopardized tissue. Either the pectoralis major or rectus abdominus muscle may be used. An *omental flap* is used rarely. The omentum, which also has a rich blood supply, is harvested from the upper abdomen and placed over the mediastinal structures. In addition to enhancing regional blood supply, the pres-

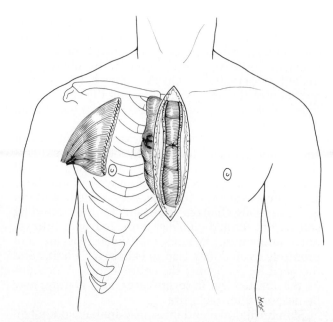

FIGURE 28-2. Pectoralis muscle flap is mobilized to reach midline and cover sternal wound. (Craver JM, Rand RP, Bostwick J III, Hatcher CR Jr, 1991: Management of postoperative mediastinitis. In Waldhausen JA, Orringer MB [eds]: Complications in Cardiothoracic Surgery, P. 128. St. Louis, Mosby—Year Book)

ence of a muscle or omental flap eradicates empty spaces within the mediastinum that could otherwise provide pockets for accumulation of purulent material.

Mediastinitis associated with sternal wound infection necessitates intensive nursing care with meticulous attention to wound management and antibiotic administration. During periods of inadequate drainage of infection and after each operative debridement, bacteremia with resultant septic shock is likely. In the presence of extensive mediastinal infection, the surgeon may elect to leave the wound open to provide adequate drainage. During the period when the wound is left open, a large protein loss can be anticipated. Multiple operative interventions may be required for debridement and eventual wound closure. Although patients are critically ill for a prolonged period, the prognosis is generally good if cardiac function is satisfactory and the infection is adequately drained.

A potential complication of mediastinitis is infection of aortic or cardiac suture lines, especially if prosthetic material, such as felt pledgets, has been implanted during the primary cardiac operation. If prosthetic material does become infected, surgical removal of the material may be necessary to eradicate the infection. A false aneurysm of the ascending aorta may also develop secondary to indolent infection. Such an infected aneurysm, termed a *mycotic aneurysm*, may occur months or years after the infection, particularly if prosthetic material has been placed on the aorta or cardiac structures (Bojar et al., 1988). Mycotic aneurysm is a particularly difficult problem to manage. Aortic rupture may occur if the aneurysm is treated conservatively. On the other hand, surgical resection of the aneurysm is technically difficult because of dense adhesions caused by infection within the mediastinum.

Superficial infection of the leg incision is an infrequent and minor problem that usually occurs in patients who are obese, are diabetic, or have compromised peripheral arterial circulation. Leg wound infections are treated with local drainage, debridement, and frequent dressing changes. Infection of the surrounding soft tissue, termed *cellulitis,* is treated with intravenous antibiotics. Wound infections that are not promptly treated may lead to extensive cellulitis and the need for reopening the entire length of incisions on the affected leg. In severe cases, skin grafting may be necessary for reclosure.

Skin breakdown and incisional drainage do not always signify infection. They may instead represent necrosis of poorly vascularized subcutaneous fat. In addition, some patients have a local inflammatory reaction to the suture material used to close subcutaneous tissue. In such cases, small openings may appear along the incision line, from which small amounts of fluid can be expressed. Occasionally, this tissue reaction continues until the incision is surgically reopened and the offending suture material removed.

An occasional late wound complication is incisional discomfort due to sternal wires or bands in the subcutaneous tissue. The patient may be able to palpate these, and they may be painful when anything is pressed against overlying skin. In cachectic patients with minimal subcutaneous tissue, the skin may erode and infection can ensue. In such cases, it may be necessary for the surgeon to reopen the incision with the patient under general anesthesia, remove the anterior portions of the wires or bands, and bury the remaining ends before reclosing the incision. Usually, this operative correction of the problem is deferred until 6 months after the original cardiac procedure to allow full healing of the sternum before removing supportive material.

URINARY TRACT COMPLICATIONS

Urinary tract infection can occur secondary to the urethral catheter inserted at the time of operation. It is particularly likely in patients with a prolonged preoperative length of hospitalization (Doebbeling et al., 1990). The majority of patients are asymptomatic, and their urine may clear spontaneously after catheter removal (Keys & Serkey, 1991). The infection is often detected by the routine urine culture obtained at the time of catheter removal. It should also be suspected if dysuria or an unexplained postoperative fever develops. Organism-specific antibiotic therapy is instituted.

Urinary retention occurs occasionally in men with preexisting prostatic hypertrophy. If a patient fails to void within 8 to 10 hours of catheter removal, the catheter is reinserted. If 500 mL or more residual urine is present in the bladder, the catheter is usually left in place. A second trial of catheter removal may be tried 24 to 48 hours later when the patient is more ambulatory. If a second recatheterization is necessary, a urologic consultation may be obtained. Sometimes a dilating procedure or transurethral prostatic resection may be necessary before successful catheter removal. If repeated catheterization or urologic instrumentation is necessary in patients with prosthetic valves, appropriate prophylactic antibiotics against infective endocarditis should be given.

MISCELLANEOUS COMPLICATIONS

Postoperative *psychological disturbances* may occur, ranging from mild depression or disorientation to agitation, hallucinations, combative behavior, or frank psychosis. Patients most likely to develop postoperative psychological sequelae include (1) those with underlying psychological disturbances, (2) those with extreme preoperative anxiety, (3) those who have a prolonged course in the intensive care unit with sleep deprivation, (4) elderly patients, and (5) those with a history of alcohol abuse. Generally, psychological complications are of a very transient nature and are treated with symptomatic management. Supportive therapy to suppress agitation and protect the patient from injury is used until the psychological disturbance resolves. If the patient has been on psychotropic medications preoperatively, the medications are generally resumed as soon as the patient is taking oral nourishment.

Because prophylactic antibiotics are given routinely, postoperative patients occasionally develop a *Clostridium difficile bowel infection* due to suppression of normal bowel flora. Protracted diarrhea with resultant dehydration can occur. Accordingly, a stool culture is obtained in postoperative patients who develop diarrhea. If the culture is positive for *C. difficile,* metronidazole (Flagyl) is generally administered to eradicate the infection. Oral vancomycin may alternatively be used.

An unusual problem after cardiac operations is development of *local tissue necrosis,* presumably due to the combination of pressure points, prolonged immobility on the operating table, and hypothermia. The most common site for development of tissue necrosis is the back of the head. Although the ulcerated tissue usually heals without complication, the affected area is generally quite painful and alopecia is common. If this problem is noted in any postoperative patients, attempts to prevent its recurrence in other patients by different intraoperative positioning of the head or placement of pillows should be promptly investigated.

Iatrogenic aortic dissection is a rare complication of cardiac operations. Injury to the aortic intima or media can occur at the site of cannulation, partial occlusion or aortic cross-clamp, or aorta–saphenous vein anastomoses. Risk factors for development of aortic dissection are cystic medial necrosis, hypertension, and atherosclerosis. Surgical repair of the aorta may be required.

DEVICE-RELATED COMPLICATIONS

Complications resulting from intraoperative CPB are unusual but can occur. *Air embolization* is the most commonly recognized complication. Numerous safety features are incorporated into the CPB system to prevent infusion of air into the arterial circulation, and various maneuvers to prevent air embolism (venting, positioning, aspiration, lung ventilation) are routinely performed by the surgeon and anesthesiologist before discontinuing CPB. However, air embolism rarely occurs and can cause catastrophic cerebral or coronary artery occlusion. A neurologic deficit known or suspected to be due to air embolism may be reversible if detected and treated in the first few postoperative hours.

The adverse physiologic effects imposed by CPB occasionally produce a clinical response known as *postperfusion syndrome*. It is characterized by pulmonary and renal dysfunction, an abnormal bleeding diathesis, increased susceptibility to infection, increased interstitial fluid, leukocytosis, fever, vasoconstriction, and hemolysis (Kirklin & Kirklin, 1990). Patients subjected to prolonged duration of CPB are most likely to experience postperfusion syndrome.

Postoperative complications can also occur as a result of implanted prosthetic devices such as cardiac valves, pacemakers, and implantable cardioverter/defibrillators. Prosthetic valves can become infected (prosthetic endocarditis), become acutely regurgitant around the sewing ring (paravalvular leak), or cause thromboembolism or anticoagulant-related hemorrhage. Pacemaker or cardioverter/defibrillator implantation can be complicated by infection, lead dislodgement, or device failure. Intra-aortic balloon counterpulsation may be complicated by limb ischemia, thromboembolism, bleeding, pseudoaneurysm, aortic dissection, or arteriovenous fistula (Finkelmeier & Finkelmeier, 1991). Ventricular assist devices may cause hemorrhage, thromboembolism, or sepsis. These prosthetic devices and their associated complications are discussed in greater detail elsewhere in the text.

REFERENCES

Anderson DR, Stephenson LW, Edmunds LH, 1991: Management of complications of cardiopulmonary bypass: Complications of organ systems. In Waldhausen JA, Orringer MB (eds): Complications in Cardiothoracic Surgery. St. Louis, Mosby–Year Book

Anderson RW, Visner MS, 1990: Shock and circulatory collapse. In Sabiston DC Jr, Spencer FC (eds): Surgery of the Chest, ed. 5. Philadelphia, WB Saunders

Bevelaqua F, Garritan S, Haas F, et al., 1990: Complications after cardiac operations in patients with severe pulmonary impairment. Ann Thorac Surg 50:602

Bojar RM, Payne DD, Sheffield AB, et al., 1988: Successful repair of postoperative ascending aortic mycotic false aneurysms using circulatory arrest. Ann Thorac Surg 46:182

Briones TL, 1991: The gastrointestinal system. In Alspach JG (ed): Core Curriculum for Critical Care Nursing, ed. 4. Philadelphia, WB Saunders

Christakis GT, Ivanov J, Weisel RD, et al., 1989: The changing pattern of coronary artery bypass surgery. Circulation 80 (Suppl I):I-151

DiSesa VJ, 1991: Pharmacologic support for low cardiac output. Semin Thorac Cardiovasc Surg 3:13

Doebbeling BN, Pfaller MA, Kuhns KR, et al., 1990: Cardiovascular surgery prophylaxis. J Thorac Cardiovasc Surg 99:981

Edwards FH, Taylor AJ, Thompson L, et al., 1991: Current status of coronary artery operation in septuagenarians. Ann Thorac Surg 52:265

Ellison N, Campbell FW, Jobes DR, 1991: Postoperative hemostasis. Semin Thorac Cardiovasc Surg 3:33

Finkelmeier BA, Finkelmeier WR, 1991: Iatrogenic arterial injuries resulting from invasive procedures. J Vasc Nurs 9:12

Franco KL, Breckenridge I, Hammond GL, 1991: The pericardium. In Baue AE, Geha AS, Hammond GL, et al. (eds): Glenn's Thoracic and Cardiovascular Surgery, ed 5. Norwalk, CT, Appleton & Lange

Geha AS, Whittlesey D, 1991: Postoperative low cardiac output. In Baue AE, Geha AS, Hammond GL, et al. (eds): Glenn's Thoracic and Cardiovascular Surgery, ed. 5. Norwalk, CT, Appleton & Lange

Grossi EA, Esposito R, Harris LJ, et al., 1991: Sternal wound infections and use of internal mammary artery grafts. J Thorac Cardiovasc Surg 102:342

Halfman-Franey M, Berg DE, 1991: Recognition and management of bleeding following cardiac surgery. Crit Care Nurs Clin North Am 3:675

Hammermeister KE, Burchfiel C, Johnson R, Grover FL, 1990: Identification of patients at greatest risk for developing major complications at cardiac surgery. Circulation 82 (Suppl IV):IV-380

Hashimoto K, Ilstrup DM, Schaff HV, 1991: Influence of clinical and hemodynamic variables on risk of supraventricular tachycardia after coronary artery bypass. J Thorac Cardiovasc Surg 101:56

Hendren WG, Higgins TL, 1991: Immediate postoperative care of the cardiac surgical patient. Semin Thorac Cardiovasc Surg 3:3

Higgins TL, Starr NJ, 1991: Risk stratification and outcome assessment of the adult cardiac surgical patient. Sem Thorac Cardiovasc Surg 3:88

Horneffer PJ, Miller RH, Pearson TA, et al., 1990: The effective treatment of postpericardiotomy syndrome after cardiac operations. J Thorac Cardiovasc Surg 100:292

Jeevanandam V, Smith CR, Rose EA, et al., 1990: Single-stage management of sternal wound infections. J Thorac Cardiovasc Surg 99:256

Jones EL, Weintraub WS, Craver JM, et al., 1991: Coronary bypass surgery: Is the operation different today? J Thorac Cardiovasc Surg 101:108

Kelleher RM, Rose AA, Ordway L, 1991: Prostaglandins for the control of pulmonary hypertension in the postoperative cardiac surgery patient: Nursing implications. Crit Care Nurs Clin North Am 3:741

Keys TF, Serkey JM, 1991: Management and control of infectious complications. Semin Thorac Cardiovasc Surg 3:71

Kirklin JW, Barratt-Boyes BG, 1993: Hypothermia, circulatory arrest, and cardiopulmonary bypass. In Cardiac Surgery, ed. 2. New York, Churchill Livingstone

Kirklin JK, Kirklin JW, 1990: Cardiopulmonary bypass for cardiac surgery. In Sabiston DC Jr, Spencer FC (eds): Surgery of the Chest, ed. 5. Philadelphia, WB Saunders

Krasna MJ, Flancbaum L, Trooskin SZ, et al., 1988: Gastrointestinal complications after cardiac surgery. Surgery 104:773

Leitch JW, Thomson D, Baird DK, Harris PJ, 1990: The importance of age as a predictor of atrial fibrillation and flutter after coronary artery bypass grafting. J Thorac Cardiovasc Surg 100:338

Loop FD, Lytle BW, Cosgrove DM, et al., 1990: Sternal wound complications after isolated coronary artery bypass grafting: Early and late mortality, morbidity, and cost of care. Ann Thorac Surg 49:179

Lorell BH, Braunwald E, 1992: Pericardial disease. In Braunwald E (ed): Heart Disease: A Textbook of Cardiovascular Medicine, ed. 4. Philadelphia, WB Saunders

Luce JM, 1987: Pathogenesis and management of septic shock. Chest 91:883

Mahfood SS, Higgins TL, Loop FD, 1991: Management of complications related to coronary artery bypass surgery. In Waldhausen JA, Orringer MB (eds): Complications in Cardiothoracic Surgery. St. Louis, Mosby–Year Book

McLaughlin JS, 1991: Positional and incisional complications of thoracic surgery. In Waldhausen JA, Orringer MB (eds): Complications in Cardiothoracic Surgery. St. Louis, Mosby–Year Book

Miller RH, Horneffer PJ, Gardner TJ, et al., 1988: The epidemiology of the postpericardiotomy syndrome: A common complication of cardiac surgery. Am Heart J 116:1323

Mills SA, Prough DS, 1991: Neuropsychiatric complications following cardiac surgery. Semin Thorac Cardiovasc Surg 3:39

Moore SL, Wilkoff BL, 1991: Rhythm disturbances after cardiac surgery. Semin Thorac Cardiovasc Surg 3:24

Moran JM, Singh AK, 1989: Cardiogenic shock. In Grillo HC, Austen WG, Wilkins EW Jr, et al. (eds): Current Therapy in Cardiothoracic Surgery. Toronto, BC Decker

Moreno-Cabral CE, Mitchell RS, Miller DC, 1988: Postoperative problems. In Manual of Postoperative Management in Adult Cardiac Surgery. Baltimore, Williams & Wilkins

Naunheim KS, Fiore AC, Wadley JJ, et al., 1988: The changing profile of the patient undergoing coronary artery bypass surgery. J Am Coll Cardiol 11:494

Neagley SR, 1991: The pulmonary system. In Alspach JG (ed): Core Curriculum for Critical Care Nursing, ed. 4. Philadelphia, WB Saunders

Ohri SK, Desai JB, Gaer JA, et al., 1991: Intraabdominal complications after cardiopulmonary bypass. J Thorac Cardiovasc Surg 52:826

Parsonnet V, Karasakalides A, Gielchinsky I, et al., 1991: Meralgia paresthetica after coronary bypass surgery. J Thorac Cardiovasc Surg 101:219

Pratter MR, Irwin RS, 1989: Pulmonary thromboembolism. In Rippe JM (ed): Manual of Intensive Care Medicine, ed. 2. Boston, Little, Brown

Reedy JE, Swartz MT, Termuhlen DT, et al., 1990: Bridge to heart transplantation: Importance of patient selection. J Heart Transplant 9: 473

Shapiro SJ, Gordon LA, 1990: General surgical complications following cardiac surgery. In Gray RJ, Matloff JM (eds): Medical Management of the Cardiac Surgical Patient. Baltimore, Williams & Wilkins

Smith PK, 1990: Postoperative care in cardiac surgery. In Sabiston DC Jr, Spencer FC (eds): Surgery of the Chest, ed. 5. Philadelphia, WB Saunders

Suchyta MR, Clemmer TP, Elliott CG, et al., 1992: The adult respiratory distress syndrome. Chest 101:1074

Tam SK, Miller JM, Edmunds LH, 1991: Unexpected, sustained ventricular tachyarrhythmia after cardiac operations. J Thorac Cardiovasc Surg 102:883

Tuman KJ, 1991: Perioperative myocardial infarction. Semin Thorac Cardiovasc Surg 3:47

Tuman KJ, McCarthy RJ, March RJ, 1992: Morbidity and duration of ICU stay after cardiac surgery. Chest 102:36

Ulicny KS Jr, Hiratzka LF, 1991: The risk factors of median sternotomy infection: A current review. J Cardiac Surg 6:338

Valta P, Takala J, Elissa T, Milic-Emili J, 1992: Effects of PEEP on respiratory mechanics after open heart surgery. Chest 102:227

Van Trigt P, Wolfe W, 1989: Pulmonary embolism. In Grillo HC, Austen WG, Wilkins EW Jr, et al. (eds): Current Therapy in Cardiothoracic Surgery. Toronto, BC Decker

Waldo AL, 1989: Arrhythmias following open heart surgery: Role of cardiac pacing and recording. In Grillo HC, Austen WG, Wilkins EW Jr, et al (eds): Current Therapy in Cardiothoracic Surgery. Toronto, BC Decker

Wareing TH, Davila-Roman VG, Barzilai B, et al., 1992: Management of the severely atherosclerotic ascending aorta during cardiac operations. J Thorac Cardiovasc Surg 103:453

Whitman GR, 1991: Hypertension and hypothermia in the acute postoperative period. Crit Care Nurs Clin North Am 3:661

Zapol WM, 1989: Adult respiratory distress syndrome. In Grillo HC, Austen WG, Wilkins EW Jr, et al. (eds): Current Therapy in Cardiothoracic Surgery. Toronto, BC Decker

29

MANAGEMENT OF CRITICALLY ILL PATIENTS

SUPPORT OF THE FAILING HEART
  Management of Heart Failure
  Implications of Mechanical Assist Devices
  Cardiopulmonary Arrest
MANAGEMENT OF RESPIRATORY FAILURE
  Acute Respiratory Distress
  Intubation and Mechanical Ventilation
  Adult Respiratory Distress Syndrome
  Weaning From Prolonged Ventilatory Support

OTHER CONSIDERATIONS IN CRITICALLY ILL
  PATIENTS
Nutritional Support
Prevention of Infection
Electrolyte and Metabolic Imbalances
Problems Associated With Immobility
SUPPORT OF THE FAMILY

One of the most challenging aspects of cardiothoracic surgical nursing is the care of patients who are critically ill. Sometimes, patients who appear to be recovering in a routine fashion develop sudden and catastrophic problems. Other patients come to operation critically ill and on life support systems. Particularly in elderly patients and in those with underlying cardiac, pulmonary, or renal impairment, serious complications can develop and evolve into multiple system organ failure. Cardiothoracic surgical nurses play a major role in determining the ultimate outcome of these critically ill patients. The most common forms of major organ system dysfunction in cardiac surgical patients are cardiogenic shock and respiratory failure.

SUPPORT OF THE FAILING HEART

MANAGEMENT OF HEART FAILURE

Acute ventricular dysfunction is a major cause of critical illness in cardiac surgical patients. Severe ventricular dysfunction, termed *cardiogenic shock*, is characterized by a cardiac index less than 2.0 L/min/m², systemic vascular resistance more than 2100 dynes·

sec·cm⁻⁵, atrial pressure greater than 20 mm Hg, and urine output less than 20 mL/h (Reedy et al., 1990). The condition is usually fatal unless temporary augmentation of cardiac function can be provided through pharmacologic or mechanical means. Cardiogenic shock may represent left ventricular, right ventricular, or biventricular dysfunction. Because coronary artery disease and valvular heart disease most commonly damage the left ventricle, left ventricular dysfunction is most common.

Standard monitoring of the patient in cardiogenic shock includes cardiac rate and rhythm, arterial pressure, central venous pressure, pulmonary artery pressure, cardiac output, and systemic vascular resistance. Measurement of these hemodynamic parameters is discussed in detail in Chapter 23, Hemodynamic Monitoring. In addition to the various intracardiac and vascular pressures and calculated indices, assessment of adequate tissue perfusion necessitates close attention to level of consciousness (cerebral blood flow), urine output (renal blood flow), and peripheral pulses and color and temperature of extremities (peripheral blood flow).

The goals of supportive therapy are to increase cardiac output and myocardial oxygen supply while reducing myocardial work, oxygen demands, and ischemia (Quaal, 1988). Interventions are focused on manipulation of those hemodynamic parameters (i.e., heart rate, preload, afterload, and contractility) that affect cardiac output. Iatrogenic alteration of hemodynamic parameters produces rapid and sometimes profound changes in the patient's cardiovascular physiologic state. Consequently, cardiothoracic surgical nurses require a thorough understanding of principles of cardiovascular physiology, the meaning and relationship of the various hemodynamic parameters, and the actions of commonly used pharmacologic agents.

Heart rate may be artificially manipulated by temporary pacing. A rate in the range of 90 to 100 beats per minute is considered optimal in most patients. Sinus bradycardia is treated with temporary atrial pacing. Atrioventricular (AV) sequential pacing is used in the presence of AV nodal dysfunction to preserve the contribution to cardiac output provided by atrial systole. The "atrial kick" (i.e., an appropriately timed atrial contraction) increases ventricular filling, allows more complete emptying of the atria, and prevents regurgitation across AV valves during ventricular systole. As compared with ventricular pacing, AV sequential pacing improves cardiac output in patients with impaired ventricular function, recent cardiac surgery, or myocardial infarction (Finkelmeier & Salinger, 1986). Ventricular pacing is used if atrial fibrillation or other supraventricular tachycardia precludes atrial or AV sequential pacing.

Antiarrhythmic medications are administered if clinically significant supraventricular tachycardia or ventricular arrhythmias occur. Tachyarrhythmias at rates greater than 120 beats per minute compromise diastolic ventricular filling time and decrease contractility by altering myocardial oxygen supply and demand (Geha & Whittlesey, 1991). Digoxin is most commonly used for ventricular rate control during supraventricular tachycardia. Use of beta-blocking agents or calcium-channel antagonists is usually precluded by their negative inotropic effects. Ventricular arrhythmias are common in patients with cardiogenic shock. Hypoxemia and hypokalemia are typical precipitants; when corrected, the ventricular ectopy generally resolves. If ventricular arrhythmias are related to myocardial ischemia or an underlying cardiac rhythm disorder, intravenous infusion of lidocaine or other antiarrhythmic agent may be required.

Preload, or filling pressure, is the end-diastolic volume in the ventricle and is measured indirectly by pulmonary artery diastolic or left atrial pressure. The relationship between end-diastolic fiber length and cardiac output is described by *Starling's law* (Hudak et al., 1990a). As preload increases, cardiac output also increases until a point is reached where a further increase in filling pressure produces a decrease in cardiac output and congestive heart failure. Preload is maintained at an optimal level for an individual patient using pulmonary artery diastolic pressure to guide volume replacement. In the presence of ventricular dysfunction, a higher preload (15–20 mm Hg) is usually required than in patients with normal ventricular function.

Left ventricular afterload, assessed by measurement of systemic vascular resistance, is usually lowered to decrease impedance to left ventricular ejection and, as a result, reduce cardiac work and oxygen consumption. Sodium nitroprusside and nitroglycerin are the mainstays of pharmacologic vasodilatation. Intra-aortic balloon counterpulsation (IABC) is often necessary to provide mechanical afterload reduction. Pulmonary vascular resistance is the clinical indicator of *right ventricular afterload.* Nitroglycerin, isoproterenol, or prostaglandin E$_1$ may be used to lower pulmonary vascular resistance in patients with right ventricular dysfunction.

Myocardial contractility may be increased using one or more of the various intravenous inotropic agents. Dopamine, dobutamine, isoproterenol, and amrinone are commonly used inotropic agents. Dopamine is often the agent of choice. In addition to its inotropic effect, dopamine at low doses stimulates renal dopaminergic receptors and thus increases renal perfusion (Greco, 1990). Usually vasodilating and inotropic agents are infused concomitantly to achieve the desired degree of afterload reduction and enhancement of myocardial contractility (DiSesa, 1991). The most effective combination and dosing of the various pharmacologic agents are determined empirically and modified by serial measurements of hemodynamic parameters.

Continuous intravenous infusions of inotropic and vasodilating agents must be performed with great attention to detail. Central venous catheters are almost always used to ensure consistent delivery of the medication and to avoid caustic effects of some agents on peripheral veins. Rate-regulating pumps are essential to maintain dosage at a constant rate. Changing intravenous solutions or tubing is performed in a manner that avoids bolusing or disruption of medication infusion with resultant precipitous hypertension or profound hypotension. Flushing a catheter through which medications are being infused is contraindicated.

Commonly, multiple drugs are administered simultaneously and doses are changed frequently. It is imperative that the nurse at the bedside knows the precise dose of each agent being infused, which catheter is being used for infusion, and which drugs can be safely infused through a single catheter or through a peripheral catheter.

Patients in cardiogenic shock are mechanically ventilated to reduce the work of respiration and, therefore, lower oxygen demand. Intravenous morphine may be administered to minimize sympathetic overstimulation due to pain or anxiety and its deleterious effects on heart rate and systemic vascular resistance (Moran & Singh, 1989). When severe hemodynamic instability is present, even routine repositioning may be precluded by the potential for inducing profound hypotension.

IMPLICATIONS OF MECHANICAL ASSIST DEVICES

Mechanical support of the failing heart is a primary modality for treating cardiogenic shock refractory to pharmacologic therapy. Most commonly used is *intra-aortic balloon counterpulsation*. The balloon-tipped catheter, usually inserted through the femoral artery in a retrograde fashion, is positioned so that the tip lies in the descending thoracic aorta, just distal to the left subclavian artery. Rhythmic inflation and deflation of the balloon in synchrony with cardiac contraction increases arterial pressure during diastole and decreases pressure during systole. IABC thus decreases myocardial oxygen consumption by reducing left ventricular afterload and improves myocardial oxygenation by augmenting coronary artery blood flow during diastole.

Interventions during IABC include monitoring and adjusting timing of balloon inflation and deflation to maximize hemodynamic benefits. Arrhythmias are treated promptly to prevent their interference with the timing of counterpulsation. Hemodynamic and clinical indicators of tissue perfusion are monitored to assess effectiveness of counterpulsation and patient readiness for weaning. Serial blood sampling (including complete blood cell count, blood urea nitrogen, creatinine, and platelet count) is performed to detect deleterious effects of IABC. An elevated white blood cell count suggests infection, increases in blood urea nitrogen and creatinine levels may represent renal dysfunction secondary to catheter-related impairment of renal artery perfusion, and a decreased platelet count (thrombocytopenia) may result from catheter-induced trauma to platelets. Antibiotics and heparin are usually administered as prophylaxis against infection and thromboembolism, respectively. The insertion site is observed for evidence of hematoma or infection.

The most common complication of IABC therapy is *limb ischemia*, which can result from thrombosis around the catheter or embolization of thrombus. Patients with underlying arterial occlusive disease and compromised blood flow to the lower extremities are at particular risk. Prevention of permanent limb dysfunction or loss is dependent on prompt detection and treatment of ischemia. The extremity distal to the balloon catheter is evaluated hourly, including palpation of peripheral pulses, and assessment of capillary refill, color, temperature, and motor and sensory function. The hallmarks of ischemia are the "six Ps": pulselessness, paresthesia, paralysis, pallor, pain, and poikilothermia (decreased temperature). Often the earliest signs are discoloration or mottling of the foot and absence of pulses. Observation of the extremity is essential since patients are typically intubated and sedated. Patients who are able to follow commands are asked to wiggle their toes and flex and extend the affected foot; the ability to do so is compared with the other foot.

Anterior compartment syndrome can develop due to edema associated with acute ischemia. The fascia surrounding the muscles in the calf is fixed in size. As the muscle becomes swollen, it is compressed and becomes ischemic. Metabolic acidosis, hyperkalemia, and elevated blood urea nitrogen and creatinine levels can all result from the toxic waste products of ischemic tissue. In addition to operative revascularization of the femoral artery, surgical *fasciotomies* (opening of the fascial compartments) may be necessary to prevent muscle necrosis (Fig. 29-1). Other complications associated with IABC include aortic dissection, hemorrhage, false aneurysm, and arteriovenous fistula (Finkelmeier & Finkelmeier, 1991).

Ventricular assist devices (VADs) are much less widely used but are available in some centers for use in patients with cardiogenic shock. A VAD is a sophisticated device designed to completely support one or both ventricles for days, weeks, or even months. Operation of a VAD is performed by a perfusionist or nurse with specialized training. Depending on the type of device, it may be attached to the patient through cannulae in the femoral vessels or cannulae inserted directly through the chest wall into the heart or great vessels. In patients requiring a VAD for postoperative cardiogenic shock, the primary complication is bleeding (Golding, 1991). Other potential complications of VADs are thromboembolism, hemolysis, and infection. IABC and VADs are discussed in more detail in Chapter 30, Mechanical Assist Devices.

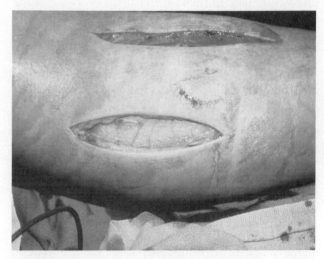

FIGURE 29-1. Fasciotomy incisions performed for relief of compartment syndrome. (Mravic PJ, Massey DM, 1992: Compartment syndrome. J Vasc Nurs 10:10)

CARDIOPULMONARY ARREST

Cardiopulmonary arrest is the cessation of spontaneous respirations and effective cardiac contractions. It can result from a respiratory arrest, a cardiac arrhythmia, or a hemodynamic catastrophe. Cardiopulmonary arrest continues to be associated with a high mortality and a significant incidence of postresuscitation neurologic impairment.

Cardiopulmonary resuscitation is initiated immediately on diagnosis of cardiac arrest. A self-inflating bag with oxygen at an FIO_2 of 100% is used to manually ventilate the patient by means of a face mask. Either oral or nasal intubation is performed to provide a secure airway, and manual ventilation through the endotracheal tube is continued. Chest compressions are performed at a rate of 80 to 100 compressions per minute (Guerci & Chandra, 1991). Electrocardiographic monitoring is established. Immediate defibrillation, using 200 joules of current, is recommended for ventricular fibrillation or ventricular tachycardia with hemodynamic instability (American Heart Association, 1990a). If unsuccessful, defibrillation is repeated a second time with 200 to 300 joules; subsequent shocks with up to 360 joules are delivered if the arrhythmia persists.

Rapid defibrillation is essential for two reasons. First, restoration of an adequate cardiac rhythm is more effective therapy than cardiopulmonary resuscitation. The outcome of cardiac arrest, with or without cardiopulmonary resuscitation, is dismal if defibrillation is not performed within 8 minutes (American Heart Association, 1990b). Second, defibrillation is most likely to be successful if performed within 1 to 2 minutes of the onset of the arrhythmia (Goldberger, 1990). Although defibrillation is not effective therapy for asystole, sometimes what appears on the electrocardiographic oscilloscope as asystole is actually a fine ventricular fibrillation that may be successfully converted with defibrillation.

Intravenous bolus doses of antiarrhythmic medications, such as lidocaine, procainamide, or bretylium, are administered to stabilize the cardiac rhythm. A continuous infusion of an appropriate antiarrhythmic medication is begun. Occasionally, the heart rhythm is so unstable that multiple episodes of ventricular tachycardia or ventricular fibrillation are occurring. In this situation, defibrillator patches may be secured to the chest wall so that defibrillation can be repeated as necessary without delay.

Most cardiac surgical patients have temporary pacing wires placed at the time of operation. If bradycardia is present, a pulse generator is connected and single- or dual-chamber pacing is performed as indicated to maintain a stable cardiac rhythm. In the absence of pacing wires, a bolus dose of atropine or an isoproterenol infusion may be given. Occasionally, electromechanical dissociation occurs; that is, a cardiac rhythm is present but no mechanical contraction is produced by the electrical depolarization (Gold-schlager, 1988). Electromechanical dissociation almost always signifies impending death.

Central venous access is usually established to ensure effective delivery of pharmacologic agents during the low flow state of artificial circulation (Smith, 1990). Generally, a central venous catheter is inserted for continuous infusion of cardiotonic medications and a peripheral catheter is used for bolus doses of drugs or fluids. Blood samples are obtained for immediate arterial blood gas and serum electrolyte analysis. In unusual situations when venous access cannot be quickly established, epinephrine or atropine can be administered through the endotracheal tube, followed by several hyperinflations of the lungs; the intracardiac route for the administration of epinephrine is considered a last resort if venous and endotracheal routes are unavailable (Bircher, 1988; American Heart Association, 1990c).

Although cardiopulmonary resuscitation may be lifesaving, external cardiac compression can cause serious complications, particularly in patients who have recently undergone sternotomy. Most common is sternal dehiscence and infection, which can lead to osteomyelitis and mediastinitis. Other complications of external cardiac massage include rib fractures, hemothorax, pneumothorax, laceration of abdominal viscera (especially the liver), and rupture of the aorta or a cardiac chamber (Goldschlager, 1988).

Circulatory support systems, such as *percutaneous cardiopulmonary bypass*, may be appropriate in selected patients. Although these devices can temporarily sustain the patient and allow time for cardiac recovery, irreversible neurologic damage related to the initial circulatory collapse all too frequently prevents long-term survival. Accordingly, portable cardiopulmonary support is generally instituted only when the arrest is witnessed, correctable underlying cardiac pathology is present, and cardiopulmonary resuscitation time is short.

MANAGEMENT OF RESPIRATORY FAILURE

ACUTE RESPIRATORY DISTRESS

Acute respiratory distress is the inability to sustain respiration that is sufficient to maintain adequate blood oxygen saturation. Tachypnea, diaphoresis, dyspnea, and tachycardia are common early manifestations. The patient often attempts to remain in a sitting position, resisting efforts to lower the head of the bed. Initially anxious and agitated, the patient gradually becomes more somnolent as the problem worsens. If not corrected, respiratory and cardiac arrest soon follow.

Immediately on noticing a deterioration in the patient's respiratory status, oxygen saturation is measured using a pulse oximeter and arterial blood gases and a portable chest roentgenogram are obtained. The lung fields are carefully auscultated. If rales are heard, intravenous diuretic therapy may be indicated to remove excess fluid. Endotracheal suctioning may be necessary if diminished breath sounds or rhonchi, representing atelectasis or the presence of secretions, respectively, are present. Suctioning must be performed with great caution in nonintubated patients with evidence of respiratory distress. Supplemental oxygenation is provided and the electrocardiogram is monitored during the procedure. Endotracheal intubation and mechanical ventilation are usually necessary to treat acute respiratory distress.

INTUBATION AND MECHANICAL VENTILATION

Endotracheal intubation is performed through the mouth or nose. Orotracheal intubation is technically easier. Also, because tubes with a larger diameter can be used for oral intubation, less airway resistance is created and more effective suctioning can be performed; nasotracheal tubes, on the other hand, are more comfortable for the patient, permit better oral hygiene, and can be more effectively stabilized (Pierson, 1988).

Endotracheal tubes are designed with a balloon that can be inflated around the tube to allow positive pressure ventilation through the tube. Almost all currently used endotracheal tubes have low pressure cuffs that are inflated to the point of a minimal leak during peak inspiration. Routine cuff deflation is generally not necessary when a minimal leak technique is used. Characteristics of a good quality endotracheal tube cuff include (1) low sealing pressure, (2) cuff pressure distributed over a large contact area, (3) large volumes of air accepted with minor increases in balloon tension, (4) maintenance of a good seal during inspiration and expiration, and (5) no distortion to the tracheal wall (Neagley, 1991).

Secure fixation of the endotracheal tube prevents dislodgement or damage to the tracheal wall and requires periodic replacement of soiled or moist tape. When intubation is prolonged, the tube is stabilized using a technique that prevents local pressure necrosis of skin on the nose or mouth. Oral hygiene measures are performed as needed. During the period that the patient is intubated, suctioning with appropriate oxygenation is performed at least every 2 hours. The injection of small amounts (2 to 3 mL) of saline into the endotracheal tube, followed by ventilation and suctioning, may facilitate loosening and mobilization of tenacious secretions.

Because of the significant complications associated with prolonged endotracheal intubation, tracheostomy is generally performed if the duration of intubation exceeds 10 to 14 days. A tracheostomy frees the patient's nose and mouth of an endotracheal tube. If level of consciousness and the swallowing mechanism are not impaired, oral feedings may be resumed.

In patients who are intubated but self-ventilating, *continuous positive airway pressure* (CPAP) may be ap-

plied to increase functional residual capacity. Occasionally, CPAP is delivered in nonintubated patients through a specially constructed, tightly fitting face mask. However, if ventilation is compromised enough to warrant a CPAP mask, intubation almost invariably becomes necessary. In addition, the masks are uncomfortable for alert patients and are often poorly tolerated.

Critically ill patients almost always require *mechanical ventilation* for support of respiratory function. Even in the presence of normal respiratory function, mechanical ventilation may be helpful in unstable patients to conserve energy that would otherwise be expended on the work of breathing. Management of ventilators is nearly always handled by respiratory therapists. However, nurses require a basic understanding of the principles and types of mechanical ventilation.

There are two components to providing adequate respiration for patients on mechanical ventilators: oxygenation (the maintenance of a satisfactory arterial oxygen pressure [Pao_2]) and ventilation (the maintenance of a satisfactory arterial carbon dioxide pressure [$Paco_2$]) (Elefteriades & Geha, 1985). Achieving adequate oxygenation is the more common problem in critically ill patients. The most common cause of hypoxemia is mismatching of ventilation to perfusion at the alveolar level (Neagley, 1991).

Oxygenation must be maintained at a level sufficient to preserve aerobic metabolism. Arterial Pao_2 can decrease to approximately 60 mm Hg before oxygen-carrying capacity begins to decrease significantly. Accordingly, a Pao_2 of 60 mm Hg is probably adequate for patients without compromised regional blood flow; a Pao_2 of 75 mm Hg is adequate for most other patients (Elefteriades & Geha, 1985). Ventilation, or the removal of carbon dioxide, is directly dependent on the minute volume (i.e., the respiratory rate times the tidal volume of each breath). For patients on mechanical ventilators, the $Paco_2$ is generally maintained at approximately 40 mm Hg. Effective CO_2 removal is rarely a problem when using mechanical ventilation in patients with respiratory failure. Common arterial blood gas abnormalities and corrective ventilator adjustments are listed in Table 29-1.

Most currently used ventilators are volume controlled; that is, a preset volume of oxygenated air is delivered by positive pressure through an endotracheal or tracheostomy tube into the tracheobronchial tree. *Intermittent mandatory ventilation* (IMV) is often used as the mode of ventilation. With IMV, the ventilator delivers a preset number of breaths each minute at a given tidal volume. Between these mandatory breaths, the patient can breathe spontaneously, generating a tidal volume that varies according to ventilatory effort.

In critically ill or cachectic patients, an *assist/control mode*, in combination with muscle paralysis with pancuronium and sedation with morphine, may be preferable to minimize energy expenditure (Moreno-Ca-

TABLE 29-1. INTERVENTIONS FOR COMMON ARTERIAL BLOOD GAS ABNORMALITIES

Abnormality	Ventilator Adjustment
High Pa_{CO_2}	Increase tidal volume Increase respiratory rate
Low Pa_{CO_2}	Decrease tidal volume Decrease respiratory rate
High Pa_{O_2}	Decrease F_{IO_2} Decrease PEEP (if >5 cm)
Low Pa_{O_2}	Increase F_{IO_2} Increase PEEP

bral et al., 1988). The assist/control mode is similar to IMV in that the ventilator delivers a preset number of breaths each minute at a given tidal volume; it differs in that spontaneous negative inspiratory pressure generated by the patient triggers delivery of the preset tidal volume (Balk, 1991).

Positive end-expiratory pressure (PEEP) is almost always used in conjunction with mechanical ventilation. PEEP is positive pressure applied at the end of expiration; it compensates for the loss of physiologic PEEP provided by the glottis in the nonintubated patient. Five centimeters H_2O pressure is the standard amount used to keep small airways open. However, because PEEP decreases intrapulmonary shunting, larger amounts may be used in selected situations to improve oxygenation and decrease the F_{IO_2} level.

An additional physiologic effect of PEEP is that it increases intrathoracic pressure, which in turn decreases venous return to the heart. Therefore, the addition of PEEP may require increasing preload to prevent a decrease in cardiac output with resultant hypotension. When high levels of PEEP are used, unilateral or bilateral pneumothoraces may develop (Fig. 29-2). Once alveolar rupture occurs, positive pressure during mechanical inhalation forces air through the rent into the pleural space. Tension pneumothorax is likely, with precipitous hypotension, tachycardia, and hypoxemia. Prompt chest tube thoracostomy is performed to relieve the tension component. Generally, the chest tube remains to suction drainage until positive pressure ventilation is discontinued.

ADULT RESPIRATORY DISTRESS SYNDROME

Adult respiratory distress syndrome (ARDS) is the most severe form of respiratory failure. It is an evolving, severe, diffuse injury of pulmonary parenchymal tissue that occurs as a response to direct or indirect injury to the lungs (Neagley, 1991). In postoperative patients, ARDS usually occurs secondary to sepsis. It is characterized by diffuse, bilateral infiltrates associated with profound hypoxemia.

A major goal of therapy in treatment of ARDS is the restoration of adequate oxygenation. Frequently, high levels of F_{IO_2} are necessary to maintain a Pa_{O_2} greater than 60 mm Hg. However, prolonged administration of an oxygen concentration greater than 50% may be complicated by clinically significant pulmonary oxygen toxicity (Irwin & Demers, 1989). Ten to 20 cm of PEEP is commonly applied when ventilating patients with ARDS. The enhanced oxygenation provided by this amount of PEEP allows the use of lower, and less toxic, F_{IO_2} levels. Bilateral prophylactic chest tubes may be inserted when high levels of PEEP are used.

High-frequency ventilation may be used in selected patients with ARDS. In this unique form of ventilation, small tidal volume breaths are delivered at high frequencies. Use of a high-frequency ventilator avoids the high airway pressures often necessary when using conventional ventilation in a patient with severe hypoxemia. Consequently, high-frequency ventilation is associated with less pulmonary barotrauma. The efficacy of high-frequency ventilation in treatment of patients with ARDS has not been definitively demonstrated, and its role remains controversial (Todd, 1994).

Diuretic therapy is used adjunctively to improve oxygenation, particularly if bilateral rales, indicative of fluid overload, are present. Even in the absence of clinical evidence of pulmonary edema, diuresis may

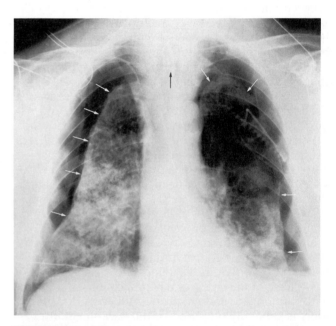

FIGURE 29-2. Anteroposterior roentgenogram demonstrating bilateral pneumothoraces secondary to mechanical ventilation with high levels of positive end-expiratory pressure. Note clearly visible edges of the partially collapsed lungs (*white arrows*) and the absence of lung markings external to lung edges. A tracheostomy tube is also apparent (*black arrow*). (Courtesy of Robert M. Vanecko, M.D.)

help by lowering the hydrostatic capillary pressure. A lower pulmonary capillary wedge pressure (that continues to provide adequate cardiac output and renal perfusion) reduces fluid movement into the interstitial tissue through capillary membranes that are made more permeable by respiratory failure (Todd, 1994). In anemic patients, oxygenation may be improved by blood replacement therapy. Although transfusion with exogenous blood can often be avoided in stable patients, blood is transfused more liberally in critically ill patients. The extra oxygen-carrying capacity provided by a normal hemoglobin level plays an important role in patients with marginal organ system function.

Hemodynamically stable patients who can tolerate repositioning are turned every 2 hours. Because pulmonary blood flow preferentially travels to dependent areas and ventilation is better in upright areas, prolonged periods in one position increase ventilation–perfusion mismatching. Especially in obese patients, oxygenation is also improved by placing the bed in a reversed Trendelenburg position (with the head elevated) so that the diaphragm is not subjected to pressure from the pendulous abdomen.

WEANING FROM PROLONGED VENTILATORY SUPPORT

Weaning is attempted when the ventilated patient demonstrates the capability for self-ventilation, as evidenced by adequate respiratory parameters. Vital capacity and negative inspiratory force are the two measurements that best represent the patient's readiness for weaning and extubation. In addition, the patient should be alert enough to protect the airway and demonstrate a gag reflex by coughing during suctioning.

In patients who have required prolonged ventilation, the weaning process often takes days or weeks. Before weaning is initiated, the patient should be receiving adequate calories to meet metabolic demands and complicating factors, such as infection or hemodynamic instability, must be under control. Impediments to weaning from mechanical ventilation are listed in Table 29-2. If the patient is otherwise stable, weaning can often be performed in an intermediate care or "step-down" unit. Nursing observation must be adequate, however, to monitor the patient's tolerance of progressive reductions in ventilatory support. Oximetry monitoring is usually performed during the weaning process to detect impending respiratory distress.

Most commonly, weaning consists of gradual reduction of the IMV rate over a period of days or weeks. The addition of *pressure support* (i.e., a preset amount of positive pressure delivered during inspiration of spontaneous breaths) may facilitate weaning (Moreno-Cabral et al., 1988). For patients who are difficult to wean, other techniques may prove more successful. Although various regimens may be used,

TABLE 29-2. IMPEDIMENTS TO WEANING FROM MECHANICAL VENTILATION

Pulmonary pathophysiology
    Atelectasis
    Retention of secretions
    Pneumonia
Fluid overload
Low cardiac output
Phrenic nerve paralysis
Nutritional depletion
Sepsis
Anemia

a consistent schedule is designed to allow periods of rest interspersed with periods in which the patient must increasingly perform the work of breathing. Nursing care and visiting periods are arranged to coincide with the weaning schedule so that the patient has adequate sleeping and resting periods. In patients who have had significant respiratory failure, weaning requires a great deal of patience and cannot be rushed to exceed the patient's endurance. Gradual retraining of the respiratory muscles is necessary before a sustained, coordinated pattern of respiratory effort is restored.

If the patient has required mechanical ventilation for more than 2 weeks, a tracheostomy tube will usually have been placed. When the patient has demonstrated the ability to sustain adequate respiration, supplemental oxygenation or humidification through a tracheostomy collar or T-shaped adaptor may be attempted. Removal of the tracheostomy tube is generally preceded by serial downsizing and changing from a cuffed to noncuffed tube. Nursing observation is essential after tracheostomy tube removal. The presence of granulation tissue due to prolonged intubation may lead to respiratory insufficiency within minutes or hours of removing the tube. Absence of a leak around the tube when the cuff is deflated is suggestive of possible upper airway obstruction. Once the tube has been removed, the stoma closes over the course of 24 to 48 hours. Insertion of another tube through the stoma is generally not possible after this time.

OTHER CONSIDERATIONS IN CRITICALLY ILL PATIENTS

NUTRITIONAL SUPPORT

Providing adequate nutrition is essential to recovery of critically ill patients. In addition to the protein and calories needed under normal circumstances, critically ill patients often need additional calories to heal wounds or combat infective processes. The altered nitrogen handling and energy requirements associated with critical illness cause muscle wasting, metabolic abnormalities, abnormal liver function, and depressed glomerular filtration (Allard & Jeejeebhoy, 1991). Malnutrition increases the risk of ventilator dependency, prolonged hospitalization, and operative mortality (Sivak, 1991). Consequently, some form of supplemental nutrition is almost always instituted in any patient who cannot be fed orally due to prolonged intubation, a diminished level of consciousness, or other factors.

Supplemental nutrition can be provided either directly into the gastrointestinal tract or intravenously. *Enteral feedings* provided via the gastrointestinal tract are generally preferred to avoid potential infectious complications associated with an indwelling central venous catheter. A small feeding tube may be placed in the duodenum or jejunum. Placing the tube distal to the pylorus avoids gastroesophageal reflux and possible aspiration associated with gastrostomy tube feedings delivered directly into the stomach.

A nasogastric route is generally chosen if feedings will be necessary for only a short time. A small-diameter tube is used with a weighted tip that aids passage into the duodenum. Proper tube position is confirmed by a chest roentgenogram before feedings are instituted. Alternatively, a jejunostomy tube is inserted through the abdominal wall, either percutaneously or through a small incision. A variety of enteral feedings are available. The feeding regimen is introduced gradually, with serial increases in volume and concentration of solution, to avoid diarrhea. Development of diarrhea necessitates temporary cessation of feedings until the problem abates. Because of the small lumen of distal feeding tubes, they become easily clogged and cannot be used for solid medications.

Central intravenous hyperalimentation is used when enteral feedings are not tolerated or advisable. A catheter in the subclavian or jugular vein is placed for continuous infusion. The solutions are hypertonic and must be infused into a central vein where rapid blood flow dilutes the solution, thus decreasing the risk of inflammation and venous thrombosis (Avunduk, 1989). Because of the risk of infection, the catheter is used solely for hyperalimentation infusion and care is taken to maintain sterility of the solution and the catheter insertion site. The catheter is changed every 5 to 7 days or if the patient develops a fever or local signs of infection at the insertion site.

PREVENTION OF INFECTION

Infection is a major problem in critically ill patients. The multitude of invasive catheters and tubes in combination with the patient's debilitated state provides a fertile setting for nosocomial pathogens. The most serious nosocomial infections in critically ill patients are bacteremia, pneumonia, and surgical wound infection (Cooper & Larson, 1992). Intravenous cathe-

ters are one of the most common sources of infection. A number of risk factors have been identified for infection related to intravenous catheters, including poor insertion technique, length of time the catheter is in place, the type of solution infused through the catheter (particularly hyperalimentation or lipid solutions), patient age, underlying disease process, and types of surgical procedures performed on the patient (Yanelli & Gurevich, 1988). To reduce the incidence of catheter-induced infections, peripheral cannulae are changed every 2 to 3 days and arterial catheters every 4 days. Central intravenous and pulmonary artery catheters are changed every 5 to 7 days.

Urethral drainage catheters are a second common source of nosocomial infection in critically ill patients. Pathogenic bacteria can enter the bladder at the time of catheterization, by retrograde migration along the outer surface of the catheter, or in urine that refluxes into the bladder from the drainage tubing (Yanelli & Gurevich, 1988). As a result, bacteriuria is thought to occur in 80% of patients who have indwelling urethral catheters for 10 days or more (Smith, 1990).

A third major source of infection is prolonged endotracheal intubation. An endotracheal tube bypasses the defense mechanisms of the nasopharynx and allows organisms to enter the sterile tracheobronchial tree. Bacterial colonization occurs after several days of endotracheal intubation, and bacterial pneumonia develops in 5% to 40% of patients (Zapol, 1989). Aspiration can also occur as a result of an altered level of consciousness, abnormal swallowing, or a depressed gag or cough reflex (Recker, 1992).

Sepsis (i.e., the presence of microorganisms or their toxins in the bloodstream) is the most serious consequence of infection. Sepsis is usually caused by a gram-negative organism, such as *E. coli, Klebsiella,* or *Aerobacter*, but may also be caused by a gram-positive pathogen, such as *Staphylococcus* or *Streptococcus* (Anderson & Visner, 1990). *Septic shock* is the body's systemic response to sepsis, manifested by hypotension, hyperthermia or hypothermia, impaired organ perfusion, metabolic abnormalities, and, if unchecked, multiple organ failure (Luce, 1987). The hallmark of septic shock is hypotension associated with a high cardiac output and low systemic vascular resistance. Sepsis also appears to produce intrinsic myocardial depression (Ognibene et al., 1988).

On clinical evidence of sepsis, attempts are made to determine the source of the infection. Blood, urine, sputum, and drainage from any wounds are cultured to identify the responsible organism. Because indwelling central intravenous catheters are a common source of sepsis, insertion sites are changed and the withdrawn catheter tip is cultured. Sometimes, the source of the infection is not easily identified. Physical findings may be masked in the critically ill patient, who typically is heavily sedated or has an impaired level of consciousness. Common covert sources of infection in such patients include sinusitis caused by nasotracheal intubation or an undetected intra-abdominal process such as acalculous cholecystitis or abscess (Zapol, 1989).

Broad-spectrum antibiotics are begun empirically and modified according to culture results as they become available. The profound vasodilatation associated with sepsis generally necessitates infusion of large volumes of fluid to maintain adequate preload and arterial pressure. In addition, a continuous intravenous infusion of a vasopressor agent, such as norepinephrine, may be necessary to increase systemic vascular resistance.

ELECTROLYTE AND METABOLIC IMBALANCES

Hypokalemia can occur secondary to urinary diuresis, diarrhea, vomiting, decreased intake, or alkalosis. Because causative factors are typically present in critically ill patients, mild to moderate hypokalemia is one of the most common metabolic imbalances in this population (Bia, 1991a). Hypokalemia is a common cause of ventricular arrhythmias. Intravenous or oral potassium supplementation is often necessary to maintain the serum potassium level in a range of 3.5 to 5.0 mEq/L.

Hyperkalemia most often occurs in association with renal failure, acidosis, or overzealous intravenous potassium supplementation. Electrocardiographic manifestations of hyperkalemia include low P wave voltage and intraventricular conduction delays that produce wide, bizarre QRS complexes (Goldschlager, 1988). The resulting cardiac rhythm may be difficult to distinguish from ventricular tachycardia.

Except for patients in renal failure, serum potassium levels between 5 and 6 mEq/L can usually be treated by withholding potassium supplementation and by diuresis. If the serum potassium level exceeds 6.0 mEq/L, if electrocardiographic manifestations of hyperkalemia are present, or if the patient's condition is deteriorating, either intravenous glucose and insulin or sodium bicarbonate is administered to shift potassium into the cells, thus lowering the serum concentration (Smith, 1990). Calcium gluconate may also be administered. Although it does not lower serum potassium levels, calcium gluconate counteracts the cardiac and neuromuscular effects of hyperkalemia (Moreno-Cabral et al., 1988).

Patients with *renal failure* may require administration of sodium polystyrene sulfonate (Kayexelate) to treat hyperkalemia. Kayexelate is a potassium-binding resin that may be given orally or in the form of a retention enema. Blood urea nitrogen and creatinine levels may also become seriously elevated in the presence of renal failure. Elective *hemodialysis* may be necessary if the blood urea nitrogen and creatinine levels reach 100 mg/dL and 10 mg/dL, respectively; indications for immediate hemodialysis include manifestations of severe uremia (neurologic disturbances or gastrointestinal bleeding), refractory hyperkalemia, severe metabolic acidosis, and fluid overload (Moreno-Cabral et al., 1988).

Continuous arteriovenous ultrafiltration may be used when pharmacologic diuresis is ineffective and the patient is too hemodynamically unstable to tolerate the rapid fluid and electrolyte shifts that occur with hemodialysis (Paradiso, 1989). In this slow form of hemodialysis, arterial and venous catheters are connected to an extracorporeal system through which the blood is circulated and exposed to a slow-flowing dialysate solution (Lawyer & Velasco, 1989). In contrast to hemodialysis, the blood is not mechanically pumped but rather is propelled through the circuit by the hydrostatic pressure of arterial blood pressure. The major advantage of continuous arteriovenous ultrafiltration is that large volumes of fluid can be removed in a manner that is better tolerated by the patient than hemodialysis; removal of nitrogenous waste products, however, is less efficient (Bia, 1991b).

Hyperglycemia can occur in critically ill patients due to diabetes, hyperalimentation, metabolic derangements, multiple resuscitative therapies, and stress (Newman, 1988). Accordingly, serial blood samples are measured to determine blood glucose levels and guide corrective therapy. Urinary ketones are also monitored. Hyperglycemia is usually treated using a sliding scale protocol for insulin administration. *Hypoglycemia* is uncommon unless iatrogenically produced; it is treated with bolus doses of intravenous glucose.

Other common metabolic disorders in critically ill patients include *hypomagnesemia*, which may cause cardiac arrhythmias, and *hypophosphatemia*, which can produce depression of ventricular function and dysfunction of white blood cells and platelets (Smith, 1990). Disturbances in the acid–base balance also occur frequently because of the many pathophysiologic processes that can increase the body's acid or base production or elimination. Inadequate alveolar ventilation that results in carbon dioxide retention is termed *respiratory acidosis*, and excessive alveolar ventilation that decreases $Paco_2$ is termed *respiratory alkalosis*; acidosis caused by a decrease in bicarbonate is called *metabolic acidosis* and alkalosis due to increased bicarbonate is *metabolic alkalosis* (Rokosky, 1989).

PROBLEMS ASSOCIATED WITH IMMOBILITY

Critically ill patients are confined to bed rest and often endure prolonged periods of passive immobility. In low cardiac output states, blood flow to the skin is marginal. Frequent turning may not be possible in hemodynamically unstable patients. As a result, *decubiti* are likely to develop on any body part that is exposed to prolonged pressure. Ulceration occurs when pressure exceeding mean capillary perfusion pressure is applied to an area of the body over time. Shearing forces, repeated injury, and infection have also been suggested as contributing factors in decubitus ulcer development (Stotts, 1988). Pressure decubiti are a source of further morbidity. Prolonged wound care is usually necessary once an ulcer develops, and skin grafting may eventually be required. Infection of a decubitus ulcer can lead to sepsis. Special oscillating mattresses, positional changes, and other nursing measures to relieve local skin pressure are an important component of caring for critically ill patients. Other consequences of immobility are deep venous thrombosis and atelectasis with resultant pneumonia. Anticoagulation with heparin and vigorous pulmonary hygiene are used to prevent deep venous thrombosis and respiratory complications, respectively.

SUPPORT OF THE FAMILY

Nurses who specialize in cardiothoracic surgical nursing routinely care for patients who are critically ill and, sometimes, dying. It is imperative that families of such patients receive adequate emotional support. Patients frequently remain critically ill for days, weeks, and sometimes even months. During this time, it is important that the family, physicians, and nursing staff all feel like they are working together in the best interest of the patient. Families require a tremendous amount of emotional support to withstand the stress of being suspended between hope for patient recovery and grief in anticipation of patient death.

Occasionally, a previously stable patient suffers a catastrophic event. This information is difficult to convey to family members. The news is profoundly shocking, and the family will need time to absorb the information. As soon as a patient has a major hemodynamic problem or suffers cardiac arrest, a team member begins communicating with the family. Often when the patient's condition is unstable, the primary physician is unable to leave the patient's bedside (or operating room) and the task is delegated to an appropriate physician or nurse member of the team. Ideally, the team member will already have an established relationship with the family. The designated liaison person remains in communication with the family until the immediate life-threatening situation resolves. Simple measures such as arranging for a priest to administer sacramental rites or contacting other family members mean a great deal to the family during this time.

Cardiothoracic surgical services often have a designated clinical nurse specialist who functions as the liaison person in communicating with families, particularly when the patient is critically ill. This individual should have excellent communication skills, including the ability to translate highly technical information into lay terms and to summarize probable outcomes in a compassionate manner. Availability of a liaison individual does not negate the need for

each nurse at the bedside to communicate openly with the family. It is natural that families seek information from those who are directly caring for the patient. At the same time, questions should be referred appropriately to the managing physician to ensure that the information that families receive is consistent and accurate. Although each person attempts to convey information as honestly and completely as possible, the same information can take on different connotations depending on what portions are stressed and the manner in which the information is communicated.

As long as aggressive supportive measures are used, it is appropriate that hope for recovery be expressed. It may be several days or sometimes weeks before it is evident whether a patient can survive. Prognostic implications should be regularly and thoroughly discussed with the family by the managing physician. When survival is no longer realistically anticipated, the managing physician discusses this openly with the family.

If critical illness and suffering of the patient has been lengthy and death becomes increasingly likely, it is natural for loved ones to want the waiting to come to an end. However, these feelings commonly evoke a great deal of guilt and it is quite difficult for family members to assume an active decision-making role in taking steps that will hasten the patient's death. Many patients have prepared *advance directives* to be followed in the event of loss of decision-making ability. Advance directives may be either of two types of documents: (1) *treatment directives* that specify what forms of medical therapy the patient wishes to receive or forego or (2) *durable power of attorney,* which designates another person to act on the patient's behalf (Wlody, 1991).

The overriding concern for the dying patient is to maximize comfort and minimize suffering. Medical and nursing care plans should reflect that a decision has been made to change the goal of therapy from prolonging life to easing death. Interventions are re-evaluated in light of whether they make the process of dying more or less difficult for the patient. Patients who die in critical care units are nearly always comatose at this stage, and it is often the family members who need emotional support and comfort. Some family members prefer to spend as much time as possible with the patient and participate actively in providing care. Although this usually means increased work for the nursing staff, this participation in care can be a highly significant and therapeutic experience for the grieving person (Hudak et al., 1990b). Others may find waiting at the hospital too stressful or have dependents at home for whom they must care. In these cases, it may be necessary to communicate by phone. This makes it more difficult to assess family members' understanding of information and the level of coping.

The nurses at the bedside play a key role in providing support for the family during and immediately after the patient's death. Assessment skills are key to providing appropriate emotional support. The manner in which families grieve varies considerably depending on a host of factors, including cultural norms, circumstances of the death, age and vitality of the patient, individual personalities of family members, and the relationship between patient and family and between the family members themselves. Although some families are effusive in their grief, others keep their emotions in check. Even when death is expected, family members sometimes react with shock and disbelief. Other common reactions include crying, screaming, hitting the wall or floor, hugging one another, sitting impassively, or abruptly leaving the area.

Occasionally, family members may become hostile or abusive to nursing or medical staff, particularly if prior relations between family and staff have been strained or if the death occurs unexpectedly. Family members who have had a strained or turbulent relationship with the patient may be unable to confront negative feelings for the deceased patient and instead direct the negativity toward staff members. It may be helpful for a patient representative or social worker who has not directly participated in the patient's care to remain available to the family. Family members may be able to verbalize feelings to these individuals that they are unable to express directly to the staff members. Value judgments should not be placed on how an individual family grieves; rather, the nurse guides the family members through the initial phase of the grieving process while allowing them to deal with the death in their own manner.

Interventions are aimed at providing comfort. Protocols should be established so that necessary administrative details can be handled with minimal bother to the family. Typical interventions include offering the services of a hospital chaplain, providing water or coffee, or sitting with the family. If the family is large or if one family member is requiring a great deal of attention, it may be necessary to have two persons available to the family during this time. For many family members, it is very important to spend a few moments with the deceased patient before leaving the hospital. Every attempt should be made to accommodate the family and to make the patient appear as natural to the family as possible.

REFERENCES

Allard JP, Jeejeebhoy KN, 1991: Nutrition in the critically ill. In Parrillo JE (ed): Current Therapy in Critical Care Medicine, ed. 2. Philadelphia, BC Decker

American Heart Association, 1990a: Electrical therapy in malignant arrhythmias. In Textbook of Advanced Cardiac Life Support, ed. 2. Dallas, American Heart Association

American Heart Association, 1990b: Advanced cardiac life support in perspective. In Textbook of Advanced Cardiac Life Support, ed. 2. Dallas, American Heart Association

American Heart Association, 1990c: Cardiovascular pharmacology I. In Textbook of Advanced Cardiac Life Support, ed. 2. Dallas, American Heart Association

Anderson RW, Visner MS, 1990: Shock and circulatory collapse. In Sabiston DC Jr, Spencer FC (eds): Surgery of the Chest, ed. 5. Philadelphia, WB Saunders

Avunduk C, 1989: Nutritional support II: Parenteral nutrition. In Rippe JM (ed): Manual of Intensive Care Medicine, ed. 2. Boston, Little, Brown & Co

Balk RA, 1991: Mechanical ventilation. In Parrillo JE (ed): Current Therapy in Critical Care Medicine, ed. 2. Philadelphia, BC Decker

Bia MJ, 1991a: Life-threatening electrolyte and metabolic disorders. In Parrillo JE (ed): Current Therapy in Critical Care Medicine, ed. 2. Philadelphia, BC Decker

Bia MJ, 1991b: Acute renal failure. In Parrillo JE (ed): Current Therapy in Critical Care Medicine, ed. 2. Philadelphia, BC Decker

Bircher DW, 1988: Access for drug administration during cardiopulmonary resuscitation. Crit Care Med 16:179

Cooper B, Larson E, 1992: Infection control issues for critical care units: An overview and challenge—physician and nurse perspective. Heart Lung 21:317

DiSesa VJ, 1991: Pharmacologic support for low cardiac output. Semin Thorac Cardiovasc Surg 3:13

Elefteriades JA, Geha AS, 1985: Respirators and respiratory management. In House Officer Guide to ICU Care: The Cardiothoracic Surgical Patient. Gaithersburg, MD, Aspen Publishers

Finkelmeier BA, Finkelmeier WR, 1991: Iatrogenic arterial injuries resulting from invasive arterial procedures. J Vasc Nursing 9:12

Finkelmeier BA, Salinger MH, 1986: Dual-chamber cardiac pacing: An overview. Crit Care Nurse 6:12

Geha AS, Whittlesey D, 1991: Postoperative complications. In Baue AE, Geha AS, Hammond GL, et al. (eds): Glenn's Thoracic and Cardiovascular Surgery, ed 5. Norwalk, CT, Appleton & Lange

Goldberger E, 1990: Defibrillation and cardioversion. In Treatment of Cardiac Emergencies, ed. 5. St. Louis, CV Mosby

Golding LA, 1991: Postcardiotomy mechanical support. Semin Thorac Cardiovasc Surg 3:29

Goldschlager NF, 1988: Cardiopulmonary arrest and resuscitation. In Luce JM, Pierson DJ (eds): Critical Care Medicine. Philadelphia, WB Saunders

Greco SA, 1990: Vasoactive drugs. In Underhill SL, Woods SL, Froelicher ES, Halpenny CJ (eds): Cardiovascular Medications for Cardiac Nursing. Philadelphia, JB Lippincott

Guerci AD, Chandra NC, 1991: Diagnostic and therapeutic techniques. In Parrillo JE (ed): Current Therapy in Critical Care Medicine, ed. 2. Philadelphia, BC Decker

Hudak CM, Gallo BM, Benz JJ, 1990a: Heart failure. In Critical Care Nursing: A Holistic Approach, ed. 5. Philadelphia, JB Lippincott

Hudak CM, Gallo BM, Benz JJ, 1990b: Caring for the patient's family. In Critical Care Nursing: A Holistic Approach, ed. 5. Philadelphia, JB Lippincott

Irwin RS, Demers RR, 1989: Oxygen therapy. In Rippe JM (ed): Manual of Intensive Care Medicine, ed. 2. Boston, Little, Brown

Lawyer LA, Velasco A, 1989: Continuous arteriovenous ultrafiltration in the ICU. Crit Care Nurse 9:29

Luce JM, 1987: Pathogenesis and management of septic shock. Chest 91:883

Moran JM, Singh AK, 1989: Cardiogenic shock. In Grillo HC, Austen WG, Wilkins EW Jr, et al (eds): Current Therapy in Cardiothoracic Surgery, Toronto, BC Decker

Moreno-Cabral CE, Mitchell RS, Miller DC, 1988: Postoperative problems. In Manual of Postoperative Management in Adult Cardiac Surgery. Baltimore, Williams & Wilkins

Neagley SR, 1991: The pulmonary system. In Alspach JG (ed): Core Curriculum for Critical Care Nursing, ed. 4. Philadelphia, WB Saunders

Newman RH, 1988: Bedside blood sugar determinations in the critically ill. Heart Lung 17:667

Ognibene FP, Parker MM, Natanson C, Shelhamer JH, Parrillo JE, 1988: Depressed left ventricular performance: Response to volume infusion in patients with sepsis and septic shock. Chest 93:903

Paradiso C, 1989: Hemofiltration: An alternative to dialysis. Heart Lung 18:282

Pierson DJ, 1988: Endotracheal intubation. In Luce JM, Pierson DJ (eds): Critical Care Medicine. Philadelphia, WB Saunders

Quaal S, 1988: Mechanical treatment of the failing heart. In Kern LS (ed): Cardiac Critical Care Nursing. Rockville, MD, Aspen Publishers

Recker D, 1992: Caring for the long-term critical care patient. Crit Care Nurse 12:40

Reedy JE, Swartz MT, Termuhlen DT, et al., 1990: Bridge to heart transplantation: Importance of patient selection. J Heart Transplant 9:473

Rokosky JS, 1989: Acid-base balance. In Underhill SL, Woods SL, Froelicher ES, Halpenny CJ (eds): Cardiac Nursing, ed. 2. Philadelphia, JB Lippincott

Sivak ED, 1991: Management of ventilator dependency following heart surgery. Semin Thorac Cardiovasc Surg 3:53

Smith PK, 1990: Postoperative care in cardiac surgery. In Sabiston DC Jr, Spencer FC (eds): Surgery of the Chest, ed. 5. Philadelphia, WB Saunders

Stotts NA, 1988: Predicting pressure ulcer development in surgical patients. Heart Lung 17:641

Todd TR, 1994: Ventilatory support of postoperative surgical patients. In Shields TW (ed): General Thoracic Surgery, ed. 4. Baltimore, Williams & Wilkins

Wlody GS, 1991: Legal and ethical aspects of critical care nursing. In Alspach JG (ed): Core Curriculum for Critical Care Nursing, ed. 4. Philadelphia, WB Saunders

Yannelli B, Gurevich I, 1988: Infection control in critical care. Heart Lung 17:596

Zapol WM, 1989: Adult respiratory distress syndrome. In Grillo HC, Austen WG, Wilkins EW Jr, et al. (eds): Current Therapy in Cardiothoracic Surgery, Toronto, BC Decker

30

MECHANICAL ASSIST DEVICES

INTRA-AORTIC BALLOON COUNTERPULSATION Principles of Counterpulsation Indications Techniques Associated Complications	**VENTRICULAR ASSIST DEVICES** Indications Types of Ventricular Assist Devices Ventricular Assist Device Function and Associated Complications **PORTABLE CARDIOPULMONARY BYPASS**

Mechanical devices that temporarily support or replace the native heart have contributed significantly to management of patients with severe ventricular dysfunction. These devices are used to treat cardiogenic shock refractory to pharmacologic therapy, primarily in one of three clinical situations: (1) after cardiac surgery, (2) after acute myocardial infarction, and (3) for support of patients awaiting cardiac transplantation, that is, as a *"bridge to transplantation."*

Use of a mechanical assist device is considered when hemodynamic data indicate persisting ventricular failure despite pharmacologic interventions to improve preload, afterload, and contractility. Types of devices range from those that augment native cardiac function to those that totally replace the ventricles. Currently available mechanical assist devices include (1) intra-aortic balloon pump, (2) ventricular assist devices (VADs), and (3) portable cardiopulmonary bypass (CPB). All must be regarded as temporary devices at this time. Thus, they are used to support cardiac function until recovery occurs or cardiac transplantation can be performed.

Decisions about patient selection for mechanical assistance, timing for initiation of therapy, and the most appropriate type of device demand a great deal of judgment on the part of the managing physician. Factors that must be considered include the nature of the underlying cardiac pathologic process, prognosis for recovery of native heart function with medical or surgical therapy, patient age, associated medical

problems, and suitability for cardiac transplantation. Because of the limited supply of donor hearts relative to demand, devices used to support patients who are transplant candidates must be suitable for maintenance of cardiac function over a period of weeks or months.

INTRA-AORTIC BALLOON COUNTERPULSATION

Intra-aortic balloon counterpulsation (IABC) was introduced into clinical use in 1968 by Kantrowitz and associates (Kantrowitz et al., 1968). Since that time, its use as a therapeutic modality has become widespread owing to development of sophisticated hemodynamic monitoring, introduction of percutaneous catheter insertion techniques, and biomedical engineering advances that improved balloon catheters and consoles (Pae & Pierce, 1991). IABC is the primary mode of circulatory assistance because of its physiologic effectiveness and relative ease and safety of applicability (Mundth, 1990).

PRINCIPLES OF COUNTERPULSATION

Counterpulsation is the phasic displacement of intra-aortic blood volume to increase arterial pressure during diastole and decrease pressure during systole. It is achieved using a balloon-tipped catheter positioned in the descending thoracic aorta just distal to the left subclavian artery (Fig. 30-1). A console attached to the catheter emits a driving gas into the balloon lumen to produce rhythmic balloon inflations and deflations in synchrony with the patient's cardiac contractions. With the use of the electrocardiographic or arterial pressure tracing, balloon inflation is timed to occur during diastole and deflation occurs during the isovolumetric phase of cardiac systole.

Counterpulsation provides two distinct hemodynamic benefits: (1) augmented diastolic arterial pressure and (2) decreased end-diastolic pressure (Fig. 30-

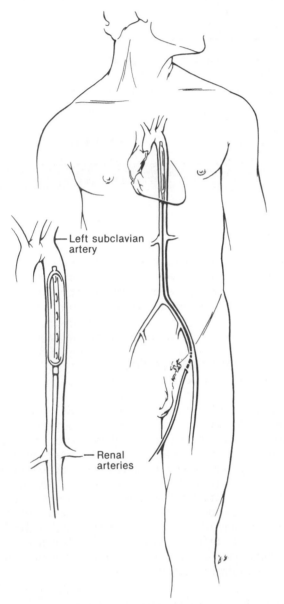

FIGURE 30-1. Intra-aortic balloon catheter positioned in descending thoracic aorta; catheter tip lies just distal to left subclavian artery. (Hudak CM, Gallo BM, Benz JJ, 1990: Intra-aortic balloon pump counterpulsation. In Critical Care Nursing, ed. 5, p. 203. Philadelphia, JB Lippincott)

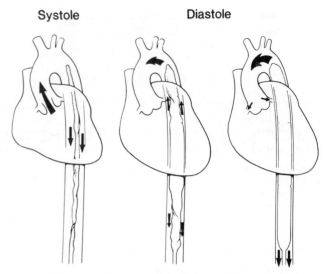

FIGURE 30-2. Hemodynamic benefits of counterpulsation. Balloon deflation decreases afterload and left ventricular work; balloon inflation augments diastolic blood flow. (Jorge E, Pierce WS, 1987: Mechanical support or replacement of the heart. In McGoon DC [ed]: Cardiac Surgery, ed. 2, p. 363. Philadelphia, FA Davis)

2). During diastole, balloon inflation mechanically displaces blood upward and downward in the aorta, producing elevation of the diastolic arterial pressure and thus augmentation of the cardiac output. Because most coronary filling occurs during diastole, coronary blood flow is particularly increased by the higher aortic root pressure.

Deflation of the balloon decreases aortic end diastolic pressure (i.e., afterload) by creating a potential space in the aorta. Consequently, less impedance to ejection exists during the subsequent left ventricular contraction. Wall tension is reduced and stroke volume is increased, providing more complete emptying of the ventricle. The resulting decrease in left ventricular end systolic volume and subsequent preload reduces cardiac work and myocardial oxygen consumption (Shinn, 1989). In addition, the lowered preload decreases resistance to coronary artery filling, allowing better subendocardial perfusion. Thus, IABC improves oxygen supply to the myocardium by augmenting coronary flow during diastole and decreases myocardial oxygen consumption by reducing the afterload against which the left ventricle must eject.

INDICATIONS

IABC is a valuable adjunct in the care of both preoperative and postoperative cardiac surgical patients (Table 30-1). It is used when pharmacologic therapy alone is unsuccessful in treatment of unstable angina, low cardiac output, or cardiogenic shock. The most frequent indication is postoperative left ventricular failure, characterized by systolic pressure less than 90 mm Hg, cardiac index less than 1.5 L/min/m^2, persis-

TABLE 30-1. INDICATIONS FOR INTRA-AORTIC BALLOON COUNTERPULSATION

Preoperative Support

Acute myocardial ischemic syndrome
Postinfarction ventricular septal defect or mitral regurgitation
Postinfarction cardiogenic shock
Irreversible cardiogenic shock, awaiting transplantation

Postoperative Support

Low cardiac output state
Reversible cardiogenic shock
Irreversible cardiogenic shock, awaiting transplantation

tent lactic acidosis, and decreased mixed venous oxygen saturation (Lee, 1990). Two to 12% of patients who undergo myocardial revascularization or valvular heart operations require IABC for postoperative augmentation of ventricular function (Naunheim et al., 1992). IABC provides temporary support while the left ventricle recovers. If ventricular dysfunction is irreversible and the patient is a suitable candidate for cardiac transplantation, IABC may provide sufficient support until a donor heart becomes available.

The most common preoperative indication for IABC is acute myocardial ischemia. Because IABC augments coronary artery perfusion, it is quite effective in treating unstable angina refractory to medical management. Particularly in patients in whom operative risk can be lessened by delaying surgery (e.g., those with postinfarction angina), IABC provides a valuable treatment alternative.

IABC may also be used to treat cardiogenic shock resulting from acute myocardial infarction. In patients with coronary artery lesions amenable to revascularization and a sufficient amount of preserved ventricular function, counterpulsation can provide life-sustaining support until reversibly damaged myocardium is revascularized by percutaneous transluminal coronary angioplasty (PTCA) or coronary artery bypass grafting. Unfortunately, IABC therapy is less useful in patients with cardiogenic shock after acute myocardial infarction if coronary artery anatomy is unsuitable for revascularization. Despite initial hemodynamic improvement with IABC, most patients remain dependent unless underlying coronary artery pathology is treated and ischemic myocardium is reperfused (Pae & Pierce, 1991). If revascularization is not possible, and cardiac transplantation is a treatment option, IABC may be used after acute myocardial infarction as a bridge to transplantation.

Another group of patients benefiting from IABC therapy are those with acute ventricular septal defect or mitral regurgitation secondary to acute myocardial infarction. The afterload reduction achieved with counterpulsation decreases left ventricular peak systolic pressure, thereby decreasing the left to right

shunt in patients with ventricular septal defect and the regurgitant flow into the left atrium in those with mitral regurgitation (Elefteriades & Geha, 1985).

IABC is contraindicated in patients with aortic regurgitation. Because balloon inflation increases intra-aortic diastolic pressure, regurgitation of blood through an incompetent aortic valve would be increased. IABC is also contraindicated in the presence of aortic dissection (Kantrowitz, 1989).

TECHNIQUES

The majority of balloon catheters are inserted into the common femoral artery using a percutaneous technique. The catheter is inserted in the femoral artery on the side with the better arterial circulation. In preoperative patients at increased risk for perioperative ventricular dysfunction, Doppler arterial pressure measurements are performed to assess arterial circulation to the lower extremities. An arterial catheter may be inserted into the femoral artery before operation to be used for pressure monitoring and to allow easy percutaneous balloon catheter insertion during the operation.

A cutdown technique is used when it is not possible to palpate femoral pulses owing to peripheral arterial occlusive disease, cardiogenic shock, or CPB, and when attempted percutaneous insertion has failed (Richenbacher & Pierce, 1991a). Formerly, a cutdown technique necessitated insertion of a graft sewn in end-to-side fashion to the artery. However, direct insertion into the artery without a graft is now possible because of the smaller diameter of currently used catheters and sheath delivery systems.

With standard femoral artery placement, the balloon catheter is positioned with the cephalad end just distal to the origin of the left subclavian artery. This places the balloon as close as possible to the aortic valve without impeding blood flow through the arch vessels. Proper positioning maximizes compartmentalization, allows peripheral flow around the balloon, and reduces the possibility of emboli to the cerebral circulation. The balloon, when inflated, should provide no more than 90% occlusion of the aorta to minimize hemolysis and prevent aortic wall damage (Quaal, 1993a). However, the balloon should not obstruct the left subclavian artery. Proper catheter position is confirmed by chest roentgenogram.

In approximately 5% of patients, femoral artery placement of a balloon catheter is precluded or contraindicated (Hazelrigg et al., 1992). Femoral artery insertion may not be possible in the presence of (1) extensive arterial occlusive disease or a previous peripheral arterial reconstructive procedure, (2) arterial injury during attempted insertion, or (3) ischemia in the ipsilateral leg. In cardiac surgical patients in whom CPB cannot be weaned and femoral cannulation fails, a balloon catheter may be inserted through the aortic arch downward into the descending thoracic aorta (Fig. 30-3). In patients awaiting cardiac

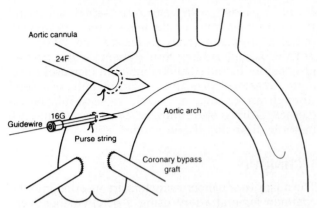

FIGURE 30-3. Balloon catheter insertion through the thoracic aorta: using the Seldinger technique, a guidewire is placed through a purestring suture in the anterior ascending aortic wall; with the aid of a dilator-sheath assembly, the balloon catheter will be passed over the wire and advanced until the balloon portion of the catheter lies just distal to the left subclavian artery; intraoperative transesophageal echocardiography may be used to guide placement. (Kaplan LJ, Weiman DS, Langan N, et al., 1992: Safe intra-aortic balloon pump placement through the ascending aorta using transesophageal ultrasound. Ann Thorac Surg 54:374. Reprinted with permission from the Society of Thoracic Surgeons)

transplantation, the balloon catheter may be placed through the subclavian artery to allow increased patient mobility during counterpulsation (Reedy et al., 1990a).

Most IABC systems use helium as the driving gas to produce balloon inflation. Optimal timing of inflation and deflation is critical to maximizing coronary artery perfusion and lowering myocardial work. Timing is adjusted by comparing arterial pressure waveform morphologies while augmenting every other cardiac cycle (i.e., a console setting of 1:2, or one counterpulsation to two cardiac contractions) (Quaal,

1988). Properly timed inflation should begin just after aortic valve closure, represented on the arterial pressure waveform by the dicrotic notch. Because of the delay between actual cardiac events and transmission of the resulting pressure changes to the arterial pressure transducer, inflation timed to appear on the oscilloscope at the onset of the dicrotic notch actually occurs correctly after valve closure. Appropriately timed inflation thus produces a V-shaped configuration at the dicrotic notch (Fig. 30-4). Early balloon inflation causes premature closing of the aortic valve, lengthening of diastole, and impedance of left ventricular ejection. Stroke volume is decreased, and left ventricular end-diastolic volume and pressure increase as a result. Late inflation produces some loss of diastolic augmentation (Shinn, 1989).

Appropriate timing of deflation is evidenced by lowering of end-diastolic pressure of the augmented cardiac cycle as compared with the patient's unassisted cardiac cycle; systolic pressure after the assisted cardiac cycle should be lower or at least not higher than unassisted systolic pressure (see Fig. 30-4) (Quaal, 1993b). Early deflation allows retrograde flow from the coronary and brachial arteries to fill the space created by balloon deflation, compromising forward flow into these vessels. In addition, the beneficial effects of afterload reduction are diminished. Late deflation impedes the subsequent left ventricular ejection and produces a great deal of intraventricular wall stress. Failure to achieve counterpulsation may indicate retention of the balloon within the sheath, incomplete unwrapping of the balloon, an empty helium tank, or mechanical failure of the console (Lee, 1990).

While the balloon catheter is in place, prophylactic antibiotics are administered to prevent infection at the insertion site with resultant bacteremia. In nonsurgical or preoperative patients, a continuous intravenous heparin or dextran infusion is usually administered to prevent clotting or platelet aggregation along the balloon catheter (Mundth, 1990). When

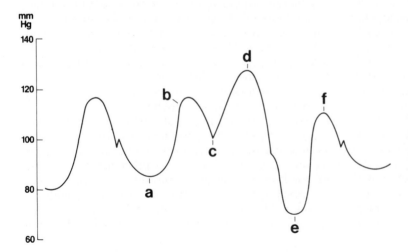

FIGURE 30-4. Arterial pressure tracing with 1:2 intra-aortic balloon counterpulsation demonstrates appropriately timed balloon inflation and deflation: *a*, unassisted aortic end diastolic pressure; *b*, unassisted systole; *c*, onset of balloon inflation; *d*, diastolic augmentation; *e*, assisted end-diastolic pressure; *f*, assisted systole. Note that both end-diastolic and systolic pressures of the assisted cardiac cycle are lower than those of the unassisted cycle. (Courtesy of Datascope Corp., Montvale, NJ)

IABC is used in the early postoperative period, anticoagulation is generally withheld until chest tube drainage subsides and clotting parameters return to normal. It is considered ill-advised to begin anticoagulant therapy immediately after cardiac surgery because blood coagulation mechanisms have been disturbed by intraoperative anticoagulation and extracorporeal circulation and because of the fresh suture lines (Elefteriades & Geha, 1985). In the absence of active bleeding, heparin infusion is generally initiated on the second or third postoperative day.

IABC is sometimes used in combination with CPB or a VAD. Counterpulsation continued during CPB may provide a pulsatile component to blood flow, although beneficial effects remain unproven. If IABC is continued during CPB, an intrinsic rate mode is used because the heart is arrested and timing from the electrocardiogram or arterial pressure is not possible. More commonly, counterpulsation is suspended during CPB. A standby mode is safe while the patient is systemically anticoagulated. IABC is occasionally used in combination with a VAD. If a nonpulsatile VAD is used (e.g., a centrifugal pump), IABC may provide a pulsatile component.

Weaning from IABC is accomplished by reducing the frequency of counterpulsations from every cardiac contraction to every other, and then to every third. When the patient is able to sustain an adequate cardiac output with a 1:3 ratio of counterpulsation or with the device momentarily in a standby mode, the balloon catheter is removed. Regardless of the patient's need for balloon augmentation, the balloon is not left motionless in the aorta; at least a 1:3 ratio of counterpulsation is continued until the catheter is removed from the aorta to reduce thrombosis along the catheter and possible embolization.

Balloon catheters inserted percutaneously can usually be removed in the intensive care unit except in cases of a high percutaneous insertion site, morbid obesity, or limb ischemia (Pae & Pierce, 1991). If the balloon catheter was inserted by direct cutdown technique, balloon catheter removal necessitates an operative procedure for repair of the femoral artery. A balloon catheter inserted through a transthoracic approach necessitates an operative procedure for catheter removal.

ASSOCIATED COMPLICATIONS

Intra-aortic balloon catheters can be associated with significant morbidity. The reported incidence of complications ranges from 8% to 21% (Naunheim et al., 1992). Risk factors for development of a major complication include female gender, diabetes mellitus, hypertension, and peripheral arterial occlusive disease (Richenbacher & Pierce, 1991a). The most common cause of morbidity is arterial injury secondary to the insertion or presence of an indwelling balloon catheter in the aorta. Complications related to arterial injury include thrombosis, embolization, aortic dissection, hemorrhage, false aneurysm, arteriovenous fistula, and embolization (Fahey & Finkelmeier, 1984; Finkelmeier & Finkelmeier, 1991).

Limb-threatening ischemia is the most common complication. Many patients who require balloon counterpulsation have atherosclerosis and are likely to have peripheral arterial (aortoiliac or femoropopliteal) occlusive lesions. Some degree of ischemia has been reported to occur in as many as 47% of patients with balloon catheters in place (Funk et al., 1989). Significant limb ischemia occurs in approximately 12% of patients (Naunheim et al., 1992). Primary mechanisms for development of ischemia include arterial injury during catheter insertion, thromboembolism, obstruction by the catheter, and artery spasm. Catheter obstruction occurs because of the catheter's large diameter and the relative lack of collateral arterial supply to the leg. The smaller caliber of arteries in women places them at higher risk for ischemic complications. Although transient ischemia may resolve with balloon catheter removal, as many as 60% of patients with significant limb ischemia require surgical intervention (Mundth, 1990).

Hemorrhage can occur due to injury to the femoral artery or perforation of the aorta, particularly if balloon advancement is traumatic. An increasing number of patients who require IABC for postinfarction angina have been treated with thrombolytic therapy or heparin. Insertion of a balloon catheter in these circumstances increases the likelihood of bleeding complications but may be unavoidable if other means of controlling ischemia are unsuccessful.

Aortic dissection can occur during insertion and advancement of the balloon catheter, particularly if repeated attempts at insertion are necessary or if the patient has associated peripheral arterial occlusive disease. Difficulty in advancing the catheter or failure to achieve counterpulsation may be indicative of aortic dissection if the balloon is lying in the false lumen. However, appropriate augmentation does not rule out the existence of dissection. Development of iatrogenic dissection necessitates prompt balloon catheter removal. False aneurysm (pseudoaneurysm) and arteriovenous fistula are other types of arterial injury that occasionally develop at the insertion site after the balloon catheter has been removed.

In addition to vascular complications, wound infection or sepsis may complicate IABC therapy. Rarely, balloon rupture occurs, evidenced by the appearance of blood in the catheter shaft (Lee, 1990). Balloon rupture is thought to be related to rough handling during insertion or prolonged contact between the balloon and a calcified atherosclerotic plaque (Richenbacher & Pierce, 1991a). Immediate removal, and if necessary, replacement with another balloon catheter, is performed to prevent helium embolization with resultant neurologic injury.

VENTRICULAR ASSIST DEVICES

Although IABC is the most commonly used mechanical assist device, it provides only augmentation of cardiac function. A *ventricular assist device* is necessary if complete support of one or both ventricles is required (Table 30-2). VADs are an evolving, highly technical, and expensive form of therapy and are available only in selected centers.

A VAD differs from CPB in that the patient's pulmonary vasculature is not bypassed. That is, blood is oxygenated by the patient, not by the device. Another difference is that VADs are designed for intermediate or long-term use. CPB is designed to be used only for the duration of a typical cardiac operation (less than 6 to 8 hours). Depending on the specific device, a VAD can be used to provide circulatory support for a few days or several months. In fact, successful VAD use for periods up to 1 year has been reported. VADs are available that provide temporary mechanical support to the left, right, or both ventricles.

Several institutions are also investigating a *total artificial heart* for use in patients with profound biventricular failure and no anticipated hope of myocardial recovery or transplantation. To date, total artificial hearts have not proven useful for permanent maintenance of the circulation but have been successful in providing a bridge to transplant in some patients.

INDICATIONS

The primary indication for VAD use is cardiogenic shock despite optimal preload, maximal drug therapy, corrected metabolism, and IABC (Table 30-3) (Reedy et al., 1990c). Unless cardiac transplantation is anticipated, the purpose of using a VAD is to allow time for recovery of cardiac function in patients with what is considered to be reversible cardiogenic shock. Several factors are taken into consideration when deciding to use a VAD. First, all of the devices can cause serious, and potentially fatal, complications (Curtis et al., 1992). Also, the devices are quite costly. More conservative, less hazardous pharmacologic therapy and IABC should be considered first. Finally, a VAD does nothing to correct underlying cardiac pathology. Therefore, VAD therapy is appropriate only in patients in whom there is a reasonable hope for cardiac recovery or transplantation.

Approximately 1% of patients who undergo cardiac operations experience postcardiotomy car-

TABLE 30-2. INDICATIONS FOR VENTRICULAR ASSIST DEVICE

Reversible cardiogenic shock after cardiac surgery
Irreversible cardiogenic shock awaiting transplantation
Acute rejection or cardiac dysfunction after transplantation

TABLE 30-3. HEMODYNAMIC INDICATIONS FOR VENTRICULAR ASSIST DEVICE*

Cardiac index < 2.0 L/min/m^2
Systemic vascular resistance > 2100 dynes·sec·cm^{-5}
Atrial pressure > 20 mm Hg
Urine output < 20 mL/h

* In the presence of optimal preload, maximal pharmacologic therapy, corrected metabolism, intra-aortic balloon counterpulsation (Reedy, 1990c)

diogenic shock that is unresponsive to IABC and inotropic pharmacologic therapy (Pae et al., 1992). Heart failure in this group of patients is often due to temporary dysfunction (i.e., *"stunned myocardium"*) and may improve with time and temporary support. Consequently, patients placed on a VAD because of inability to wean from CPB after a cardiac operation should be those in whom a technically satisfactory repair of underlying cardiac pathology has been accomplished (Magovern & Pierce, 1989). With appropriate candidate selection, VADs provide a valuable treatment modality to increase survival in this moribund group of patients.

Approximately 45% of patients who would probably otherwise die can be successfully weaned from ventricular support, and 55% of weaned patients are discharged from the hospital; the overall survival rate is 25% (Pae et al., 1992). Patients most likely to recover are those with isolated left ventricular failure or predominant right with only mild left ventricular failure; acute perioperative myocardial infarction, on the other hand, is a strong deterrent to myocardial recovery (Pennington et al., 1988).

VADs also provide a safe and effective way of supporting hemodynamic function in critically ill patients who have already been or who are likely to be accepted as candidates for heart transplantation. As waiting time for transplantation has increased, availability of devices designed for long-term support has become more important. However, proper patient selection for VAD bridging is crucial to survival outcomes (Kanter et al., 1988). In general, patients receiving mechanical support as a bridge to transplant should meet the same criteria as for heart transplant candidacy (Reedy et al., 1990c). Indications and predictions for survival are being refined as more experience is gained in the use of VADs (Emery & Joyce, 1991).

TYPES OF VENTRICULAR ASSIST DEVICES

Several types of VADs are in clinical use or under investigation. Some are designed for external use, and others are implantable. VADs are generally categorized according to whether they provide pulsatile or nonpulsatile flow and by the type of pump (i.e., centrifugal, pneumatic, electrical, or axial-flow). Of damage to the native atrium, which will be anastomosed to the transplanted heart. It also decompresses the left ventricle more completely (Ruzevich, 1991). The cannulae exit the chest below the costal margin and are connected to the pneumatic pump, which is attached by tubing to an external control console. If biventricular support is necessary, two pneumatic pumps, with appropriate cannulation, may be used (Fig. 30-6).

The Heartmate is also a pneumatic VAD but differs from Abiomed and Thoratec VADs in that the pump is implantable and the device is designed for left ventricular assistance only (Frazier et al., 1992; Seche, 1992). Major advantages of pneumatic pumps are that the potential for thromboembolism and trauma to blood elements is minimal (Pae & Pierce, 1991).

Electrical Pump

The *Novacor Left Ventricular Assist System* (Novacor Division, Baxter Healthcare, Oakland, CA) is an electrical VAD. The Novacor pump is an implantable device, placed in the abdominal wall and connected to an external console by a cable (Fig. 30-7) (Reedy et al., 1990a). It is designed exclusively for support of the left ventricle, and its inflow and outflow cannulae are inserted in the apex of the left ventricle and aorta, respectively. Because the Novacor VAD is designed for direct cannulation of the left ventricle, it is used for bridging to transplantation (i.e., when the ventricle is not expected to recover).

Axial-Flow Pump

The *Hemopump* Cardiac Assist System (Johnson and Johnson Interventional Systems, Rancho Cordova, CA) is a device that uses an axial flow pump to augment left ventricular cardiac output. The device contains a small archimedean screw that rotates at a high speed, drawing blood through a cannula in the left ventricle and propelling it into the aorta. It is connected by a flexible cable to an externally positioned electric motor (Golding, 1991). The Hemopump is capable of generating up to 3.5 L/min of nonpulsatile blood flow and does not require synchronization with left ventricular contractions (Wampler et al., 1991; Fields & Mentzer, 1992).

A primary advantage of the Hemopump is that a major surgical procedure is not required for its insertion (Baldwin et al., 1992). Instead, a cutdown technique is performed to expose the femoral artery. Then, using fluoroscopy, the device is advanced in a retrograde fashion through the aorta into the left ventricle. Intravascular insertion allows rapid institution of ventricular assistance and reduces the risks of infection, bleeding, and other complications of a thoracic surgical procedure (Rountree et al., 1991). In addition, placement of the device directly in the left ventricle provides significant chamber decompression. Because retrograde passage through the aortic valve is required, the device is not used in patients with aortic valve disease or an aortic valvular prosthesis.

VENTRICULAR ASSIST DEVICE FUNCTION AND ASSOCIATED COMPLICATIONS

Most acquired forms of cardiac pathology affect left ventricular function predominantly. Consequently, it is the left ventricle that more often requires mechanical support. While a left-sided VAD (LVAD) is operational, the heart can continue to contract. Pharmacologic agents that affect myocardial contractility, preload, and afterload may be used to maximize in-

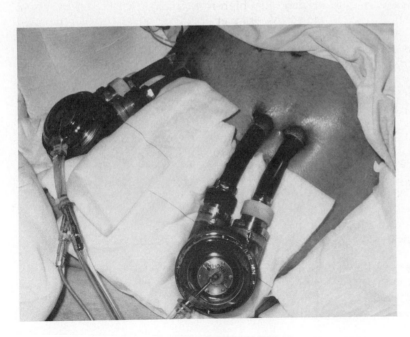

FIGURE 30-6. Right and left Thoratec ventricular assist devices in patient awaiting cardiac transplantation. (Courtesy of Robert M. Mentzer, Jr., M.D.)

the various devices, only several are available for general use; the others remain under investigation and their use is limited to approved centers (Noon, 1991).

Centrifugal Pump

Centrifugal pump systems (Bio-Medicus, Medtronic Bio-Medicus, Eden Prairie, MN, or Sarns, Sarns/3M, Ann Arbor, MI) are used most commonly for short-term postoperative support of cardiac surgical patients. The centrifugal pump, which provides non-pulsatile flow, is also used for intraoperative CPB in many centers (Fig. 30-5). When used for prolonged postoperative circulatory support, the system provides partial CPB (i.e., blood is oxygenated by the patient rather than the device). The primary advantage of a centrifugal pump is its easy applicability, widespread availability, and familiarity to surgeons and perfusionists in institutions where cardiac surgery is performed routinely.

Centrifugal pumps are not well suited for use longer than 7 to 10 days (Richenbacher & Pierce, 1991b). They necessitate continuous monitoring and are associated with significant morbidity when use is prolonged. Bleeding, sepsis, and thromboembolism are the primary complications (Killen et al., 1991). In addition, patients are essentially limited to bed rest. Sustained immobility increases risk for respiratory infections or other problems that may preclude eventual cardiac transplantation (McCarthy et al., 1991).

In patients who are candidates for transplantation, it is preferable to use a device that is more suited to the prolonged waiting period typically associated with organ transplantation. Devices with pneumatic or electrical pumps are more complex and costly but are better designed for long-term support and generally do not necessitate bed rest. The increased cardiac output provided by the VAD often allows discontinuance of intravenous inotropic support and the patient can increase exercise tolerance in preparation for transplantation (Reedy et al., 1990c).

Pneumatic Pump

Pneumatic pumps are air-driven devices that provide pulsatile blood flow. Examples of pneumatically driven, pulsatile VADs include (1) the *Pierce-Donachy Thoratec VAD* (Thoratec, Berkeley, CA), (2) the *Abiomed Bi-Ventricular Support (BVS) System* (Abiomed Cardiovascular, Danvers, MA), and (3) the *HeartMate VAD* (Thermo Cardiosystems, Woburn, MA). The Thoratec and Abiomed systems have external, pulsatile pumping chambers and can provide complete temporary left, right, or biventricular support. The pulsatile pumping chambers of both devices lie close to the thorax and are connected by transcutaneous cannulae to the inflow and outflow sites; the Thoratec system has a single pumping chamber for each ventricle, and the Abiomed uses a prosthetic atrium and ventricle in combination (Fields & Mentzer, 1992)

Implantation of a pneumatic VAD necessitates a major operation. To provide mechanical support to the left ventricle, the inflow cannula is placed in either the left atrium or the left ventricle. Left atrial cannulation avoids further injury to an already damaged left ventricle and is associated with less bleeding from the cannulation site (Magovern & Pierce, 1989). Ventricular cannulation, on the other hand, may be advantageous in transplant candidates since it avoids

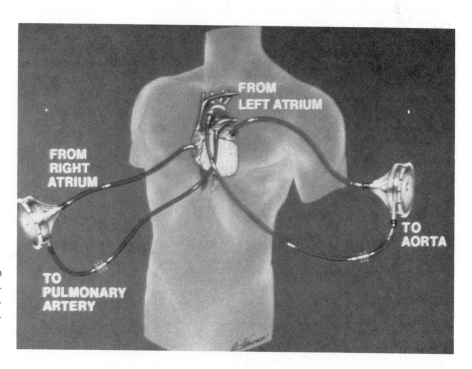

FIGURE 30-5. A centrifugal pump may be used for short-term left ventricular, right ventricular, or biventricular support of the heart. (Courtesy of Medtronic Bio-medicus, Inc., Eden Prairie, MN)

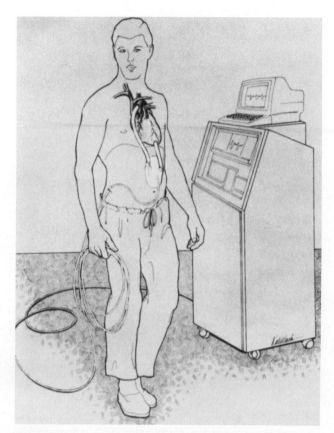

FIGURE 30-7. Schematic of Novacor Left Ventricular Assist System (Novacor division (Oakland, CA) of Baxter Healthcare). (Reedy JE, Ruzevich SA, Noedel NR, et al., 1990: Nursing care of the ambulatory patient with a mechanical assist device. J Heart Transplant 9:100)

trinsic cardiac function. Cardiac output, as measured by thermodilution technique with a pulmonary artery catheter, reflects the combined output by the LVAD and the ventricle itself. Acceptable cardiac output when a LVAD is in place depends on adequate filling (determined by right ventricular function and adequate intravascular volume) and proper emptying (affected by afterload). Although there is no way to synchronize LVAD function with right-sided cardiac activity, filling of a left-sided VAD (or left ventricle in the case of a Hemopump) is usually not a problem unless the patient has elevated pulmonary vascular resistance and right ventricular failure. If so, a right VAD (RVAD) or right-sided CPB may be used to provide biventricular support. A VAD is unlikely to sustain a patient successfully if inadequate filling is due to significant hemorrhage.

Although VADs can effectively enhance hemodynamic stability, they are associated with significant morbidity regardless of the type of device or support used (Pae et al., 1992). Excessive bleeding can be a major problem, particularly in patients who require VAD use in the early postoperative period when hemostasis is impaired. Bleeding is of less concern

when VADs are used for long-term support in patients waiting for transplantation. Infectious complications that may occur with VAD use include local infection around cannulation sites, mediastinitis, pneumonia, or generalized sepsis (Vaska, 1991). Thromboembolism is a potential problem because of the large artificial surface in contact with blood (Reedy et al, 1990a). In patients waiting for cardiac transplantation, some form of anticoagulation or antiplatelet therapy is desirable because thromboembolism may have catastrophic consequences for the patient or preclude transplantation. Use of a mechanical assist device for bridging to transplantation may also make implantation of a transplanted heart more difficult because of adhesions from the prolonged presence of prosthetic materials (Emery et al., 1991).

PORTABLE CARDIOPULMONARY BYPASS

Portable cardiopulmonary bypass (PCPB) describes a system that allows rapid institution and temporary provision of total cardiac and pulmonary support for the patient. The *Bard CPS System* (CR Bard, Billerica, MA) is a CPB system similar to that used for cardiac operations, except that it is designed for use outside the operating room. The device is mounted on a wheeled cart and is equipped with a battery pack so that it can be moved easily to the patient's location, and so that the patient on PCPB can be safely transported to an intensive care unit, catheterization laboratory, or operating room.

Indications for use of PCPB are still evolving. Clinical application of the device is composed of two categories: (1) as an emergency resuscitative tool for patients in cardiogenic shock or cardiac arrest and (2) as an elective hemodynamic support device in patients undergoing high-risk cardiac catheterization procedures (Mooney et al., 1991). PCPB is not well suited for chronic circulatory support. Patients who cannot be weaned but who are acceptable transplant candidates are transferred to a form of mechanical assistance suitable for long-term support (Reedy et al., 1990b).

PCPB has been used primarily to provide CPB to patients with catastrophic hemodynamic instability in a variety of settings within the hospital. It appears most promising for stabilization of patients who are severely hypotensive but who still have some cardiac function. For those who suffer cardiac arrest, survival is influenced by location of the patient at the time of cardiac arrest. Survival is most likely after PCPB resuscitation of patients who experience cardiac arrest in a cardiac catheterization laboratory (Mooney et al., 1991). Possible reasons for increased survival in patients who experience cardiac arrest in a cardiac catheterization laboratory include (1) the rapidity of instituting CPR, PCPB, and definitive therapy in this setting and (2) the greater likelihood in this group of patients of underlying cardiac pathology amenable to PCPB resuscitation.

Emergent PCPB has not been effective in increasing survival in patients who have experienced unwitnessed cardiac arrest before initiation of extracorporeal circulation with PCPB (Hartz et al., 1990; Hill et al., 1992). Both irreversible neurologic and cardiac damage have been primary factors in the demise of this group of patients.

PCPB is used electively in some centers for selected patients undergoing high-risk cardiac catheterization, PTCA, or aortic valvuloplasty. PCPB has also been reported in patients sustaining massive cardiothoracic trauma to allow time to establish a diagnosis and initiate treatment (Attar & Hankins, 1990). However, its use is limited in trauma victims because of the need for systemic anticoagulation with currently available PCPB systems.

The PCPB system can be prepared and ready for use in 5 to 10 minutes. Femoral artery and vein cannulation is generally performed by a surgeon, using a cutdown technique. In the presence of shock or cardiac arrest, proper identification of the vessels is difficult and precludes a percutaneous insertion technique. Percutaneous insertion may be performed in elective situations but is more likely to be associated with injury to the femoral artery or vein.

A venous cannula is inserted into the femoral vein and advanced through the inferior vena cava into the right atrium (Fig. 30-8). The arterial cannula is inserted in the femoral artery, and anticoagulation with heparin is begun. The venous cannula allows diversion of blood from the right side of the heart to the PCPB system. A centrifugal pump within the system circulates the blood through the tubing to a heat exchanger, where it can be warmed, and then through the system's oxygenator where gas exchange occurs. The blood is then returned to the systemic circulation through the femoral artery cannula.

Management of the PCPB system is usually performed by a perfusionist or critical care nurse. As with standard CPB machines, a regulator on the console of the machine determines the speed of the centrifugal pump and thus the rate of blood flow through the system. Systemic anticoagulation, guided by intermittent measurements of activated clotting time, is maintained with intravenous bolus doses of heparin (Cone et al., 1992).

Several differences exist between PCBP and intraoperative CPB. Unlike standard CPB, the PCPB system has no reservoir. Therefore, flow rate to the patient is more dependent on minute to minute changes in venous return from the patient. Intravascular volume is manipulated to optimize blood flow. That is, preload is increased by administering fluids and decreased using diuretic agents. Vasodilating agents may be administered to decrease afterload. Another important difference between portable and intraoperative CPB is that PCPB cannulation does not provide the same degree of cardiac decompression as

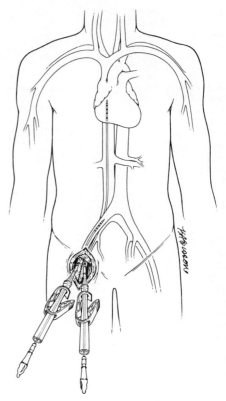

FIGURE 30-8. Diagram illustrating cutdown and femoral artery and vein cannulation for portable cardiopulmonary support. (Hartz RS, LoCicero J III, Sanders JH Jr., et al., 1990: Clinical experience with portable cardiopulmonary bypass in cardiac arrest patients. Ann Thorac Surg 50:438. Reprinted with permission of the Society of Thoracic Surgeons)

does direct cannulation of the right atrium. PCPB also differs in that it does not provide for cooling of body temperature. The device does have a heat exchanger so that the blood can be warmed as it circulates through the tubing circuit.

The most common complication of PCPB is injury to the femoral artery and vein during cannulation. Significant bleeding or femoral arterial damage are particularly problematic when a percutaneous insertion technique has been used. Surgical repair of the femoral artery, vein, or both may be necessary.

REFERENCES

Attar S, Hankins JR, 1990: Heart assist devices in cardiothoracic trauma. In Turney SZ, Rodriguez A, Cowley RA (eds): Management of Cardiothoracic Trauma. Baltimore, Williams & Wilkins

Baldwin RT, Radovancevic B, Duncan JM, et al., 1992: Management of patients supported on the Hemopump Cardiac Assist System. Texas Heart Inst J 19:81

Cone M, Hoffman M, Jessen D, et al., 1992: Cardiopulmonary support in the intensive care unit. Am J Crit Care 1:98

Curtis JJ, Walls JT, Schmaltz R, et al., 1992: Experience with the Sarns centrifugal pump in postcardiotomy ventricular failure. J Thorac Cardiovasc Surg 104:554

Elefteriades JA, Geha AS, 1985: The intra-aortic balloon pump. In House Officer Guide to ICU Care: The Cardiothoracic Surgical Patient. Gaithersburg, MD, Aspen Publishers

Emery RW, Eales F, Joyce LD, et al., 1991: Mechanical circulatory assistance after heart transplantation. Ann Thorac Surg 51:43

Emery RW, Joyce LD, 1991: Directions in cardiac assistance. J Cardiac Surg 6:400

Fahey VA, Finkelmeier BA, 1984: Iatrogenic arterial injuries. Am J Nurs 84:448

Fields BL, Mentzer RM Jr, 1992: Extended circulatory support for cardiac failure. Cardiac Surg: State Art Rev 6:439

Finkelmeier BA, Finkelmeier WR, 1991: Iatrogenic arterial injuries resulting from invasive procedures. J Vasc Nurs 9:12

Frazier OH, Duncan M, Radovancevic B, et al., 1992: Successful bridge to heart transplantation with a new left ventricular assist device. J Heart Lung Transplant 11:530

Funk M, Gleason J, Foell D, 1989: Lower limb ischemia related to use of the intra-aortic balloon pump. Heart Lung 18:542

Golding LA, 1991: Postcardiotomy mechanical support. Semin Thorac Cardiovasc Surg 3:29

Hartz RS, LoCicero J III, Sanders JH Jr, et al., 1990: Clinical experience with portable cardiopulmonary bypass in cardiac arrest patients. Ann Thorac Surg 50:437

Hazelrigg SR, Auer JE, Seifert PE, 1992: Experience in 100 transthoracic balloon pumps. Ann Thorac Surg 54:528

Hill JG, Bruhn PS, Cohen SE, et al., 1992: Emergent applications of cardiopulmonary support: A multi-institutional experience. Ann Thorac Surg 54:699

Kanter KR, McBride LR, Pennington DG, et al., 1988: Bridging to cardiac transplantation with pulsatile ventricular assist devices. Ann Thorac Surg 46:134

Kantrowitz A, 1989: Intra-aortic balloon pumping: Clinical aspects and prospects. In Unger F (ed): Assisted Circulation 3. Berlin, Springer-Verlag

Kantrowitz A, Tjonneland S, Freed PS, et al., 1968: Initial clinical experience with intra-aortic balloon pumping in cardiogenic shock. JAMA 203:113

Killen DA, Piehler JM, Borkon AM, Reed WA, 1991: Bio-Medicus ventricular assist device for salvage of cardiac surgical patients. Ann Thorac Surg 52:230

Lee ME, 1990: Mechanical support of the circulation. In Gray RJ, Matloff JM (eds): Medical Management of the Cardiac Surgical Patient, Baltimore, Williams & Wilkins

Magovern JA, Pierce WS 1989: Support of the failing left heart: Left heart assistance. In Grillo HC, Austen WG, Wilkins EW, et al. (eds): Current Therapy in Cardiothoracic Surgery. Toronto, BC Decker

McCarthy PM, Portner PM, Tobler HG, et al., 1991: Clinical experience with the Novacor ventricular assist system. J Thorac Cardiovasc Surg 102:578

Mooney MR, Arom KV, Joyce LD, 1991: Emergency cardiopulmonary bypass support in patients with cardiac arrest. J Thorac Cardiovasc Surg 101:450

Mundth ED, 1990: Assisted circulation. In Sabiston DC, Spencer FC (eds): Surgery of the Chest, ed. 5. Philadelphia, WB Saunders

Naunheim KS, Swartz MT, Pennington DG, et al., 1992: Intraaortic balloon pumping in patients requiring cardiac operations. J Thorac Cardiovasc Surg 104:1654

Noon GP, 1991: Bio-Medicus ventricular assistance. Ann Thorac Surg 52:230

Pae WE Jr, Miller CA, Matthews Y, Pierce WS, 1992: Ventricular assist devices for postcardiotomy cardiogenic shock. J Thorac Cardiovasc Surg 104:541

Pae WE Jr, Pierce WS, 1991: Intra-aortic balloon counterpulsation, ventricular assist pumping, and the artificial heart. In Baue AE, Geha AS, Hammond GL, et al. (eds): Glenn's Thoracic and Cardiovascular Surgery, ed. 5. Norwalk, CT, Appleton & Lange

Pennington DG, McBride LR, Kanter KR, et al., 1988: Effect of perioperative myocardial infarction on survival of postcardiotomy patients supported with ventricular-assist devices. Circulation 78(Suppl III):III-110

Quaal SJ, 1988: Mechanical treatment of the failing heart. In Kern LS (ed): Cardiac Critical Care Nursing. Gaithersburg, MD, Aspen Publishers

Quaal SJ, 1993a: Basic principles of IABC. In Comprehensive Intra-aortic Balloon Counterpulsation, ed. 2. St. Louis, CV Mosby

Quaal SJ, 1993b: Conventional timing using the arterial waveform. In Comprehensive Intra-aortic Balloon Counterpulsation, ed. 2. St. Louis, CV Mosby

Reedy JE, Ruzevich SA, Noedel NR, et al., 1990a: Nursing care of the ambulatory patient with a mechanical assist device. J Heart Transplant 9:97

Reedy JE, Swartz MT, Raithel SC, et al., 1990b: Mechanical cardiopulmonary support for refractory cardiogenic shock. Heart Lung 19:514

Reedy JE, Swartz MT, Termuhlen DT, et al., 1990c: Bridge to heart transplantation: Importance of patient selection. J Heart Transplant 9:473

Richenbacher WE, Pierce WS, 1991a: Management of complications of intraaortic balloon counterpulsation. In Waldhausen JA, Orringer MB (eds): Complications in Cardiothoracic Surgery. St. Louis, Mosby–Year Book

Richenbacher WE, Pierce WS, 1991b: Management of complications of mechanical circulatory assistance. In Waldhausen JA, Orringer MB (eds): Complications in Cardiothoracic Surgery. St. Louis, Mosby–Year Book

Rountree WD, Rutan PM, McClure A, 1991: The Hemopump cardiac assist system: Nursing care of the patient. Crit Care Nurse 11:46

Ruzevich SA, 1991: Heart assist devices: State of the art. Crit Care Nurs Clin North Am 3:723

Seche LA, 1992: The Thermo Cardiosystems implantable left ventricular assist device as a bridge to cardiac transplantation. Heart Lung 21:112

Shinn JA, 1989: Circulatory assist devices. In Underhill SL, Woods SL, Froelicher ES, Halpenny CJ (eds): Cardiac Nursing, ed. 2. Philadelphia, JB Lippincott

Vaska PL, 1991: Biventricular assist devices. Crit Care Nurse 11:52

Wampler RK, Frazier OH, Lansing AM, et al., 1991: Treatment of cardiogenic shock with the Hemopump left ventricular assist device. Ann Thorac Surg 52:506

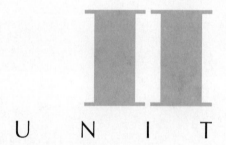

UNIT II

CARDIOTHORACIC TRANSPLANTATION AND TRAUMA

31

HEART, LUNG, AND HEART-LUNG TRANSPLANTATION

HEART TRANSPLANTATION	LUNG AND HEART-LUNG TRANSPLANTATION
Recipient Selection and Management	Development of Lung and Heart-Lung
Donor Selection and Management	Transplantation
Transplant Procedure	Indications for Transplantation
Postoperative Considerations	Operative Procedures
	Results

Current accomplishments in transplantation of the heart and lungs are the result of research dating back to the beginning of the 20th century. As early as 1905, Alexis Carrel performed experimental heart transplantation in a dog (Kirklin & Barratt-Boyes, 1993). Investigations regarding technical and immunologic aspects of transplant have continued since that time. Although many researchers have contributed to the field, Norman Shumway is generally credited for current success in cardiac transplantation because of his sustained research and clinical contributions. James Hardy and Joel Cooper have been pioneers in the field of lung transplantation. Growth in thoracic transplantation is demonstrated by the official report from the registry of the International Society for Heart and Lung Transplantation. In the 25 years since thoracic transplantation in a human was first successfully accomplished, nearly 20,000 heart and more than 2000 lung or heart-lung transplantations have been performed (Kaye, 1992).

HEART TRANSPLANTATION

The first successful heart transplant was performed by Christiaan Barnard in 1966 (Kirklin & Barratt-Boyes, 1993). Despite technical accomplishment of the procedure, organ rejection prevented long-term survival of patients. It was not until the early 1980s that results improved dramatically due to availability of the immunosuppressive agent cyclosporine. Since that time, both the number of facilities in which cardiac transplantation is performed and the number of transplant operations performed have increased substantially. *Cardiac transplantation* is currently a standard modality for treatment of end-stage heart disease. It is performed not only in adults but also in newborns and children with severe, uncorrectable forms of congenital heart disease.

RECIPIENT SELECTION AND MANAGEMENT

Candidates for cardiac transplantation are those individuals with a terminal cardiac condition who are unable to perform minimal activities of an acceptable life-style and who cannot achieve palliation or prolongation of life with conventional medical or surgical therapy (Gay & O'Connell, 1990). Life expectancy is often 1 year or less, and patients typically have a New York Heart Association class IV functional status. Most transplant programs limit candidates to those younger than 60 to 65 years of age who have no other irreversible medical problems, such as malignancy or hepatic or renal failure.

The vast majority of cardiac transplantations in adults are performed in patients with cardiomyopathy or ischemic heart disease (Fig. 31-1). Most cardiac transplantations are performed for dilated cardiomyopathy, the most common form of cardiomyopathy in this country. Dilated cardiomyopathy may be idiopathic or occur secondary to viral infection or pregnancy. It is characterized primarily by dilatation and impaired systolic function of the left ventricle. However, patients with dilated cardiomyopathy severe enough to warrant transplantation generally have right ventricular failure as well.

Ischemic heart disease is the other major indication and accounts for an increasing number of heart transplants in adults. Transplant candidates with ischemic heart disease usually have irreversible left ventricular or biventricular dysfunction. However, in unusual instances transplantation may be indicated primarily for relief of angina or arrhythmias that are refractory to pharmacologic therapy or not amenable to surgical correction (Gay & O'Connell, 1990). Cardiac transplantation is also a therapeutic modality for adults with selected types of valvular or uncorrectable congenital heart disease.

Heart transplantation is contraindicated in the presence of factors that make success unlikely. One of the primary contraindications is severe, irreversible pulmonary hypertension. Because a transplanted heart has a normal, thin-walled right ventricle, it may not function adequately in a recipient with fixed, elevated pulmonary vascular resistance (Bahnson et al., 1991b). Patients with pulmonary vascular resistance greater than six Wood units are therefore excluded from consideration for heart transplantation. They may, however, be suitable candidates for combined heart-lung transplantation.

The necessity for life-long immunosuppression precludes cardiac transplantation in other patients. For example, recent pulmonary infarction (i.e., within 2 to 3 months) is a contraindication because it can evolve into a necrotizing pneumonia or lung abscess when immunosuppression is initiated. Active infection also eliminates candidacy since perioperative immunosuppression would lead to overwhelming sepsis. Active peptic ulcer disease is a contraindication because immunosuppressive therapy is likely to exacerbate gastrointestinal irritation and produce gastrointestinal bleeding.

Other factors are relative contraindications when allocating a resource as limited as donor hearts. Individuals with diffuse, advanced peripheral or cerebral arterial occlusive disease are generally not suitable candidates for cardiac transplantation. In some centers, insulin-dependent diabetes is considered a contraindication because corticosteroid immunosuppression can exacerbate diabetes (Hudak et al., 1990). In addition, diabetic individuals have a propensity for accelerated atherosclerosis that could cause progressive coronary artery disease in the transplanted heart. However, other centers have demonstrated good long-term survival in carefully selected diabetic patients with a relatively low risk of diabetic complications (Munoz et al., 1992).

Psychological stability and ability to comply with the management protocol after transplantation are important considerations. Candidacy is precluded in persons with active drug or alcohol abuse and in those with significant psychological pathology. Addiction to drugs, alcohol, or cigarettes is indicative of inability to comply with the complex medical regimen that is essential after transplantation. Although organ dysfunction (e.g., kidney, liver, or brain) secondary to cardiac disease is frequently present in potential recipients, it is usually considered reversible with successful transplantation and therefore does not necessarily preclude candidacy. Table 31-1 lists typical criteria for heart transplant recipients.

Patients who meet screening criteria for candidacy undergo an extensive evaluation. Most will have already undergone coronary angiography or endomyocardial biopsy to detect conditions that may be treated with more conservative forms of therapy. Additional components of transplant evaluation usually include right-sided heart catheterization; echocardiography; pulmonary function testing; renal, hepatic, hematologic, and general metabolic laboratory

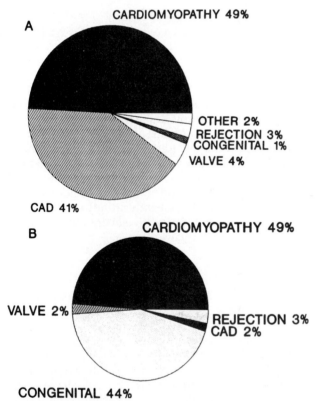

FIGURE 31-1. Indications for cardiac transplantation in adult patients older than 18 years of age **(A)** and in children from birth to 18 years of age **(B)**. *CAD,* coronary artery disease. (Kaye MP, 1992: The registry of the International Society for Heart and Lung Transplantation: Ninth official report—1992. J Heart Lung Transplant 11:600)

TABLE 31-1. RECIPIENT CRITERIA FOR HEART TRANSPLANTATION

Acceptance Criteria

End-stage heart disease unresponsive to more conventional therapy
Age < 65 years
Strong family support system
Ability to adhere to complex medical regimen

Exclusion Criteria

Irreversible renal or hepatic failure
Active substance abuse
Pulmonary vascular resistance > 6 Wood units
Malignancy
Recent pulmonary infarction
Active infection
Active peptic ulcer disease
Psychological instability

Relative Contraindications

Advanced peripheral atherosclerosis
Diabetes mellitus

---

evaluations; and a psychological profile (Futterman, 1988a).

The commitment to undergo cardiac transplantation is a major undertaking that involves not only the recipient but also the entire family support system. Implications for the pretransplant waiting period and post-transplant life-style are profound. Development of a close, supportive relationship between the transplant team and the candidate is essential. Extensive teaching and counseling are integral components and are initiated as soon as transplantation is considered.

Once candidacy is determined, relevant data are obtained for matching the recipient with an appropriate donor, including ABO blood group, weight, size, tissue typing, and current clinical status. United Organ Sharing Network (UNOS) is the organization responsible for registering recipients and allocating hearts and other organs donated for transplantation. The patient's name, weight, ABO blood type, and urgency of need for a donor organ are entered into a national database (Futterman, 1988a).

During the waiting period, pharmacologic therapy (e.g., afterload reduction, inotropic, and diuretic agents) is used to support hemodynamic function. Antiarrhythmic medications may be necessary because malignant ventricular arrhythmias and sudden cardiac death commonly occur in association with severe left ventricular dysfunction (Wenger et al., 1990). In patients with arrhythmias that are refractory to pharmacologic suppression, implantable cardioverter/defibrillators have proven efficacious in preventing sudden death during the waiting period (Bolling et al., 1991). Anticoagulant therapy is also recommended to reduce the risk of pulmonary or systemic embolization arising from thrombus associated with atrial fibrillation, poorly contractile ventricles, or peripheral venous stasis.

Mechanical support of the heart may become necessary if pharmacologic therapy alone is inadequate. Devices that act as a *"bridge to transplant"* provide an important treatment modality because of the long waiting time for donor organs and the successful outcomes of transplantation in this population of patients. Intra-aortic balloon counterpulsation is the most commonly used mechanical assist device, but it only augments cardiac function. Occasionally, profound heart failure during the waiting period necessitates use of a ventricular assist device until a donor heart is located. Favorable survival results in this high-risk group of patients are dependent on judicious candidate selection. As experience is gained in use of mechanical devices to provide a bridge to transplant, indications and predictions for survival are becoming more refined (Emery & Joyce, 1991). Ventricular assist devices are generally not used in patients who have undergone previous cardiac surgery. Because the devices necessitate anticoagulation, perioperative bleeding may be significantly increased in those in whom the transplant procedure is a reoperation.

DONOR SELECTION AND MANAGEMENT

One of the most significant limiting features in cardiac transplantation is the inadequate number of donors in comparison with the number of patients waiting for transplant. Currently, the number of patients added to the waiting list each month is consistently higher than the number of patients receiving transplanted hearts (Stevenson et al., 1992). Because of the scarcity of acceptable donors, the mortality rate in most programs is higher among patients waiting for transplant than in those undergoing the procedure. As many as 30% of candidates accepted for cardiac transplantation may die before suitable donor hearts become available (McCarthy et al., 1991).

Allocation of available donor hearts is complex and sometimes controversial. Survival after transplantation is maximized when donor hearts are used for eligible candidates who are stable enough to wait as outpatients; conversely, death before transplantation is minimized by allocating donor hearts first to patients dependent on intravenous inotropic agents or mechanical assist devices (Stevenson et al., 1992).

Donors are most often young adults who die of closed-head trauma, anoxia, or intracerebral hemorrhage. Because of the prevalence of coronary artery disease in this country, donor age is generally restricted to younger than 40 years in males and younger than 45 years in females. However, these age criteria are at times relaxed as a result of the organ shortage. Older donors are occasionally accepted, particularly for older recipients, if absence of coronary artery disease or other cardiac abnormality is demonstrated by coronary angiography or echocardiography, respectively.

Suitable donors include those who have normal cardiac function, as demonstrated by echocardiography or nuclear scintigraphy, and adequate hemodynamic parameters without excessive doses of inotropic medications. A donor must have a compatible ABO blood type (Rh factor not important) and be of similar size and weight to the recipient. If the recipient has tested positive for cytotoxic antibodies, donor-specific cross-matching is performed to ensure that recipient serum does not destroy the donor organ (Hudak et al., 1990). Severe chest trauma, major systemic illness, malignancy, or active infection in the donor precludes use of the heart (Funk, 1986).

Appropriate donor management before organ harvest is essential and must be directed at protecting all usable organs. Ideally, the lungs, kidneys, liver, and pancreas are harvested in addition to the heart. Arterial and central venous pressure monitoring, as well as a urethral drainage catheter, are important to titrate therapy to preserve function of potential donor organs. Mechanical ventilation is maintained to support respiratory function and ensure adequate blood oxygen saturation levels. Blood, urine, and sputum cultures are obtained from the donor to detect active infection (Reitz, 1989).

Physiologic stability is tenuous and of limited duration in a brain-dead donor; common problems that require careful management include hypotension and hypokalemia due to diabetes insipidus, hypothermia, anemia, and neurogenic pulmonary edema (Bahnson et al., 1991a). Volume replacement and vasopressor agents are usually required to manage the diabetes insipidus associated with severe neurologic injury. However, prolonged administration of large doses of vasopressors may be detrimental to myocardial function. The need for such agents may also reflect underlying ventricular dysfunction in the donor heart. Many potential donors will have had short periods of cardiopulmonary resuscitation and defibrillation, but prolonged periods of hypotension or cardiac arrest exclude use of the heart for transplantation (Baldwin, 1991).

TRANSPLANT PROCEDURE

Organ harvest is often performed at a distant hospital and, almost always, the heart is only one of several organs procured. The various organs are not only used for separate recipients but are generally harvested by separate teams of transplant surgeons for use in different facilities. Another team is used for recipient preparation to expedite the process and reduce donor organ ischemic time. Therefore, coordination of timing among the various harvest teams and between each of the harvest and recipient teams is essential. If organ procurement is well coordinated between the multiple transplant teams and the donor coordinator, a maximal number of recipients can benefit from each donor with good results for all.

Harvest of the heart is performed through a median sternotomy incision. The donor heart is carefully inspected for injury or congenital abnormality before and after being removed from the chest of the donor. After systemic anticoagulation with heparin, cardioplegic solution is administered into the coronary circulation. The donor heart is then excised. When cardiac function ceases, so does the supply of oxygenated blood to myocardial tissue. The heart remains without oxygen until circulation to coronary arteries is restored after implantation of the organ in the recipient. Therefore, the transplant procedure must be accomplished expediently. Cardioplegic arrest, along with immersing the heart in cold saline to provide topical hypothermia, provides adequate protection against ischemic damage for 4 to 6 hours (Baldwin, 1991).

Over 95% of currently performed cardiac transplantations are *orthotopic transplantations*. In an orthotopic transplant, the recipient's heart is removed and the donor heart is inserted in its place in normal anatomic position in the thorax (Fig. 31-2). With the use of cardiopulmonary bypass, circulation and oxygenation are preserved in the recipient while the native heart is excised by transecting the pulmonary artery, aorta, and atria. Posterior and lateral walls of the atria and the atrial septum are left intact to serve as cuffs for the donor heart (Hudak et al., 1990). The donor heart is implanted with atrial, pulmonary artery, and aortic anastomoses. Because the transplanted heart has no innervation from the autonomic nervous system, normal cardiac responses to various reflexes, such as vagal or Valsalva stimulation, do not occur. Initially, intravenous catecholamines, such as isoproterenol or dopamine, are often necessary to increase heart rate and support cardiac function until the ventricle adjusts to the absence of autonomic innervation (Futterman, 1988a).

Rarely, a *heterotopic transplantation* is performed. A heterotropic transplant is one in which the recipient heart is left in place and the donor heart is inserted into the thorax adjacent to the native heart (Fig. 31-3). A synthetic graft is implanted between the native and donor pulmonary arteries to allow the two hearts to function together. Heterotopic transplantation may be indicated when there is a size mismatch between recipient and donor hearts or in the presence of moderate to severe pulmonary hypertension.

The International Registry reports an operative mortality rate (i.e., within 30 days) of 9% to 10% (Kaye, 1992). Operative mortality for patients undergoing cardiac transplantation has remained stable in recent years despite expansion of indications to include higher-risk patients (e.g., those on mechanical assist devices or with associated medical illnesses). Operative risk is increased in patients undergoing heterotopic transplantation (25%) or retransplantation (34%) and in those who require preoperative

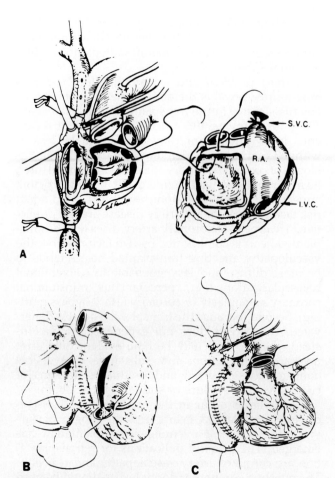

cardiac surgery. Inotropic and vasodilating drugs are frequently required in the early postoperative hours to support cardiac function. Because of the serious consequences of infection in immunosuppressed patients, efforts are made to reduce those factors that increase the risk of infection. Reverse isolation is usually practiced for the first several days. Intravenous and other invasive catheters are removed as soon as possible, and antibiotics are used sparingly to avoid overgrowth of more resistant bacteria (Futterman, 1988b). One of the most important considerations in postoperative care is the immunosuppression regimen. Organ rejection remains a significant problem despite immunosuppression because of immunologic differences between donor and recipient hearts. A careful balance must be maintained between adequate suppression of the patient's immunologic defense mechanisms and prevention of overwhelming infection. Because each of the immunosuppressive agents is associated with significant adverse effects, multiple agents are administered so that adequate immunosuppression can be achieved using low doses of individual agents. Most transplant centers administer three drugs prophylactically to suppress the body's immunologic defenses: cyclosporine, azathioprine, and corticosteroids.

FIGURE 31-2. Orthotopic cardiac transplantation. **(A)** Recipient heart has been removed (*left*) and donor heart is ready for implantation (*right*); left atrial anastomosis is begun at recipient left superior pulmonary vein and donor left atrial appendage (S.V.C., superior vena cava; R.A., right atrium; L.A., left atrium, I.V.C., inferior vena cava). **(B)** Left atrial anastomosis has been completed and right atrial anastomosis is begun; note that incision in donor right atrium begins through the inferior vena cava and then curves anteromedially to avoid injury to the sinus node. **(C)** The atrial anastomoses are completed, and the aortic anastomosis is near completion; the pulmonary arterial anastomosis is performed last, after removal of the aortic clamp. (Baldwin JD, 1991: Cardiac transplantation. In Baue AE, Geha AS, Hammond GL, et al [eds]: Glenn's Thoracic and Cardiovascular Surgery, ed. 5, p. 1618. Norwalk, CT, Appleton & Lange)

hospitalization or mechanical support (14%) (Kriett & Kaye, 1991). The most common early complication of cardiac transplantation and a leading cause of operative death is perioperative cardiac dysfunction (Bahnson et al., 1991b).

POSTOPERATIVE CONSIDERATIONS

Early postoperative care of cardiac transplant patients is similar to that of patients undergoing other types of

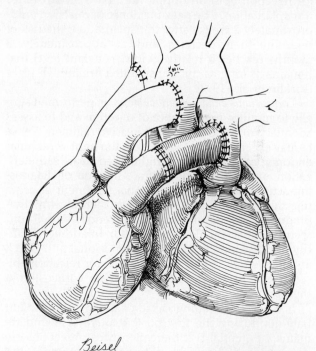

Beisel

FIGURE 31-3. Heterotopic cardiac transplantation. An anastomosis is constructed between the donor and recipient left atria. The ascending aorta of the donor heart is anastomosed to the ascending aorta of the recipient heart, the donor superior vena cava to the recipient superior vena cava, and the donor pulmonary artery to the recipient pulmonary artery, using a synthetic graft. (Waldhausen JA, 1985: Transplantation of the heart and lungs. In Johnson's Surgery of the Chest, ed. 5, p. 523. Chicago, Year Book Medical Publishers)

The primary complications of cyclosporine therapy are renal failure and hypertension. Many patients require chronic antihypertensive therapy. Cyclosporine can also cause hepatotoxicity, neurologic disturbances, and hirsuitism (Baldwin, 1991). Corticosteroids can lead to infection, hyperlipidemia, hypertension, and diabetes (Lee et al., 1991). In addition, large corticosteroid doses given repeatedly to treat rejection can cause severe side effects, particularly osteoporosis, metabolic abnormalities, and infection (Wahlers et al., 1990). As in all immunosuppressed patients, the risk of malignancy, particularly lymphoma, is increased after heart transplantation (Baldwin, 1991).

Current 1- and 5-year survival rates after heart transplantation are 78% and 67%, respectively (Kaye, 1992). The three major complications of heart transplantation are rejection, infection, and coronary artery vasculopathy. *Hyperacute rejection* is a rejection episode that occurs almost immediately after reperfusion of the transplanted heart. Although uncommon, hyperacute rejection is usually so severe that retransplantation is necessary. The more common form of rejection (i.e., *acute rejection*) has become less prevalent with the addition of cyclosporine to the immunosuppressive regimen. Still, most patients have a major rejection episode during the first 3 months after transplantation. The peak incidence of rejection is approximately 2 weeks after transplantation; the risk of rejection then declines and at approximately 3 months reaches a relatively low, constant level that remains as long as the transplanted organ is in place (Kirklin et al., 1992).

Transvenous endomyocardial biopsy is performed serially to monitor for evidence of rejection and to assess adequacy of the immunosuppressive regimen. These biopsy specimens, obtained from the right ventricular endomyocardium during right-sided heart catheterization, provide a very accurate method of diagnosing acute rejection. Conventional treatment of acute rejection is bolus doses of corticosteroids (methylprednisolone), administered intravenously on 3 consecutive days (Wahlers et al., 1990). In addition, antithymocyte globulin (ATG) or monoclonal anti–T-cell antibodies (OKT3) are administered for rejection episodes that recur or are refractory to corticosteroid therapy.

Infection is a leading cause of death in transplant patients during the first postoperative year and remains a potential risk thereafter. Most infections are not acquired from the external environment but result from opportunistic organisms within the individual, such as *Staphylococcus epidermidis*, enteric bacteria, and latent viruses (Lange et al., 1992). In addition to the early postoperative period, patients are most susceptible to infection during treatment of acute rejection when higher doses of immunosuppressive drugs are administered (Futterman, 1988b). A wide spectrum of bacterial, viral, fungal, or protozoal infections may occur (Reitz, 1989). Most common

are bacterial pneumonia and cytomegalovirus infections (Bahnson et al., 1991b). Because of the immunosuppressed state, clinical manifestations of infection are often subtle.

A third problem and a major limiting factor in long-term survival is the development of *coronary artery vasculopathy* in the transplanted heart (Gao et al., 1989). As many as 40% of cardiac transplant recipients have angiographically demonstrable lesions within 3 years of transplantation (Baldwin, 1991). Etiology of coronary artery disease in transplanted hearts is not yet well defined, but multiple factors appear to be involved (Johnson, 1992). Traditional risk factors for coronary artery disease are not predictive. Treatment of coronary artery disease in a transplanted heart is complicated by two factors. First, the vasculopathy affecting transplanted hearts tends to be more diffuse and less amenable to conventional revascularization (i.e., percutaneous transluminal coronary angioplasty or coronary artery bypass grafting). Second, because the transplanted heart is denervated, the patient does not experience angina. Instead, the problem may become evident only after myocardial infarction and substantial irreversible damage have occurred and produce symptoms of congestive heart failure or sudden cardiac death.

As increases occur in the number of patients receiving transplanted hearts and the length of survival, the need for eventual retransplantation has emerged. The primary indications for retransplantation are coronary artery vasculopathy and rejection. The question of whether donor hearts should be used preferentially for first-time transplantation or for retransplantation raises difficult ethical issues. Repeat transplantation is associated with a markedly increased mortality rate as compared with primary transplantation, especially in patients with a shorter interval between transplants, rejection as the cause of allograft failure, or the need for preoperative mechanical assistance (Ensley et al., 1992).

LUNG AND HEART-LUNG TRANSPLANTATION

DEVELOPMENT OF LUNG AND HEART-LUNG TRANSPLANTATION

Availability of cyclosporine, improvements in donor preservation, and refinement of surgical techniques have allowed development of other forms of thoracic transplantation. Although still evolving, these forms of thoracic transplantation offer the potential for prolonged survival and improved quality of life in otherwise terminally ill patients. However, because the procedures continue to be associated with significant morbidity and mortality, they are reserved for patients who have a life expectancy of less than 1 to 2 years with conventional forms of therapy.

The first human lung transplant was performed by

Hardy in 1963 (Hardy et al., 1963). As with cardiac transplantation, long-term patient survival was not achieved despite technical accomplishment of the operation. In contrast to other types of organ transplants, however, progress lagged in transplant procedures involving the lung even after improved immunosuppression with cyclosporine. A number of factors unique to the lung retarded experimental and clinical progress of lung transplantation. These include (1) fragility of lung tissue, such that a minor insult can produce severe dysfunction; (2) the necessary interruption of bronchial vessels at the time of transplant, leading to bronchial anastomosis ischemia; (3) a greater risk of infection due to exposure of the tracheobronchial tree to the atmosphere; (4) the

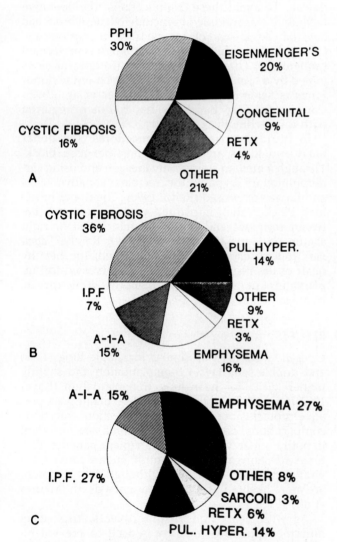

FIGURE 31-4. Indications for heart-lung transplantation **(A)**, double lung transplantation **(B)**, and single lung transplantation **(C)**. *PPH,* primary pulmonary hypertension; *RETX,* retransplantation; *I.P.F.,* idiopathic pulmonary fibrosis; *PUL, HYPER,* pulmonary hypertension; *A-1-A,* α_1-antitrypsin deficiency. (Kaye MP, 1992: The registry of the International Society for Heart and Lung Transplantation: Ninth official report—1992. J Heart Lung Transplant 11:602)

TABLE 31-2. RECIPIENT CRITERIA FOR LUNG TRANSPLANTATION

Acceptance Criteria

End-stage pulmonary disease unresponsive to more conventional therapy
<60 years of age
Oxygen dependency
Strong family support system
Ability to adhere to complex medical regimen

Exclusion Criteria

Ventilator dependency
Corticosteroid dependency
Diabetes mellitus
Active infection
Malignancy
Renal or hepatic failure
Substance abuse
Psychological instability

lack of an experimental model analogous to the clinical situation; and (5) difficulty in definitively diagnosing causes of early dysfunction of the transplanted lung (Cooper, 1991). In addition to these factors, lung and heart-lung transplantation are limited by the lack of suitable donor lungs. Because of susceptibility of the lungs to infection and edema, especially in the event of donor brain death, only about 15% of cardiac donors are also suitable lung donors (Aziz & Jamieson, 1991; Cooper, 1991).

INDICATIONS FOR TRANSPLANTATION

The current era of successful lung transplantation was introduced by Cooper in 1983 (Toronto Lung Transplant Group, 1986). Since that time, technical aspects of the procedure have been refined and the success rate has improved steadily (Haydock et al., 1992). Lung transplantation is performed for treatment of end-stage restrictive or obstructive pulmonary disease (Fig. 31-4). Patients considered for transplantation must demonstrate progressive lung disease, as evidenced by decreased exercise tolerance or deteriorating pulmonary function studies, increasing oxygen requirements, or increasing complications such that estimated survival time is less than 12 to 18 months (Kaiser et al., 1992). Typical criteria for lung transplant candidacy are displayed in Table 31-2.

Initial clinical success was achieved with *single lung transplantation* in patients with restrictive lung disease, most commonly pulmonary fibrosis. Replacing one of the diseased lungs dramatically improves pulmonary function in patients with restrictive lung disease. The poor compliance and increased vascular resistance in the remaining native lung cause the transplanted lung to be preferentially ventilated and perfused (Cooper, 1991).

Single lung transplantation was considered not applicable for the more common obstructive form of pulmonary disease. Transplant surgeons believed that the remaining native lung would be preferentially ventilated, resulting in air-trapping, mediastinal shift, and crowding of the transplanted lung (Kaiser et al., 1991). Perfusion, on the other hand, would be directed preferentially to the transplanted lung because of its lower pulmonary vascular resistance. Consequently, double lung transplantation was developed to provide a treatment alternative for patients with obstructive lung disease.

However, with increased clinical experience, single lung transplantation has proven successful in patients with obstructive as well as restrictive pulmonary disease (Marinelli et al., 1992). As a result, single lung transplantation is now being performed in patients with obstructive lung disease, granulomatous lung disease, and pulmonary hypertension (Mohiaddin et al., 1991; Pasque et al., 1992). Emphysema is the most frequently occurring form of obstructive pulmonary disease. It typically develops secondary to smoking in older persons who would not be candidates for a transplant procedure. However, patients afflicted with end-stage emphysema at an early age, such as those with an inherited alpha-1-antitrypsin deficiency, are considered ideal candidates because of their young age and lack of involvement of other organs (Kaiser et al., 1991).

Double, or *bilateral, lung transplantation* is recommended for patients with cystic fibrosis or bilateral pulmonary sepsis from another cause (see Fig. 31-4) (Pasque et al., 1990). Single lung transplantation is not appropriate in septic pulmonary diseases because the native, diseased lung would provide a continued focus of sepsis, particularly once the patient began immunosuppressive therapy after transplantation (Patterson et al., 1988). Double lung transplantation also continues to be used selectively for obstructive disease in younger patients and in those with a large bullous component to their disease (Pasque et al., 1990; Kaiser et al., 1992).

Heart-lung transplantation is performed for pulmonary or cardiac diseases associated with irreversible pulmonary hypertension (see Fig. 31-4). The three most common diagnoses for which heart-lung transplantation is performed are primary pulmonary hypertension, Eisenmenger's syndrome, and cystic fibrosis (Kaye, 1992). However, the number of heart-lung transplantations appears to be decreasing as applicability of single and double lung transplantation has broadened to include more forms of pulmonary and pulmonary vascular disease.

OPERATIVE PROCEDURES

Donor preservation and operative techniques for lung and heart-lung transplantation are evolving rapidly as more experience is gained. Single lung trans-

plantation is performed through a thoracotomy incision and using single lung anesthesia. The native lung is excised and the donor lung implanted with bronchial, left atrial (containing the pulmonary vein orifices), and pulmonary artery anastomoses.

Double lung transplantation was initially performed by implanting both donor lungs as a block. Through a median sternotomy incision and using cardiopulmonary bypass, the recipient lungs were removed and the donor lungs implanted by performing anastomoses of the trachea, pulmonary artery, and left atrial cuff. The first double lung transplant procedures were associated with considerable morbidity. Airway problems related to the tracheal anastomosis (e.g., dehiscence and stenosis) were common late sequelae. To avoid these complications, the operative technique was modified to include bilateral bronchial anastomoses instead of a single tracheal anastomosis. Currently, bilateral lung transplantation is performed sequentially. Through bilateral thoracotomy incisions joined by a transverse sternotomy, each of the donor lungs is separately implanted (Kaiser et al., 1992). Cardiopulmonary bypass is not routinely required with this technique.

In heart-lung transplant procedures, the donor heart and lungs are removed together as a block. Through a median sternotomy incision and using cardiopulmonary bypass, the recipient's native heart and lungs are excised (Reitz, 1990). The donor heart-lung block is then implanted with anastomoses between recipient and donor trachea (airway), right atrium (inflow), and aorta (outflow). Rarely, "domino" transplantation may be performed; the healthy heart of the heart-lung recipient is harvested for implantation in a second recipient awaiting cardiac transplantation (Smith, 1991).

RESULTS

Operative mortality is similar for single lung (13%) and double lung (14%) transplantation and slightly higher (20%) for heart-lung transplantation (Kaye, 1992). As with heart transplantation, major postoperative problems are infection and rejection. Infectious complications, particularly pneumonia, are prevalent in both lung and heart-lung transplant patients. Bacterial infections are most common but are rarely fatal; viral and fungal infections, although less common, are more likely to lead to the patient's death (Maurer et al., 1992).

As with heart transplant recipients, triple-drug immunosuppressive therapy is used to prevent rejection. Lung rejection is manifested initially by a deterioration in arterial oxygen tension, minimal temperature elevation, and perihilar infiltrates (Kaiser et al., 1991). However, the diagnosis of rejection in a transplanted lung remains imprecise. It is sometimes only the response to therapy that enables the clinician to diagnose rejection. In patients who have undergone heart-lung transplantation, the heart and lungs can reject separately. Often, the lung rejects before and without cardiac rejection (Wallwork, 1989).

REFERENCES

Aziz S, Jamieson S, 1991: Combined heart and lung transplantation. In Baue AE, Geha AS, Hammond GL, et al. (eds): Glenn's Thoracic and Cardiovascular Surgery, ed. 5. Norwalk, CT, Appleton & Lange

Bahnson HT, Griffith BP, Armitage JM, et al., 1991a: Organ procurement and preservation. In Baue AE, Geha AS, Hammond GL, et al. (eds): Glenn's Thoracic and Cardiovascular Surgery, ed. 5. Norwalk, CT, Appleton & Lange

Bahnson HT, Hardesty RL, Griffeth BP, et al., 1991b: Management of complications related to cardiac transplantation. In Waldhausen JA, Orringer MB (eds): Complications in Cardiothoracic Surgery. St. Louis, Mosby–Year Book

Baldwin JC, 1991: Cardiac transplantation. In Baue AE, Geha AS, Hammond GL, et al. (eds): Glenn's Thoracic and Cardiovascular Surgery, ed. 5. Norwalk, CT, Appleton & Lange

Bolling SF, Deeb GM, Morady F, et al., 1991: Automatic internal cardioverter defibrillator: A bridge to heart transplantation. J Heart Lung Transplant 10:562

Cooper JD, 1991: Lung transplantation. In Baue AE, Geha AS, Hammond GL, et al. (eds): Glenn's Thoracic and Cardiovascular Surgery, ed. 5. Norwalk, CT, Appleton & Lange

Emery RW, Joyce LD, 1991: Directions in cardiac assistance. J Cardiac Surg 6:400

Ensley RD, Hunt S, Taylor DO, et al., 1992: Predictors of survival after repeat heart transplantation. J Heart Lung Transplant 11:S142

Funk M, 1986: Heart transplantation: Postoperative care during the acute period. Crit Care Nurs 6:27

Futterman LG, 1988a: Cardiac transplantation: A comprehensive nursing perspective: I. Heart Lung 17:499

Futterman LG, 1988b: Cardiac transplantation: A comprehensive nursing perspective: II. Heart Lung 17:631

Gao SZ, Schroeder JS, Alderman EL, 1989: Prevalence of accelerated coronary artery disease in heart transplant survivors. Circulation 80 (Suppl III):III-100

Gay WA, O'Connell JB, 1990: Cardiac transplantation. In Sabiston DC Jr, Spencer FC (eds): Surgery of the Chest, ed. 5. Philadelphia, WB Saunders

Hardy JD, Webb WR, Dalton TL Jr, Walker GR Jr, 1963: Lung homotransplantation in man: Report of the initial case. JAMA 186:1063

Haydock DA, Trulock EP, Kaiser LR, et al., 1992: Lung transplantation. J Thorac Cardiovasc Surg 103:329

Hudak CM, Gallo BM, Benz JJ (eds), 1990: Cardiac surgery and heart transplantation. In Critical Care Nursing: A Holistic Approach, ed. 5. Philadelphia, JB Lippincott

Johnson MR, 1992: Transplant coronary disease: Nonimmunologic risk factors. J Heart Lung Transplant 11:S124

Kaiser LR, Cooper JD, Trulock EP, et al., 1991: The evolution of single lung transplantion for emphysema. J Thorac Cardiovasc Surg 102:333

Kaiser LR, Pasque MK, Trulock EP, et al., 1992: Bilateral sequential lung transplantation: The procedure of choice for double-lung replacement. Ann Thorac Surg 52:438

Kaye MP, 1992: The registry of the International Society for Heart and Lung Transplantation: Ninth official report—1992. J Heart Lung Transplant 11:599

Kirklin JW, Barratt-Boyes BG, 1993: Primary cardiomyopathy and cardiac transplantation. In Cardiac Surgery, ed. 2. New York, Churchill Livingstone

Kirklin JK, Naftel DC, Bourge RC, et al., 1992: Rejection after cardiac transplantation. Circulation 86 (Suppl II):II-236

Kriett JM, Kaye MP, 1991: The registry of the International Society for Heart and Lung Transplantation: Eighth official report—1991. J Heart Lung Transplant 10:491

Lange SS, Prevost S, Lewis P, Fadol A, 1992: Infection control practices in cardiac transplant recipients. Heart Lung 21:101

Lee KF, Pierce JD, Hess ML et al., 1991: Cardiac transplantation with corticosteroid-free immunosuppression: Long-term results. Ann Thorac Surg 52:211

Marinelli WA, Hertz MI, Shumway SJ, et al., 1992: Single lung transplantation for severe emphysema. J Heart Lung Transplant 11:577

Maurer JR, Tullis DE, Grossman RF, et al., 1992: Infectious complications following isolated lung transplantation. Chest 101:1056

McCarthy PM, Portner PM, Tobler HG, et al., 1991: Clinical experience with the Novacor ventricular assist system. J Thorac Cardiovasc Surg 102:578

Mohiaddin RH, Paz R, Theodoropoulous S, et al., 1991: Magnetic resonance characterization of pulmonary arterial blood flow after single lung transplantation. J Thorac Cardiovasc Surg 101:1016

Munoz E, Lonquist JL, Radovancevic B, et al., 1992: Long-term results in diabetic patients undergoing heart transplantation. J Heart Lung Transplant 11:943

Pasque MK, Cooper JD, Kaiser LR, et al., 1990: Improved technique for bilateral lung transplantation: Rationale and initial clinical experience. Ann Thorac Surg 49:785

Pasque MK, Kaiser LR, Dresler CM, et al., 1992: Single lung transplantation for pulmonary hypertension. J Thorac Cardiovasc Surg 103:475

Patterson GA, Cooper JD, Goldman B, et al., 1988: Technique of successful clinical double-lung transplantation. Ann Thorac Surg 45:626

Reitz BA, 1989: Cardiac transplantation. In Grillo HC, Austen WG, Wilkins EW (eds): Current Therapy in Cardiothoracic Surgery. Toronto, BC Decker

Reitz BA, 1990: Heart and lung transplantation. In Sabiston DC Jr, Spencer FC (eds): Surgery of the Chest, ed. 5. Philadelphia, WB Saunders

Smith JA, Cochrane AD, Esmore DS, 1991: Technique and results of cardiac transplantation using "domino-donor" hearts. J Cardiac Surg 6:381

Stevenson LW, Warner SL, Hamilton MA, et al., 1992: Modeling distribution of donor hearts to maximize early candidate survival. Circulation 86 (Suppl II):II-224

Toronto Lung Transplant Group, 1986: Unilateral lung transplantation for pulmonary fibrosis. N Engl J Med 314:1140

Wahlers T, Heublein B, Cremer J, et al., 1990: Treatment of rejection after heart transplantation: What dose of pulsed steroids is necessary. J Heart Transplant 9:568

Wallwork J, 1989: Indications for operation, patient selection and assessment. In Heart and Heart-Lung Transplantation. Philadelphia, WB Saunders

Wenger NK, Abelman WH, Roberts WC, 1990: Cardiomyopathy and specific heart muscle disease. In Hurst JW (ed): The Heart, ed. 7. New York, McGraw-Hill

32

CHAPTER

CARDIAC AND THORACIC TRAUMA

TYPES OF INJURIES
  Bony Injuries
  Aortic Transection
  Cardiac Injuries
  Tracheal and Bronchial Injuries
  Pulmonary Injuries

Pneumothorax and Hemothorax
Esophageal Perforation
Injury to the Diaphragm
ACUTE MANAGEMENT OF THE CHEST
  TRAUMA VICTIM

The incidence of chest trauma continues to increase, largely owing to the prevalence of accidents associated with high speed and rapid deceleration and with violent acts of aggression. Motor vehicle accidents account for nearly half of traumatic deaths, followed by suicide (28%) and homicide (22%) (LoCicero & Mattox, 1989). In addition to the increased number of trauma victims, improvements in emergency transport systems allow more patients to reach hospitals where appropriate diagnosis and treatment can occur.

Chest trauma is categorized as either blunt or penetrating. *Blunt chest trauma* consists of those injuries to thoracic structures that are caused by application of external force to the thorax without penetration of the chest wall. Blunt trauma is most often associated with motor vehicle accidents but can also result from falling or crushing accidents (Hood, 1990). In high speed accidents, injury results from the application of shearing force to contiguous fixed and nonfixed intrathoracic structures as the person rapidly decelerates. In low speed accidents, the injury is likely to be caused by localized crushing. *Penetrating chest trauma* consists of injuries to thoracic structures caused by an object that penetrates the chest wall. The incidence of penetrating thoracic injuries, and gunshot wounds in particular, appears to be increasing at an alarming rate (Follette, 1991).

TYPES OF INJURIES

BONY INJURIES

Rib fractures are the most common chest injury, particularly in older individuals with more brittle bones. Fractures frequently occur in the fifth through ninth ribs, often at the posterior angle (Rodriguez, 1990a; McElvein & Novick, 1991). Clinical manifestations of rib fracture are pain, point tenderness, and splinting. The diagnosis is confirmed by posteroanterior and lateral chest roentgenograms. Treatment is palliative; pain medications are prescribed, and, if necessary, intercostal nerve blocks may be used to provide local anesthesia. It is important that pain control is adequate to prevent hypoventilation with resultant atelectasis and retention of secretions. Healing of rib fractures takes 3 to 6 weeks.

If more than one rib is fractured, respiratory function may be compromised. Elderly patients in particular may develop significant atelectasis and pneumonitis (Hood, 1990). Such patients may require admission to the hospital for observation, supplemental oxygenation, pulmonary hygiene, or ventilatory support. Contrary to popular belief, application of a chest binder or taping of the chest wall is not indicated because these splinting devices impede deep breathing and predispose to atelectasis (Baker, 1990; Hood, 1990).

Clinical significance is attached to fracture of the first or second rib. A great deal of force is required to fracture these ribs because they are well protected by the clavicle, scapula, humerus, and soft tissue (Rodriguez, 1990a). For this reason, the possibility of associated internal injuries must be considered. Serious injury to intrathoracic structures is also more likely when multiple ribs are fractured. Upper rib fractures may be associated with aortic injury; spleen and liver injuries are frequently associated with fracture of multiple lower ribs.

Flail chest is the term used to describe an injury in which two or more ribs or costal cartilages are fractured in several places (Fig. 32-1). The dislocated segments move paradoxically to the remainder of the bony structure of the chest wall during respiration; that is, the flail segment moves inward during inspiration as the remainder of the rib cage moves outward, and vice versa. Usually the injured ribs heal without treatment. If the size of the flail segment is large, the lung on the injured side may be significantly hypoventilated. Mechanical ventilation with positive end-expiratory pressure (PEEP) may be necessary for stabilization of the bony thorax if the injury is associated with respiratory insufficiency. In such cases, it is usually underlying pulmonary contusion, rather than abnormal chest movements, that causes the respiratory failure.

Fracture of the sternum is usually caused by impact of a victim's chest against a steering wheel (Rodriquez, 1990a). The fracture may be detected by palpation, local swelling and discoloration, pain, and its appearance on a lateral roentgenogram (McElvein & Novick, 1991). Unless the fracture produces severe displacement of the sternal edges, open reduction and fixation are generally not required. Sternal fracture is most significant because of its frequent association with myocardial contusion. Accordingly, patients are usually admitted for observation and cardiac monitoring. Less commonly, sternal fracture is accompanied by tracheobronchial or great vessel injury.

Fractures of the scapula and clavicle are relatively uncommon. Although treatment for both is palliative, they are often associated with injury to underlying structures. In contrast to other fractures of the bony thorax, a fractured clavicle is treated with an external support brace. A figure-of-eight soft harness is generally applied for 6 to 8 weeks to produce sustained hyperextension of the shoulders.

AORTIC TRANSECTION

Aortic transection describes traumatic laceration of the aorta. The injury is most often caused by severe blunt chest trauma associated with rapid deceleration or severe chest compression. It is a leading cause of immediate death in motor vehicle accidents and falls (Turney & Rodriguez, 1990). Traumatic aortic injury almost always occurs at one of two sites: (1) the thoracic isthmus, just distal to the left subclavian artery at the location of the ligamentum arteriosum, or (2) just distal to the aortic valve (Fig. 32-2). Injury is more likely at these locations because the segment of aorta between the aortic valve and thoracic isthmus is not tethered. The heart and descending aorta, on the other hand, are relatively fixed in position by contiguous structures. Transection just distal to the left subclavian artery is most often produced by rapid horizontal deceleration, such as occurs with high-speed motor vehicle accidents. Rapid vertical deceleration, as occurs with a fall from a building or airplane, is likely to cause disruption of the ascending aorta.

Eighty percent of persons with aortic transection, and almost all of those with transection of the ascending aorta, die at the scene of the accident. However, if aortic adventitia or periaortic fibrous tissue remains intact, blood is contained in the aorta and the victim may survive for a period of time. The prognosis for these early survivors depends on timely diagnosis of the injury. Precipitous adventitial rupture within hours or days is common. Death from exsanguination is most likely in the first few hours after injury; initial survivors die at a rate of 2% to 10% per hour (Turney & Rodriguez, 1990). Therefore, it is essential to con-

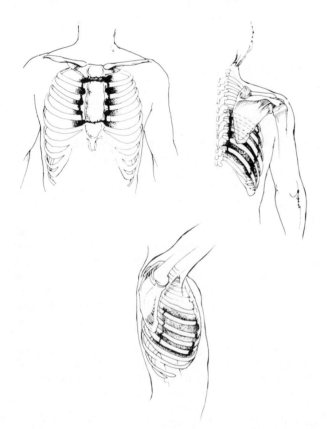

FIGURE 32-1. Typical sites of flail chest injury. (Campbell DB, 1992: Trauma to the chest wall, lung, and major airways. Semin Thorac Cardiovasc Surg 4:235)

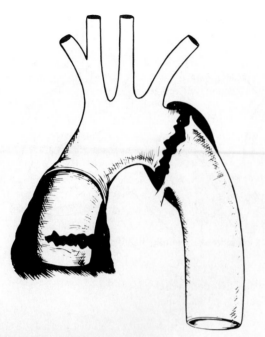

FIGURE 32-2. Schematic representation of aorta demonstrating the two common sites of aortic transection. (Turney SZ, Rodriquez A: Injuries to the great thoracic vessels. In Turney SZ, Rodriquez A, Cowley RA [eds]: Management of Cardiothoracic Trauma, p. 232. Baltimore, Williams & Wilkins)

sider the diagnosis of aortic transection in any victim of a deceleration-type injury, particularly if other injuries indicative of major chest trauma are present.

A fracture of the sternum, clavicle, first rib, or multiple ribs suggests that there has been a blow to the chest forceful enough to tear the aorta. Additional evidence of aortic transection is provided by roentgenographic signs of bleeding into the pericardial or pleural spaces. Mediastinal widening is the most common radiographic finding (Merrill et al., 1988). Obliteration of the aortic knob, pleural effusion (hemothorax), and tracheal deviation may also be present. Interpretation of roentgenographic mediastinal widening is difficult because the chest radiograph is almost always obtained with portable equipment using an anteroposterior projection. In anteroposterior chest films, there is some magnification of the mediastinal shadow due to technique. Also, the absence of a widened mediastinum does not rule out the diagnosis. Other signs and symptoms of aortic transection that may be present include shock, a systolic murmur, and a differential in blood pressure measurements between upper and lower extremities.

Aortography remains the gold standard for diagnosis of aortic transection. If aortic injury is suggested by the type of accident, clinical manifestations, or radiographic findings, an aortogram is obtained to confirm the diagnosis. If aortography is not immediately available and the patient is hemodynamically stable, computed tomography of the chest may be used to aid in diagnosis by revealing the presence of a periaortic hematoma. However, the accuracy of chest computed tomography is inadequate for using the study to rule out the diagnosis (McLean et al., 1991). The role of transesophageal echocardiography in diagnosing aortic transection is still being defined.

Often, the diagnosis of aortic transection is delayed because of associated injuries, some of which may require urgent operative treatment. Failure to establish the diagnosis usually results in precipitous death of the patient. Once the diagnosis is established, surgical repair of the aorta is performed immediately, unless severe associated injuries take precedence. If hemothorax is present, repair of the aortic transection is of highest priority. If no hemothorax is present and there is evidence of active bleeding elsewhere (e.g., in the abdomen), other surgical interventions may take priority, particularly since systemic anticoagulation will be necessary if cardiopulmonary bypass is used during the aortic repair.

Surgical repair of the aorta is performed through a left thoracotomy incision for aortic transection in the classic location. The aorta is clamped above and below the area of transection, and the injured segment is resected and replaced with a prosthetic graft. Cardiopulmonary bypass is generally not used because it necessitates systemic anticoagulation, which is contraindicated in the presence of active bleeding or associated injuries. Prognosis for patient survival is good if repair is undertaken before adventitial rupture. Complications of the operative repair include bleeding, renal failure, and paraplegia due to ischemic injury to the spinal cord during the time that blood flow through the descending aorta is interrupted. Several techniques are described in the surgical literature for intraoperative protection of spinal cord blood flow and monitoring of spinal cord ischemia. Despite these measures, the development of paraplegia as an operative complication remains unpredictable, occurring in 5% to 14% of patients who undergo operative repair of the descending thoracic aorta (Mattox, 1989; Cowley et al., 1990).

Rarely, in patients with undiagnosed aortic transection, the adventitia remains intact and a chronic traumatic aneurysm develops at the site of the transection. The aneurysm may exist for many years before it is detected when a chest roentgenogram is performed for another reason or the patient develops symptoms of aneurysm enlargement. Because of the propensity for sudden rupture, operative repair of chronic traumatic aneurysm is recommended, even in the absence of symptoms (Finkelmeier et al., 1982).

CARDIAC INJURIES

Penetrating Wounds

Cardiac injuries are usually the result of penetrating wounds that occur during acts of aggression. The

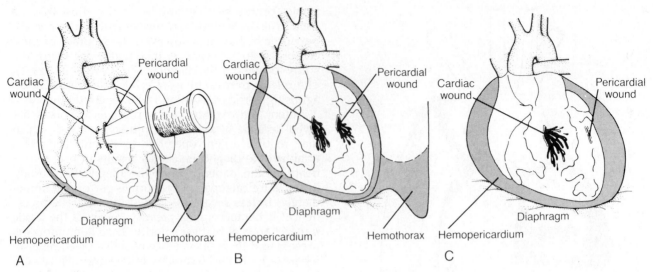

FIGURE 32-3. Penetrating injury to the heart **(A)**, with open **(B)** and sealed **(C)** pericardial wound. (Symbas PN, 1989: Contusion of the heart. In Cardiothoracic Trauma, p. 31. Philadelphia, WB Saunders)

most common cause is gunshot wounds, followed by stabbing. Gunshot wounds are more often lethal because they produce a larger defect in the pericardium and more destruction of myocardial tissue. As a result, exsanguination is more likely than with stab wounds, which cause a small pericardial rent that is likely to seal off and cause cardiac tamponade (Attar et al., 1991) (Fig. 32-3). Cardiac injuries can also result from blunt chest trauma. Any portion of the heart can be damaged by traumatic injury. Right ventricular laceration is most common because of its anterior location, followed by left ventricular injury (Attar et al., 1991). Frequently, more than one cardiac chamber is involved. As with aortic transection, individuals with injuries to the heart frequently die due to tamponade or exsanguination before reaching the hospital.

If the patient arrives at the hospital with cardiac arrest or in extremis (i.e., with severe hypotension refractory to volume resuscitation), it may be necessary for the surgeon to open the patient's chest in the emergency department. A left anterolateral thoracotomy incision is made, and a rib retractor is used to separate the ribs. Because massive hemorrhage is likely, digital or clamp compression of the bleeding site and rapid infusion of large volumes of blood or other fluid is mandatory. In the event of severe internal damage to the heart, the likelihood of survival is remote. If bleeding cannot be quickly controlled, exsanguination, tamponade, or cardiac failure results in the patient's death.

In hemodynamically stable patients, cardiac injury should be considered in any individual with a history of a penetrating wound to the chest, upper abdomen, or neck. A heart wound is particularly likely if the entrance wound of a penetrating object is between the two midclavicular lines (Rodriguez et al., 1990b)

(Fig. 32-4). Blood in the left pleural space provides further evidence of cardiac or vascular injury. In all patients who have suffered major chest trauma, the heart is carefully auscultated for the presence of murmurs.

An echocardiogram is performed if internal cardiac injury is suspected. Availability of transesophageal

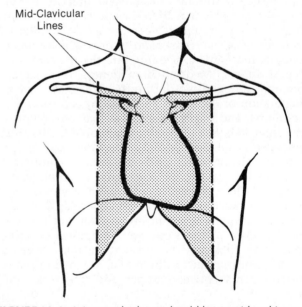

FIGURE 32-4. Injury to the heart should be considered in any patient with a penetrating wound between the anterior midclavicular lines (*shaded area*). (Rodriquez A, 1990: Initial patient evaluation and indications for thoracotomy. In Turney SZ, Rodriquez A, Cowley RA [eds]: Management of Cardiothoracic Trauma, p. 9. Baltimore, Williams & Wilkins)

echocardiography has enhanced rapid and accurate diagnosis of cardiac injuries. Transesophageal echocardiography can be performed in the emergency department, can be accomplished in approximately 15 minutes, provides information that can be immediately interpreted, has minimal risks, and does not necessitate administration of contrast medium (Shapiro et al., 1991). Using this bedside technique, intracardiac septal defects, valvular damage, or the presence of foreign bodies can be diagnosed (Follette, 1991).

If the patient survives long enough to be transported to the operating room, surgical exploration is performed with repair of the traumatic defect. A median sternotomy incision is generally used since it provides excellent exposure of the heart and great vessels. Repair of injured cardiac valves, coronary arteries, or septa requires trained personnel and equipment for providing extracorporeal circulation (cardiopulmonary bypass) during the operation. However, most individuals with cardiac injuries who survive to be transported to a hospital do not have internal cardiac damage but rather have a laceration confined to the atrial or ventricular wall. This type of cardiac injury can often be repaired without cardiopulmonary bypass by clamping the injured tissue and suturing the laceration. Delay in operation, rather than lack of cardiopulmonary bypass capability in the institution, is the major cause of mortality in these patients (Lockhart, 1986).

Patients who undergo repair of a lacerated cardiac chamber wall should also be carefully assessed for injury to internal structures of the heart. Occasionally, a penetrating object perforates the atrial or ventricular septum or damages one of the cardiac valves without producing hemodynamic compromise. The internal injury may not be detected when the external laceration is repaired. If an internal cardiac defect is identified but the patient demonstrates no adverse hemodynamic effects, the surgeon may elect to defer intracardiac repair for several weeks until tissues surrounding the lacerated area have matured and become more firm. This makes the repair technically easier and safer for the patient. Foreign bodies that penetrate the heart and are free-floating in one of the cardiac chambers should be removed. However, if the object is embedded in myocardium, operative removal may not be necessary unless its presence causes arrhythmias, infection, or pericardial effusion.

Myocardial Contusion

Myocardial contusion is injury of the heart muscle secondary to blunt trauma. It is particularly likely in accidents in which there is a blow to the anterior chest, such as when an individual is propelled against the steering wheel of a car (Fig. 32-5). Because the right ventricle is the most anterior chamber of the heart, it is most often injured. Myocardial contusion usually does not produce hemodynamic dysfunction. Instead, it is detected by the same electrocardiographic, echocardiographic, and enzymatic changes representative of acute myocardial infarction. A pericardial rub may also be present.

If myocardial contusion is suspected, the patient is observed in the hospital with continuous electrocardiographic monitoring. Although no specific electrocardiographic abnormality is pathognomonic for myocardial contusion, nearly any type of electrocardiographic change can occur as a result of the injury (Unkle et al., 1989). Treatment is similar to that for myocardial infarction, including electrocardiographic monitoring, rest, supplemental oxygen, and mild fluid restriction. Serial measurement of creatine ki-

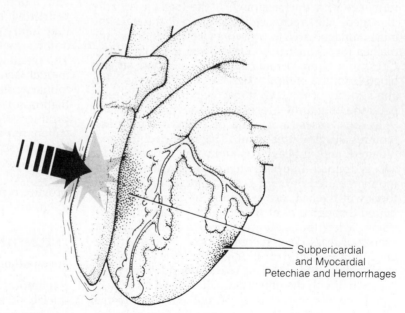

FIGURE 32-5. Blunt trauma to the anterior chest resulting in myocardial contusion. (Symbas PN, 1989: Contusion of the heart. In Cardiothoracic Trauma, p. 57. Philadelphia, WB Saunders)

Subpericardial
and Myocardial
Petechiae and Hemorrhages

nase isoenzyme levels is done. In severe cases, contusion can produce significant clinical sequelae, including conduction disturbances, arrhythmias, pericardial effusion, myocardial rupture, or cardiogenic shock. Late complications of myocardial contusion include constrictive pericarditis and ventricular aneurysm.

TRACHEAL AND BRONCHIAL INJURIES

Laceration or *transection of the trachea* or a *major bronchus* is uncommon but can be lethal. The injury is most often due to blunt trauma. Severity of tracheal or bronchial injury can vary from a partial tear to complete disruption. The majority of tracheobronchial injuries occur within 2.5 cm of the carina; the cervical trachea is affected in 10% to 15% of patients (Weissberg & Utkin, 1991).

Patients with complete tracheal transection present with profound respiratory distress, stridor, hemoptysis, hoarseness, and cyanosis. The injury causes a massive air leak that is likely to produce a tension pneumothorax. A continuous air leak remains after chest tube placement, and significant subcutaneous emphysema is generally present. Hypoventilation, with resultant impaired carbon dioxide removal, occurs because an effective tidal volume of air cannot be moved in and out of the tracheobronchial tree (Elefteriades & Geha, 1985). Hypoxemia is usually present as well secondary to associated pulmonary contusion or the marked reduction in minute volume. The chest roentgenogram reveals pneumothorax, hemothorax, and mediastinal emphysema. Bronchoscopy is performed to confirm the diagnosis and to define the location and extent of the injury (Weissberg & Utkin, 1991).

The first priority in the treatment of tracheal or bronchial injury is establishment of a patent airway using an endotracheal tube or, if necessary, by performance of a tracheostomy. If the trachea is badly damaged, the tracheostomy is placed through the most damaged area to conserve viable portions of the trachea for reconstruction (Mathisen & Grillo, 1991). Chest tube thoracostomy is used to evacuate air and blood from the pleural space. Depending on location and severity of the tear, it may be impossible to reexpand the lung until integrity of the airway is restored.

In most cases, a tracheal or bronchial laceration requires surgical treatment. The lacerated tissue is repaired, and, if heavy contamination is present, the area is drained. Injuries to the upper trachea are commonly repaired through a cervical incision. Injuries to the lower trachea, carina, and right bronchus are repaired through a right posterolateral thoracotomy incision; a left thoracotomy approach is used for left bronchial tears (Weissberg & Utkin, 1991). With severe injuries, survival is most likely in young persons, who better tolerate the profound hypoxemia associated with the injury and who have a more resilient tracheobronchial tree. Severe tracheobronchial injuries are frequently associated with injury to surrounding structures (e.g., the esophagus, thoracic great vessels, larynx, cervical spine, or recurrent laryngeal nerves) (Mathisen & Grillo, 1991).

PULMONARY INJURIES

There are two types of pulmonary injuries: laceration and contusion. *Laceration,* or tearing of the parenchyma (lung tissue), is associated with leakage of air and blood into the pleural space. Pulmonary lacerations can often be treated by placement of a chest tube to drain the pleural space until the laceration heals. In fact, only 10% to 20% of penetrating thoracic injuries require surgical intervention (Mandal & Oparah, 1989).

However, if significant bleeding or a large air leak persists, surgical exploration is performed to repair the laceration and to explore for other intrathoracic injuries. Most parenchymal injuries can be repaired by simple oversewing of the lung; massive tissue destruction or uncontrolled hemorrhage occasionally necessitates lobectomy or pneumonectomy (Robison et al., 1988). Sometimes a lung laceration is caused by a penetrating object, such as a bullet, that remains in the parenchyma. Surgical removal of the object may be necessary if it is large or sharp and centrally located or if it causes infection or hemoptysis.

Pulmonary contusion is injury of the lung parenchyma itself. Contusion occurs most often in association with a blast injury, such as an explosion, or with rapid deceleration. The injury, which may affect one or both lungs, occurs when hemorrhage and interstitial edema obliterate alveolar spaces, producing consolidation of large areas of lung tissue (Hood, 1990). A localized infiltrate is usually apparent on the initial chest roentgenogram, tends to progress over the next several days, and resolves within 1 week.

Treatment of pulmonary contusion includes fluid restriction, diuresis, antibiotics, pulmonary hygiene, and, if necessary, mechanical ventilation. The goal of restricting hydration is not always achieved since lung injury is often accompanied by other major body injuries that necessitate vigorous fluid resuscitation. The resultant early overhydration is the most detrimental factor associated with worsening of the pulmonary contusion (Lockhart, 1986). Diminished ventilation of the contused portions of lung tissue produces significant arteriovenous shunting with resultant hypoxemia. Severe pulmonary contusion may be followed by *adult respiratory distress syndrome.* Mechanical ventilation with adjunctive PEEP is generally considered to be the most effective method for improving functional residual capacity, keeping alveoli open, and improving oxygenation.

PNEUMOTHORAX AND HEMOTHORAX

Pneumothorax

Pneumothorax and hemothorax are common sequelae of intrathoracic injuries. *Pneumothorax* (i.e., the presence of air in the pleural space) occurs when air enters one of the pleural cavities, either from the lung or from outside the body. Pneumothorax associated with blunt chest trauma is most often due to laceration of the pulmonary parenchyma by the sharp ends of fractured rib segments. With penetrating trauma, it is generally the penetrating object that injures the lung. Rarely, pneumothorax is caused by a bronchial or tracheal tear.

The abnormal communication between the airways and pleural space allows inspired air to leak through the opening and become trapped between visceral and parietal pleurae. The degree of pneumothorax is determined by the rate of air leakage. The size of a pneumothorax is described according to the estimated percent of lung collapse (e.g., a 100% pneumothorax denotes complete collapse of the lung). Chest tube thoracostomy is almost always necessary unless the pneumothorax is small (less than 15% to 20%) and does not increase in size over time. If mechanical ventilation is necessary because of associated injuries, the increased airway pressure and use of PEEP may aggravate or perpetuate air leakage (Wiles, 1990).

A large or untreated air leak can produce a *tension pneumothorax* (i.e., complete collapse of the ipsilateral lung and shifting of the mediastinum to the opposite side). Tension pneumothorax can be fatal if untreated. The increased intrathoracic pressure compresses the superior and inferior vena cavae, compromising venous return to the heart and thereby decreasing cardiac output. Treatment of tension pneumothorax is immediate thoracentesis or chest tube thoracostomy.

Less commonly, parenchymal air leakage does not produce pneumothorax; instead, air travels along the pleural surfaces to enter the mediastinum or subcutaneous tissue. The abnormal presence of air in these locations is termed *mediastinal emphysema* or *subcutaneous emphysema*, respectively.

Fractured rib segments or penetrating objects can also create a perforation in the chest wall. *Sucking chest wound* describes a chest wall injury that allows air to move freely in and out of the pleural space during respiration. The injury significantly disturbs the normal physiology of ventilation. Pleural and atmospheric pressures equilibrate, removing the gradient responsible for moving air in and out of the tracheobronchial tree. If the pressure changes produce "to and fro" movement of the mediastinum, venous return to the heart may also be compromised. A sucking chest wound, which is uncommon except in military trauma, can be life threatening. Treatment includes chest tube thoracostomy to evacuate the pneumothorax and an occlusive dressing over the open wound to prevent continued entry of air into the pleural cavity.

Hemothorax

Hemothorax is the presence of blood in the pleural space. Some degree of hemothorax occurs in virtually all cases of chest trauma. Significant hemothorax can result from injury to the heart, one of the major vascular structures within the thorax, or pulmonary parenchymal or intercostal blood vessels. Massive hemorrhage into one or both pleural spaces is the most common cause of shock in patients with chest trauma. It is usually caused by laceration of the heart or great vessels. Because nearly the entire blood volume can be emptied into one hemithorax, death from exsanguination occurs unless the bleeding source is tamponaded (Elefteriades & Geha, 1985).

Hemothorax appears on a chest roentgenogram as an opacity at the base of the lung if the film is taken with the patient in an erect position. When the film is taken with the patient in a supine position, as is often the case with victims of chest trauma, hemothorax produces a hazy shadow superimposed over the entire lung field. Except in cases of significant bleeding, hemothorax can often be treated with chest tube drainage. Only 10% of patients require thoracotomy (Rodriguez, 1990a). However, if blood loss from the chest tube does not diminish within several hours of tube placement, exploratory thoracotomy is generally performed to identify and ligate the bleeding vessel or vessels.

It is important that accumulated blood in the pleural space be thoroughly evacuated. If a moderate amount of blood remains in the pleural space, it becomes fibrous, entrapping the lung and inhibiting full lung expansion. In addition, blood provides an excellent medium for the growth of bacteria and may lead to *empyema* (i.e., infection of the pleural space). Blood that is not drained within 1 week after occurrence of a hemothorax is usually too gelatinous to be evacuated by tube thoracostomy. A thoracotomy may be necessary for removal of the clotted blood. *Decortication*, or removal of the fibrinous, visceral pleura, is often required as well, to allow full reexpansion of the lung.

ESOPHAGEAL PERFORATION

Esophageal perforation is a tear or disruption in the wall of the esophagus. It may be caused by penetrating wounds of the chest, ingestion of a caustic substance or foreign body, instrumentation, or severe vomiting. Rarely, it results from blunt chest trauma. Classic manifestations of esophageal perforation are severe chest pain and the presence of mediastinal or subcutaneous air on the roentgenogram. Other signs and symptoms include subcutaneous emphysema, dysphagia, fever, shock, neck swelling, pleural effusion, hemoptysis, and hematemesis.

Diagnosis is based on these findings and a corroborative clinical history. A contrast swallow study or esophagoscopy is performed to confirm the diagnosis. Treatment of esophageal perforation is surgical exploration to drain the area of infection and repair the perforation. Saliva and gastric contents are diverted by nasogastric suction catheters placed above and below the anastomosis or by surgical division of the esophagus. Appropriate antibiotic therapy is essential to control mediastinal infection.

If diagnosis of esophageal perforation is delayed, mediastinitis soon develops from leakage of esophageal contents into the mediastinum. Sepsis ensues and death is likely unless surgical treatment is promptly undertaken. Primary repair of the esophagus is rarely possible when surgical intervention is performed more than 24 hours after injury. In these cases, the esophagus is divided and an *esophagostomy* is performed; the proximal esophageal segment is brought through the skin of the neck as a fistula so that saliva can drain into an esophagostomy pouch. The distal esophageal lumen is sutured closed and a drainage catheter placed. Enteral or intravenous alimentation is necessary until the infection has cleared and the esophagus can be reconstructed.

INJURY TO THE DIAPHRAGM

Laceration of the diaphragm can result from either blunt or penetrating chest or abdominal trauma. It is commonly caused by rib fractures or by rapid deceleration associated with increased intra-abdominal pressure. In most cases, abdominal injuries are also present. Injury to the diaphragm almost always occurs on the left side, probably because the liver protects the right diaphragm and because of the preponderance of right-handed assailants who are most likely to cause left-sided wounds in their victims. The primary symptom associated with diaphragmatic injury is abdominal, chest, or shoulder pain. If the rent is large enough to allow herniation of an abdominal viscus, the stomach, colon, or small bowel may migrate through the rent into the thorax, producing symptoms of gastrointestinal distress. Auscultation of the chest may reveal diminished breath sounds on the side of the tear or the presence of bowel sounds in the chest.

On a supine chest roentgenogram, abdominal viscera may be apparent in the thorax. If the patient has a nasogastric tube in place, its tip may appear in the thorax as well. Diaphragmatic injury should also be suspected when there is unexplained difficulty in maintaining adequate ventilation. Sometimes positive pressure mechanical ventilation prevents herniation of abdominal viscera through the diaphragmatic injury. Respiratory decompensation may occur when mechanical ventilation is terminated and normal negative pressure ventilation precipitates herniation (Wiles, 1990). If the diagnosis is made soon after the injury, repair of a diaphragmatic laceration can be performed through a laparotomy incision. An abdominal approach allows the surgeon to thoroughly explore the abdomen for associated injuries, which are frequently present (Rodriguez, 1990c).

Small diaphragmatic perforations may remain undetected because they produce no associated signs and symptoms at the time of injury. However, the pressure of abdominal contents against the weakened diaphragmatic site of injury can produce gradual enlargement of the opening with eventual herniation of abdominal contents into the thorax. As the volume of herniated contents increases, the patient may develop chest or abdominal pain, shortness of breath, or acute bowel obstruction.

In such cases, or if the diagnosis is missed for other reasons, a traumatic diaphragmatic hernia may be detected months or years after the injury. A gastrointestinal contrast study is often performed before late operative repair to determine which portion of the gastrointestinal tract has herniated through the diaphragmatic opening. If colon is present in the thorax, a cleansing bowel preparation may be performed preoperatively to reduce the risk of intrathoracic contamination should bowel perforation occur during the operative procedure.

A thoracotomy is used for repair of a delayed traumatic diaphragmatic hernia because adhesions are usually present between intrathoracic segments of abdominal viscera and lung (Ganzel & Gray, 1991). A thoracotomy incision allows structures to be safely mobilized and returned through the diaphragmatic rent to the abdominal cavity. The diaphragm is then repaired.

ACUTE MANAGEMENT OF THE CHEST TRAUMA VICTIM

Most chest injuries require only conservative therapy, such as chest tube insertion for evacuation of pneumothorax or hemothorax. Exploratory thoracotomy and operative repair of internal structures are necessary only in a small percentage of cases. However, when life-threatening internal injuries are present, survival depends on rapid diagnosis and immediate interventions to maintain airway patency, adequate ventilation, and hemodynamic stability.

Chest trauma can produce a number of life-threatening physiologic abnormalities (Fig. 32-6). *Airway obstruction* can be caused by a foreign object or by laceration or transection of the trachea or a major bronchus. *Massive hemothorax* or *cardiac tamponade* may result from injury to the heart or a major blood vessel. *Tension pneumothorax* can occur secondary to tracheobronchial or pulmonary parenchymal disruption. *Severe impairment of ventilation* can occur if a penetrating object creates a sucking chest wound.

General resuscitation principles are implemented in providing immediate care to the victim of chest trauma. These include (1) establishing and maintaining a reliable airway, (2) providing adequate ventilation, and (3) supporting circulation. With severe injuries, it is frequently necessary to begin cardiopulmonary resuscitation in the field. If spinal cord injury is suspected, the head and neck are immobilized to prevent further damage. In unconscious or severely injured patients, intubation is performed to ensure a patent airway. An emergency tracheostomy may be

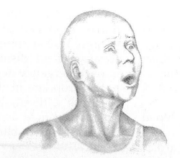

UPPER AIRWAY (LARYNGEAL) OBSTRUCTION

Marked restlessness
Anxious facies
Ashen-gray color or cyanosis
Stridor (crowing respiration)
Indrawing at suprasternal notch, around clavicles,
    in intercostal spaces, and at epigastrium

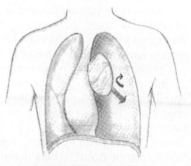

TENSION PNEUMOTHORAX

Progressive cyanosis
Respiratory embarrassment
Tracheal displacement away from affected side
Hyperresonant percussion note
Distant or absent breath sounds
Shock

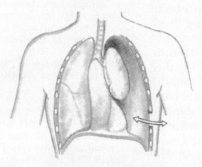

OPEN PNEUMOTHORAX

Cyanosis
Respiratory embarrassment
Sucking wound of the chest
Shock

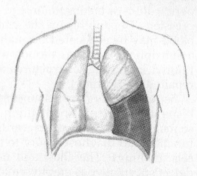

MASSIVE HEMOTHORAX

Cyanosis
Respiratory embarrassment
Dullness of percussion
Absent or distant breath sounds
Unrelenting shock if hemothorax increases

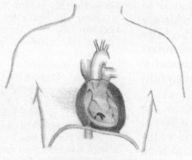

CARDIAC TAMPONADE

Neck veins distended
Falling or absent blood pressure
Patient in variable degrees of shock or in extremis
Venous pressure elevated (pathognomonic)
Muffled or distant heart tones

FIGURE 32-6. The major life-threatening injuries associated with thoracic trauma and associated manifestations. (Hood RM, 1989: Pre-hospital management, initial evaluation, and resuscitation. In Hood RM, Boyd AD, Culliford AT [eds]: Thoracic Trauma, p. 14. Philadelphia, WB Saunders)

necessary if upper airway obstruction is present or intubation fails (Hood, 1990). A self-inflating bag or mechanical volume respirator is used to provide ventilation to patients who are unable to adequately sustain self-ventilation.

Chest compressions are begun if cardiac arrest has occurred. At the same time, maneuvers are initiated to correct the cause of the cardiovascular collapse. Cardiac arrest associated with chest trauma is usually due to hemorrhagic shock or cardiac tamponade.

Chest compressions alone are of little value until intravascular volume is restored or cardiac tamponade is relieved.

Hemorrhagic shock is manifested by hypotension, low cardiac output, low central venous pressure, and decreased urine output (Rodriguez, 1990b). Rapid volume replacement, autotransfusion, and control of bleeding are the mainstays of correcting hemorrhagic shock. A crystalloid solution, such as lactated Ringer's solution, is infused through one or more large-bore intravenous catheters until compatible blood for transfusion is available. Chest tube drainage systems with autotransfusion capabilities are used to salvage and transfuse blood drained from the chest. Direct pressure is used to control external hemorrhage. Emergent thoracotomy may be necessary to control massive intrathoracic bleeding.

Cardiac tamponade occurs when accumulated blood in the pericardial sac or mediastinal cavity causes equalization of fluid pressures within the cardiac chambers. Because blood flow into and through the heart is dependent on the interchamber pressure gradients that normally exist, adequate filling of the heart cannot occur when these gradients disappear (Elefteriades & Geha, 1985). Recognition of acute cardiac tamponade is essential. The diagnosis is suggested by hypotension that (1) is out of proportion to blood loss, (2) is associated with distended neck veins, and (3) persists despite volume replacement and vasopressive medications. Other signs include distant heart sounds and pulsus paradoxus. Cardiac tamponade is treated by a procedure to drain the pericardium or mediastinum and relieve cardiac compression. Depending on the clinical circumstances, blood may be evacuated through pericardiocentesis, a subxiphoid incision, sternotomy, or thoracotomy. Injured intrathoracic structures are then operatively repaired as indicated.

Because the organs responsible for circulation and respiration are contained within the thorax, it is essential to rapidly evaluate cardiac and pulmonary function and diagnose injury to the heart, great vessels, or lungs. The chest and neck are palpated to detect subcutaneous emphysema. The lung fields are auscultated to detect tension pneumothorax and the need for emergency tube thoracostomy. Chest tubes are inserted in either or both sides of the thorax if absent breath sounds suggest the presence of significant air or fluid in the pleural spaces.

Life-threatening injuries to internal viscera are sometimes present without evidence of any external wounds (blunt trauma) or with only a small entry wound (penetrating trauma). Both the chest and back should be carefully examined for a penetrating wound. Identification of entry and exit sites suggest the path through the chest of a penetrating object and which internal structures are likely to be injured. Chest trauma is frequently accompanied by other injuries, such as head injury, long bone fractures, and injury to abdominal viscera, particularly the spleen or liver (Hood, 1990). Therefore, initial medical management includes identification and prioritization of severity of the various injuries with consultation with appropriate surgical specialists.

In moribund trauma victims, a thoracotomy is sometimes performed in the emergency department as a therapeutic measure to control hemorrhage or relieve tamponade. Although thoracotomy in the emergency department can be life-saving in some patients, in others it offers no realistic probability of salvaging the patient and exposes physicians and nurses at the bedside to infectious risks (e.g., hepatitis and human immunodeficiency virus infection). Because of the dismal survival results, thoracotomy in the emergency department is generally considered not appropriate in the following groups of patients: (1) those without signs of life at the time of initial prehospital field assessment and (2) those with cardiac arrest after blunt chest trauma (Lorenz et al., 1992).

REFERENCES

Attar S, Suter CM, Hankins JR, et al., 1991: Penetrating cardiac injuries. Ann Thorac Surg 51:711

Baker JL, 1990: Management of thoracic trauma by the emergency physician. In Turney SZ, Rodriguez A, Cowley RA (eds): Management of Cardiothoracic Trauma. Baltimore, Williams & Wilkins

Cowley RA, Turney SZ, Hankins JR, et al., 1990: Rupture of the thoracic aorta caused by blunt trauma. J Thorac Cardiovas Surg 100:652

Elefteriades JA, Geha AS, 1985: Chest trauma. In House Officer Guide to ICU Care: The Cardiothoracic Surgical Patient. Gaithersburg, MD, Aspen Publishers

Finkelmeier BA, Mentzer RM Jr, Kaiser DL, et al., 1982: Chronic traumatic aneurysm. J Thorac Cardiovas Surg 84:257

Follette DM, 1991: Penetrating cardiac injuries—a look to the future. Ann Thorac Surg 51:701

Ganzel BL, Gray LA, 1991: Diaphragmatic injuries. In Webb WR, Besson A (eds): Thoracic Surgery: Surgical Management of Chest Injuries, Vol. 7. St. Louis, Mosby–Year Book

Hood M, 1990: Trauma to the chest. In Sabiston DC Jr, Spencer FC (eds): Surgery of the Chest, ed. 5. Philadelphia, WB Saunders

LoCicero J III, Mattox KL, 1989: Epidemiology of chest trauma. Surg Clin North Am 69:15

Lockhart CG, 1986: Thoracic trauma. Crit Care Q 9:32

Lorenz HP, Steinmetz B, Lieberman J, et al., 1992: Emergency thoracotomy: Survival correlates with physiologic status. J Trauma 32:780

Mandal AK, Oparah SS, 1989: Unusually low mortality of penetrating wounds of the chest. J Thorac Cardiovasc Surg 97:119

Mathisen DJ, Grillo HC, 1991: Airway trauma: Laryngotracheal trauma. In Webb WR, Besson A (eds): Thoracic Surgery: Surgical Management of Chest Injuries, Vol. 7. St. Louis, Mosby–Year Book

Mattox KL, 1989: Fact and fiction about management of aortic transection. Ann Thorac Surg 48:1

McElvein RB, Novick WM, 1991: Chest wall fractures. In Webb WR, Besson A (eds): Thoracic Surgery: Surgical Management of Chest Injuries, Vol. 7. St. Louis, Mosby–Year Book

McLean TR, Olinger GN, Thorsen MK, 1991: Computed tomography in the evaluation of the aorta in patients sustaining blunt chest trauma. J Trauma 31:254

Merrill WH, Lee RB, Hammon JW, et al., 1988: Surgical treatment of acute traumatic tear of the thoracic aorta. Ann Surg 207:699

Robison PD, Harman PK, Trinkle JK, Grover FL, 1988: Management of penetrating lung injuries in civilian practice. J Thorac Cardiovasc Surg 95:184

Rodriguez A, 1990a: Injuries of the chest wall, the lungs, and the pleura. In Turney SZ, Rodriguez A, Cowley RA (eds): Management of Cardiothoracic Trauma. Baltimore, Williams & Wilkins

Rodriguez A, 1990b: Initial patient evaluation and indications for thoracotomy. In Turney SZ, Rodriguez A, Cowley RA (eds): Management of Cardiothoracic Trauma. Baltimore, Williams & Wilkins

Rodriguez A, 1990c: Injuries to the diaphragm. In Turney SZ, Rodriguez A, Cowley RA (eds): Management of Cardiothoracic Trauma. Baltimore, Williams & Wilkins

Shapiro MJ, Yanofsky SD, Trapp J, et al., 1991: Cardiovascular evaluation in blunt thoracic trauma using transesophageal echocardiography (TEE). J Trauma 31:835

Turney SZ, Rodriguez A, 1990: Injuries to the great thoracic vessels. In Turney SZ, Rodriguez A, Cowley RA (eds): Management of Cardiothoracic Trauma. Baltimore, Williams & Wilkins

Unkle DW, Smejkal R, O'Malley KF, 1989: Myocardial contusion without creatine kinase-MB elevation. Heart Lung 18:539

Weissberg D, Utkin V, 1991: Airway trauma: Tracheobroncial trauma. In Webb WR, Besson A (eds): Thoracic Surgery: Surgical Management of Chest Injuries, Vol. 7. St. Louis, Mosby–Year Book

Wiles CE III, 1990: Critical care of chest trauma. In Turney SZ, Rodriguez A, Cowley RA (eds): Management of Cardiothoracic Trauma. Baltimore, Williams & Wilkins

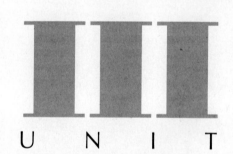

UNIT III

THORACIC SURGERY

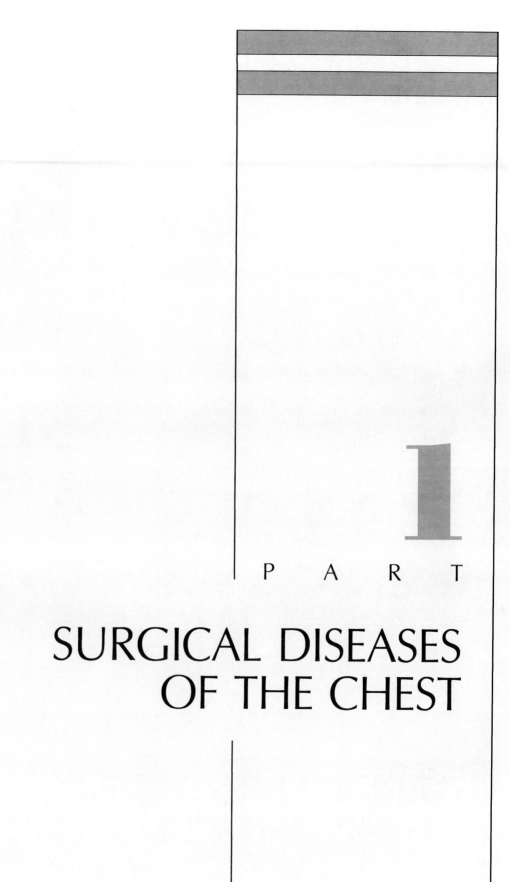

1

P A R T

SURGICAL DISEASES
OF THE CHEST

33

PULMONARY, TRACHEAL, AND PLEURAL DISEASES

LUNG CANCER

Carcinoma of the lung was relatively uncommon until the early part of the 20th century. Since that time, however, the incidence has increased dramatically. It is currently one of the most common malignant diseases in the United States and the most common reason for operations performed on the lung. The disease can occur in young adults but is most often seen in late middle age or in elderly persons. Although lung cancer continues to occur more frequently in men, the incidence in women has been climbing steadily. A decade ago, the ratio of men to women was 8:1; it is now less than 2:1 (Shields et al., 1994). In contrast to the stable or decreasing death rates occurring with other forms of cancer, the death rate from lung cancer continues to increase (Carter & Matthay, 1991). Lung cancer has been the leading cause of

death from cancer in men for many years. It has recently replaced breast cancer as the leading cause of death from cancer in women.

ETIOLOGIC FACTORS

A number of factors are associated with an increased incidence of lung cancer. Cigarette smoking is believed to be the primary and most significant etiologic factor (Sabiston, 1990). The increased risk associated with smoking applies to several types of lung cancer and is related to both the number of cigarettes smoked per day and the duration of smoking years (Shields et al., 1994). Prospective epidemiologic studies have demonstrated a 9- to 10-fold increased risk in average cigarette smokers and a 10- to 25-fold increased risk in heavy smokers (Carter & Matthay, 1991). In addition, cigarette smoking markedly increases risk imposed by other environmental carcinogens. Although cessation of smoking is associated with a progressively declining risk, previous smokers continue to be at higher risk for the remainder of their lives (Mulshine & Tockman, 1992).

Industrial exposure also predisposes to lung cancer. Specifically identified agents include asbestos, radioactive material, arsenic, and nickel (Shields et al., 1994). The role played by air pollution is not well determined, but lung cancer is more common in urban areas and in persons with chronically diseased and scarred lungs. Genetic factors also contribute to development of lung cancer. Epidemiologic studies consistently demonstrate an excess of lung cancer in some families that cannot be accounted for by chance or common environmental exposure (Sellers et al., 1991). It is likely that smoking and other environmental carcinogens exert additive or synergistic effects while genetic characteristics probably augment susceptibility to these carcinogens in the environment (Carter & Matthay, 1991). Individuals who develop lung cancer are at increased risk for developing a second and third primary lung tumor.

HISTOLOGIC CELL TYPES

Bronchogenic carcinoma, which arises from the epithelial lining of the bronchi, is by far the most common form of lung cancer and accounts for approximately 90% of cases. Far less common are bronchoalveolar carcinoma, originating in the lung parenchyma itself, and mesothelioma, which arises in the pleura. Bronchogenic carcinoma is categorized into four histologic cell types: (1) adenocarcinoma, (2) squamous or epidermoid carcinoma, (3) small cell carcinoma, and (4) large cell carcinoma. Some lung tumors have a mixed histologic type (e.g., both squamous and adenocarcinomatous features).

Adenocarcinoma comprises approximately 40% of lung tumors. Its increasing incidence has caused it to surpass squamous cell carcinoma in recent years as the most common form of lung cancer. Adenocarcinoma occurs more commonly in women. It is also the histologic subtype most likely to occur in nonsmokers who develop lung cancer (Sridhar & Raub, 1992). Adenocarcinoma usually originates in the lung periphery, arising from the epithelium of distal bronchi to form a small nodule. The tumors characteristically grow at an intermediate rate, more slowly than small cell tumors but faster than squamous cell lesions (Shields et al., 1994). Adenocarcinoma tends to metastasize to liver, brain, bone, and adrenal glands, as well as to lymph nodes (Sabiston, 1990). Some adenocarcinomas occur in conjunction with areas of scarring or chronic interstitial fibrosis. These so-called scar carcinomas most frequently arise in the peripheral portions of the upper lobes, particularly in the apical segment (Auerbach & Garfinkel, 1991).

Bronchoalveolar cancer is an unusual form of lung cancer that spreads along alveolar walls. It may represent a highly differentiated form of adenocarcinoma, although many pathologists regard it as a separate and distinct histologic form of lung cancer (Shields et al., 1994). Although its features overlap with those of adenocarcinoma and both cancers can coexist in the same patient, the prognosis in patients with bronchoalveolar cancer is generally better and more influenced by extent of lung involvement than by lymph node metastasis (Daly et al., 1991). Like adenocarcinoma, the incidence of bronchoalveolar carcinoma appears to be increasing in comparison to other cell types. Some researchers postulate that this actually represents a decrease in those cell types strongly linked to smoking (squamous cell and small cell) owing to the increased use of filters and decreased nicotine content in cigarettes and a decrease in the quantity of smoking (Auerbach & Garfinkel, 1991; Sridhar & Raub, 1992). Bronchoalveolar carcinoma is also referred to as *alveolar cell carcinoma, bronchioloalveolar carcinoma,* and *bronchiolar carcinoma.*

Squamous cell carcinoma comprises 30% to 35% of lung cancer. It almost always occurs in individuals with a long smoking history. Squamous cell tumors are generally centrally located in major bronchi and are relatively slow growing. They often remain within the thorax, spreading by direct extension and invasion of hilar, mediastinal, and supraclavicular lymph nodes. The tumor is frequently detected late in the course of the disease when bronchial obstruction leads to atelectasis or pneumonia (Carter & Matthay, 1991). Distant metastasis occurs less frequently than with other forms of lung cancer.

Small cell carcinoma accounts for 20% to 25% of lung tumors. It consists of several subtypes, the most common of which is *oat cell carcinoma.* Most individuals who develop small cell tumors have a smoking history. Small cell lung cancer is highly malignant and is characterized by early and widespread dissemination, rapid growth, and relatively short patient survival (Meyer, 1989). The majority of tumors are located centrally. Brain, liver, bone, and adrenal metastases are common (Neagley, 1991). Because of the rapid systemic spread, surgical resectability is uncommon.

Large cell carcinoma, comprising 7% to 10% of lung cancer, includes giant cell and undifferentiated tumors. *Giant cell tumors* occur in the lung periphery and are quite malignant (Carter & Matthay, 1991). *Undifferentiated large cell tumors* usually involve large bronchi. Both types are characterized by large, bulky tumors with areas of necrosis.

Rarely, patients develop multiple primary lung carcinomas. *Synchronous tumors* are separate primary lung tumors occurring simultaneously in different locations. They may have differing histologic cell types or the same cell type. However, it is difficult to distinguish with certainty synchronous tumors of the same cell type from a single primary tumor with an intrapulmonary metastasis. *Metachronous tumors* are primary lung tumors that develop as separate occurrences separated by an interval of time. Given the prevalence of bronchogenic cancer and the fact that inhaled carcinogens affect large areas of respiratory epithelium, it is presumed that metachronous tumors would occur more commonly if survival from primary lung cancer were not so low (Fleisher et al., 1991). The predominant histologic cell type in patients with synchronous or metachronous lung tumors is squamous cell (Rosengart et al., 1991).

TUMOR LOCATION AND ROUTES OF EXTENSION

Lung neoplasms occur more commonly in the right lung, and usually in the upper lobes (Shields et al., 1994). The location of the tumor is generally categorized as central, peripheral, or apical. Lesions are termed *central* if they involve the mainstem, lobar, or segmental bronchi and *peripheral* if they originate in distal bronchi, bronchioles, or lung parenchyma. Central lesions are associated with a poorer prognosis because the tumor often spreads to hilar and mediastinal lymph nodes before detection. Peripheral lesions are occasionally detected on a routine chest roentgenogram while the patient is still without symptoms. A tumor in the apex of either lung is referred to as a *Pancoast* or *superior sulcus tumor*. Because of their location, superior sulcus tumors are likely to invade the mediastinum, brachial plexus, and cervical sympathetic nerves (Sabiston, 1990).

There are three routes by which lung tumors metastasize. The first is by direct extension. Tumors can grow directly into pulmonary parenchyma, across fissures, along a bronchus, and into adjacent structures in the thorax, such as the pleura, chest wall, or mediastinal organs. Second, lung tumors spread through the lymphatic system. Lymph nodes in close proximity and likely to be invaded by malignant lung tumors include those in the pulmonary hila, the mediastinum, and the paratracheal, paraesophageal, supraclavicular, and cervical regions (Sabiston, 1990). Undifferentiated small cell lesions are most likely to spread in this manner, followed by undifferentiated large cell, adenocarcinoma, and squamous cell tumors (Shields et al., 1994). Even small tumors may be associated with hilar or mediastinal lymph node metastasis (Shields, 1990a). The third route of metastasis is hematologic spread. Tumor cells invade branches of the pulmonary veins within the lung and are disseminated to distant structures through the vascular system. The most common sites of lung cancer metastasis are demonstrated in Figure 33-1.

CLINICAL MANIFESTATIONS

Occasionally, a lung neoplasm is detected before development of symptoms when a chest roentgenogram taken for another purpose displays an abnormal shadow. However, 90% to 95% of patients with lung cancer are symptomatic at the time of diagnosis

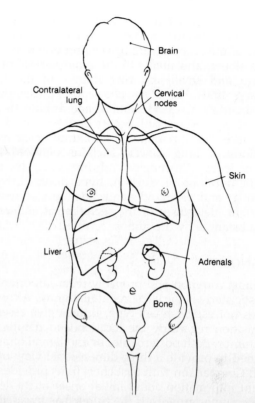

FIGURE 33-1. Common sites of metastasis in patients with carcinoma of the lung. (Beahrs OH, Myers MH [eds], 1992: American Joint Committee on Cancer: Manual for Staging of Cancer, ed. 4, p. 122. Philadelphia, JB Lippincott)

(Shields, 1991). The clinical signs and symptoms depend on size and location of the tumor, extent of spread to adjacent or distant structures, and occurrence of associated hormonal syndromes. Most common are pulmonary symptoms secondary to irritation, obstruction, or ulceration of a bronchus (Shields, 1991). Cough occurs in a majority of patients. Patients often develop persistent upper respiratory tract infections or pneumonia due to bronchial obstruction. Other common symptoms include hemoptysis, chest pain, and wheezing. Nonspecific symptoms associated with lung cancer include weight loss, anorexia, and malaise.

If the tumor has spread beyond the lung itself to involve pleura, chest wall, mediastinal structures, or nerves, the patient may experience corresponding symptoms. Compression of the recurrent laryngeal nerve may cause hoarseness; brachial nerve compression may produce persistent arm or shoulder pain; esophageal compression may result in dysphagia; pleural invasion may cause pleural effusion; and extensive mediastinal spread can produce superior vena cava syndrome, manifested by swelling of the face and upper extremities and venous distention in the neck and anterior chest wall.

Pancoast's syndrome describes the characteristic clinical manifestations associated with superior sulcus tumors (i.e., severe pain and Horner's syndrome). Localized pain begins in the shoulder and vertebral border of the scapula, later extending down the arm to the elbow, and finally to the ulnar surface of the forearm and small and ring fingers of the hand (Paulson, 1991). *Horner's syndrome* (i.e., ptosis, pupillary constriction, vasodilatation, and anhidrosis [absence of sweat secretion]) occurs on the affected side of the face and upper extremity. Extrathoracic manifestations of lung cancer, such as elevated liver enzyme levels, Cushing's syndrome, excessive antidiuretic hormone production, hypercalcemia, hypoglycemia, and carcinoid syndrome, can occur due to distant metastases or the secretion of endocrine-like substances by the tumor.

DIAGNOSIS

The most common and probably most important diagnostic study is the chest roentgenogram. Although it does not establish cell type, it does give essential information regarding the location and nature of a lung tumor. Both posteroanterior and lateral films are obtained to provide a three-dimensional view of the chest. Comparison with past chest films provides important information about initial onset of the lesion and its rate of growth. If the tumor has invaded the chest wall, the chest roentgenogram may demonstrate rib destruction (Allen et al., 1991). Tomograms, which are special roentgenograms in which individual planes are in focus while the remainder of details are blurred, may be useful in selected situations to better visualize suspicious lesions.

Computed tomography, a technique for imaging cross-sectional anatomy, is often beneficial in evaluation of suspected mediastinal adenopathy (i.e., abnormal enlargement of mediastinal lymph nodes) that may represent malignant invasion. Computed tomography may also demonstrate invasion of the soft tissues or vertebral bodies. When a chest computed tomographic scan is obtained for evaluation of a patient with lung cancer, the upper abdomen is usually included in the scan so that occult liver or adrenal metastasis may be detected.

Direct evaluation of the tracheobronchial tree is performed with a fiberoptic bronchoscope. Bronchoscopy allows a thorough examination of segmental and subsegmental bronchi. Bronchoscopic visualization of the affected area may reveal the tumor itself exposed in bronchial mucosa or changes in the bronchial wall or lumen size caused by tumor infiltration or external compression (Shields, 1991). In addition, tissue may be obtained for histologic evaluation by (1) biopsy of a small piece of bronchial tissue, (2) brushing the surface of the lesion, or (3) aspirating fluid washed over the suspicious area.

Cytologic evaluation of sputum (sputum cytology) may be performed in patients with large tumors involving a main bronchus. Tumors most likely to produce a positive sputum cytology are those that are centrally located, greater than 2 cm in diameter, or a squamous cell type (Shields, 1991). A transthoracic needle biopsy is occasionally performed to obtain tissue from lesions located in the lung periphery. Although transthoracic needle biopsy is often successful in establishing a diagnosis, there is a significant incidence of false-negative results. Thoracotomy is usually necessary to prove absence of malignancy.

If the chest roentgenogram or computed tomographic scan suggests mediastinal lymph node involvement, mediastinoscopy or mediastinotomy may be performed for biopsy of mediastinal lymph nodes. Fine-needle aspiration of lymph nodes in the supraclavicular fossa (scalene nodes) is performed to obtain tissue for histologic examination if the nodes are palpable. Thoracoscopy may occasionally be used to obtain tissue if less invasive diagnostic efforts have been unsuccessful and pulmonary resection is not anticipated. Brain, liver, or bone scans may be performed in patients in whom distant metastasis is suspected. If none of these diagnostic measures yields a definitive diagnosis or if surgical exploration is likely in any case, an exploratory thoracotomy may be performed without definitive confirmation of malignancy. Diagnostic studies used in the evaluation of thoracic surgical diseases are described in further detail in Chapter 36, Diagnostic Evaluation of Thoracic Disease.

STAGING OF LUNG CANCER

To classify extent of disease, direct therapy, and provide better prognostic information, standard nomenclature for pathologic classification was developed by the American Joint Committee on Cancer Staging and End Results Reporting (Beahrs & Myers, 1978). It has since been expanded and revised into the currently used International Staging System, which consists of a three-letter code: the first letter "T" categorizes tumor size; the second, "N," the presence and extent of nodal involvement; and the third, "M," the presence of distant metastases (Table 33-1) (Mountain, 1986).

Depending on *TNM designation*, the stage of the patient's disease is categorized (Table 33-2). *Occult lung cancer* is present when cytologic examination of sputum reveals malignant cells but there is no identifiable lesion on the chest roentgenogram. Occult neoplasm is rare and nearly always represents in situ or early invasive squamous cell carcinoma (Pairolero et al., 1989). The other stages signify progressively larger and more invasive tumors (Fig. 33-2A through D). *Stage I lung cancer* is considered early disease with a favorable prognosis after surgical resection; *stage II tumors* are intermediate; and *stage III and IV tumors* are considered advanced with a poor prognosis (Martini et al., 1992).

Although the TNM staging system provides useful prognostic information about non–small cell lung tumors, it is not generally used for small cell lung cancer. Instead, small cell tumors are often categorized as localized or extensive. *Localized small cell cancer* is

TABLE 33-1. INTERNATIONAL STAGING SYSTEM FOR LUNG CANCER: TNM DEFINITIONS

Primary Tumor (T)

TX   Tumor proven by the presence of malignant cells in bronchopulmonary secretions but not visualized roentgenographically or bronchoscopically, or any tumor that cannot be assessed

T0   No evidence of primary tumor

TIS   Carcinoma in situ

T1   A tumor that is 3.0 cm or less in greatest dimension, surrounded by lung or visceral pleura, and without evidence of invasion proximal to a lobar bronchus at bronchoscopy

T2   A tumor more than 3.0 cm in greatest dimension, or a tumor of any size that either invades the visceral pleura or has associated atelectasis or obstructive pneumonitis extending to the hilar region. At bronchoscopy, the proximal extent of demonstrable tumor must be within a lobar bronchus or at least 2.0 cm distal to the carina. Any associated atelectasis or obstructive pneumonitis must involve less than the entire lung.

T3   A tumor of any size with direct extension into the chest wall, diaphragm, or the mediastinal pleura or pericardium without involving the heart, great ves-

Primary Tumor (T) (*Continued*)

sels, trachea, esophagus, or vertebral body, or a tumor in the main bronchus within 2.0 cm of the carina without involving the carina

T4   A tumor of any size with invasion of the mediastinum or involving heart, great vessels, trachea, esophagus, vertebral body, or carina or presence of malignant pleural effusion

Nodal Involvement (N)

N0   No demonstrable metastasis to regional lymph nodes

N1   Metastasis to lymph nodes in peribronchial or ipsilateral hilar region, or both, including direct extension

N2   Metastasis to ipsilateral mediastinal and subcarinal lymph nodes

N3   Metastasis to contralateral mediastinal lymph nodes, contralateral hilar nodes, ipsilateral or contralateral scalene or supraclavicular nodes

Distant Metastasis (M)

M0   No (known) distant metastasis

M1   Distant metastasis present

(Mountain CF, 1986: A new international staging system for lung cancer. Chest 89:2255)

defined as tumor confined to one hemithorax with or without involvement of supraclavicular lymph nodes; *extensive small cell lung cancer* signifies that tumor is present beyond the ipsilateral hemithorax (Shields, 1991).

TREATMENT

Survival prognosis for patients with lung cancer continues to be poor. Despite intensive research and treatment efforts, the diagnosis is still associated with

TABLE 33-2. INTERNATIONAL STAGING SYSTEM FOR LUNG CANCER: STAGE GROUPING

Stage	TNM Classification		
Occult	TX	N0	M0
0	TIS	Carcinoma in situ	
I	T1	N0	M0
	T2	N0	M0
II	T1	N1	M0
	T2	N1	M0
IIIA	T3	N0	M0
	T3	N1	M0
	T1–3	N2	M0
IIIB	Any T	N3	M0
	T4	Any N	M0
IV	Any T	Any N	M1

(Mountain CF, 1986: A new international staging system for lung cancer. Chest 89:2255)

a near 90% mortality rate (Mulshine & Tockman, 1992). For non–small cell lung cancer, the treatment of choice is surgical resection of the tumor and surrounding lymphatic tissue. The selection of the specific operative procedure depends on location and size of the tumor, whether spread to regional lymph nodes has occurred, involvement of extraparenchymal structures, and the patient's age and general medical condition, particularly cardiovascular and respiratory function.

Successful surgical treatment of lung cancer necessitates a pulmonary resection that completely eradicates the tumor yet leaves the patient with adequate lung function. If the lesion is small and located in the periphery, it may be possible to accomplish complete resection with removal of only the tumor itself and minimal surrounding lung tissue. This procedure, termed a *wedge resection*, sacrifices the least amount of normal lung tissue. If an entire segment of a lobe is removed, the procedure is termed a *segmentectomy*. More commonly, lung tumors are positioned in such a way that it is necessary to remove an entire lobe (*lobectomy*) to perform a curative resection.

Removal of an entire lung, or *pneumonectomy*, may be necessary if the tumor is centrally located or involves more than one lobe. A pneumonectomy sacrifices considerably more lung tissue but is generally well tolerated in patients with adequate pulmonary function. However, patients with moderate impairment of pulmonary function may be unable to withstand loss of an entire lung. A *sleeve resection* (i.e., removal of a lobe with its attaching bronchus and

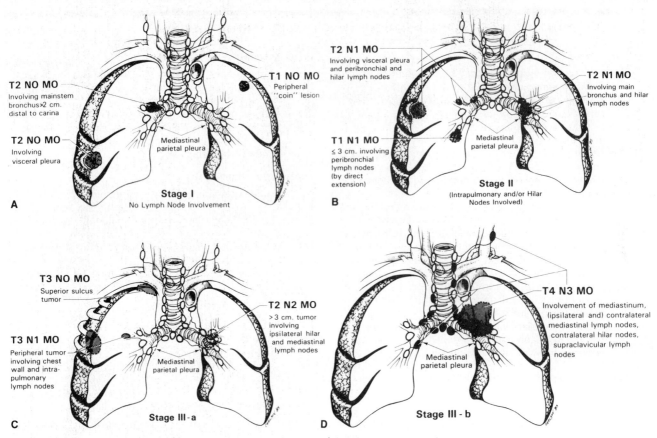

FIGURE 33-2. Categorization of lung cancer using International Staging System: **(A)** Stage I. **(B)** Stage II. **(C)** Stage IIIA. **(D)** Stage IIIB. (Mountain CF, 1986: A new international staging system for lung cancer. Chest 4:230S–S231S)

reimplantation of the remaining lobe) is performed in selected situations, such as when (1) a tumor is centrally located, (2) metastatic lymph nodes are present near a main bronchus, or (3) compromised pulmonary function precludes pneumonectomy (Van Schil et al., 1991).

If a tumor has invaded structures adjacent to the lung, an *extended resection*, including the chest wall or diaphragm, may be performed concomitantly with the pulmonary resection. In patients with chest wall invasion, prognosis appears to be less influenced by spread to the chest wall than by the presence of tumor in lymph tissue (Allen et al., 1991). Consequently, in patients with no evidence of mediastinal lymph node (N2) involvement, surgical resection of the tumor, overlying parietal pleura, and an *en bloc chest wall resection* may be performed (Albertucci et al., 1992). Depending on the size and location of the defect created by the removal of rib segments, plastic reconstruction of the chest wall with placement of prosthetic material may be necessary. A *pneumonectomy* may include removal of a portion of the pericardium if tumor has invaded the pericardium. If the tumor encroaches on the carina of the mainstem tra-

chea, curative resection is generally considered not technically feasible. However, in a few institutions with extensive experience with tracheal surgery, carinal resection and reconstruction in combination with pneumonectomy is being performed (Mathisen & Grillo, 1991).

Long-term results of surgical treatment are primarily dependent on the stage of the tumor at the time of operation. Five-year survival after surgical resection of stage I (T1,N0,M0 or T2,N0,M0) lung cancer is approximately 70% (Flehinger et al., 1992). Stage II (T1,N1,M0 or T2,N1,M0) disease is associated with a 49% five-year survival after surgical resection (Burt & Martini, 1991). Curative surgical resection is possible in some stage IIIA lung tumors (e.g., peripheral tumors that have invaded the parietal pleura, pericardium, diaphragm, or chest wall or which are located in the main bronchus within 2 cm of the carina). However, in stage IIIA tumors with N2 (ipsilateral mediastinal or subcarinal lymph node) involvement, surgical resection is possible in only 3% to 6% of patients (Shields, 1990b). Pulmonary resection procedures are discussed in more detail in Chapter 38, Surgical Treatment of Pulmonary Disease.

In many patients with lung cancer, the extent of tumor at the time of diagnosis precludes surgical resection. Evidence of extrapulmonary tumor spread, such as paralysis of the recurrent laryngeal nerve, superior vena cava syndrome, phrenic nerve paralysis, pleural effusion containing malignant cells, extrathoracic metastases, or involvement of the main pulmonary artery, precludes curative resection. Small cell lung cancer is seldom treated with surgical resection, except as one component of multimodal therapy in patients with localized disease. Finally, operative risk may preclude surgical therapy in patients with marginal pulmonary reserve, recent myocardial infarction, unstable angina, arrhythmias, or congestive heart failure.

Radiation therapy may be used adjunctively with surgical resection or as the primary treatment if pulmonary resection is not a viable option. For most types of lung cancer, radiation therapy alone is unlikely to be curative. Preoperative radiation is seldom performed because it delays operation and increases operative morbidity. However, in patients with Pancoast tumors, preoperative radiation may be successful in converting a nonresectable tumor into one that can be surgically removed. Radiation therapy is often administered after surgical resection if histologic examination of lymph nodes sampled at the time of operation reveals malignant cells. Brain irradiation is sometimes performed prophylactically in patients with small cell tumors because it has proven efficacious in preventing brain metastasis.

Brachytherapy may be considered for tumors that prove to be surgically nonresectable at thoracotomy due to invasion of adjacent structures or inability of the patient to tolerate the necessary pulmonary resection. It consists of the intraoperative implantation of radioactive material into the tumor. The advantage of brachytherapy as opposed to external-beam radiation is that high doses of radiation can be delivered to the tumor itself with little damage to surrounding tissue (Martini, 1989). However, it remains unproven whether brachytherapy increases survival more effectively than conventional external radiation therapy (Lewis et al., 1990).

Chemotherapy is generally reserved for those patients with small cell or stage II or III non–small cell tumors. Often, a combination of chemotherapeutic agents is given. In patients with small cell lung cancer, chemotherapy is usually combined with thoracic irradiation. The large bulk of the tumor at the primary site and the mediastinal lymph nodes are irradiated, and the disseminated component is treated with intensive chemotherapy (Meyer, 1989). Commonly used chemotherapeutic agents include cyclophosphamide, doxorubicin, vincristine, cisplatin, and etoposide. Some surgeons also include surgical resection with the other two modalities for patients with resectable small cell tumors and no distant metastases (Muller et al., 1992).

OTHER INTRATHORACIC MALIGNANCIES

Primary tumors of the trachea are rare. The majority are malignant and are usually squamous cell carcinoma or adenoid cystic carcinoma. Tracheal tumors can extend up and down the trachea and metastasize into regional lymph nodes, mediastinal structures, and lung parenchyma. They are not easily visible on the chest roentgenogram; as a result, the diagnosis is often not made until the patient develops airway obstruction from the tumor (Grillo, 1989). Common manifestations of tracheal tumors are cough, hemoptysis, and signs of progressive airway obstruction (Grillo & Mathisen, 1991). Surgical resection and tracheal reconstruction may be performed if the tumor is not extensive and has not metastasized. Radiation therapy may also be used.

Mesothelioma is an unusual neoplasm that originates in the pleura. Any portion of the parietal, visceral, or mediastinal pleura may be the site of origin of the tumor, which grows selectively along the pleural surfaces (Shields, 1989). Extension into the lung parenchyma is unusual. Benign mesothelioma and localized malignant mesothelioma are rare. Most common is a diffuse, malignant variety that is often associated with a history of asbestos exposure. Common clinical manifestations include dyspnea from associated pleural effusion and chest wall pain caused by tumor invasion (Kittle, 1989). Although abnormalities on the chest roentgenogram or CT scan may be suggestive of mesothelioma, definitive diagnosis is based on histologic examination of pleural tissue obtained by pleural needle biopsy, thoracoscopy, or thoracotomy.

All forms of treatment for mesothelioma, and particularly the role of surgical resection, are controversial because none has proven efficacy (Rusch et al., 1991). One of two surgical procedures may be performed: *pleurectomy* (removal of the parietal pleura) or *extrapleural pneumonectomy* (resection of the parietal pleura and ipsilateral lung). Of the two procedures, pleurectomy carries a lower operative risk but does not provide complete removal of all gross disease as does extrapleural pneumonectomy. Neither procedure has been shown to definitively increase survival (Rusch et al., 1991). Isolated radiation and chemotherapy have also been ineffective in curing mesothelioma, but one or both are sometimes used as an adjunct to surgical resection. Regardless of therapy, malignant mesothelioma is usually a fatal disease. Most patients die within 1 to 2 years of diagnosis.

BENIGN LUNG NEOPLASMS

Benign lung neoplasms are uncommon. The most frequently occurring benign tumor is *hamartoma*, which is also referred to as *chondroma*. It occurs more often in men, and in 90% of cases it arises in the lung periphery (Shields & Robinson, 1994). The vast majority of hamartomas do not produce symptoms, and although they may increase in size, growth is usually slow (Hansen et al., 1992). The tumor is usually detected as an incidental finding on a chest roentgenogram. Hamartomas do not require treatment except in the rare instance of symptoms due to bronchial compression, such as atelectasis or infection. However, surgical removal is often undertaken to definitively differentiate hamartoma from a malignant tumor. Other less common benign lung neoplasms include fibroma, pulmonary hemangioma, leiomyoma, and papilloma.

INFECTIOUS PROBLEMS

PULMONARY INFECTION

Widespread availability of broad-spectrum antibiotics has greatly decreased the incidence of serious *pulmonary infections*. Consequently, pulmonary infections requiring surgical intervention are unusual except in patients who are immunocompromised by disease or because of immunosuppressive therapy. However, the population of individuals with compromised immune function has grown, principally due to three factors: (1) an increased number of organ transplant recipients who must take immunosuppressive medications to prevent rejection of a transplanted organ, (2) aggressive chemotherapy protocols used to treat lymphoproliferative and neoplastic disorders, and (3) the significant incidence of acquired immunodeficiency syndrome (AIDS) (Van Trigt, 1990). Immunocompromised individuals are subject to a variety of bacterial, fungal, and parasitic infections.

Individuals who abuse intravenous drugs are also at greater risk for pulmonary infections. Several factors directly related to intravenous substance abuse contribute to development of pulmonary infections, including (1) vomiting and aspiration due to the respiratory depression associated with drug overdose; (2) septic pulmonary emboli secondary to tricuspid valve endocarditis or injection site thrombophlebitis; and (3) the frequently associated problems of alcoholism, malnourishment, substandard housing, and the increasing incidence of AIDS in this population (Hoover et al., 1988). The most common type of pulmonary infection is *pneumonia*. Community-acquired pneumonia is usually attributable to bacterial infection, commonly with pneumococcus; hospital-acquired pneumonia is more often caused by aerobic gram negative bacilli (e.g., *Escherichia coli, Serratia marcescens,* or *Klebsiella pneumoniae*) or *Pseudomonas* (Mark & Baldwin, 1991). Pneumonia is treated with organism-specific antibiotic therapy. A pneumonitis that does not resolve is suggestive of bronchial obstruction secondary to tumor. Uncommonly, pneumonia leads to development of a lung abscess.

Tuberculosis, once thought to be nearly eradicated, is reemerging in urban areas, particularly in immunocompromised patients. Pulmonary tuberculosis is caused by the organism *Mycobacterium tuberculosis.* The bacilli responsible for pulmonary tuberculosis are most often airborne, and the disease is highly contagious, especially in closed populations of susceptible individuals (Shields, 1994). In adults, tuberculosis typically begins as a pneumonia in the apical or posterior segment of an upper lobe or the superior segment of a lower lobe; the pneumonic infiltrate progresses to caseous necrosis, cavity formation, drainage into an adjacent bronchus, and expectoration of debris and viable mycobacteria from the cavity (Moran, 1990).

The most common symptoms of tuberculosis are a persistent cold and cough, night sweats, chest pain, weight loss, and hemoptysis (McMillan, 1991). The diagnosis is confirmed by isolating *M. tuberculosis* from sputum or lung tissue. Medical treatment consists of various antituberculous chemotherapeutic agents, administered in combination. The purpose of combined therapy is to produce an effective bactericidal combination with minimal side effects, while avoiding development of resistance to a particular agent (McMillan, 1991). An example of an appropriate pharmacologic regimen is isoniazid and rifampin for 9 months with ethambutol or streptomycin for the first 2 to 8 weeks (Shields, 1994). Surgical therapy may be required for drug-resistant infections or to treat complications of tuberculosis, such as massive hemoptysis or empyema.

The most commonly occurring *pulmonary fungal infections* are aspergillosis (fungus ball), blastomycosis, coccidioidomycosis, cryptococcosis, and histoplasmosis (Takaro, 1989). Several types of fungal infections can produce a pulmonary nodule similar in appearance to a malignant lesion. Although most pulmonary infections are treated medically, bronchoscopy or open-lung biopsy through thoracoscopy may be necessary for diagnostic purposes.

LUNG ABSCESS

The formation of a local area of infection and tissue destruction in the pulmonary parenchyma is termed a *lung abscess* (Fig. 33-3). Lung abscess can develop as a result of (1) aspiration of esophageal contents or other foreign matter into the tracheobronchial tree, (2) pneumonia, (3) infection elsewhere in the body, (4) pulmonary embolism, or (5) bronchial obstruction by tumor or a foreign body.

Aspiration is the most common cause of lung abscess, especially in the presence of alcohol abuse, seizure disorders, general anesthesia, or prolonged intubation. Oral or gastric feeding of patients with diminished levels of consciousness or who are in a supine position also predisposes to aspiration and lung abscess. Because aspiration usually occurs when the patient is supine, lung abscesses typically develop in the right upper lobe or left or right lower

FIGURE 33-3. Schematic of chest computed tomographic scan demonstrating difference between **(A)** empyema, an extrapulmonary process, and **(B)** lung abscess, an intrapulmonary process. (DeMeester TR, Lafontaine E, 1990: The pleura. In Sabiston DC Jr, Spencer FC [eds]: Surgery of the Chest, ed. 5, p. 469. Philadelphia, WB Saunders)

lobes. The responsible pathogens, derived from the mixed flora of the mouth, are most commonly *Staphylococcus*, fusiform bacilli, alpha-nonhemolytic *Streptococcus*, *Peptococcus*, or *Bacteroides fragilis* (Hood, 1994a).

Unchecked necrosis of infected tissue in a lung abscess eventually produces erosion into a bronchus or the pleural space. Communication with a bronchus allows the lung abscess to be partially drained by expectoration of suppurative material. Erosion into the pleural space (i.e., a *bronchopleural fistula*) produces an empyema. Lung abscesses are usually treated with pulmonary hygiene interventions and organism-specific antimicrobial therapy. Surgical procedures to drain infected material or remove necrotic lung tissue are rarely required.

EMPYEMA THORACIS

Empyema thoracis is infection of the pleural space (see Fig. 33-3). More than 50% of empyemas result from pyogenic pneumonia; other common causes are infection after an operation on the esophagus, lungs, or mediastinum and extension of a subphrenic abscess (Miller, 1990). In most patients, the pleural space is infected with more than one organism. *Staphylococcus aureus* is most common, but *Pseudomonas aeruginosa*, *Klebsiella pneumoniae*, *Escherichia coli*, *Aerobacter aerogenes*, *Proteus,* and *Salmonella* are also typical (Miller, 1990). Common clinical manifestations of empyema include fever, chest pain, dyspnea, and cough (Smith et al., 1991).

Treatment encompasses two primary objectives: (1) adequate drainage of infected material and (2) lung reexpansion (Ali & Unouh, 1990). Chest tube thoracostomy or rib resection and open drainage may be performed to drain the pleural space. *Thoracoscopy* is sometimes performed for direct visualization and debridement of the empyema cavity, followed by cyclic irrigation and drainage (Ridley & Braimbridge, 1991). *Decortication* (i.e., an operation to remove infected or constrictive pleura) may be necessary to achieve lung reexpansion. Failure of the lung to reexpand leaves a residual space that invariably becomes

reinfected. Occasionally, it may be necessary to surgically obliterate a residual space. A *thoracoplasty* is the surgical collapsing of the chest wall to obliterate the space surrounding the nonexpanded lung. Alternatively, a *pectoralis muscle flap* may be performed, in which extrathoracic muscle is transposed to fill the residual space. Although antibiotics are important in treating pneumonia that might lead to empyema, their value in treating established empyema is unproven (Ridley & Braimbridge, 1991).

BRONCHIECTASIS

Bronchiectasis is a disease characterized by localized or diffuse dilatation and destruction of bronchi. Pathogenesis of the condition is infection, followed by obstruction, followed by destruction of the involved bronchi (Sealy, 1989). The diagnosis is suggested by a clinical history of multiple respiratory infections with cough, abundant sputum production, or hemoptysis. Bronchoscopy and bronchography are performed to confirm the diagnosis and identify bronchiectatic segments. The mainstay of medical treatment is vigorous pulmonary hygiene, including postural drainage. Surgical resection of the involved portions of lung may be indicated in patients with recurrent pneumonia; complications of pulmonary infections; continuing, copious sputum; hemoptysis; and, in children, significant failure of growth or development (Mark & Baldwin, 1991).

ABNORMALITIES OF THE PLEURAL SPACE

PNEUMOTHORAX

Pneumothorax is the abnormal accumulation of air in the pleural space. It can occur (1) as an spontaneous event, (2) secondary to blunt or penetrating chest trauma, (3) as a result of an invasive intrathoracic procedure (e.g., central venous catheter placement, transthoracic needle biopsy, or thoracentesis), (4) due to parenchymal disruption associated with pulmonary resection procedures, or (5) secondary to the use of high levels of positive end-expiratory pressure in mechanically ventilated patients. Pneumothorax most often results from the rupture of an air-filled pseudocyst within the lung. *Pseudocysts* may be characterized as blebs or bullae, depending on size and structure (Wakabayashi et al., 1990). A *bleb* is a small group of alveoli with abnormally thin walls usually located in the lung periphery. Large pseudocysts, or *bullae,* commonly develop in individuals with emphysematous lung disease. A disruption in the visceral covering of the pseudocyst allows air from the tracheobronchial tree to leak into the pleural space. As air accumulates in the pleural space, the ipsilateral lung is increasingly compressed. If air continues to fill the pleural space, it eventually compresses mediastinal structures, shifting them toward the opposite hemithorax. This condition is termed *tension pneumothorax.* Unrelieved tension pneumothorax causes severe hemodynamic compromise due to inability of the compressed vena cavae to deliver blood into the heart. Cardiac filling decreases, causing decreased cardiac output and profound hypotension.

Primary spontaneous pneumothorax is presumed to occur due to idiopathic rupture of a peripheral bleb. The condition most often occurs in healthy young men with an asthenic (slight) body build and is manifested by pleuritic chest pain. Smoking substantially increases the risk of developing a spontaneous pneumothorax, particularly in men (Bense, 1992). A small spontaneous pneumothorax may be treated with activity restriction and observation, but more often chest tube thoracostomy and the application of negative suction to the pleural space is necessary. If a tension component is present, immediate evacuation of air from the pleural space may be accomplished by thoracentesis (followed by chest tube thoracostomy) or emergent chest tube insertion. Usually, the alveolar rent gradually seals and the air leak abates within 1 to 2 days.

A patient who has experienced a spontaneous pneumothorax is at increased risk to develop another one subsequently. Approximately 20% of patients experience recurrent pneumothorax, usually within 2 years and on the same side as the first (Deslauriers et al., 1991). Once a second pneumothorax has occurred, the risk for a third is even greater. The most common treatment for recurrent pneumothoraces is *surgical pleurodesis* or mechanical abrasion of the pleural surfaces to produce inflammation with resultant adhesion formation. Pleurodesis can often be accomplished through video-assisted thoracoscopy. If pseudocysts are detected at the time of operation, they may be surgically resected. Occasionally, pleurodesis is performed after the first episode of spontaneous pneumothorax if the air leak persists despite conservative measures or the patient's life-style is such that a subsequent pneumothorax could be life threatening (e.g., working in a hyperbaric chamber, scuba diving, or piloting small aircraft requiring use of a pressurized mask).

Secondary spontaneous pneumothorax, or that which develops secondary to another condition, occurs most commonly in older persons with emphysema or other forms of chronic obstructive pulmonary disease. The predominant symptom in this group of patients is acute shortness of breath, which, because of impaired pulmonary function, can progress to frank respiratory failure (Deslauriers et al., 1991). Chest tube drainage is promptly initiated and may be necessary for several weeks until the air leak resolves.

Patients receiving mechanical ventilation with high levels (15–20 cm) of positive end-expiratory pressure are also at risk for secondary spontaneous pneumothoraces, which may develop bilaterally. Such patients are generally critically ill and are likely to succumb to the hemodynamic sequelae of tension pneumothorax if the air is not promptly evacuated. A vigorous air leak may persist and chest tube drainage with negative suction is usually required until mechanical ventilation is discontinued.

In patients with AIDS, pneumothoraces occur frequently in association with *Pneumocystis carinii* pneumonia (Fleisher et al., 1988). Treatment of pneumothorax in the presence of an immunocompromised state requires special considerations. Healing of visceral pleura and resolution of the air leak is very slow. Chest tube drainage is frequently required for weeks, or even months. Under most other circumstances, pneumothorax is treated with closed water-seal drainage until the air leak completely resolves. However, because of the persistence of air leaks and the often limited life-expectancy in patients with AIDS, a *Heimlich valve* may be used in place of a conventional water-seal drainage system so that the patient can be discharged from the hospital. Heimlich valves, chest tubes, and drainage systems are described in further detail in Chapter 42, Pleural Thoracostomy Drainage.

Surgical pleurodesis is undesirable for prevention of recurrent pneumothorax in patients with AIDS because of the significant morbidity associated with an operation. *Chemical pleurodesis,* also called *pleural sclerosis,* may be performed instead. Installation of a talc solution through a chest tube (*talc poudrage*) has been used successfully in patients with AIDS and *P. carinii* pneumonia to prevent pneumothorax recurrence (Tunon-de-Lara et al., 1992). The installation of the caustic solution produces an inflammatory response that causes the visceral and parietal pleural surfaces to become adherent. Such adherence, termed *pleural symphysis,* serves to obliterate the potential pleural space so that the lung is unable to collapse.

PLEURAL EFFUSION

Pleural effusion is the abnormal accumulation of fluid between the parietal pleura, which lines the inside of the chest wall, and the visceral pleura, which covers the lungs. Under normal conditions, 5 to 10 L of fluid flows from systemic capillaries in the parietal pleura into the pleural space each day (DeMeester & LaFontaine, 1990). The fluid is rapidly absorbed, mostly by pulmonary capillaries in the visceral pleura and to a much smaller extent by pulmonary lymphatics. Only several milliliters of fluid are normally present in the pleural cavity. If a disturbance in the normal equilibrium of fluid entering and leaving the pleural space occurs, the pleural space fills with fluid and the ipsilateral lung is compressed.

Thoracentesis is commonly performed for diagnostic purposes. The fluid obtained is categorized as either transudative or exudative, primarily according to the total protein and lactate dehydrogenase content of the fluid. *Transudative pleural effusions* are caused by an imbalance in formation and reabsorption of pleural fluid. Congestive heart failure and pulmonary embolism are examples of conditions that cause transudative pleural effusions. Transudative pleural effusion is managed primarily by treating the underlying disease process.

Exudative pleural effusions are caused by pathologic processes that either increase permeability of the pleural surface to protein or decrease lymphatic flow. Although lymphatic drainage plays a minor role in removal of fluid from the pleural space, it is important in clearing protein that normally enters the space from the parietal and visceral pleural surfaces (DeMeester & LaFontaine, 1990). Consequently, exudative effusions have a higher pleural fluid-to-serum protein ratio. Other descriptive information that may help determine etiology of a pleural effusion includes the color, odor, and character of the fluid as well as analysis of the fluid for white blood cell count and differential, glucose, and pH values. Gram and acid-fast bacillus stains and pleural fluid cultures are performed if infection is suspected; if malignancy is likely, pleural fluid cytology or a pleural biopsy is performed (Sahn, 1989).

Pleural effusion can result from a number of non-malignant disease processes but more often occurs secondary to malignancy (Table 33-3). Several types of malignant diseases are associated with pleural effusion, most commonly lung cancer, breast cancer, and lymphoma (Flye, 1989). Local inflammation and increased capillary permeability associated with tumor implants increase fluid transudation, while lymphatic obstruction impairs its resorption (Deslauriers et al., 1991). The occurrence of pleural effusion secondary to malignancy is an ominous sign. Average patient survival after its development is only 3 months (Ponn et al., 1991).

Palliative treatment of malignant pleural effusion is undertaken to relieve the associated respiratory distress, which is often the only or most troublesome symptom in a patient who is otherwise able to remain fairly active. Evacuation of fluid by thoracentesis or chest tube thoracostomy is most often performed to provide symptomatic relief. A thoracoscopy may be performed if loculated areas of fluid are present. Through the thoracoscope, adhesions that are pre-

---

TABLE 33-3. CAUSES OF PLEURAL EFFUSION

Malignancy
Congestive heart failure
Pulmonary embolism
Cirrhosis of the liver with ascites
Nephrotic syndrome
Infections
    Tuberculosis
    Histoplasmosis
Immunologic diseases
    Rheumatoid disease
    Systemic lupus erythematosus
Postpericardiotomy syndrome
Chylothorax
Hemothorax

---

venting free drainage of fluid can be disrupted. Prompt evacuation of the effusion is important to achieving lung reexpansion. Because malignant effusions are exudative, the visceral pleura becomes coated with a proteinaceous material. If the effusion remains for an extended period, the lung becomes trapped and incapable of reexpansion.

Because of the underlying malignancy, fluid can be expected to reaccumulate. Intermittent thoracentesis or tube thoracostomy is uncomfortable for the patient and can cause pneumothorax, hypoproteinemia, or empyema (Flye, 1989). Chemical pleural sclerosis is often performed to prevent reaccumulation of fluid. Although pleural sclerosis does not affect progression of disease, it provides palliation from the dyspnea produced by recurring effusions. As in treatment of pneumothorax, the objective of pleural sclerosis is inflammation of the pleural surfaces with resultant pleural symphysis so that fluid accumulation cannot recur.

Chemical sclerosis is typically performed through the chest tube by injection of a caustic agent after the effusion has been drained and the lung has reexpanded. Full lung expansion is important so that visceral and parietal pleural layers can become adherent to one another. Formerly, tetracycline was the standard agent used for chemical sclerosis. Because it is no longer commercially available, other agents, such as doxycycline (an antibiotic in the tetracycline class), bleomycin (a chemotherapeutic agent), or talc may be selected. After fluid instillation, the chest tube is clamped for several hours. During this period, the patient is repositioned from side to back to side to allow distribution of the sclerosing solution over the entire pleural surface.

Despite pleural sclerosis, effusions recur in 15% to 20% of patients (Ponn et al., 1991). Surgical procedures for prevention of effusion recurrence include mechanical abrasion (pleurodesis) or removal of the parietal pleura (pleurectomy). These procedures are generally not performed for treatment of malignant effusions because of the significant morbidity associated with a thoracic operation in a patient with a limited life expectancy.

An alternative therapy for intractable pleural effusion is the implantation of a pleuroperitoneal shunt. The *Denver pleuroperitoneal shunt* (Denver Biomaterial, Evergreen, CO) consists of a pumping chamber that contains a one-way valve and connects fenestrated catheters placed in the pleural space and peritoneum (Fig. 33-4). The shunt drains fluid from the pleural space into the peritoneal cavity, where it is reabsorbed. Because pleural pressure is lower than peritoneal pressure, drainage of fluid through the shunt requires frequent manual compression of the pumping chamber, which is placed in subcutaneous tissue over the anterolateral costal margin of the chest wall (Ponn et al., 1991). Placement of the shunt can usually be performed using local anesthesia and sedation.

CHYLOTHORAX

Chylothorax is the presence of *chyle* (i.e., lymphatic fluid that originates in the intestines) in the pleural space. Chyle can enter the pleural space when the *thoracic duct,* which courses through the thorax in proximity to the esophagus, becomes disrupted or obstructed. The primary function of the thoracic duct is the transport of digestive fat from the liver and intestinal tract into the venous system (Miller, 1994).

FIGURE 33-4. Schematic illustrating pleuroperitoneal shunt. (Ponn RB, Blancaflor J, D'Agostino RS, et al., 1991: Pleuroperitoneal shunting for intractable pleural effusions. Ann Thorac Surg 51:606. Reprinted with permission of the Society of Thoracic Surgeons)

Chylothorax can occur as a complication of thoracic operations, caused by laceration of the thoracic duct or its major divisions. It can also result from obstructed lymphatic flow secondary to lymphoma or other malignancy. Chylothorax is distinguished from other types of pleural effusions by the characteristic milky appearance of the fluid.

Treatment of chylothorax consists of chest tube thoracostomy drainage and limitation of chyle formation through dietary management. Reducing the dietary intake of long-chain fatty acids and replacement of normal dietary fat by medium-chain triglycerides decreases lymphatic flow through the thoracic duct (Simpson, 1990). Parenteral nutrition is generally instituted to replete fluid, electrolytes, and protein. In postoperative thoracic surgical patients, reexploration of the thorax with ligation of the thoracic duct may occasionally be necessary if significant chylous drainage persists.

OTHER DISORDERS

HEMOPTYSIS

Hemoptysis, or expectoration of blood, can occur as a manifestation of a number of pathologic cardiovascular and pulmonary conditions. Most often, it occurs in small quantities. Occasionally, *massive hemoptysis,* defined as expectoration of more than 600 mL of blood over a 24-hour period, occurs. Massive hemoptysis is a life-threatening condition. If untreated, the patient is likely to die of suffocation secondary to hemorrhage into the tracheobronchial tree. The patient usually succumbs to impaired oxygenation before enough bleeding occurs to cause hemodynamic instability.

Bronchoscopy is performed, preferably during the period of active bleeding and under general anesthesia (Garzon, 1989). This allows identification of the bleeding origin and insertion of a *bronchial blocker* in the affected bronchial orifice. The bronchial blocker, which consists of a balloon-tipped catheter, is used to occlude the lumen of the affected bronchus, thus preventing blood from spilling into other parts of the tracheobronchial tree. Emergent pulmonary angiography may be performed with selective embolization of the responsible artery. Thoracotomy with resection of involved pulmonary parenchyma may also be necessary because of the significant incidence (80%) of recurrent massive hemoptysis (Garzon, 1989).

FOREIGN BODY ASPIRATION

Aspiration of foreign bodies is relatively uncommon in adults except in persons in whom the ability of the glottis to protect the airway is diminished. Specifically, aspiration is most likely after heavy ingestion of alcohol or other consciousness-altering drug and in persons with decreased levels of consciousness. Aspirated items are usually organic material, such as gum, hard candy, nuts, or boluses of food. Inorganic items include such things as needles, teeth, dental plates, beer can tabs, or other objects that may be placed in the mouth.

A large, solid object lodged in the trachea or a major bronchus may produce airway obstruction. Rigid bronchoscopy is performed if there is suspicion of a lodged foreign object. If the object has sharp edges, perforation of the airway can occur before or during removal. A small object in a distal airway can produce pneumonia, either from contamination or airway obstruction and atelectasis. Sometimes aspiration is a presumptive diagnosis based on clinical history and the type of pneumonia that is present. Because the most direct pathway into the tracheobronchial tree is through the right mainstem bronchus, aspiration pneumonia occurs typically in the right upper lobe.

PULMONARY ARTERIOVENOUS MALFORMATION

A *pulmonary arteriovenous malformation* is a congenital anomalous communication between a pulmonary artery and vein. Symptoms of this disorder, which include dyspnea, clubbing, and cyanosis, usually appear in early adulthood (Wallenhaupt & D'Souza, 1988). Arterial blood gases reveal lower than normal oxygen saturation. A pulmonary arteriovenous malformation is generally apparent on the chest roentgenogram as a solitary pulmonary nodule, usually with two large vascular markings (Miller, 1991). Surgical repair is indicated because of the known complications of this malformation, including massive hemoptysis, hemothorax, cerebral abscess, bacterial endocarditis, and systemic embolization (Wallenhaupt & D'Souza, 1988).

BRONCHOLITHIASIS

Broncholithiasis is an unusual disorder in which hilar lymph nodes become enlarged and calcified. The cause of calcification is most often a prior granulomatous infection, particularly histoplasmosis or tuberculosis (Faber, 1989). Cough and hemoptysis are common manifestations, caused by bronchial compression or erosion by a calcified lymph node. The patient may expectorate fragments of the eroding *broncholith* (calcified lymph node) (Hood, 1994b). In selected patients, bronchoscopy may be performed for removal or laser eradication of a broncholith. However, because the broncholith is frequently imbedded in bronchial tissue with intense inflammation and fibrosis, removal through bronchoscopy can result in significant bleeding or bronchial perforation. Thoracotomy may be required for removal of the broncholith and the surrounding bronchial and lung tissue.

REFERENCES

Albertucci M, DeMeester TR, Rothberg M, et al., 1992: Surgery and the management of peripheral lung tumors adherent to the parietal pleura. J Thorac Cardiovasc Surg 103:8

Ali I, Unouh H, 1990: Management of empyema thoracis. Ann Thorac Surg 50:355

Allen MS, Mathisen DJ, Grillo HC, et al., 1991: Bronchogenic carcinoma with chest wall invasion. Ann Thorac Surg 51:948

Auerbach O, Garfinkel L, 1991: The changing pattern of lung carcinoma. Cancer 68:1973

Beahrs OH, Myers MH (eds), 1978: The Manual for Staging Cancer, ed. 2. American Joint Committee on Cancer. Philadelphia, JB Lippincott

Bense L, 1992: Spontaneous pneumothorax. Chest 101:891

Burt M, Martini N, 1991: Surgical treatment of lung carcinoma. In Baue AE, Geha AS, Hammond GL, et al. (eds): Glenn's Thoracic and Cardiovascular Surgery, ed. 5. Norwalk, CT, Appleton & Lange

Carter D, Matthay RA, 1991: Lung cancer: Epidemiology, etiology, and pathology. In Baue AE, Geha AS, Hammond GL, et al. (eds): Glenn's Thoracic and Cardiovascular Surgery, ed. 5. Norwalk, CT, Appleton & Lange

Daly RC, Trastek VF, Pairolero PC, et al., 1991: Bronchoalveolar carcinoma: Factors affecting survival. Ann Thorac Surg 51:368

DeMeester TR, Lafontaine E, 1990: The pleura. In Sabiston DC Jr, Spencer FC (eds): Surgery of the Chest, ed. 5. Philadelphia, WB Saunders

Deslauriers J, Beauchamp G, Desmeules M, 1991: Benign and malignant disorders of the pleura. In Baue AE, Geha AS, Hammond GL, et al. (eds): Glenn's Thoracic and Cardiovascular Surgery, ed. 5. Norwalk, CT, Appleton & Lange

Faber LP, 1989: Broncholithiasis. In Grillo HC, Austen WG, Wilkins EW, et al. (eds): Current Therapy in Cardiothoracic Surgery. Toronto, BC Decker

Flehinger BJ, Kimmel M, Melamed MR, 1992: The effect of surgical treatment on survival from early lung cancer. Chest 101:1013

Fleisher AG, McElvaney G, Lawson L, et al., 1988: Surgical management of spontaneous pneumothorax in patients with acquired immunodeficiency syndrome. Ann Thorac Surg 45:21

Fleisher AG, McElvaney G, Robinson CL, 1991: Multiple primary bronchogenic carcinomas: Treatment and follow-up. Ann Thorac Surg 51:48

Flye MW, 1989: Malignant pleural effusion. In Grillo HC, Austen WG, Wilkins EW, et al. (eds): Current Therapy in Cardiothoracic Surgery. Toronto, BC Decker

Garzon AA, 1989: Massive hemoptysis: Surgical and tamponade therapy. In Grillo HC, Austen WG, Wilkins EW, et al. (eds): Current Therapy in Cardiothoracic Surgery. Toronto, BC Decker

Grillo HC, 1989: Benign and malignant diseases of the trachea. In Shields TW (ed): General Thoracic Surgery, ed. 3. Philadelphia, Lea & Febiger

Grillo HC, Mathisen DJ, 1991: The trachea: Tumors, strictures, and tracheal collapse. In Baue AE, Geha AS, Hammond GL, et al. (eds): Glenn's Thoracic and Cardiovascular Surgery, ed. 5. Norwalk, CT, Appleton & Lange

Hansen CP, Holtveg H, Francis D, et al., 1992: Pulmonary hamartoma. J Thorac Cardiovasc Surg 104:674

Hood RM, 1994a: Bacterial infections of the lung. In Shields TW (ed): General Thoracic Surgery, ed. 4. Baltimore, Williams & Wilkins

Hood RM, 1994b: Bronchial compressive diseases. In Shields TW (ed): General Thoracic Surgery, ed. 4. Baltimore, Williams & Wilkins

Hoover EL, Hsu H, Webb H, et al., 1988: The surgical management of empyema thoracis in substance abuse patients: A 5-year experience. Ann Thorac Surg 46:563

Kittle CRF, 1989: Pleural mesothelioma. In Grillo HC, Austen WG, Wilkins EW, et al. (eds): Current Therapy in Cardiothoracic Surgery. Toronto, BC Decker

Lewis JW, Ajlouni M, Kvale PA, et al., 1990: Role of brachytherapy in the management of pulmonary and mediastinal malignancies. Ann Thorac Surg 49:728

Mark JB, Baldwin JC, 1991: Pneumonia, lung abscess, and bronchiectasis. In Baue AE, Geha AS, Hammond GL, et al. (eds): Glenn's Thoracic and Cardiovascular Surgery, ed. 5. Norwalk, CT, Appleton & Lange

Martini N, 1989: Unresectable neoplasms of the lung. In Grillo HC, Austen WG, Wilkins EW, et al. (eds): Current Therapy in Cardiothoracic Surgery. Toronto, BC Decker

Martini N, Burt ME, Bains MS, et al., 1992: Survival after resection of stage II non–small cell lung cancer. Ann Thorac Surg 54:460

Mathisen DJ, Grillo HC, 1991: Carinal resection for bronchogenic carcinoma. J Thorac Cardiovasc Surg 102:16

McMillan IK, 1991: Surgical treatment of tuberculosis. In Baue AE, Geha AS, Hammond GL, et al. (eds): Glenn's Thoracic and Cardiovascular Surgery, ed. 5. Norwalk, CT, Appleton & Lange

Meyer JA, 1989: Small-cell carcinoma. In Grillo HC, Austen WG, Wilkins EW, et al. (eds): Current Therapy in Cardiothoracic Surgery. BC Decker

Miller JI, 1994: Chylothorax. In Shields TW (ed): General Thoracic Surgery, ed. 4. Baltimore, Williams & Wilkins

Miller JI, 1990: Empyema thoracis. Ann Thorac Surg 50:343

Miller JI, 1991: Benign tumors of the lower respiratory tract. In Baue AE, Geha AS, Hammond GL, et al. (eds): Glenn's Thoracic and Cardiovascular Surgery, ed. 5. Norwalk, CT, Appleton & Lange

Moran JF, 1990: Surgical treatment of pulmonary tuberculosis. In Sabiston DC Jr, Spencer FC (eds): Surgery of the Chest, ed. 5. Philadelphia, WB Saunders

Mountain CF, 1986: A new international staging system for lung cancer. Chest 89:2255

Muller LC, Salzer GM, Huber H, et al., 1992: Multimodal therapy of small cell lung cancer in TNM stages I through IIIA. Ann Thorac Surg 54:493

Mulshine ML, Tockman MS, 1992: Considerations in population-based screening for the early detection of lung cancer. In Bernal SD, Hesketh PJ (eds): Lung Cancer Differentiation: Implications for Diagnosis and Treatment. New York, Marcel Dekker

Neagley SR, 1991: The pulmonary system. In Alspach JG (ed): Core Curriculum for Critical Care Nursing, ed. 4. Philadelphia, WB Saunders

Pairolero PC, Trastek VF, Payne WS, 1989: Occult neoplasia. In Grillo HC, Austen WG, Wilkins EW, et al. (eds): Current Therapy in Cardiothoracic Surgery. Toronto, BC Decker

Paulson DL, 1991: Superior sulcus tumors. In Baue AE, Geha AS, Hammond GL, et al. (eds): Glenn's Thoracic and Cardiovascular Surgery, ed. 5. Norwalk, CT, Appleton & Lange

Ponn RB, Blancaflor J, D'Agostino RS, et al., 1991: Pleuroperitoneal shunting for intractable pleural effusions. Ann Thorac Surg 51:605

Ridley PD, Braimbridge MV, 1991: Thoracoscopic debridement and pleural irrigation in the management of empyema thoracis. Ann Thorac Surg 51:461

Rosengart TK, Martini N, Ghosn P, Burt M, 1991: Multiple primary lung carcinomas: Prognosis and treatment. Ann Thorac Surg 52:773

Rusch VW, Piantadosi S, Holmes EC, 1991: The role of extrapleural pneumonectomy in malignant mesothelioma. J Thorac Cardiovasc Surg 102:1

Sabiston DC Jr, 1990: Carcinoma of the lung. In Sabiston DC Jr, Spencer FC (eds): Surgery of the Chest, ed. 5. Philadelphia, WB Saunders

Sahn SA, 1989: Benign and malignant pleural effusions. In Shields TW (ed): General Thoracic Surgery, ed. 3. Philadelphia, Lea & Febiger

Sealy WC, 1989: Bronchiectasis. In Grillo HC, Austen WG, Wilkins EW, et al., (eds): Current Therapy in Cardiothoracic Surgery. Toronto, BC Decker

Sellers TA, Potter JD, Bailey-Wilson JE, et al., 1991: Lung cancer detection and prevention: Evidence for an interaction between smoking and genetic predisposition. Cancer Res 52 (Suppl):2694S

Shields TW, Robinson PG, Radosevich JA, 1994: Lung Cancer: Etiology, carcinogenesis, molecular biology, and pathology. In Shields TW (ed): General Thoracic Surgery, ed. 4. Baltimore, Williams & Wilkins

Shields TW, 1989: Primary tumors of the pleura. In General Thoracic Surgery, ed. 3. Philadelphia, Lea & Febiger

Shields TW, 1994: Pulmonary tuberculosis and other mycobacterial infections of the lung. In General Thoracic Surgery, ed. 4. Baltimore, Williams & Wilkins

Shields TW, 1990a: Behaviors of small bronchial carcinomas. Ann Thorac Surg 50:691

Shields TW, 1990b: The significance of ipsilateral mediastinal lymph node metastasis (N2 disease) in non-small cell carcinoma of the lung. J Thorac Cardiovasc Surg 99:48

Shields TW, 1991: Lung cancer: Diagnosis and staging. In Baue AE, Geha AS, Hammond GL, et al. (eds): Glenn's Thoracic and Cardiovascular Surgery, ed. 5. Norwalk, CT, Appleton & Lange

Shields TW, Robinson PG, 1994: Benign tumors of the lung. In Shields TW (ed): General Thoracic Surgery, ed. 4. Baltimore, Williams & Wilkins

Simpson L, 1990: Chylothorax in adults: Pathophysiology and management. In Deslauriers J, Lacquet LK (eds): Thoracic Surgery: Surgical Management of Pleural Diseases. St. Louis, CV Mosby

Smith JA, Mullerworth MH, Westlake GW, Tatoulis J, 1991: Empyema thoracis: A 14-year experience in a teaching center. Ann Thorac Surg 51:39

Sridhar KS, Raub WA, 1992: Present and past smoking history and other predisposing factors in 100 lung cancer patients. Chest 101:19

Takaro T, 1989: Fungal infection. In Grillo HC, Austen WG, Wilkins EW, et al. (eds): Current Therapy in Cardiothoracic Surgery. BC Decker

Tunon-de-Lara JM, Constans J, Vincent MP, et al., 1992: Spontaneous pneumothorax associated with *Pneumocystis carinii* pneumonia. Chest 101:1177

Van Schil PE, de la Riviere AB, Knaepen PJ, et al., 1991: TNM staging and long-term follow-up after sleeve resection for bronchogenic tumors. Ann Thorac Surg 52:1096

Van Trigt P, 1990: Lung infections and diffuse interstitial lung disease. In Sabiston DC Jr, Spencer FC (eds): Surgery of the Chest, ed. 5. Philadelphia, WB Saunders

Wakabayashi A, Brenner M, Wilson AF, et al., 1990: Thoracoscopic treatment of spontaneous pneumothorax using carbon dioxide laser. Ann Thorac Surg 50:786

Wallenhaupt SL, D'Souza V, 1988: Combined radiological and surgical management of arteriovenous malformation of the lung. Ann Thorac Surg 45:213

34

ESOPHAGEAL DISEASES

NORMAL ESOPHAGEAL FUNCTION
BENIGN DISORDERS
    Motility Disorders
    Esophageal Diverticulum
    Hiatal Hernia
    Gastroesophageal Reflux
    Esophageal Stricture
    Other Benign Disorders

ESOPHAGEAL INJURIES
    Caustic Injury
    Perforation
    Foreign Body Obstruction
ESOPHAGEAL CANCER

NORMAL ESOPHAGEAL FUNCTION

The esophagus is a hollow tube that extends from the oropharynx to the stomach, passing through the neck, through the thoracic cavity, and into the abdomen. Typically, it is described as having upper (cervical), middle (thoracic), and lower (abdominal) portions, which have different sources of arterial blood supply and lymphatic drainage. The organ has an outer longitudinal and inner circular layer of muscle and differs from muscle in other locations in that it has no serosal layer. Like each of the other compartments of the gastrointestinal tract, the esophagus has its own distinctive pH environment, enzyme content, and propulsive ability and is coupled to its adjoining compartments by a unique valve (Stein et al., 1992a).

The esophagus serves three physiologic functions: (1) transmission of food from the oropharynx to the stomach, (2) control of reflux of stomach contents into the lower esophagus, and (3) prevention of aspiration of esophageal contents into the tracheobronchial tree. Sphincters located at the upper and lower ends control movement of food and fluids into and out of the esophagus. The upper esophageal sphincter (UES), also called the cricopharyngeal sphincter, is composed primarily of the cricopharyngeus muscle. The UES maintains constant closure of the esophageal entrance except during swallowing (Wilkins, 1989). The lower esophageal sphincter (LES) is not anatomically distinct. However, esophageal muscle at the junction of the stomach clearly acts as a physiologic sphincter, maintaining closure of the distal esophagus except during swallowing, vomiting, or belching.

The esophagus is innervated by both the parasympathetic and sympathetic systems. Parasympathetic innervation, particularly that from the vagus nerves, controls opening and closing of the sphincters as well as peristalsis of ingested material. Sympathetic innervation, composed of mediastinal branches from the thoracic sympathetic trunk and recurrent sympathetic branches from the celiac axis, appears to have little functional importance (Orringer, 1991).

Normal esophageal function is dependent on complex coordination of neural and muscular activity. Contraction of the UES during swallowing begins an orderly downward wave of positive pressure that propels ingested food through the length of the esophagus and into the stomach. Intraluminal pressure reaches 40 to 80 mm Hg and is somewhat more forceful in the lower than in the upper esophagus (Ellis, 1990).

BENIGN DISORDERS

Disorders of the esophagus are among the most poorly understood and difficult to treat diseases of the thorax. Common among the "benign" or nonmalignant diseases of the esophagus are motility disorders, or forms of dysfunctional peristalsis.

MOTILITY DISORDERS

Motility disorders are pathologic conditions characterized by abnormal peristalsis, sphincter dysfunction, or a combination of the two. Failure of the propulsive ability of the esophagus hampers the forward movement of food and enhances regurgitation; sphincter dysfunction exposes the esophagus to the luminal contents of the stomach, causing symptoms and eventual mucosal injury (Stein et al., 1992a). Primary motility disorders of the esophagus may involve the swallowing mechanism, the UES, the body of the esophagus, or the LES (Naunheim & Baue, 1991). Impaired esophageal motility may also occur secondary to various collagen disorders (e.g., scleroderma), alcohol abuse, and diabetes or as a response to infection or caustic injury of the esophagus (Duranceau et al., 1991; Wilkins, 1994).

Achalasia is the esophageal motility disorder most commonly treated with surgical therapy. It is characterized by absent peristalsis in the body of the esophagus, excessive pressure in the LES, and a failure of the LES to relax in response to swallowing (Ellis, 1990). It is a disorder of unknown etiology that occurs most often in young and middle-aged adults. Because the LES fails to relax appropriately, undigested food is retained in the esophagus.

The predominant symptom is dysphagia, which occurs in almost all patients. Regurgitation, epigastric discomfort, and weight loss are also common. Nocturnal regurgitation may cause aspiration and respiratory sequelae (Ellis, 1990). In the early stage, solids are typically tolerated better than liquids and warm foods better than cold foods (Naunheim & Baue, 1991). Halitosis is typically present because of undigested food in the esophagus. Achalasia is a progressive disease; the most serious potential complication in untreated patients is the development of esophageal cancer (Ellis, 1990).

Diagnosis of achalasia is accomplished by esophageal manometry studies, contrast radiologic examination (barium swallow), and esophagoscopy. Manometry studies demonstrate a zone of high intraesophageal pressure in the LES and aperistalsis in the body of the esophagus. The barium contrast study reveals dilatation of the upper esophagus and a narrowed distal esophagus (Fig. 34-1).

Pharmacologic therapy is largely unsuccessful in relieving symptoms of achalasia (Naunheim & Baue, 1991). Instead, two primary therapies are used to mechanically relieve obstructive symptoms. The first is forceful dilatation of the LES, which is often performed with a pneumatic dilating instrument. A balloon-tipped dilator is advanced into the esophagus under fluoroscopic guidance and positioned so that the balloon is astride the gastroesophageal junction. Once properly positioned, the balloon is inflated,

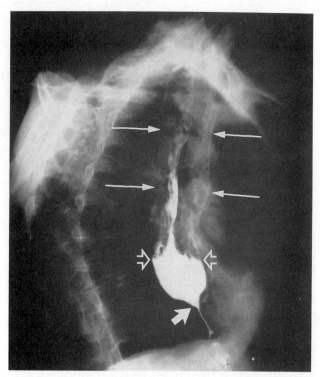

FIGURE 34-1. Barium contrast study demonstrating typical features of achalasia. Note dilated esophageal body (*long arrows*), fluid level of barium in esophagus (*short open arrows*), and characteristic "bird's beak" deformity (*short solid arrow*) produced by distal esophageal narrowing. (Courtesy of Robert M. Vanecko, M.D.)

producing sharp, localized, severe pain as evidence of proper dilatation (Wilkins, 1994). Pneumatic dilatation relieves dysphagia and regurgitation in approximately 70% of patients (Stein et al., 1992b). Iatrogenic perforation of the esophagus is an occasional complication of the procedure. It is suggested by prolonged pain or blood on the dilator; if suspected, a contrast esophageal swallow study is promptly performed to confirm the diagnosis (Wilkins, 1994).

The second form of treatment for achalasia is a surgical procedure, esophagomyotomy. An *esophagomyotomy* consists of division of the outer, muscular layer of the gastroesophageal junction to allow more complete emptying of the esophagus. Some surgeons recommend performance of a concomitant antireflux procedure to prevent iatrogenic gastroesophageal reflux through the newly dilated sphincter. A variety of operative techniques comprise the "antireflux procedures." They are delineated in Chapter 39, Surgical Treatment of Esophageal Disease.

Diffuse esophageal spasm is another form of impaired esophageal motility. In this disorder, sphincter relaxation occurs appropriately in response to swallowing, but high-amplitude, nonperistaltic, repetitive contractions occur in the body of the esophagus (Ellis, 1990). Esophageal spasm typically causes chest pain that mimics pain produced by myocardial ischemia. Particularly since both types of pain are relieved with nitroglycerin, esophageal spasm is sometimes mistaken for angina. Dysphagia, regurgitation, and weight loss are other common manifestations of esophageal spasm (Wilkins, 1994). Calcium-channel antagonist medications are often effective in relieving associated symptoms. Occasionally, an esophagomyotomy, extended for the length of the segment of abnormal motility, is necessary to relieve spasm.

Impaired function of the swallowing mechanism or UES (i.e., *oropharyngeal dysphagia*) is usually caused by a neuromuscular disorder, such as Parkinson's disease, cerebral vascular accident, muscular dystrophy, or myasthenia gravis. Clinical manifestations of oropharyngeal dysphagia include hesitancy in initiating swallow, food or liquids sticking in the throat, a cough after swallowing, and aspiration (Ellis, 1990). Medical therapy is based on treatment of the underlying disorder. Surgical therapy is not helpful for most forms of oropharyngeal dysfunction.

ESOPHAGEAL DIVERTICULUM

Esophageal motility disorders are thought to contribute to development of esophageal diverticula. An *esophageal diverticulum* is an epithelial-lined blind pouch leading from the main lumen of the esophagus (Trastek, 1994). The three major types of esophageal diverticula are (1) pharyngoesophageal pulsion or Zenker's diverticulum, (2) epiphrenic pulsion diverticulum, and (3) parabronchial traction diverticulum. *Pulsion diverticula* develop as a result of forces within the esophageal mucosa acting against an area of resistance, and *traction diverticula* are caused by forces exerted from outside the esophagus, such as inflammatory adhesions (Ferguson, 1991).

Zenker's diverticulum is the most common type of esophageal diverticulum and the form most likely to necessitate surgical therapy. Zenker's diverticula originate near the cricopharyngeus muscle. The cause of the lesion is unknown. Early in its development, the diverticulum is small and varies in size with the phase of swallowing. Once established, a diverticulum enlarges rapidly and descends dependently due to constant distention with ingested material (Trastek, 1994). In severe cases, the sac may retain several hundred milliliters of undigested food and fluid and extend to or below the level of the aortic arch (Skinner & Belsey, 1988a).

Progressive symptoms occur due to esophageal obstruction and unimpeded emptying of the diverticulum into the upper esophagus. Characteristic symptoms include high esophageal dysphagia, foul breath, noisy deglutition (swallowing), and spontaneous regurgitation with or without coughing or choking episodes (Trastek, 1994). If untreated, continuous saliva and food spillage may cause aspiration pneumonia; local complications, such as inflammation, perforation, abscess formation, or tracheoesophageal fistula,

may also occur (Duranceau et al., 1991). Zenker's diverticulum is treated surgically. For small diverticula, *cricopharyngeal esophagomyotomy* is usually sufficient to relieve symptoms. Diverticulopexy or diverticulectomy may be performed for larger diverticula. *Diverticulopexy* consists of suspending the diverticulum in an inverted position so that it does not fill but rather drains easily into the esophagus (Naunheim & Baue, 1991). *Diverticulectomy* is surgical resection of the diverticulum.

HIATAL HERNIA

The esophagus normally passes from the thorax into the abdomen through an opening in the diaphragm known as the esophageal hiatus. The distal esophagus is tethered in place by the phrenoesophageal membrane, which extends from the transversus abdominus muscle and the diaphragm to connective tissue of the intrathoracic esophageal submucosa (Skinner, 1994). *Hiatal hernia* is an anatomic deformity of the esophageal hiatus that allows translocation of the gastroesophageal junction or part of the stomach into the thorax. It is thought to occur in as many as 10% of adults in the United States (Skinner, 1994).

Most common is type I, or *sliding hiatal hernia* (Fig. 34-2). It is characterized by stretching of the phrenoesophageal membrane, resulting in protrusion of a small portion of gastric cardia through the esophageal hiatus (Skinner, 1994). Type I hiatal hernia produces no symptoms or complications in and of itself. However, it is often associated with regurgitation of acidic gastric contents into the distal esophagus, a condition termed gastroesophageal reflux and described in detail below. Treatment of type I hiatal hernia is not necessary except for complications of the condition.

In type II, or *paraesophageal hernia*, a defect in the phrenoesophageal membrane allows herniation of peritoneum with protrusion of a portion or all of the stomach into the thoracic pressure compartment (see Fig. 34-2). In contrast to sliding hiatal hernias, paraesophageal hernias may cause symptoms even without associated gastroesophageal reflux, including early satiety, vomiting after a full meal, epigastric distress, dysphagia, and gurgling within the chest (Skinner, 1990). Surgical repair of paraesophageal hernias is recommended because of the risk of (1) gastric obstruction, infarction, or strangulation; (2) bleeding; or (3) acute intrathoracic dilatation (Skinner, 1994).

GASTROESOPHAGEAL REFLUX

Gastroesophageal reflux is the regurgitation of acidic gastric contents into the distal esophagus. Some degree of reflux occurs normally and is considered physiologic; the refluxed material quickly returns to the stomach, producing no symptoms or injury to esophageal mucosa (Skinner, 1994). The mechanism for pathologic gastroesophageal reflux remains ill defined. Whatever the mechanism, pathologic reflux is

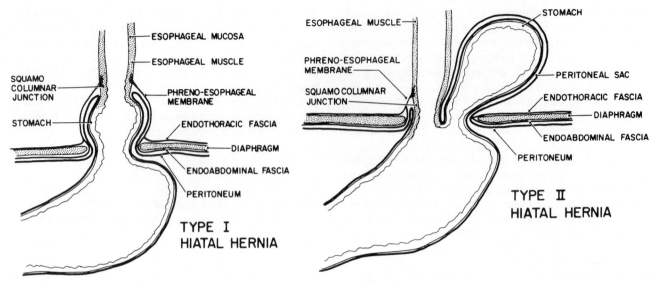

FIGURE 34-2. Diagrammatic representation of type I and type II hiatal hernia. In a type I hiatal hernia, the phrenoesophageal membrane is intact; in a type II hiatal hernia, a defect in the phrenoesophageal membrane permits herniation of the peritoneal sac. (Skinner DB, 1981: Hiatal hernia and gastroesophageal reflux. In Sabiston DC Jr [ed]: Davis-Christopher Textbook of Surgery, ed. 12, p. 823. Philadelphia, WB Saunders)

said to exist when the increased frequency and degree of reflux, and delayed clearing of refluxed material, are sufficient to produce symptoms or esophageal injury.

Pathologic gastroesophageal reflux accounts for approximately 75% of esophageal pathology and affects 0.4% of individuals in the United States (Stein et al., 1992c). The condition was formerly believed to develop principally in persons with a sliding hiatal hernia, but gastroesophageal reflux is now known to occur in many other conditions (Ellis, 1990). Probably most common of these is scleroderma, a progressive systemic disease that produces fibrosis of esophageal smooth muscle, resulting in absence of peristalsis in the lower two thirds of the esophagus (Mansour & Malone, 1988).

The predominant symptom of gastroesophageal reflux is epigastric or substernal discomfort, commonly termed *heartburn*. Two distinct patterns of reflux are observed. Some patients have an increased amount of reflux during daytime activities but do not experience it while reclining at night; in others, the regurgitation of gastric contents occurs primarily when they are reclining (Skinner, 1994). The most sensitive and specific diagnostic study for detection of gastroesophageal reflux is ambulatory esophageal pH monitoring (Stein et al., 1992c).

Treatment of esophageal reflux is aimed at relieving symptoms and reducing damaging effects of regurgitated gastric juice on the esophagus (Ellis, 1990). Modification of diet, sitting upright during and after meals, and keeping the head of the bed elevated are measures that often help reduce the degree of reflux.

Pharmacologic therapy usually consists of cimetidine or ranitidine to suppress gastric acid secretion and metoclopramide to enhance gastric emptying. Antacids also provide symptomatic relief. If medical therapy is unsuccessful in eliminating persistent symptoms of reflux, an antireflux operation may be necessary to restore competency to the LES.

Continued reflux of gastric contents into the esophagus eventually causes tissue ulceration that can lead to bleeding, perforation, or stricture formation. Gastroesophageal reflux can also result in development of *Barrett's esophagus*, a phenomenon in which columnar epithelium replaces the normally occurring squamous cell lining in the distal esophagus (Backer & LoCicero, 1986). The cellular dysplasia is thought to occur as a response to reflux of gastric acid into the esophagus. As squamous epithelium is destroyed by inflammation, it is replaced by columnar epithelium (Ellis, 1990). However, Barrett's esophagus is not simple reepithelialization of injured esophageal lining but rather the development of a heterogeneous collection of cell types and patterns, some resembling gastric body and cardia mucosa and others resembling gastric mucosa that has undergone intestinal metaplasia (Shahian & Ellis, 1989). The mucosal abnormality is significant because of the increased incidence of esophageal adenocarcinoma after its development. Patients with Barrett's esophagus are also at increased risk for progression of the mucosal abnormality up the esophagus, stricture formation, or hemorrhage from a Barrett's ulcer (Stein et al., 1992c). Accordingly, detection of Barrett's esophagus warrants medical therapy and, if necessary, a mentation, respectively. Rarely, undiagnosed esophageal perforation produces a localized, contained periesophageal abscess rather than mediastinitis. In such patients, the abscess may cause manifestations of chronic infection (anemia, weight loss, inanition) that lead to its eventual diagnosis and treatment.

FOREIGN BODY OBSTRUCTION

Foreign body obstruction occurs most frequently in young children. Occasionally, a foreign object becomes lodged in the esophagus of an adult. Common items that may inadvertently be swallowed and remain in the esophagus include chicken and fish bones, coins, large boluses of meat, safety pins, and dentures (Boyd, 1990). The esophagus is vulnerable to retention of a swallowed foreign body because of weak peristalsis and multiple narrowings (Holinger & Bowes, 1989). Objects usually lodge in one of the three normal areas of esophageal narrowing: (1) at the esophageal entrance in the area of the cricopharyngeus muscle; (2) in the midportion where the esophagus is indented by the crossing of the left mainstem bronchus and aortic arch; or (3) at the LES (Rothberg et al., 1994). Often, an object becomes lodged because a sharp edge impinges on esophageal mucosa (Henderson, 1989).

Clinical manifestations include chest pain, dysphagia, and a sensation of having "something stuck." If the esophagus is totally obstructed, drooling of saliva or aspiration may occur. The presence of a foreign object can usually be demonstrated radiographically, either with a plain chest roentgenogram or a contrast swallow study. Although the object sometimes disimpacts itself and passes into the stomach without sequelae, it may perforate the pleura or aorta or eventually lead to stricture formation (Henderson, 1989). Removal of foreign bodies is usually performed using a rigid esophagoscope with the patient under general anesthesia. Particular care is used if the object has sharp edges to avoid iatrogenic esophageal perforation during the removal procedure (Boyd, 1990). Prolonged impaction of a foreign object may lead to abscess formation or aspiration pneumonia.

ESOPHAGEAL CANCER

Esophageal cancer is relatively rare in the United States but is common in other parts of the world, such as China. Malignant neoplasms may occur in the upper, middle, or lower esophagus (Fig. 34-5). The histologic cell type is, with rare exception, either *squamous cell carcinoma* (most common in the upper and middle esophagus) or *adenocarcinoma* (most common in the distal esophagus). Unusual neoplasms of the esophagus include oat cell carcinoma, melanoma, and sarcoma (Caldwell et al., 1991). The etiology of esophageal cancer appears to be multifactorial and varies with geography and culture (Steiger, 1991). Smoking

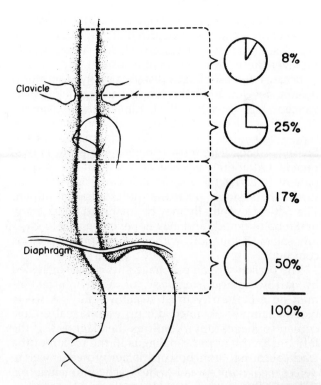

FIGURE 34-5. Distribution of esophageal carcinoma by anatomic location: upper (8%), middle (25%), and lower (17%) esophagus and gastroesophageal junction (50%). (Ellis FH Jr, 1990: Disorders of the esophagus in the adult. In Sabiston DC Jr, Spencer FC [eds]: Surgery of the Chest, ed. 5, p. 872. Philadelphia, WB Saunders)

and heavy alcohol ingestion are identified risk factors for squamous carcinoma; Barrett's epithelium in the distal esophagus predisposes to adenocarcinoma (Skinner & Belsey, 1988c). Conditions that produce chronic esophageal irritation or metaplastic strictures, such as lye burns, achalasia, and peptic reflux esophagitis, are also thought to predispose to esophageal carcinoma (Bains & Shields, 1994). The disease is more prevalent in men between 50 and 70 years of age and in African-Americans.

Cancer of the esophagus is a devastating illness, both because of its lethal nature and its profound impact on quality of life. The tumor spreads by direct invasion of surrounding structures and through lymphatic and hematogenous routes to distant structures. Neoplasms in the cervical esophagus are likely to invade the vagal nerves, trachea, vertebrae, carotid vessels, or thyroid; those in the thoracic portion invade the trachea, bronchi, pericardium and heart, pulmonary vessels, vertebrae, or aorta (Steiger, 1991). The depth of tumor invasion through the esophageal wall and the presence of tumor cells in regional lymph nodes are both predictive factors in determining prognosis in patients with esophageal cancer. Because the esophagus has no serosa, or outer protective layer, and because of its extensive submucosal lymphatic connections, local, regional, or distant spread has often occurred at the time of initial diagnosis (Backer & LoCicero, 1986). Metastasis to the liver, lung, or bone is not unusual.

Because the esophagus distends easily, symptoms do not develop until the tumor has reached an advanced stage (Steiger, 1991). Clinical manifestations of esophageal cancer are identical whether the cell type is squamous cell or adenocarcinoma (Skinner & Belsey, 1988c). The most common symptom is dysphagia. Often there is a history of weight loss and the patient is cachectic. As the disease progresses, the tumor increasingly obstructs the esophageal lumen. The patient eventually may be unable to tolerate any oral food or liquids and may not even be able to swallow saliva. Aspiration, with resultant pneumonia, is common.

The presence of an esophageal tumor is suggested by narrowing and irregularity of the esophageal lumen on a barium contrast swallow study. A tissue biopsy sample, obtained during esophageal endoscopy (esophagoscopy), confirms the diagnosis. If the lesion is in the upper esophagus in the region of the tracheal carina, bronchoscopy is performed as well to detect malignant spread to the tracheobronchial tree (Ellis, 1990).

Therapy for esophageal cancer remains somewhat controversial because no particular treatment or combination of treatments has proven effective in improving survival rates. Prognosis for survival is poor, particularly if the tumor is located in the upper one third of the esophagus. Because dysphagia is a late symptom, it is frequently accompanied by advanced disease and no other symptom is consistently present at an early stage of the disease (Skinner & Belsey, 1988c). It is estimated that cure is possible in fewer than 10% of patients with carcinoma of the esophagus (Ginsberg & Waters, 1994).

Surgical intervention may be undertaken for one of several purposes: (1) to surgically resect the tumor for curative purposes, (2) to restore the patient's ability to eat and drink, or (3) to divert esophageal contents (saliva) through an esophageal fistula and to provide an alternative route for alimentation. *Esophagogastrectomy with esophagogastrostomy* (removal of the diseased esophageal segment and reattachment of stomach to proximal esophagus) is considered to be the surgical procedure with the best relief of dysphagia and possibility of cure (Lund et al., 1990). Alternatively, resected esophagus may be replaced with a harvested segment of large bowel (*esophagogastrectomy with colon interposition*). These procedures are discussed further in Chapter 39, Surgical Treatment of Esophageal Disease.

Irradiation, chemotherapy, or both may be used as adjuncts to surgical therapy. Some surgeons use adjunctive therapy before surgical resection to reduce tumor size and increase the probability of technical success in removing all malignant cells (Naunheim et al., 1992). Others believe it is preferable to proceed initially with surgical resection and follow with adjunctive therapy. Enteral or parenteral alimentation is usually an important supplemental component of therapy because of the inevitable nutritional depletion associated with the disease.

Whether or not cure is possible, palliative therapy is important to relieve bothersome symptoms produced by esophageal obstruction. However, patients with incurable esophageal cancer have markedly limited life spans. Average survival without treatment or with palliation is only 4 months (Ellis, 1990). Therefore, palliative interventions must be carefully planned to restore swallowing capability and improve quality of life without exposing the patient to excessive morbidity from the treatment and lengthy hospitalization (Kratz et al., 1989). Ideally, palliative therapy maximizes the number of days that a patient is able to both swallow and be at home with family (Pagliero, 1991).

A number of palliative therapies may be useful to lessen obstruction and restore swallowing. In selected situations, tumor resection with restoration of esophageal continuity may be performed to relieve dysphagia and associated aspiration and to prevent hemorrhage from an ulcerating tumor or septic intoxication from one that is infected (Skinner & Belsey, 1988d). A procedure to bypass the obstructed esophagus without resection of the tumor (*retrosternal gastric bypass*) may be performed if the tumor is technically not resectable because of local extension to adjacent structures. Palliative surgical procedures are associated with considerable morbidity.

Alternatively, *esophageal dilatation* may be performed or a plastic tube (e.g., a *Celestin tube*) may be placed in the lumen of the esophagus through an endoscope to stent open the obstructed segment. Other palliative procedures performed by endoscopic means include photodynamic laser therapy and brachytherapy. *Photodynamic therapy* consists of intravenous infusion of a photosensitive substance; *laser therapy* is then performed by means of esophagoscopy to create an opening in the occluded esophagus large enough for the passage of secretions and ingested food. *Brachytherapy* is a form of radiation therapy in which radioactive isotopes are implanted directly into the tumor. *Radiation therapy,* alone or in combination with *chemotherapy*, may be used for palliation. However, radiation may lead to lung damage, esophageal necrosis or stricture, or tracheoesophageal fistula; chemotherapy has also proved disappointing in prolonging complication-free survival (Skinner & Belsey, 1988d).

REFERENCES

Backer CL, LoCicero III J, 1986: Surgical management of esophageal disorders. Crit Care Q 9:12
Bains MS, Shields TW, 1994: Squamous cell carcinoma of the esophagus. In Shields TW (ed): General Thoracic Surgery, ed. 4. Baltimore, Williams & Wilkins

Boyd AD, 1990: Endoscopy: Bronchoscopy and esophagoscopy. In Sabiston DC Jr, Spencer FC (eds): Surgery of the Chest, ed. 5. Philadelphia, WB Saunders

Caldwell CB, Bains MS, Burt M, 1991: Unusual malignant neoplasms of the esophagus. J Thorac Cardiovasc Surg 101:100

Duranceau A, Lafontaine ER, Deschamps C, 1991: Complications of operations for esophageal motor disorders. In Waldhausen JA, Orringer MB (eds): Complications in Cardiothoracic Surgery. St. Louis, Mosby–Year Book

Ellis FH Jr, 1990: Disorders of the esophagus in the adult. In Sabiston DC Jr, Spencer FC (eds): Surgery of the Chest, ed. 5. Philadelphia, WB Saunders

Ferguson MK, 1991: Evolution of therapy for pharyngoesophageal (Zenker's) diverticulum. Ann Thorac Surg 51:848

Ginsberg RJ, Waters PF, 1994: Surgical palliation of inoperable carcinoma of the esophagus. In Shields TW (ed): General Thoracic Surgery, ed. 4. Baltimore, Williams & Wilkins

Gustafson RA, Murray GF, 1989: Benign tumor. In Grillo HC, Austen WG, Wilkins EW, et al. (eds): Current Therapy in Cardiothoracic Surgery. Toronto, BC Decker

Henderson RD, 1989: Benign strictures of the esophagus. In Shields TW (ed): General Thoracic Surgery, ed. 3. Philadelphia, Lea & Febiger

Henderson RD, Henderson RF, 1990: Surgical management of 100 consecutive esophageal strictures. J Thorac Cardiovasc Surg 99:1

Holinger LD, Bowes AK, 1989: Management of foreign bodies of the upper aerodigestive tract. In Shields TW (ed): General Thoracic Surgery, ed. 3. Philadelphia, Lea & Febiger

Kratz JM, Reed CE, Crawford FA, et al., 1989: A comparison of endoesophageal tubes. J Thorac Cardiovasc Surg 97:19

Lund O, Kimose HK, Aarogaard MT, et al., 1990: Risk stratification and long-term results after surgical treatment of carcinomas of the thoracic esophagus and cardia. J Thorac Cardiovasc Surg 99:200

Mansour KA, Malone CE, 1988: Surgery for scleroderma of the esophagus: A 12 year experience. Ann Thorac Surg 46:513

Naunheim KS, Baue AE, 1991: Esophageal dysmotility. In Baue AE, Geha AS, Hammond GL, et al. (eds): Glenn's Thoracic and Cardiovascular Surgery, ed. 5. Norwalk, CT, Appleton & Lange

Naunheim KS, Petruska PJ, Roy TS, et al., 1992: Preoperative chemotherapy and radiotherapy for esophageal carcinoma. J Thorac Cardiovasc Surg 103:887

Orringer MB, 1991: Complications of esophageal resection and reconstruction. In Waldhausen JH, Orringer MB (eds): Complications in Cardiothoracic Surgery. St. Louis, Mosby–Year Book

Pagliero KM, 1991: Palliative treatment for carcinoma of the esophagus. In Baue AE, Geha AS, Hammond GL, et al. (eds): Glenn's Thoracic and Cardiovascular Surgery, ed. 5. Norwalk, CT, Appleton & Lange

Rothberg M, Johnson S, DeMeester TR, 1994: Anatomy of the esophagus. In Shields TW (ed): General Thoracic Surgery, ed. 4. Baltimore, Williams & Wilkins

Shahian DM, Ellis FH Jr, 1989: Barrett's esophagus. In Shields TW (ed): General Thoracic Surgery, ed. 3. Philadelphia, Lea & Febiger

Skinner DB, 1994: Gastroesophageal reflux. In Shields TW (ed): General Thoracic Surgery, ed. 4. Baltimore, Williams & Wilkins

Skinner DB, 1990: Esophageal hiatal hernia—the condition: Clinical manifestations and diagnosis. In Sabiston DC Jr, Spencer FC (eds): Surgery of the Chest, ed. 5. Philadelphia, WB Saunders

Skinner DB, Belsey RH, 1988a: The pharynx, cricopharyngeus, and Zenker's diverticulum. In Management of Esophageal Disease. Philadelphia, WB Saunders

Skinner DB, Belsey RH, 1988b: Spontaneous rupture and Boerhaave's syndrome. In Management of Esophageal Disease. Philadelphia, WB Saunders

Skinner DB, Belsey RH, 1988c: Esophageal malignancies: Incidence, etiology, presentation, and diagnosis. In Management of Esophageal Disease. Philadelphia, WB Saunders

Skinner DB, Belsey RH, 1988d: Palliation for advanced esophageal cancer. In Management of Esophageal Disease. Philadelphia, WB Saunders

Steiger Z, 1991: Esophageal cancer. In Baue AE, Geha AS, Hammond GL, et al. (eds): Glenn's Thoracic and Cardiovascular Surgery, ed. 5. Norwalk, CT, Appleton & Lange

Stein HJ, DeMeester TR, Hinder RA, 1992a: The concept of outpatient physiologic monitoring to diagnose functional foregut disorders. Curr Probl Surg 24:425

Stein HJ, DeMeester TR, Hinder RA, 1992b: Evaluation and surgical management of motor disorders of the esophageal body and lower esophageal sphincter. Curr Probl Surg 24:447

Stein HJ, DeMeester TR, Hinder RA, 1992c: Evaluation and surgical management of the gastroesophageal reflux disease. Curr Probl Surg 24:482

Stirling MC, Orringer MB, 1988: The combined Collis-Nissen operation for esophageal reflux strictures. Ann Thorac Surg 45:148

Trastek VF, 1994: Esophageal diverticula. In Shields TW (ed): General Thoracic Surgery, ed. 4. Baltimore, Williams & Wilkins

Vanecko RM, Shields TW, 1994: Esophageal trauma. In Shields TW (ed): General Thoracic Surgery, ed. 4. Baltimore, Williams & Wilkins

Wilkins EW Jr, 1989: Motor disturbances of deglutition. In Shields TW (ed): General Thoracic Surgery, ed. 3. Philadelphia, Lea & Febiger

Wilkins EW Jr, 1994: Motor disturbances of deglutition. In Shields TW (ed): General Thoracic Surgery, ed. 4. Baltimore, Williams & Wilkins

Witte J, Pratschke E, 1991: Esophageal perforation. In Baue AE, Geha AS, Hammond GL, et al. (eds): Glenn's Thoracic and Cardiovascular Surgery, ed. 5. Norwalk, CT, Appleton & Lange

35

DISEASES OF THE MEDIASTINUM AND CHEST WALL

DISORDERS OF THE MEDIASTINUM
    Mediastinal Masses
    Superior Vena Cava Syndrome
    Fibrosing Mediastinitis
MYASTHENIA GRAVIS
    Clinical Manifestations
    Diagnosis and Treatment

CHEST WALL DISORDERS
    Tumors of the Chest Wall
    Pectus Deformities

DISORDERS OF THE MEDIASTINUM

The mediastinum is an extrapleural space that lies between the right and left thoracic cavities and contains vital structures of the cardiovascular, pulmonary, enteric, and nervous systems (Ewing & Hardy, 1991). It is surrounded by the thoracic inlet (superior), the diaphragm (inferior), the parietal pleura (lateral), the sternum (anterior), and the vertebral column (posterior). The mediastinum is commonly described as being composed of three anatomic subdivisions: anterosuperior, middle, and posterior. Structures contained within each of the three areas are listed in Table 35-1.

MEDIASTINAL MASSES

Although most mediastinal masses represent metastatic spread of tumors originating elsewhere, *primary neoplasms* and *cysts* of the mediastinum can occur and are the focus of this discussion. The most common primary mediastinal masses are cysts, neurogenic tumors, thymomas, lymphomas, and germ cell tumors (Davis et al., 1990) (Table 35-2). The incidence of these various mediastinal tumors and cysts differs with the age of the patient group under consideration (Shields, 1991a).

Most mediastinal masses arise in the anterosuperior subdivision. Of these, thymoma, lymphoma, and germ cell tumors are most common. Masses occurring in the middle mediastinum are usually lymphomas or cysts (Cohen et al., 1991). Tumors that originate in the posterior mediastinum are usually neurogenic, arising from intercostal nerves, sympathetic ganglia, or paraganglia cells (Davis, 1990). Less commonly occurring posterior mediastinal masses include thymic and bronchogenic cysts. The majority of primary mediastinal masses in adults are benign. However, the number of adults with malignant mediastinal lesions, specifically lymphomas and neurogenic tumors, has increased in the past 2 decades (Cohen et al., 1991).

Clinical Manifestations

Symptoms are present in approximately 56% of adults diagnosed with mediastinal lesions (Cohen et al., 1991). They are usually related to compression or invasion of structures adjacent to the mass (Davis et al., 1990). In the adult, most normal mediastinal structures are mobile enough to conform to distortion from pressure; malignant disease, on the other hand, is often accompanied by both distortion and fixation of vital structures (Shields, 1991a). Consequently,

TABLE 35-1. STRUCTURES CONTAINED IN THE THREE ANATOMIC SUBDIVISIONS OF THE MEDIASTINUM

Anterosuperior Mediastinum

Thymus gland
Aortic arch and branches
Great veins
Lymphatics
Fatty areolar tissue

Middle Mediastinum

Heart
Pericardium
Phrenic nerves
Tracheal bifurcation
Main bronchi
Pulmonary hila
Lymph nodes

Posterior Mediastinum

Esophagus
Vagus nerves
Sympathetic nervous chain
Thoracic duct
Descending aorta
Azygous and hemiazygous systems
Paravertebral lymph nodes
Fatty areolar tissue

symptoms of obstruction and compression are more commonly observed in association with malignant lesions.

The most common symptoms of large tumors are pain, cough, and dyspnea. Other manifestations of local invasion or compression include recurrent respiratory infections, hemoptysis, dysphagia, hoarseness, Horner's syndrome, superior vena cava (SVC)

TABLE 35-2. MOST COMMON PRIMARY MEDIASTINAL CYSTS AND NEOPLASMS

Cysts
  Bronchogenic
  Pericardial
  Enteric
Neurogenic tumors
  Neurilemoma
  Ganglioneuroma
  Neuroblastoma
  Neurofibroma
Thymoma
Lymphoma
  Hodgkin's
  Non-Hodgkin's
Germ cell tumors
  Teratoma
  Seminoma
  Nonseminoma

syndrome, and cardiac arrhythmias (Ewing & Hardy, 1991). Tumor location affects the type of presenting symptoms. Anterosuperior masses often lead to SVC syndrome, middle lesions to cardiac tamponade, and posterior lesions to spinal cord compression (Davis et al., 1990). Signs and symptoms that occur are also related to the lesion's size and the presence of infection or associated disease states (Shields, 1991a).

Mediastinal tumors sometimes produce hormones or antibodies that cause systemic syndromes (e.g., thyrotoxicosis due to mediastinal goiter or hypercalcemia caused by mediastinal parathyroid adenoma) (Davis et al., 1990). Serum levels of human chorionic gonadotropin may be elevated in the presence of malignant germ cell tumors, and serum alpha-fetoprotein elevation indicates a tumor that contains nonseminomatous elements (Hainsworth & Greco, 1991). Constitutional symptoms, such as fatigue, weight loss, fever, and chills, are sometimes associated with malignant lesions.

Diagnosis and Treatment

Mediastinal lesions are generally detected because of an abnormal shadow or mediastinal configuration on the chest roentgenogram. Because primary mediastinal masses are often associated with a characteristic location, identification of the anatomic subdivision within which a mass is found provides important descriptive information and is often helpful in differential diagnosis. Posteroanterior and lateral chest films are used to determine the lesion's location in the anterosuperior, middle, or posterior portion of the mediastinum. The chest roentgenogram also provides useful information about lesion size and relative density (solid or cystic), the presence and pattern of calcification, and displacement or alteration of normal mediastinal structures (Davis et al., 1990).

Computed tomography provides a sensitive method of distinguishing between fatty, vascular, cystic, and soft tissue masses (Shields, 1991a). Accordingly, a computed tomographic scan is almost always obtained to define more accurately the character and size of the mass, its location, and the proximity or involvement of contiguous structures. Magnetic resonance imaging may also be useful in evaluation of mediastinal masses, particularly to provide definition of posterior mediastinal tumors when spinal cord compression is suspected.

For most mediastinal tumors, surgical resection is the primary therapy, regardless of benignancy or malignancy. However, definitive diagnosis of a mediastinal tumor before surgical exploration is desirable because some tumors are treated primarily with other modalities. Tissue for histologic examination may be obtained by mediastinotomy, mediastinoscopy, video-assisted thoracoscopy, or thoracotomy. Fine-needle aspiration biopsy can sometimes provide a definitive cytologic diagnosis.

Specific Neoplasms and Cysts

Thymomas are tumors derived from thymic epithelial cells. They occur most often in adults in their fifth or sixth decade of life (Shields, 1991b). Thirty to 50% of patients with thymoma have associated myasthenia gravis, and 10% to 15% of patients with myasthenia have a thymoma (Kirschner, 1991). Myasthenia gravis is discussed later in the chapter.

Thymomas may be either benign or malignant. In contrast to most neoplasms, benignancy or malignancy of a thymoma cannot be established by histologic examination of tumor cells. Instead, the determination of malignancy is made primarily by gross examination of the tumor at the time of surgical resection. Pathologic staging is based on the extent of the tumor's invasive characteristics (i.e., absence of an enclosing capsule or invasion of adjacent mediastinal fat, pleura, pericardium, great vessels, or lung) (Wilkins et al., 1991). Staging by the surgeon is supplemented by histologic examination of the tissue to detect microscopic spread not evident under gross inspection. Complete surgical resection is the treatment of choice for all patients, except those with grossly nonresectable disease or with evidence of tumor spread beyond the thorax (Shields, 1991b). Radiation therapy is used adjunctively in patients with thymomas that are considered malignant.

Lymphomas are malignant tumors of the lymphoid tissues. They are broadly categorized as *Hodgkin's lymphoma* or *non-Hodgkin's lymphoma*. In most patients with lymphoma, the mediastinum is involved at some point during the course of the disease; it is infrequently the sole site at the time of diagnosis (Davis et al., 1990). Lymphoma differs from most other mediastinal tumors in that it is treated primarily with radiation therapy and chemotherapy (Ewing & Hardy, 1991). Mediastinoscopy, mediastinotomy, or thoracotomy may be necessary to obtain adequate tissue for histologic diagnosis.

Germ cell tumors include teratoma, seminoma, and nonseminomatous germ cell tumor. *Teratoma* is a benign neoplasm composed of multiple tissues foreign to the area in which the tumor is found (Ewing & Hardy, 1991). Mediastinal teratomas are usually cystic and frequently contain skin, hair, smooth muscle, teeth, bone, or fat. Teratoma is treated by surgical resection of the tumor. Complete excision is usually possible, and prognosis after tumor removal is excellent (Trastek & Pairolero, 1991).

Malignant germ cell tumors are categorized histologically as seminoma or nonseminomatous germ cell tumor. The great majority occur in men between 20 and 35 years of age (Hainsworth & Greco, 1991). *Seminoma* is histologically identical to malignant germinal tumor of testicular origin. Surgical resection is performed infrequently since radiation therapy or chemotherapy can produce cure in many instances. *Nonseminomatous germ cell tumors* are those that con-

tain areas of embryonal carcinoma, teratocarcinoma, choriocarcinoma, or endodermal sinus tumor (Hainsworth & Greco, 1991). They are more aggressive than seminomas and are associated with a less favorable prognosis. Recommended therapy for this form of germ cell tumor includes intensive chemotherapy and aggressive surgical resection of residual disease (Wright et al., 1990).

Mediastinal cysts may be bronchogenic, pericardial, or enteric. Bronchogenic cysts are most common. They are closed sacs thought to result from an abnormal budding process that occurs during early development of the foregut (St.-Georges et al., 1991). Despite the benignancy of mediastinal cysts, they frequently produce symptoms such as chest pain, dyspnea, or cough. Surgical resection is recommended to establish a definitive tissue diagnosis, alleviate symptoms, and prevent complications (Duranceau & Deslaurier, 1991).

Neurogenic tumors include (1) neurilemomas (schwannomas), (2) ganglioneuromas and neuroblastomas, (3) neurofibromas, and (4) paraganglionic tumors (Ewing & Hardy, 1991). Although the majority of neurogenic tumors arising in children are malignant, those that occur in adults are most often benign (Davis et al., 1990). Because of the characteristic shape, the term *dumbbell tumor* is commonly used to denote neurogenic tumors that extend into the spinal canal. Neurogenic tumors are generally treated with surgical resection. Adjunctive treatment, usually radiation therapy, is recommended for malignant tumors.

SUPERIOR VENA CAVA SYNDROME

The SVC is the major vessel draining venous blood from the head, neck, upper extremities, and upper thorax (Stea & Kinsella, 1991). It is confined in a tight compartment in the superior mediastinum, immediately adjacent and anterior to the trachea and right mainstem bronchus and surrounded by lymph nodes draining the entire right and lower portion of the left chest (McFadden & Jamplis, 1994). *Superior vena cava syndrome* is a condition in which venous flow through the SVC is obstructed either as a result of extrinsic compression of the vessel or internal occlusion from thrombus or a foreign body.

In approximately 90% of cases, SVC syndrome occurs secondary to malignant disease (Doty & Jones, 1991). By far the most common etiology is bronchogenic cancer, usually originating in the right upper lobe. Mediastinal tumors, lymphoma, or metastatic disease from other organs can also cause SVC syndrome. Nonmalignant conditions that can lead to SVC syndrome include granulomatous diseases, such as histoplasmosis or tuberculosis; mediastinal infection; mediastinal goiter; and the presence of an indwelling central venous catheter or pacemaker lead.

Clinical Manifestations

SVC obstruction causes increased pressure in veins that normally drain into the vessel. It also stimulates the formation of extensive venous collateral circulation; most important is the azygous venous collateral pathway in the chest wall (Doty & Jones, 1991). SVC syndrome usually develops insidiously over a period of weeks or months (Stea & Kinsella, 1991). The most prominent feature is swelling of the face, neck, and upper extremities, caused by engorgement of veins that normally empty into the SVC. Venous distention is usually apparent in the neck vessels, as well as in those of the anterior chest wall. Plethora (i.e., red, florid complexion) and cyanosis of the face may be apparent, particularly when the patient is recumbent (Stea & Kinsella, 1991). Other manifestations of SVC syndrome include hoarseness, stridor, tongue swelling, nasal congestion, epistaxis, dysphagia, headaches, dizziness, syncope, lethargy, and chest pain (Doty & Jones, 1991). Severity of symptoms is affected by the rapidity with which obstruction occurs and, therefore, the degree to which collateral pathways have developed. Because venous drainage through the inferior vena cava is not impeded, the trunk and lower extremities are not affected by SVC syndrome.

Diagnosis and Treatment

If extrinsic compression due to malignancy is the presumed cause, a percutaneous needle or incisional biopsy is performed to obtain a histologic diagnosis (Davis et al., 1990). Invasive diagnostic procedures, such as bronchoscopy or mediastinoscopy, may also be necessary and can usually be performed safely despite increased venous pressure. Radiation therapy or chemotherapy is generally used to treat SVC syndrome of malignant etiology. Even if the diagnosis of malignancy is only presumptive, SVC syndrome is considered by some to be one of the rare indications for instituting radiation therapy in the absence of a definitive tissue diagnosis of cancer. Others advocate a tissue diagnosis in all patients before initiating therapy (Gordon & Kies, 1991). Chemotherapy has proven preferable to radiation therapy in selected patients with chemosensitive tumors. However, in the presence of edema, it carries the hazard of inducing vomiting, resulting in potential airway obstruction. The malignant processes that cause SVC syndrome are usually inoperable.

In patients with SVC syndrome secondary to benign disease, bed rest with head elevation is helpful in producing gradual improvement of symptoms. Diuretics and corticosteroids may also be administered, particularly to reduce cerebral edema that may lead to central nervous system dysfunction. If the cause of venous obstruction is thrombus, thrombolytic therapy may be effective in restoring blood flow through the SVC. Venous thrombectomy or a surgical procedure to bypass the obstructed SVC may also be considered. SVC syndrome is usually not life-threatening unless it develops rapidly or is associated with neurologic sequelae (Davis et al., 1990). In such unusual cases, emergent treatment, usually radiation therapy, is performed.

FIBROSING MEDIASTINITIS

Fibrosing mediastinitis is an uncommon entity that appears to occur when a specific agent or agents produce a granulomatous reaction and immune response in the mediastinum, resulting in varying degrees of sclerosis (Ewing & Hardy, 1991). It is thought to occur most often in association with the fungal infection histoplasmosis. However, in many cases, no histologic diagnosis other than fibrosis can be established (Hood, 1994). The process typically begins with a granulomatous reaction in mediastinal lymph nodes and surrounding tissue and can progress to more generalized inflammation and fibrosis. A biopsy of mediastinal tissue is usually performed for diagnostic purposes.

Extensive fibrosis can lead to compression of structures contained in the mediastinum, including the vena cavae, trachea, bronchi, or esophagus (Davis et al., 1990). Associated clinical manifestations include signs of SVC syndrome, chest pain, dysphagia, or dyspnea (Van Trigt, 1990). Treatment of fibrosing mediastinitis is primarily supportive. Surgical therapy may become necessary to treat SVC syndrome, bronchial or esophageal strictures, constrictive pericarditis, or other complications (Ewing & Hardy, 1991).

MYASTHENIA GRAVIS

Myasthenia gravis is a disease caused by impaired neuromuscular transmission in voluntary muscles. The disorder, which is thought to have an autoimmune origin, results from an imbalance in the interaction of acetylcholine released from presynaptic terminals and acetylcholine receptors on the postsynaptic terminals (Olanow & Wechsler, 1990).

CLINICAL MANIFESTATIONS

Myasthenia gravis is characterized by progressive weakness and easy fatigability of voluntary muscles. Almost any muscle group in the body can be involved. Most commonly affected are the ocular, shoulder, and upper extremity muscles (Ewing & Hardy, 1991). Ptosis and diplopia are frequent presenting symptoms and eventually occur in the great majority of patients. The involvement of bulbar and skeletal muscle groups can produce symptoms of dysphagia, respiratory distress, impaired chewing, dysarthria, nasal speech, facial weakness (transverse smile or involuntary grimace), atrophic tongue, difficulty supporting the head with neck muscles, and symmetric weakness of the extremities (Olanow & Wechsler, 1990). The most serious symptoms are those of respiratory distress, requiring mechanical ventilatory support (Kirschner, 1991).

Clinical manifestations of the disease may develop insidiously or appear precipitously. Symptoms typically fluctuate throughout the day and from day to day, with exacerbation after exercise and as the day progresses (Ewing & Hardy, 1991). Pregnancy, stress, allergies, or menses may also affect the degree of symptoms. Although the disorder may be confined to the ocular muscles, most patients develop generalized weakness within 1 year of onset of the ocular form (Olanow & Wechsler, 1990).

DIAGNOSIS AND TREATMENT

Diagnostic confirmation of myasthenia gravis is achieved by performing a *Tensilon test*, which consists of administering intravenous edrophonium (Tensilon), a short-acting anticholinesterase agent. Ninety-five percent of patients with myasthenia gravis experience immediate improvement after receiving the drug (Ewing & Hardy, 1991).

Medical therapy for myasthenia gravis includes medications (anticholinesterase, corticosteroid, and immunosuppressive agents) and plasmapheresis. The clinical course of the disease and response to treatment are difficult to predict and episodic remissions do occur. For reasons that are incompletely understood, significant clinical improvement can be achieved in some cases with surgical removal of the thymus gland from the mediastinum (Fig. 35-1).

Thymectomy is always performed in patients with myasthenia gravis if a thymoma is present. In the absence of thymoma, the indications and timing for thymectomy are somewhat controversial. It is most commonly performed in patients with generalized symptoms of the disease, including ptosis, dysarthria, dysphagia, and weakness of the respiratory muscles. Clinical improvement occurs in 60% to 85% of patients after thymectomy; complete remission is reported in 20% to 35% (Ewing & Hardy, 1991). Sometimes clinical improvement does not occur for 3 to 5 years from the time of operation (Olanow & Wechsler, 1990).

CHEST WALL DISORDERS

TUMORS OF THE CHEST WALL

Tumors of the chest wall are unusual. Those that do occur may involve the soft tissues, the bony structures, or both and may arise from any of a variety of cell types (Table 35-3). Approximately half are benign and half are malignant.

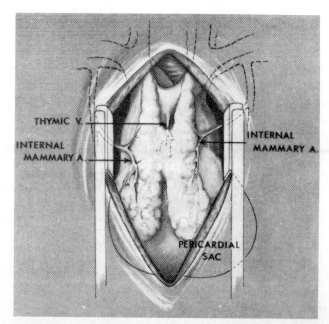

FIGURE 35-1. Anatomic location of thymus gland in anterior mediastinum overlying pericardium and great vessels. (Trastek VF, Payne WS, 1989: Surgery of the thymus gland. In Shields TW [ed]: General Thoracic Surgery, ed. 3, p. 1124. Philadelphia, Lea & Febiger)

Benign Tumors

Benign bony tumors include fibrous dysplasia, chondroma, osteochondroma, and eosinophilic granuloma. *Fibrous dysplasia* is most common, usually affecting posterior and lateral ribs. It generally produces a lesion that expands slowly and painlessly until the periosteum is stretched or the rib is fractured (McCormack, 1991). *Chondroma*, a tumor of the costal cartilage, usually occurs as a small, slowly enlarging, sometimes painful lesion in the anterior chest wall. Although benign, chondromas can recur after excision and sometimes undergo malignant degeneration. *Osteochondroma*, which arises from the rib cortex, causes a painless protuberance of the rib. *Eosinophilic granuloma* is a painful bony lesion, frequently accompanied by constitutional symptoms of fever and mal-

TABLE 35-3. PRIMARY CHEST WALL TUMORS

Benign	Malignant
Bony skeleton	Bony skeleton
Fibrous dysplasia	Chondrosarcoma
Chondroma	Osteogenic sarcoma
Osteochondroma	Myeloma
Eosinophilic granuloma	Ewing's sarcoma
Soft tissue	Soft tissue
Fibroma	Fibrous histiocytoma
Lipoma	Rhabdomyosarcoma

aise. Benign tumors that may originate in the chest wall soft tissue include *fibroma* and *lipoma*.

Malignant Tumors

Malignant neoplasms may originate in the chest wall or may represent metastases from lung, pleura, mediastinum, muscle, or breast (Pairolero, 1994). The most common primary malignant tumor of the chest wall is *chondrosarcoma*. It occurs most often in the anterior chest wall and in young adults, usually men. Less common are *myeloma,* which usually occurs in older individuals and *Ewing's sarcoma,* which is predominantly seen in children and particularly boys. *Osteogenic sarcoma* is rare. It is more virulent and is associated with early hematogenous spread and a poor prognosis (McCormack, 1991). *Fibrous histiocytoma* and *rhabdomyosarcoma* are examples of malignant soft tissue tumors.

Diagnosis and Treatment

The first indication of a chest wall tumor is a visible or palpable mass that is often asymptomatic. As the neoplasm enlarges, approximately two thirds of benign and almost all malignant lesions become painful (Pairolero, 1990). Computed tomography is particularly useful in defining the extent of the tumor and determining the presence of extension into adjacent structures. Magnetic resonance imaging may also be helpful in delineating spinal cord involvement (McCormack, 1991). Definitive diagnosis is made by needle or incisional biopsy if the planned surgical treatment is extensive. In other cases, a definitive diagnosis may be made at the time of tumor resection.

Surgical resection is the treatment of choice for most benign tumors because of pain and a mass effect produced by the lesion or the potential for some benign lesions to undergo malignant degeneration. Most primary and some secondary malignant neoplasms are also treated with surgical resection. Even if cure is not anticipated, palliative resection may be performed to reduce pain caused by the lesion or to remove an infected, bleeding, or ulcerated tumor that is malodorous or disfiguring. A wide excision is performed for malignant lesions. If a significant portion of chest wall is removed, chest wall reconstruction may be necessary to maintain adequate respiratory function and to protect the thoracic viscera (Pairolero, 1994). In some cases, a muscle flap alone may provide adequate coverage of soft tissues. In others, a synthetic prosthesis may be necessary to adequately restore the chest wall. Depending on the type of tumor, radiation therapy or chemotherapy may be used adjunctively.

PECTUS DEFORMITIES

Pectus deformities are structural abnormalities of the anterior chest wall. The etiology of the deformities is unknown but is thought to be multifactorial (Welch & Shamberger, 1989). An increased familial incidence exists and pectus deformities are slightly more common in boys. *Pectus excavatum* (funnel chest) is the most common developmental deformity of the chest. It is characterized by inward depression of the lower sternum and adjacent cartilages (Fig. 35-2). The deformity is usually apparent soon after birth, progresses during childhood, and becomes even more pronounced during adolescence (Fonkalsrud, 1991).

Pectus excavatum primarily affects posture, typically producing slouching, sunken chest, and rounded shoulders. The degree of deformity varies from slight to severe. Moderate to severe pectus excavatum causes displacement of the heart into the left chest and impingement of pulmonary expansion during inspiration (Fonkalsrud, 1991). However, the significance of the deformity in producing physiologic alterations in cardiorespiratory function is a matter of some controversy (Wynn et al., 1990).

Less common is *pectus carinatum* (pigeon breast), a deformity consisting of outward protrusion of the sternum. Pectus carinatum produces a rigid chest with increased anteroposterior diameter locked into a position of nearly full inspiration; respiratory efforts

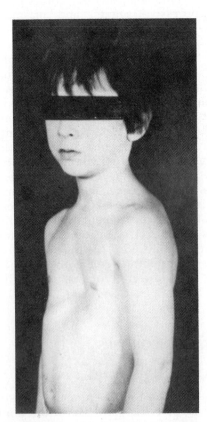

FIGURE 35-2. Child with pectus excavatum deformity. (Sandza JF Jr, Clark RE, 1982: The chest wall. In Ellis FH Jr, Goldsmith HS [eds]: Goldsmith Practice of Surgery, rev. ed, p. 22. Philadelphia, Harper & Row)

are less efficient and gradual loss of lung compliance, progressive emphysema, and pulmonary infection may result (Fonkalsrud, 1991).

In both types of pectus deformity, the primary consequence is the psychological effect of cosmetic disfigurement. However, pectus deformities are progressive and, when severe, are believed by some to contribute to cardiac arrhythmias and exercise intolerance. Currently, many pectus deformities are repaired in early childhood (ages 2–5 years) and most are repaired before the adolescent growth spurt. Rarely, a pectus repair is performed during adolescence or early adulthood.

REFERENCES

Cohen AH, Thompson L, Edwards FH, Bellamy RF, 1991: Primary cysts and tumors of the mediastinum. Ann Thorac Surg 51:378

Davis RD, Oldham HN Jr, Sabiston DC Jr, 1990: The mediastinum. In Sabiston DC Jr, Spencer FC (eds): Surgery of the Chest, ed. 5. Philadelphia, WB Saunders

Doty DB, Jones KW, 1991: Superior vena cava syndrome. In Baue AE, Geha AS, Hammond GL, et al. (eds): Glenn's Thoracic and Cardiovascular Surgery, ed. 5. Norwalk, CT, Appleton & Lange

Duranceau AC, Deslauriers J, 1991: Foregut cysts of the mediastinum in the adult. In Shields TW (ed): The Mediastinum. Philadelphia, Lea & Febiger

Ewing HP, Hardy JD, 1991: The mediastinum. In Baue AE, Geha AS, Hammond GL, et al. (eds): Glenn's Thoracic and Cardiovascular Surgery, ed. 5. Norwalk, CT, Appleton & Lange

Fonkalsrud EW, 1991: Chest wall abnormalities. In Baue AE, Geha AS, Hammond GL, et al. (eds): Glenn's Thoracic and Cardiovascular Surgery, ed. 5. Norwalk, CT, Appleton & Lange

Gordon LI, Kies MS, 1991: Diagnosis and treatment of mediastinal lymphomas. In Shields TW (ed): The Mediastinum. Philadelphia, Lea & Febiger

Hainsworth JD, Greco FA, 1991: General features of malignant germ cell tumors and primary seminomas of the mediastinum. In Shields TW (ed): The Mediastinum. Philadelphia, Lea & Febiger

Hood RM, 1994: Bronchial compressive diseases. In Shields TW (ed): General Thoracic Surgery, ed. 4. Baltimore, Williams & Wilkins

Kirschner PA, 1991: Myasthenia gravis. In Shields TW (ed): The Mediastinum. Philadelphia, Lea & Febiger

McCormack P, 1991: Chest wall tumors. In Baue AE, Geha AS, Hammond GL, et al. (eds): Glenn's Thoracic and Cardiovascular Surgery, ed. 5. Norwalk, CT, Appleton & Lange

McFadden PM, Jamplis RW, 1994: Superior vena cava syndrome. In Shields TW (ed): General Thoracic Surgery, ed. 4. Baltimore, Williams & Wilkins

Olanow CW, Wechsler AS, 1990: Surgical management of myasthenia gravis. In Sabiston DC Jr, Spencer FC (eds), 1990: Surgery of the Chest, ed. 5. Philadelphia, WB Saunders

Pairolero PC, 1994: Chest wall tumors. In Shields TW (ed): General Thoracic Surgery, ed. 4. Baltimore, Williams & Wilkins

Pairolero PC, 1990: Surgical management of neoplasms of the chest wall. In Sabiston DC Jr, Spencer FC (eds): Surgery of the Chest, ed. 5. Philadelphia, WB Saunders

Shields TW, 1991a: Primary mediastinal tumors and cysts and their diagnostic investigation. In Shields TW (ed): The Mediastinum. Philadelphia, Lea & Febiger

Shields TW, 1991b: Thymic tumors. In Shields TW (ed): The Mediastinum. Philadelphia, Lea & Febiger

St.-Georges R, Deslauriers J, Duranceau A, et al., 1991: Clinical spectrum of bronchogenic cysts of the mediastinum and lung in the adult. Ann Thorac Surg 52:6

Stea B, Kinsella TJ, 1991: Superior vena cava syndrome: Clinical features, diagnosis, and treatment. In Shields TW (ed): The Mediastinum. Philadelphia, Lea & Febiger

Trastek VF, Pairolero PC, 1991: Benign germ cell tumors of the mediastinum. In Shields TW (ed): The Mediastinum. Philadelphia, Lea & Febiger

Van Trigt P, 1990: Lung infections and diffuse interstitial lung disease. In Sabiston DC Jr, Spencer FC (eds), 1990: Surgery of the Chest, ed. 5. Philadelphia, WB Saunders

Welch KJ, Shamberger RC, 1989: Chest wall deformities. In Shields TW (ed): General Thoracic Surgery, ed. 3. Philadelphia, Lea & Febiger

Wilkins EW, Grillo HC, Scannell JG, et al., 1991: Role of staging in prognosis and management of thymoma. Ann Thorac Surg 51:888

Wright CD, Kesler KA, Nichols CR, et al., 1990: Primary nonseminomatous germ cell tumors. J Thorac Cardiovasc Surg 99:210

Wynn SR, Driscoll DJ, Ostrom NK, et al., 1990: Exercise cardiorespiratory function in adolescents with pectus excavatum. J Thorac Cardiovasc Surg 99:41

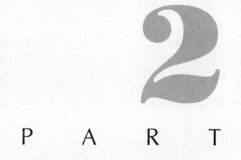

P A R T

PREOPERATIVE EVALUATION AND PREPARATION

36

DIAGNOSTIC EVALUATION OF THORACIC DISEASE

ROENTGENOGRAPHIC STUDIES
  Chest Roentgenograms
  Tomography
  Other Roentgenographic Studies
LABORATORY PROCEDURES
FUNCTIONAL ASSESSMENT STUDIES
  Pulmonary Function Testing
  Esophageal Manometry

ENDOSCOPIC EXAMINATIONS
  Bronchoscopy
  Esophagoscopy
INVASIVE PROCEDURES FOR TISSUE
    SAMPLING
  Mediastinal Lymph Node Biopsy
  Transthoracic Needle Biopsy
  Thoracentesis and Pleural Biopsy
  Video-Assisted Thoracoscopy
  Incisional Biopsies

Thoracic diseases encompass a wide variety of neoplastic, infectious, and acquired disorders. Any of a number of diagnostic modalities may be important in establishing diagnoses. Those studies most commonly used in patients who undergo thoracic surgical procedures are the focus of this chapter.

ROENTGENOGRAPHIC STUDIES

CHEST ROENTGENOGRAMS

The *chest roentgenogram* is the most common diagnostic study used to evaluate diseases of the thorax. In patients with pulmonary tumors, it is the primary diagnostic imaging modality. It also plays an important role in detection of less common intrathoracic tumors occurring in the mediastinum or chest wall. Although the roentgenogram does not distinguish malignancy and benignancy or determine histologic cell type, it provides essential information about location and characteristics of a tumor and involvement of adjacent structures. Lesion size, relative density (solid or cystic), the presence and pattern of calcifica-

tion, and displacement or alteration of normal structures are demonstrated (Davis et al., 1990). Comparison with previous chest roentgenograms can help determine onset of an abnormality and its rate of growth. The chest roentgenogram is also useful in determining the extent of benign, diffuse pulmonary disease (Hyers & Bedrossian, 1991). It may detect other intrathoracic abnormalities as well, such as thoracic aortic aneurysm, pleural effusion, or pneumothorax.

The standard method for obtaining a chest roentgenogram is with the patient in an upright position and during a full inspiration. The diaphragms are lower when the patient is upright and the lungs are more fully expanded than when the patient is in a supine position and the diaphragms are pushed upward by abdominal viscera (Matthay & Sostman, 1990). *Posteroanterior* and *lateral* projections are obtained to provide a three-dimensional view of the chest. The lateral roentgenogram demonstrates certain areas of the thorax better than the posteroanterior projection. It may reveal findings not apparent on the posteroanterior roentgenogram, such as small mediastinal lesions, masses in the anterior portions of the lung adjacent to the mediastinum, and lesions in the vertebral column or behind the heart (Miller, 1994). An *expiration* posteroanterior roentgenogram may be helpful in the diagnosis of small pneumothoraces. A pneumothorax appears larger during expiration because lung volume is reduced; expiration also increases density of the lung, thus enhancing the contrast between the appearance of lung tissue and air (DeMeester & LaFontaine, 1990).

Other projections may be useful in specific situations. *Oblique* roentgenograms are those in which the beam is focused obliquely at the patient's chest. Oblique views are useful in projecting lesions free from overlying structures (e.g., determining whether a lesion is in the lung or chest wall) (Miller, 1994). A *lordotic* projection, obtained by angling the patient's chest backward, is useful in demonstrating apical lesions that may be obscured by the clavicle or first rib in the posteroanterior projection. A *lateral decubitus* roentgenogram is taken with the patient lying on the right or left side. It is primarily used to demonstrate the presence and mobility of fluid in the pleural space (Freundlich & Bragg, 1992).

TOMOGRAPHY

A *tomogram* is a type of roentgenogram in which individual planes are in focus and adjacent planes are blurred. It provides more precise definition of a lesion's morphologic characteristics than a plain roentgenogram and is used primarily to determine the presence, size, number, and location of pulmonary nodules (Matthay & Sostman, 1990). Tomography demonstrates more nodules than the plain chest roentgenogram, and calcification is better demonstrated (Shields & Wolverson, 1991). Therefore, a tomogram may be helpful in evaluating pulmonary lesions in certain locations or in detecting the presence of lesions not apparent on the plain roentgenogram in patients likely to have multiple lesions (e.g., those with metastatic pulmonary tumors).

Conventional tomography has largely been replaced by *computed tomography* (CT), a technique for imaging cross-sectional anatomy. In patients with lung tumors, CT scanning is generally accepted as the most accurate, noninvasive method of evaluating mediastinal lymph nodes (Ratto et al., 1990). Consequently, a CT scan is almost always performed if the plain chest roentgenogram is suggestive of mediastinal lymphadenopathy (i.e., enlarged lymph nodes) that might represent mediastinal metastasis and preclude surgical resection of a tumor. Although the CT scan does not establish the presence of malignant cells in mediastinal lymph tissue, it illustrates enlarged or multiple lymph nodes that are suggestive of tumor invasion. CT scanning is also helpful in demonstrating malignant invasion of vertebral bodies or soft tissue. Chest CT scans in patients with suspected lung cancer usually include imaging the upper abdomen to detect occult adrenal or liver metastasis.

CT scanning is also the imaging method of choice in patients with primary mediastinal tumors because it accurately localizes and characterizes pathologic processes within the mediastinum (McLoud, 1989). It provides a sensitive method of distinguishing between fatty, vascular, cystic, and soft tissue masses (Shields, 1991a). Depending on the indication, intravenous contrast medium may be administered to enhance the distinction between vascular structures and surrounding tissue.

OTHER ROENTGENOGRAPHIC STUDIES

Magnetic resonance imaging (MRI) may be performed in selected patients with mediastinal abnormalities. MRI uses radio waves modified by a magnetic field to produce somewhat different images than those obtained by CT scanning (Miller, 1994). Although CT scanning more clearly delineates a mediastinal mass from surrounding structures, it is limited to the axial plane; MRI can supply images on the coronal and sagittal planes (Fig. 36-1) (Ricci et al., 1990). It is particularly useful in evaluation of some mediastinal masses (e.g., neurogenic tumors in the posterior mediastinum). It is also helpful in delineating vascular abnormalities, such as coarctation of the aorta.

Contrast swallow studies are performed to evaluate esophageal abnormalities, such as tumor, stricture, or diverticulum. Radiopaque barium sulfate is swallowed by the patient, and fluoroscopic images are obtained. The esophageal lumen is outlined by the barium, allowing detection of esophageal abnormalities (e.g., tumor or achalasia) or esophageal displacement by adjacent mediastinal structures, such as enlarged lymph nodes or an enlarged left atrium (Matthay & Sostman, 1990). Cine or videotape recordings of the barium swallow and swallowing of both a solid and a liquid bolus may be performed to increase accuracy of the study (DeMeester & Watson, 1991). *Cinefluorography* is particularly helpful to detect pharyngeal or upper esophageal abnormalities because of the rapidity with which swallowing occurs.

Bronchography consists of imaging the chest after injecting contrast medium into the trachea and insufflating it into the dependent lung by manual pulmonary inflation (Le Roux & Rocke, 1989). The procedure, which requires the use of general anesthesia, is performed infrequently in the United States except to define the extent and distribution of bronchiectasis before surgical resection.

LABORATORY PROCEDURES

Cytologic examination of body fluid or exudate is performed to detect and identify malignant cells. Sputum cytology is often performed in patients with large bronchogenic tumors. Lung tumors most likely to yield malignant cells in a sputum sample are those that are centrally located, greater than 2 cm, and of a

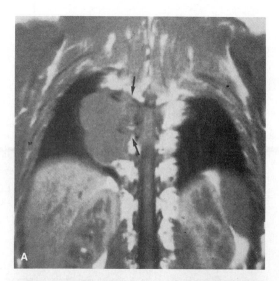

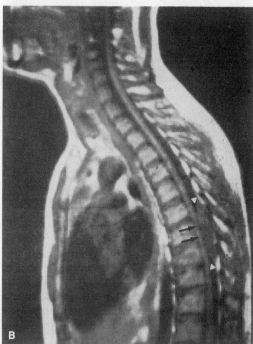

FIGURE 36-1. Magnetic resonance imaging in a patient with a malignant schwannoma. Coronal **(A)** and sagittal **(B)** planes allow evaluation of the intraspinal component (*arrows*) of this neurogenic tumor of the posterior mediastinum. (Ricci C, Rendina EA, Venuta F, et al., 1990: Diagnostic imaging and surgical treatment of dumbbell tumors of the mediastinum. Ann Thorac Surg 50:588)

squamous cell type (Shields, 1991b). To obtain sputum samples, the patient is asked to expectorate into a specimen cup, usually immediately on arising in the morning. Samples are obtained on 3 consecutive days to increase accuracy.

A *culture* of sputum, lung tissue, or pleural fluid may be performed if an infectious pulmonary disease is suspected. Sputum cultures are most frequently performed. A cooperative patient with a productive cough is usually able to expectorate adequate sputum for culture preparation. In others, aerosol treatments or endotracheal suctioning may be necessary to obtain an adequate sputum sample for culture. Lung tissue is obtained by needle or incisional biopsy, and pleural fluid is obtained by thoracentesis. In addition to routine culture studies, smears of exudate or fluid may be prepared using special staining techniques for detection of tuberculosis, fungi, or parasites (Sommers & Sommers, 1994). A *Gram stain* is usually performed in conjunction with a culture to provide a preliminary estimation of the quantity and type of bacteria present in a specimen. Gram stain findings allow initiation of appropriate antimicrobial therapy before availability of the culture results.

Skin tests may be applied for detection of several infectious pulmonary diseases. The most commonly used skin test is the Mantoux, performed as a screening test for tuberculosis. A small amount of Tween 80 *purified protein derivative* is injected intradermally (McMillan, 1991). The degree of induration at the injection site after a period of 48 to 72 hours is visually assessed and measured with a ruler. Ten millimeters or greater of induration is considered a positive result. However, conclusive diagnosis of tuberculosis can only be made by isolating *Mycobacterium tuberculosis* from a clinical specimen (Everett, 1989). Skin tests may also be performed to detect fungal pulmonary infections, such as coccidioidomycosis or histoplasmosis. As with tuberculosis, a positive skin test is suggestive only; definitive diagnosis must be established by culture isolation of the organism.

FUNCTIONAL ASSESSMENT STUDIES

PULMONARY FUNCTION TESTING

Pulmonary function testing is often performed preoperatively to assess lung function and predict a patient's ability to withstand a planned thoracic operation, particularly pulmonary resection. The most frequently performed test is *forced vital capacity* (FVC), measured using a spirometer. The FVC maneuver is a means of quantifying both volume and flow of respiration. FVC is the maximal volume of air expelled by forced exhalation after maximal inspiration. Flow is represented by *forced expiratory volume in 1 second* (FEV_1), which is the average flow exhaled in the first second (Enright & Hodgkin, 1991). Reliability of results is dependent on the patient's ability to cooperate fully with the various breathing maneuvers.

FVC and FEV_1 are each compared with a "normal" value for the patient derived from studies of large groups of individuals with normal pulmonary function and taking into account the patient's age, sex, height, and race (Siddiqui & Knight, 1989). The measured value is then expressed as a percentage of the predicted normal value for that patient. In addition, a ratio is derived by comparing FEV_1 to FVC (i.e., FEV_1:FVC ratio). FEV_1, FVC, and the FEV_1:FVC ratio are commonly measured because they are the best indicators of chronic obstructive pulmonary disease, the most prevalent form of lung disease (Kanarek, 1989) (Table 36-1).

Arterial blood gases are sometimes measured during pulmonary function testing to identify arterial hypoxemia or carbon dioxide retention. In preoperative patients, arterial blood gas measurements provide baseline values for comparison with postoperative measurements. *Diffusion capacity* is a useful measurement in evaluation of patients in whom interstitial pulmonary disease, such as sarcoidosis or pulmonary fibrosis, is suggested. It is a measure of the capacity of the pulmonary membrane to transfer gas between alveolar air and pulmonary capillary blood (Boomsma & Glassroth, 1994).

ESOPHAGEAL MANOMETRY

Esophageal manometry is the recording of intraluminal pressures within the esophagus. It is primarily used for definition of esophageal motility disorders, particularly achalasia, scleroderma, and esophageal spasm (DeMeester & Watson, 1991). Before the development of esophageal manometry, the esophagus was considered to be basically an anatomic conduit; development of manometric studies increased understanding of its physiologic function (Ellis, 1990).

Manometric testing consists of recording pressures simultaneously at various levels within the esophagus to evaluate the esophageal body and upper and lower sphincters (Duranceau, 1994) (Fig. 36-2). The study is commonly performed using a multiple-lumen, water-perfused catheter assembly. Lateral sideholes spaced at measured intervals from the catheter tip connect each lumen to an external pressure trans-

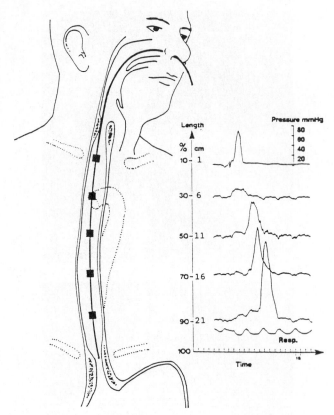

FIGURE 36-2. Diagrammatic representation demonstrating position of transducers during standard esophageal manometry and typical pressure response in the esophageal body during swallowing. Transducers are 5 cm apart, and the proximal transducer is 1 cm below the upper esophageal sphincter. (Stein HJ, DeMeester TR, Hinder RA, 1992: Evaluation and surgical management of motor disorders of the esophageal body and lower esophageal sphincter. Curr Probl Surg 24:460)

ducer. Alternatively, a catheter assembly with a series of electronic pressure transducers on the catheter itself may be used. Baseline pressures are recorded at the lower and upper esophageal sphincters and in the esophageal body, and various swallowing and provocative maneuvers are performed to assess esophageal peristalsis and sphincter function.

The diagnostic value of standard manometry is limited by the intermittent and unpredictable occurrence of motor abnormalities and symptoms in patients with esophageal motility disorders (Stein et al., 1992). As a result, *ambulatory esophageal motility monitoring* was developed. A catheter containing two or more electronic pressure transducers is placed in the esophagus and connected to a digital data recorder. Intraluminal pressures are recorded for 24 hours, during which time the patient maintains a diary of activities and oral intake. By using ambulatory manometry, evaluation of esophageal motility can be based on more than 1000 contractions monitored under a variety of physiologic conditions (Stein et al., 1992).

TABLE 36-1. INTERPRETATION OF SPIROMETRY VALUES

Obstructive Pulmonary Disease

FEV_1/FVC < 70% *and*:

FEV₁ (% of Predicted)	*Degree of Obstruction*
>80	None
65–69	Mild
50–64	Moderate
35–49	Severe
<35	Very severe

Restrictive Pulmonary Disease

FEV_1/FVC > 70% *and*:

FEV₁ and FVC < 80% of predicted = restrictive pulmonary disease. Lung volume measurements are necessary to categorize severity.

(Adapted from Siddiqui AK, Knight L, 1989: Pulmonary function tests. In Braun SR [ed]: Concise Textbook of Pulmonary Medicine. New York, Elsevier)

Esophageal pH measurement is an important component of motility studies. Because of the distinct differences in esophageal and gastric pH levels, pH measurements in the distal esophagus, in combination with various provocative maneuvers, are used to diagnose gastroesophageal reflux and evaluate the patient's response to medical therapy. The pH measurements provide information about competence of the lower esophageal sphincter, as well as the ability of the esophagus to clear refluxed material. In patients with complex esophageal disorders thought to be associated with reflux, *24-hour ambulatory pH monitoring* may be performed (DeMeester & Watson, 1991).

ENDOSCOPIC EXAMINATIONS

BRONCHOSCOPY

Bronchoscopy, or endoscopic inspection of the tracheobronchial tree, is useful in the diagnosis of many types of pulmonary disease. Bronchoscopy is most commonly performed in patients with primary carcinoma of the lung to assist with diagnosis and staging. In patients with central lung lesions that are presumed to be endobronchial, bronchoscopy allows visual inspection of abnormal bronchial mucosa and procurement of tissue for histologic evaluation. Bronchoscopic inspection may reveal a visible tumor in the bronchial mucosa or changes in the bronchial wall or lumen size that suggest tumor infiltration or external compression (Shields, 1991b). Bronchoscopy is also widely used to establish a diagnosis in patients with nonspecific symptoms of pulmonary disease, such as persistent cough, hemoptysis, or unilateral wheezing (McElvein, 1991).

There are two types of bronchoscopes: the fiberoptic bronchoscope, which is almost always used for diagnostic bronchoscopy, and the rigid bronchoscope. *Fiberoptic bronchoscopy* may be performed with the patient awake, using local anesthesia and intravenous sedation. Before the procedure, oral intake is withheld for 6 to 8 hours. An anticholinergic agent and cough suppressant are often administered in addition to a sedating medication. A topical anesthetic agent is sprayed into the back of the throat and may also be injected through the neck directly into the trachea.

The bronchoscope is passed through the nose, mouth, or an endotracheal tube into the trachea and advanced into the right and left bronchi. Segmental and subsegmental bronchi may be directly visualized. Recently, computer-assisted imaging during bronchoscopy has become available. A micro camera incorporated into the bronchoscope allows intraluminal images to be projected on a screen in the operating room. Photographs of endobronchial abnormalities can be taken during the procedure to document the appearance of identified abnormalities (Fig. 36-3).

Depending on the presumptive diagnosis, tissue or cells are obtained for histologic or cytologic analysis and for culture. Three methods are available for obtaining specimens from the endobronchial surface: (1) biopsy, (2) brushing, or (3) lavage. A *biopsy* is performed using a forceps passed through the bronchoscope to pluck a small piece of bronchial mucosa.

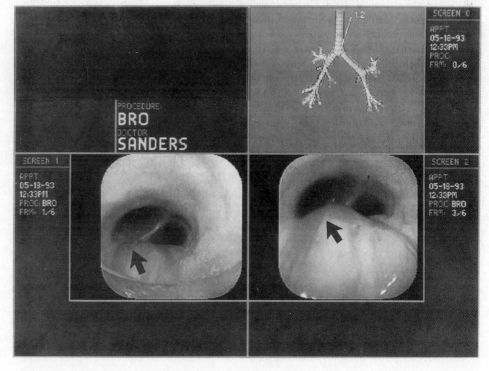

FIGURE 36-3. Images recorded during video-assisted bronchoscopy. The diagrammatic representation of the tracheobronchial tree in screen 0 (*upper right*) is used to designate the location of the endobronchial images displayed in screens 1 (*bottom left*) and 2 (*bottom right*). The endobronchial images reveal an abnormal area (*arrows*) at the bifurcation of the right and left mainstem bronchi. Histologic examination of tissue obtained from this area revealed adenocarcinoma. (Courtesy of Axel W. Joob, M.D.)

Because the surface of the tumor may be necrotic, several pieces of tissue are sampled to obtain enough tissue for histologic detail (Sommers & Sommers, 1994). *Bronchial brushing* consists of rubbing a brush over the surface of a lesion to gather cellular material. A *bronchial lavage* is performed by instilling sterile saline over a suspicious lesion and aspirating the fluid into a collection receptacle.

A *transbronchial needle biopsy* may be performed through bronchoscopy to obtain lung tissue in patients with suspected sarcoidosis or pulmonary infection (LoCicero & Shields, 1989). A flexible needle is passed through the bronchoscope and used to penetrate the trachea or bronchus to aspirate cells from within the lung. Successful biopsy through a transbronchial approach obviates the need for diagnostic open-lung biopsy, a procedure associated with considerable morbidity in patients with acute forms of pulmonary disease. Lymph nodes in the subcarinal area or adjacent to the trachea and mainstem bronchi may also be sampled using a transbronchial technique.

In addition to its diagnostic value, bronchoscopy is frequently used therapeutically for (1) serial deep bronchial lavage and suctioning in patients with persistent atelectasis or copious secretions, (2) removal of an aspirated foreign body, (3) facilitation of endotracheal intubation, and (4) control of bleeding in the presence of massive hemoptysis. Fiberoptic bronchoscopy rarely causes complications. Those that do occur are usually related to preoperative medications, cardiopulmonary dysfunction, technical difficulties, or biopsy (Kirby & Ginsberg, 1991). *Rigid bronchoscopy* is performed infrequently, primarily for therapeutic procedures. Indications for rigid bronchoscopy include massive hemoptysis, aspirated foreign bodies, tracheal stenosis, and emergency airway control in patients with tumors obstructing the trachea or mainstem bronchi (Mathisen, 1989). General anesthesia is used for rigid bronchoscopy or for bronchoscopy performed concomitantly with thoracotomy.

ESOPHAGOSCOPY

Esophagoscopy, or endoscopic inspection of the esophagus, is performed to directly examine the esophagus and biopsy tissue in patients with symptoms of esophageal disease. Esophagoscopy allows diagnostic evaluation of esophageal masses, strictures, and mucosal abnormalities, such as esophagitis, Barrett's mucosa, and candidiasis (fungal infection) (Heitmiller & Mathisen, 1989). Suggestive data from fluoroscopic or manometric studies may be confirmed and tissue biopsy samples may be extracted for histologic evaluation (Ellis, 1990). Esophagoscopy is also useful in diagnosis of esophageal perforation and for determination of severity of damage after caustic injuries of the esophagus. Two major differences between the esophagus and tracheobronchial tree distinguish esophagoscopy from bronchoscopy: (1) the esophagus is more friable and therefore more prone to endoscopic injury, such as perforation, and (2) the esophagus is subject to a broader spectrum of pathologic conditions, many of which can be managed with endoscopic techniques (Faber & Warren, 1989).

Before esophagoscopy, food and fluids are withheld for 6 to 8 hours. A longer period of fasting may be required in patients with disorders that interfere with esophageal emptying, such as achalasia or gastric outlet obstruction. The patient is generally premedicated with an anticholinergic agent (e.g., atropine) to decrease secretions and vasovagal response and with an antiemetic, sedative agent (Holscher & Siewart, 1991). A flexible, fiberoptic esophagoscope is most commonly used. Fiberoptic esophagoscopic evaluation is usually performed with the patient lying in a left lateral decubitus position with the knees, spine, and neck flexed (Stein et al., 1992). As the endoscope is advanced into the esophagus, the interior of the esophagus and gastroesophageal junction are directly visualized.

Rigid esophagoscopy (i.e., using a rigid rather than fiberoptic esophagoscope) may be preferable in selected situations, such as assessing abnormalities of the cricopharyngeus (primary muscle of the upper esophageal sphincter) and upper esophagus or procuring deep biopsy samples (DeMeester & Watson, 1991). Rigid esophagoscopy is performed using general anesthesia. In addition to diagnostic uses, esophagoscopy is sometimes performed for therapeutic purposes, such as removal of foreign bodies lodged in the esophagus, sclerosing of esophageal varices, dilatation of strictures, and placement of intraluminal tubes (Heitmiller & Mathisen, 1989). Major complications occur rarely; aspiration is most common (Kirby & Ginsberg, 1991) and is best prevented by an adequate length of fasting before the procedure. Less frequently, esophagoscopy causes esophageal perforation. The most common site of esophageal perforation is just above the cricopharyngeus secondary to difficult esophageal intubation (Faber & Warren, 1989).

INVASIVE PROCEDURES FOR TISSUE SAMPLING

MEDIASTINAL LYMPH NODE BIOPSY

The lymph nodes draining the lungs may be divided into two groups: (1) pulmonary lymph nodes, or those contained within the visceral pleura, and (2) mediastinal lymph nodes (Nohl-Oser, 1989). In patients with lung cancer, the presence of tumor cells in mediastinal lymph nodes represents extrapulmonary spread. It is the most important factor in predicting survival outcome in patients who do not have metastases outside the chest (Jolly et al., 1991).

Mediastinal lymph node biopsy is indicated when lymph node adenopathy is suggested by a chest

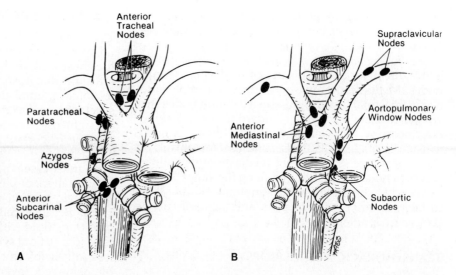

FIGURE 36-4. Mediastinal lymph nodes. **(A)** Nodes accessible through mediastinoscopy. **(B)** Nodes requiring incisional biopsy (mediastinotomy, thoracoscopy, thoracotomy). (LoCicero J, Shields TW, 1989: Surgical diagnostic procedures. In Shields TW [ed]: General Thoracic Surgery, ed. 3, p. 270. Philadelphia, Lea & Febiger)

roentgenogram or CT scan. It is performed before thoracotomy because pulmonary resection is usually not performed if metastasis to mediastinal lymphatic tissue has already occurred. Mediastinal lymph node biopsy may also be performed to definitively diagnose a suspected malignant tumor before institution of nonsurgical therapies, such as irradiation or chemotherapy. Depending on location of the tumor and its presumed anatomic lymphatic drainage, lymph node tissue may be procured from the mediastinum by mediastinoscopy, by mediastinotomy, or occasionally by video-assisted thoracoscopy, which is discussed later in the chapter (Fig. 36-4).

Transcervical mediastinoscopy is performed using general anesthesia. A small incision is made just above the supraclavicular notch. The surgeon primarily uses finger dissection to create a tunnel in the pretracheal fascia through which the mediastinoscope is advanced (Fig. 36-5) (McElvein, 1991). By using instruments passed through the mediastinoscope, lymph nodes along the trachea and either main bronchus can be dissected bluntly and removed in total; alternatively, a piece of lymph tissue can be extracted using a forceps (LoCicero & Shields, 1989). Although complications are uncommon, mediastinoscopy can cause hemorrhage, injury to a major

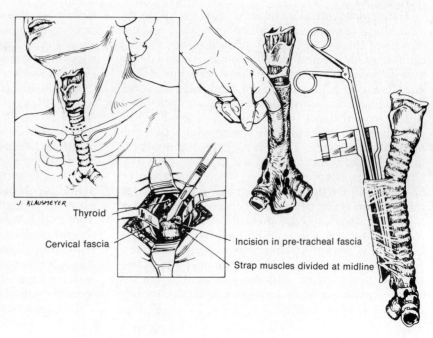

FIGURE 36-5. Mediastinoscopy. A transverse incision is made just above the sternum. Finger dissection is used to create a tunnel within the pretracheal fascia through which the mediastinoscope is advanced. Identified lymph nodes are biopsied with an instrument passed through the mediastinoscope. (Mackenzie JW, Riley DJ, 1991: Diagnostic procedures: Mediastinal evaluation—scalene lymph node biopsy, mediastinoscopy, and mediastinotomy. In Baue AE, Geha AS, Hammond GL, et al. [eds]: Glenn's Thoracic and Cardiovascular Surgery, ed. 5, p. 163. Norwalk, CT, Appleton & Lange)

airway, esophageal perforation, pneumothorax, or recurrent laryngeal nerve injury (Kirby & Ginsberg, 1991).

Mediastinotomy, also called a *Chamberlain procedure,* is the direct surgical exposure of mediastinal lymph nodes. Mediastinotomy is performed to sample anterior mediastinal or aortopulmonary lymph nodes that are inaccessible through a standard transcervical mediastinoscopy (Mackenzie & Riley, 1991a). A small incision is made over the second costal cartilage on the appropriate side. A right mediastinotomy allows access to nodes at the hilus or along the superior vena cava and trachea; a left mediastinotomy allows access to hilar, anterior, paratracheal, and subaortic nodes (LoCicero & Shields, 1989).

TRANSTHORACIC NEEDLE BIOPSY

A *transthoracic needle biopsy* is a procedure performed to obtain lung tissue for histologic examination in patients with lesions located in the lung periphery. It may also be performed for biopsy of hilar or mediastinal masses (Shields & Wolverson, 1991). Except for pulmonary lesions fixed to the chest wall, transthoracic needle biopsy is almost always performed by an invasive radiologist and guided by fluoroscopy or CT scanning. Fluoroscopy is used for easily visualized lesions, especially when the lesion is located in the lower lung fields; CT scanning is used when lesions are not well localized on the chest roentgenogram or are located in close proximity to the heart, major blood vessels, or hilum of the lung (Shields & Wolverson, 1991). A needle is inserted through the chest wall and guided into the lesion. As the needle tip is moved within the lesion, cells are aspirated for cytologic evaluation. A chest roentgenogram is obtained after the procedure to detect iatrogenic pneumothorax.

Transthoracic needle biopsy is most useful for establishing a diagnosis in those patients who, because of type of disease or general medical status, are not candidates for surgical resection but in whom a definitive diagnosis is necessary to direct nonsurgical therapy. Its use in patients who are candidates for surgical resection is controversial. Because there is a significant incidence of false-negative results, the procedure does not eliminate the possibility of a pulmonary malignancy. Therefore, thoracotomy for definitive identification and removal of the lesion is usually considered necessary even when needle biopsy has yielded no diagnosis of malignancy. Since surgical resection is the treatment of choice in the event of a positive diagnosis, the procedure rarely alters the course of therapy. Contraindications to needle biopsy of the lung include pulmonary hypertension, suspected arteriovenous fistula, pulmonary cysts or bullae, and hemorrhagic diathesis (LoCicero & Shields, 1989). Complications include pneumothorax and hemoptysis (McLoud, 1989).

THORACENTESIS AND PLEURAL BIOPSY

Thoracentesis is aspiration of fluid or air from the pleural space using a needle or catheter inserted through the chest wall. In the presence of unexplained pleural effusion, diagnostic thoracentesis may be performed to obtain pleural fluid for laboratory analysis. Measurement of lactate dehydrogenase, total protein, pH, glucose, white blood cell count, and amylase provide important clues about etiology of a pleural effusion.

In most cases of malignant pleural effusion, cytologic analysis of pleural fluid determines the site and histologic type of the primary tumor (Serre et al., 1990). Because cells in fluid swell and degenerate over time, fluid withdrawn during an initial thoracentesis in a patient with suspected malignant disease is less satisfactory for cytologic study than a fluid sample removed several days later (Sommers & Sommers, 1994). *Needle biopsy of pleural tissue* is performed percutaneously in a similar manner to that used for thoracentesis. A biopsy needle device is used to entrap and withdraw a small piece of pleura.

VIDEO-ASSISTED THORACOSCOPY

Video-assisted thoracoscopy is a recent addition to the armamentarium of procedures for diagnosis of intrathoracic diseases. It consists of using endoscopic instruments and micro cameras to provide visualization of and access to intrathoracic organs without a thoracotomy incision (Lewis et al., 1992). Diagnostic procedures that may be performed through thoracoscopy include biopsies of pleura, mediastinal lymph nodes or neoplasms, and lung. Although thoracoscopy was performed as early as 1910 by Jacobaeus, its uses were limited by inadequate visibility and instrumentation. Applications for the procedure have expanded rapidly as a result of two developments: (1) micro cameras and solid-state systems that project anatomic images on a screen and (2) special instruments that allow more precise operative techniques (Lewis et al., 1992; McKeown et al., 1992).

In patients with pleural abnormalities, thoracoscopy is thought to achieve a higher degree of accuracy than needle biopsy of the pleura because pleural metastases can vary in location according to the type of tumor (Armengod et al., 1990). Thoracoscopy allows direct visualization of all pleural surfaces. It may also be performed for definitive diagnosis of idiopathic pleural effusions when thoracentesis fails to establish a diagnosis (Mack et al., 1992). Thoracoscopy may be used instead of mediastinotomy for biopsy of mediastinal lymph nodes located in the aortopulmonary window. Biopsy of lung parenchyma through thoracoscopy may be performed in patients with undiagnosed pulmonary disease that is likely to require medical as opposed to surgical therapy.

Thoracoscopy is performed using general anesthesia and a scope similar to that used for mediastinoscopy. Patients are usually informed and prepared for possible thoracotomy if the desired procedure cannot be accomplished through thoracoscopy. The patient is placed in a lateral decubitus position. Usually three small incisions are necessary for insertion of the thoracoscope and operating instruments. One incision is made in the sixth or seventh intercostal space in the midaxillary line for insertion of the thoracoscope; the second and third incisions are made in the third to sixth intercostal spaces along the anterior and posterior axillary lines to allow insertion and manipulation of instruments (Fig. 36-6) (Lewis et al., 1992). Strategic positioning of the thoracoscopic camera and endoscopic instruments is important to maximizing visualization and ensuring success of the procedure (Landreneau et al., 1992).

A single lung ventilation technique is used; that is, the patient is intubated with a double-lumen endotracheal tube and only the contralateral lung is ventilated. Single lung ventilation allows collapse of the lung on the operative side, thereby providing maximal exposure and avoiding injury to intrathoracic structures. At the conclusion of the biopsy, the ipsi-

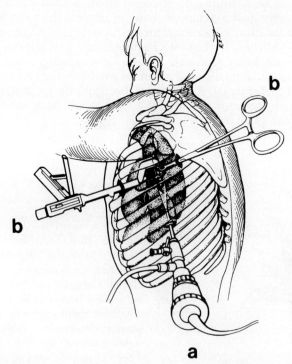

FIGURE 36-6. Imaged thoracoscopy. Thoracoscope is inserted through 6th or 7th intercostal space in midaxillary line (a); two additional incisions are created for passage and manipulation of instruments (b). (Lewis RJ, Caccavale RJ, Sisler GE, McKenzie JW, 1992: One hundred consecutive patients undergoing video-assisted thoracic operations. Ann Thorac Surg 54:423. Reprinted with permission of the Society of Thoracic Surgeons)

lateral lung is reinflated. Chest tube thoracostomy drainage is required for several days after the procedure.

Thoracoscopy is used therapeutically for procedures such as pleurodesis in the treatment of spontaneous pneumothorax, thoracic sympathectomy, empyema evacuation, creation of a pericardial window, and wedge resection. It is contraindicated in two groups of patients: (1) those who are unable to tolerate single lung anesthesia and (2) those with complete obliteration of the pleural space due to adhesions (Lewis et al., 1992).

INCISIONAL BIOPSIES

Open-lung biopsy is a technique for obtaining lung tissue for examination through a small thoracotomy incision (Fig. 36-7). It is most often used to diagnose persistent diffuse pulmonary infiltrates of unknown etiology (Mackenzie & Riley, 1991b). Typically, candidates for open-lung biopsy are patients in whom surgical therapy through a conventional thoracotomy is not anticipated but in whom less-invasive procedures have failed to establish a diagnosis. An incisional biopsy allows procurement of larger tissue samples than can be obtained through needle aspiration techniques. The need for open-lung biopsy through thoracotomy has been reduced substantially by the ability to procure adequate lung tissue samples by thoracoscopy. However, it remains a valuable diagnostic modality in patients who are unable to undergo thoracoscopy because of an inability to tolerate single lung anesthesia or the presence of an obliterated pleural space.

Open-lung biopsy is performed using general anesthesia. A short submammary incision through the fifth intercostal space is commonly used. This incision provides excellent exposure to the lateral aspects of the upper and lower lobes, produces minimal postoperative discomfort, and avoids the need to divide the pectoralis major muscle (LoCicero & Shields, 1989). Although open-lung biopsy is a relatively minor surgical procedure, it necessitates general anesthesia and an incision in the thorax. It may be associated with significant morbidity because of the serious illnesses typically present in patients who require the procedure.

Pericardial biopsy is indicated for diagnosis of unexplained pericardial effusion or pericarditis. The procedure is performed through a small thoracotomy or subxiphoid incision. A small portion of pericardial tissue may be resected concomitantly to allow drainage of associated pericardial effusion. However, in the presence of persistent, recurring pericardial effusion, an extensive pericardiectomy performed through thoracoscopy or thoracotomy is generally necessary to ensure chronic drainage.

Scalene lymph node biopsy is performed for diagnosis of suspected lung carcinoma or sarcoidosis in patients

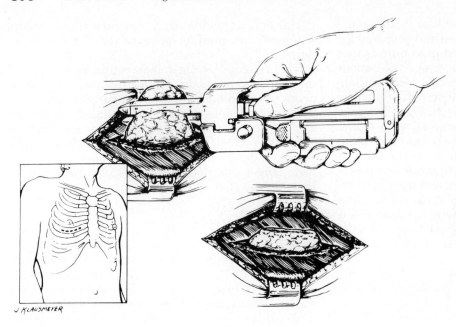

FIGURE 36-7. Open lung biopsy. Through a small anterior thoracotomy incision, a piece of peripheral lung parenchyma is excised using a mechanical stapler. (Mackenzie JW, Riley DJ, 1991: Diagnostic procedures: Pulmonary biopsy—fine needle aspiration, open-lung biopsy, and thoracoscopy. In Baue AE, Geha AS, Hammond GL, et al [eds]: Glenn's Thoracic and Cardiovascular Surgery, ed. 5, p. 174. Norwalk, CT, Appleton & Lange)

who have palpable supraclavicular lymph nodes. Lymph nodes in the anterior scalene fat pad may contain pathologic tissue because these paratracheal lymphatics at the base of the neck drain lymphatic fluid from the lungs and mediastinum (LoCicero & Shields, 1989). A small supraclavicular incision, using local anesthesia, allows access to the scalene fat pad, which is excised from the anterior surface of the anterior scalene muscle (Fig. 36-8).

Exploratory thoracotomy may be necessary in se-lected instances when less invasive procedures fail to provide definitive diagnosis of an intrathoracic abnormality or if a diagnosis will not obviate the need for thoracotomy. For example, exploratory thoracotomy is indicated in the case of a lung tumor that is thought to be malignant and surgically resectable, even if prior diagnostic studies fail to establish the certainty of malignancy. Exploratory thoracotomy for diagnosis is generally avoided if a lung lesion does not appear to be resectable (Shields, 1989).

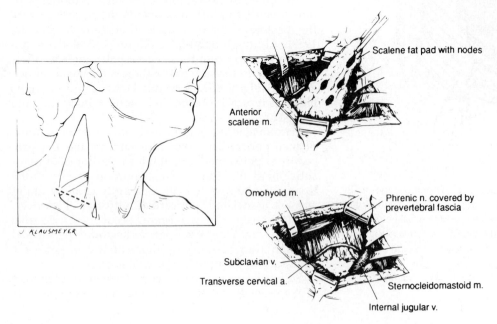

Scalene fat pad with nodes

Anterior scalene m.

Omohyoid m.

Phrenic n. covered by prevertebral fascia

Subclavian v.

Transverse cervical a.

Sternocleidomastoid m.

Internal jugular v.

FIGURE 36-8. Scalene node biopsy is performed through a 2-to 3-cm incision above the clavicle (**left**); fat pad containing scalene lymph nodes is excised (**top right**) guided by anatomic landmarks (**bottom right**). (Makenzie JW, Riley DJ, 1991: Diagnostic procedures: Mediastinal evaluation—scalene lymph node biopsy, mediastinoscopy, and mediastinotomy. In Baue AE, Geha AS, Hammond GL, et al [eds]: Glenn's Thoracic and Cardiovascular Surgery, ed. 5, p. 161. Norwalk, CT, Appleton & Lange)

REFERENCES

Armengod AC, Saumench J, Moya J, 1990: Points to consider when choosing a biopsy method in cases of pleuritis of unknown origin, with special reference to thoracoscopy. In Deslauriers J, Lacquet LK (eds): Thoracic Surgery: Surgical Management of Pleural Diseases. St. Louis, CV Mosby

Boomsma JD, Glassroth J, 1994: Pulmonary gas exchange. In Shields TW (ed): General Thoracic Surgery, ed. 4. Baltimore, Williams & Wilkins

Davis RD, Oldham HN Jr, Sabiston DC Jr, 1990: The mediastinum. In Sabiston DC Jr, Spencer FC (eds): Surgery of the Chest, ed. 5. Philadelphia, WB Saunders

DeMeester TR, Lafontaine E, 1990: The pleura. In Sabiston DC Jr, Spencer FC (eds): Surgery of the Chest, ed. 5. Philadelphia, WB Saunders

DeMeester TR, Watson A, 1991: The esophagus: Anatomy and functional evaluation. In Baue AE, Geha AS, Hammond GL, et al. (eds): Glenn's Thoracic and Cardiovascular Surgery, ed. 5. Norwalk, CT, Appleton & Lange

Duranceau A, 1994: Physiology and physiologic studies of the esophagus. In Shields TW (ed): General Thoracic Surgery, ed. 4. Baltimore, Williams & Wilkins

Ellis FH Jr, 1990: Disorders of the esophagus in the adult. In Sabiston DC Jr, Spencer FC (eds): Surgery of the Chest, ed. 5. Philadelphia, WB Saunders

Enright PL, Hodgkin JE, 1991: Pulmonary function tests. In Respiratory Care, ed. 3. Philadelphia, JB Lippincott

Everett ED, 1989: Mycobacterial infections of the lung. In Braun SR (ed): Concise Textbook of Pulmonary Medicine. New York, Elsevier

Faber LP, Warren WH, 1989: Endoscopic examinations. In Shields TW (ed): General Thoracic Surgery, ed. 3. Philadelphia, Lea & Febiger

Freundlich IM, Bragg DG, 1992: Introduction. In Freundlich IM, Bragg DG (eds): A Radiologic Approach to Diseases of the Chest. Baltimore, Williams & Wilkins

Heitmiller RF, Mathisen DJ, 1989: Esophagoscopy. In Grillo HC, Austen WG, Wilkins EW, et al. (eds): Current Therapy in Cardiothoracic Surgery. Toronto, BC Decker

Holscher AH, Siewart JR, 1991: Diagnostic procedures: Endoscopy and esophagoscopy. In Baue AE, Geha AS, Hammond GL, et al. (eds): Glenn's Thoracic and Cardiovascular Surgery, ed. 5. Norwalk, CT, Appleton & Lange

Hyers TM, Bedrossian CW, 1991: The diagnosis of benign, diffuse pulmonary disease. In Baue AE, Geha AS, Hammond GL, et al. (eds): Glenn's Thoracic and Cardiovascular Surgery, ed. 5. Norwalk, CT, Appleton & Lange

Jolly PC, Hutchinson CH, Detterbeck F, et al., 1991: Routine computed tomographic scans, selective mediastinoscopy, and other factors in evaluation of lung cancer. J Thorac Cardiovasc Surg 102:266

Kanarek DJ, 1989: Evaluation for pulmonary resection. In Grillo HC, Austen WG, Wilkins EW, et al. (eds): Current Therapy in Cardiothoracic Surgery. Toronto, BC Decker

Kirby TJ, Ginsberg RJ, 1991: Complications of endoscopy: Bronchoscopy, esophagoscopy, and mediastinoscopy. In Waldhausen JA, Orringer MB (eds): Complications in Cardiothoracic Surgery. St. Louis, Mosby–Year Book

Landreneau RJ, Mack MJ, Hazelrigg SR, et al., 1992: Video-assisted thoracic surgery: Basic technical concepts and intercostal approach strategies. Ann Thorac Surg 54:800

Le Roux BT, Rocke DA, 1989: Bronchography. In Grillo HC, Austen WG, Wilkins EW, et al. (eds): Current Therapy in Cardiothoracic Surgery. Toronto, BC Decker

Lewis RJ, Caccavale RJ, Sisler GE, McKenzie JW, 1992: One hundred consecutive patients undergoing video-assisted thoracic operations. Ann Thorac Surg 54:421

LoCicero J, Shields TW, 1989: Surgical diagnostic procedures. In Shields TW (ed): General Thoracic Surgery, ed. 3. Philadelphia, Lea & Febiger

Mack MJ, Aronoff RJ, Acuff TE, et al., 1992: Present role of thoracoscopy in the diagnosis and treatment of diseases of the chest. Ann Thorac Surg 54:403

Mackenzie JW, Riley DJ, 1991a: Diagnostic procedures: Mediastinal evaluation—scalene lymph node biopsy, mediastinoscopy, and mediastinotomy. In Baue AE, Geha AS, Hammond GL, et al. (eds): Glenn's Thoracic and Cardiovascular Surgery, ed. 5. Norwalk, CT, Appleton & Lange

Mackenzie JW, Riley DJ, 1991b: Diagnostic procedures: Pulmonary biopsy-fine needle aspiration, open lung biopsy, and thoracoscopy. In Baue AE, Geha AS, Hammond GL, et al. (eds): Glenn's Thoracic and Cardiovascular Surgery, ed. 5. Norwalk, CT, Appleton & Lange

Mathisen DJ, 1989: Bronchoscopy. In Grillo HC, Austen WG, Wilkins EW, et al. (eds): Current Therapy in Cardiothoracic Surgery. Toronto, BC Decker

Matthay RA, Sostman HD, 1990: Chest imaging. In George RB, Light RW, Matthay MA, Matthay RA (eds): Chest Medicine, ed. 2. Baltimore, Williams & Wilkins

McElvein RB, 1991: Bronchoscopy, transbronchial biopsy, and bronchoalveolar lavage. In Baue AE, Geha AS, Hammond GL, et al. (eds): Glenn's Thoracic and Cardiovascular Surgery, ed. 5. Norwalk, CT, Appleton & Lange

McKeown PP, Conant P, Hubbel DS, 1992: Thoracoscopic lung biopsy. Ann Thorac Surg 54:490

McLoud TC, 1989: Radiologic assessment. In Grillo HC, Austen WG, Wilkins EW, et al. (eds): Current Therapy in Cardiothoracic Surgery. Toronto, BC Decker

McMillan IK, 1991: Surgical treatment of tuberculosis. In Baue AE, Geha AS, Hammond GL, et al. (eds): Glenn's Thoracic and Cardiovascular Surgery, ed. 5. Norwalk, CT, Appleton & Lange

Miller WT, 1994: Roentgenographic evaluation of the lungs and chest. In Shields TW (ed): General Thoracic Surgery, ed. 4. Baltimore, Williams & Wilkins

Nohl-Oser HC, 1989: Lymphatics of the lung. In Shields TW (ed): General Thoracic Surgery, ed. 3. Philadelphia, Lea & Febiger

Ratto GB, Frola C, Cantoni S, Motta A, 1990: Improving clinical efficacy of computed tomographic scan in the preoperative assessment of patients with non-small cell lung cancer. J Thorac Cardiovasc Surg 99:416

Ricci C, Rendina EA, Venuta F, et al., 1990: Diagnostic imaging and surgical treatment of dumbbell tumors of the mediastinum. Ann Thorac Surg 50:586

Serre G, Daste G, Vincent C, et al., 1990: Diagnostic approach to the patient with pleural effusion: Cytologic analysis of pleural fluid. In Deslauriers J, Lacquet LK (eds): Thoracic Surgery: Surgical Management of Pleural Diseases. St. Louis, CV Mosby

Shields JB, Wolverson MK, 1991: Thoracic imaging. In Baue AE, Geha AS, Hammond GL, et al. (eds): Glenn's Thoracic and Cardiovascular Surgery, ed. 5. Norwalk, CT, Appleton & Lange

Shields TW, 1989: Carcinoma of the lung. In Shields TW (ed): General Thoracic Surgery, ed. 3. Philadelphia, Lea & Febiger

Shields TW, 1991a: Primary mediastinal tumors and cysts and their diagnostic investigation. In Shields TW (ed): The Mediastinum. Philadelphia, Lea & Febiger

Shields TW, 1991b: Lung cancer: Diagnosis and staging. In Baue AE, Geha AS, Hammond GL, et al. (eds): Glenn's Thoracic and Cardiovascular Surgery, ed. 5. Norwalk, CT, Appleton & Lange

Siddiqui AK, Knight L, 1989: Pulmonary function tests. In Braun SR (ed): Concise Textbook of Pulmonary Medicine. New York, Elsevier

Sommers HM, Sommers KE, 1994: Laboratory investigations in the diagnosis of pulmonary diseases. In Shields TW (ed): General Thoracic Surgery, ed. 4. Baltimore, Williams & Wilkins

Stein HJ, DeMeester TR, Hinder RA, 1992: Evaluation and surgical management of motor disorders of the esophageal body and lower esophageal sphincter. Curr Probl Surg 24:447

PREOPERATIVE MANAGEMENT AND COUNSELING

PREOPERATIVE EVALUATION
    Patient Interview
    Physical Assessment
    Diagnostic Studies

PREOPERATIVE REGIMEN
    General Guidelines
    Special Considerations
PREOPERATIVE COUNSELING

Preoperative management of thoracic surgical patients includes both physical and psychological preparation for the planned operation. Although much of the preparatory management is standard, some important differences exist depending on the specific disease necessitating surgical intervention. The various thoracic surgical pathologies can be broadly categorized into three groups: (1) diseases of the lungs, (2) esophageal diseases, and (3) diseases of the mediastinum. Because patients are generally admitted to the hospital on the day of a planned thoracic operation, most of the evaluation and preparation for surgery must be completed on an outpatient basis or during a previous admission.

PREOPERATIVE EVALUATION

The preoperative nursing evaluation complements that performed by the physician and provides baseline information that enhances interpretation of postoperative findings. It also allows the nurse to establish a relationship with the patient and family and identify potential problems that may occur during the perioperative period. Information for the preoperative evaluation is obtained from the patient record, interview with and physical examination of the patient, and diagnostic studies.

PATIENT INTERVIEW

The *preoperative assessment* begins with an interview to gain information about the clinical history and to assess the patient's understanding of the illness, emotional readiness for the planned procedure, and family support system. Several components of the clinical history are of particular importance in preoperative patients: (1) the current illness and associated symptoms, (2) the presence of coexisting medical diseases, (3) the current medication regimen and any known allergies, and (4) the patient's functional status.

Factors that influence perioperative risk may also be identified during the preoperative interview. A history of cigarette smoking is pertinent in any patient undergoing a thoracic operation. Because cigarette smoking is an etiologic factor in both lung and esophageal cancer, a long smoking history is typical. Alcohol abuse (a risk factor for esophageal cancer) or its sequelae (e.g., hepatic or cardiovascular disease) may be present in patients with esophageal tumors. Exposure to environmental carcinogens or tuberculosis and travel to areas endemic for specific pulmonary infections are other relevant features of the clinical history.

Current Illness and Associated Symptoms

Most patients who undergo thoracic operations have malignant disease of the lungs, esophagus, or mediastinum. Associated constitutional symptoms, such as weight loss, anorexia, and malaise, are frequently present. Other significant signs and symptoms may be noted, depending on the type of underlying disease (Table 37-1). Lung cancer is the most common diagnosis in preoperative thoracic surgical patients. Ninety to 95% of patients with lung cancer are symptomatic at the time of diagnosis (Shields, 1991). Typical clinical manifestations include cough, persistent upper respiratory tract infections, pneumonia, hemoptysis, and chest pain.

Patients with benign or malignant esophageal disease commonly have some degree of dysphagia. They may experience pain, choking, or vomiting with eating; may need to eat very slowly or take liquids with food; and may have difficulty in maintaining body weight (Stein et al., 1992). In those patients with esophageal cancer, nutritional depletion has often occurred and cachexia may be evident. Associated symptoms are also common in adults with primary mediastinal neoplasms or cysts (Cohen et al., 1991). Lesions in the mediastinum typically produce manifestations related to compression or invasion of structures adjacent to the mass (Davis et al., 1990). Symptoms may also result from endocrine or other biochemical products secreted by the tumor.

Associated Medical Diseases

Associated medical diseases are common in patients who require thoracic surgery and can significantly affect operative outcome (Table 37-2). Most thoracic operations are performed in middle-aged and elderly individuals. Pulmonary and cardiovascular disease are prevalent in this population. Systemic diseases, such as diabetes, hypertension, peripheral atherosclerosis, and renal insufficiency are also frequently present (Pairolero & Payne, 1991).

The presence and severity of existing pulmonary disease has a major impact on operative risk, particularly in patients who will undergo pulmonary resection. Chronic obstructive pulmonary disease is the most common form of pulmonary impairment in thoracic surgical patients. Less commonly, pulmonary function is impaired by pulmonary fibrosis or a previous pulmonary resection for lung cancer (Kanarek, 1989).

Coexistent cardiovascular pathology, present in many older patients, can also increase operative risk significantly. Manifestations of organic heart disease that are well tolerated before surgery may become more serious with the alterations in gas exchange that occur during the perioperative period (Wilson, 1991). Patients at increased risk for complications include those with unstable angina, recent myocardial infarction, congestive heart failure, uncontrolled hypertension, or severe aortic stenosis (Hillis et al., 1992).

TABLE 37-1. COMMON CLINICAL MANIFESTATIONS IN PREOPERATIVE THORACIC SURGICAL PATIENTS

Pulmonary Disease

Cough
Sputum production
Hemoptysis
Pneumonia
Shortness of breath
Wheezing
Chest pain
Hoarseness
Weight loss

Esophageal Disease

Dysphagia
Weight loss
Heartburn
Regurgitation

Mediastinal Masses

Chest pain
Cough
Dyspnea
Dysphagia
Superior vena cava syndrome
Hoarseness

TABLE 37-2. COMMON ASSOCIATED MEDICAL PROBLEMS IN THORACIC SURGICAL PATIENTS

Chronic obstructive pulmonary disease
Coronary artery disease
Peripheral arterial occlusive disease
Hypertension
Diabetes mellitus

Other Relevant Data

During the preoperative interview, the nurse also assesses the patient's understanding of the clinical problem and planned therapy, level of anxiety, and coping ability. Appropriate preoperative counseling is based on this assessment. The patient's living arrangements and social support system are reviewed so that suitable discharge planning can be initiated. Early identification of discharge needs helps alleviate patient anxiety during the perioperative period and facilitates efficient use of hospital and community support resources.

PHYSICAL ASSESSMENT

Physical examination of the thoracic surgical patient focuses particularly on the pulmonary and cardiovascular systems. The lungs are auscultated to provide baseline data regarding respiratory rate, breath sounds, or the presence of adventitious sounds. Heart sounds are auscultated, and the cardiac rate, rhythm, and any extra sounds or murmurs are noted. Blood pressure, temperature, and weight are measured, and peripheral pulses are palpated. The carotid arteries are auscultated to detect bruits that might represent carotid arterial occlusive disease. In patients who will undergo thymectomy, baseline respiratory parameters are measured. The findings from this preoperative examination provide important baseline values for comparison with postoperative findings.

Functional status is assessed to evaluate the patient's ability to increase activity appropriately in the postoperative period. Functional capacity is particularly important in patients who will undergo pulmonary resection. It facilitates the surgeon's determination of the patient's ability to withstand removal of a portion of lung or an entire lung. Functional status in patients with lung disease is typically categorized using the *Karnofsky Scale of Performance* (Table 37-3). A clinical stair climbing test may also be performed to provide a subjective estimation of a patient's cardiopulmonary reserve (Shields, 1989). The patient is asked to climb one or more flights of stairs, accompanied by a surgeon or nurse who can directly evaluate the presence and severity of dyspnea on exertion. This subjective assessment may provide helpful supplemental information to data obtained from standard pulmonary function or exercise testing.

DIAGNOSTIC STUDIES

Standard laboratory studies obtained before operations on the thorax include a complete blood cell count, urinalysis, blood clotting studies, blood chemistry survey, electrocardiogram, and chest roentgenogram. These baseline studies are typically performed within 1 week of the planned operation and are essential to detect any abnormalities that could increase risk of the operation or alter the plan of therapy. In

patients with signs or symptoms of ischemic heart disease, exercise stress testing may be performed to detect myocardial ischemia before proceeding with a planned thoracic operation. Arrhythmias or congestive heart failure may also require diagnostic evaluation before operation.

In selected patients, room air arterial blood gases may be measured to identify arterial hypoxemia or carbon dioxide retention and to provide a baseline for comparison with postoperative measurements. In patients with pulmonary neoplasms, a stool specimen may be obtained to test for the presence of blood. Occult blood in the stool might indicate that the lung lesion is not a primary tumor but rather an adenocarcinoma of the bowel that has metastasized to the lung.

In patients who will undergo pulmonary resection, *pulmonary function testing* is generally performed to assess the patient's ability to withstand removal of a portion of functional lung tissue. Pulmonary function testing identifies patients at higher risk for pulmonary complications and allows implementation of prophylactic interventions in the preoperative period (Lumb, 1990). The most commonly measured parameters are *forced vital capacity* (FVC) and *forced expiratory volume* (FEV), which quantitate volume and flow of respiration. FVC measures the total volume of air that can be forcefully expelled after maximal inspiration. Forced expiratory volume in 1 second (FEV_1) measures the average flow exhaled in the first second (Enright & Hodgkin, 1991). FEV_1, FVC, and the FEV_1:FVC ratio are the best indicators of obstructive lung disease. Although no single value can determine inability to tolerate pulmonary resection, an FEV_1 of less than 1 L, or 40% of predicted normal, is generally considered to contraindicate a major pulmonary resection (Shields, 1989).

Patients with intrathoracic abnormalities will often have previously undergone bronchoscopy, chest computed tomography, or magnetic resonance imaging as part of the diagnostic evaluation. In patients with diseases of the esophagus, esophagoscopy, contrast swallow studies, or esophageal manometry may have been performed. These diagnostic modalities are described in detail in Chapter 36, Diagnostic Evaluation of Thoracic Disease.

TABLE 37-3. KARNOFSKY SCALE OF PERFORMANCE

Clinical Status	Percentage
Normal, no evidence of disease	100
Minor signs or symptoms of disease	90
Normal activity with effort	80
Cares for self, cannot do normal activities	70
Cares for self with occasional assistance	60
Requires frequent assistance and medical care	50
Disabled, requires special care and assistance	40
Severely disabled, hospitalization indicated	30
Hospitalization with active supportive treatment	20
Moribund, fatal processes progressing rapidly	10

(Adapted from Shields TW, 1994: Presentation, diagnosis, and staging of bronchial carcinoma and of the asymptomatic solitary pulmonary nodule. In Shields TW [ed]: General Thoracic Surgery, ed. 4. Baltimore, Williams & Wilkins)

PREOPERATIVE REGIMEN

GENERAL GUIDELINES

Most medications, with the exception of anticoagulant and antiplatelet agents, are continued throughout the preoperative period until the time of surgery. This includes maintenance antihypertensive, antiarrhythmic, antianginal, and antiseizure agents (Reves et al., 1990). Digoxin is sometimes administered prophylactically before major pulmonary or esophageal resection procedures because of the prevalence of postoperative supraventricular tachycardia. Although the etiology is unclear, postoperative supraventricular tachycardia is common, particularly in elderly patients (Shields, 1994). Achieving a therapeutic serum digoxin level before operation may not prevent occurrence of tachyarrhythmias, but it is believed by some to facilitate control of the ventricular response rate during supraventricular tachycardia.

Preoperative antibiotic prophylaxis is generally performed to reduce the likelihood of perioperative infection. Wound contamination is most likely to occur during the operation. Potential sources of microorganisms include a preexisting infection, the patient's skin, and operating room personnel and equipment. The most frequently encountered causative pathogens for infection of surgical wounds are *Staphylococcus aureus* and *S. epidermidis* (Doebbling et al., 1990). Pulmonary infections after noncardiac thoracic operations are usually due to *Hemophilus influenzae*, pneumococcus, or *S. aureus* (Kaiser, 1990). A broad-spectrum agent, such as a cephalosporin, is administered intramuscularly just before transporting the patient to the operating room or intravenously when the patient arrives in the operating room. One or two subsequent doses may be given in the postoperative period. If the patient is allergic to penicillin, an alternative agent, such as vancomycin, is used.

Generally, 2 units of cross-matched blood are reserved for potential intraoperative use. Transfusion of homologous blood is performed judiciously. Blood is a limited commodity and despite testing of donors, a small risk exists for transmitting hepatitis B, hepatitis C (non-A, non-B hepatitis), or human immunodeficiency virus infection through homologous transfusion. Blood transfusions can also cause allergic reactions and sensitization to blood products (Scott et al., 1990).

Patients are instructed to abstain from any oral intake after midnight on the evening before the planned procedure. A preoperative shower, using an antibacterial soap, is prescribed for the evening before and morning of the operation. The patient is instructed to thoroughly cleanse the chest and axillae. Shaving of the chest is usually performed in the operating room. A preoperative enema is generally not necessary.

Before transporting the patient to the operating room, a preoperative medication is administered to reduce anxiety, provide perioperative amnesia, suppress physiologic stress responses, and facilitate induction of anesthesia. One or more of several types of drugs may be administered, including (1) sedatives, hypnotics, and tranquilizers; (2) opioids; (3) anticholinergic agents; or (4) antihistamines and antacids (Wong & Brunner, 1994). The type and dosage are generally prescribed by the anesthesiologist, based on the patient's age, underlying pulmonary disease, associated medical diseases, and level of anxiety. Administration of the preoperative medication is carefully timed to reduce patient apprehension at the time of transfer yet maintain a level of consciousness sufficient for the patient to cooperate with preparatory interventions on arrival in the operating room.

SPECIAL CONSIDERATIONS

In patients with underlying pulmonary disease, the preoperative regimen may include interventions that are instituted several weeks before a planned operation. Particularly if pulmonary resection is planned, therapies such as smoking cessation, bronchial hygiene treatments, or administration of bronchodilating medications may significantly improve pulmonary function. Smoking cessation is of prime importance. It permits recovery of mucociliary function and allows bronchitic effects of tobacco smoke to abate (Metzler, 1989). Even a smoke-free period of 1 to 2 weeks increases a patient's ability to clear secretions during the postoperative period. An aggressive bronchial hygiene regimen, which may include bronchodilating medications, will also aid in removing retained secretions. Occasionally, pulmonary function that is initially considered inadequate for surgical removal of lung tissue can be improved enough to allow tolerance of pulmonary resection.

In diabetic patients, insulin dosage is reduced on the day of operation. Typically, one half of the usual dose is given and glucose-containing intravenous fluids are administered to prevent hypoglycemia. In patients who have been receiving chronic corticosteroid therapy, parenteral corticosteroids are administered immediately before the operation and are continued postoperatively until oral corticosteroid therapy is resumed. A parenteral corticosteroid regimen prevents acute adrenal insufficiency that can result from abrupt cessation of corticosteroid therapy in corticosteroid-dependent patients (Gotch, 1991). Patients undergoing thymectomy for treatment of myasthenia gravis require careful titration of pharmacologic therapy during the preoperative period. Achieving relative stability of the disease before thymectomy is important to minimize postoperative complications (Mathisen, 1991). Usually, a neurologist directs the patient's preoperative medication regimen.

For selected procedures, such as esophageal resection with colon interposition, a special preoperative regimen is necessary to cleanse the bowel of fecal material and normal bacterial flora. Bowel cleansing reduces the likelihood of perioperative infection caused by bacteria normally present in the bowel. The regimen generally consists of several days of dietary restrictions and oral antibiotics.

PREOPERATIVE COUNSELING

A wide continuum of learning needs and emotional responses are encountered in preoperative patients. Although typically described as "preoperative teaching," the purpose of preoperative counseling is two-fold: (1) provision of adequate information about the perioperative course and (2) provision of psychological support sufficient to allay anxiety and promote effective coping. Two factors merit special consideration in thoracic surgical patients. First, most patients are admitted to the hospital on the morning of the planned operation. Second, many patients who undergo thoracic surgical procedures have been diagnosed with, or face the possibility of, a malignant disease. Thus, the time available for preoperative instruction after hospital admission is limited and patients are likely to have significant anxiety.

Ideally, preoperative counseling is initiated before admission. It is best performed by a staff nurse or clinical specialist from the unit where the patient will recover postoperatively. Preoperative teaching is designed to complement information the patient receives from the surgeon and anesthesiologist regarding the planned operation and its potential benefits and risks. Specific content varies depending on protocols for the particular operation, surgeon, and institution. Preoperative instruction typically includes a description of the projected events that will occur during each phase of the hospitalization, with special emphasis on the perioperative period (Table 37-4). Information about discharge from the hospital and recovery at home are best deferred until after the operation. Often, the teaching session is supplemented with written materials, particularly if the patient and family have differing needs for information. Audiovisual materials are also helpful adjuncts to teaching and provide a reference throughout the patient's hospitalization. Because they involve more than one sense in the learning process, they are thought to increase knowledge retention (Scalzi & Burke, 1989).

TABLE 37-4. CONTENT OF PREOPERATIVE EDUCATION

Preoperative Phase

Members of the team
Dietary restrictions
Antibacterial shower
Preparatory shave
Disposition of belongings
Preoperative sedation
Time and length of operation
Waiting room for family

Postoperative Phase

Units in which patient will stay
Visiting for family
Overview of attached catheters and monitoring devices
Expectations for patient participation in recovery process
Pulmonary hygiene measures
Pain control
Activity guidelines
Progression of ambulation

During preoperative counseling, expectations for the patient's participation in the recovery process are discussed. Patient instruction about the pulmonary hygiene regimen, progressive ambulation, and pain management is particularly important in thoracic surgical patients. Adequate lung expansion and clearing of secretions is essential to prevent atelectasis, pneumonia, or respiratory failure. Usually an incentive spirometry device is used in the postoperative period to facilitate effective lung expansion (Fig. 37-1). Typically, the patient is instructed to use the device every 1 to 2 hours to take and sustain a series of deep inspirations. Allowing the patient to practice breathing exercises in the preoperative period improves postoperative cooperation and strengthens respiratory musculature (Wolfe & Smith, 1990).

Patients are also informed about the planned progression of activity after surgery. Early and progressive ambulation is important to reduce the morbidity associated with immobility. If adequately prepared, the patient can participate more effectively in this regimen. It is also important to discuss postoperative pain management before thoracic operations. Because major chest wall muscles are generally divided, thoracotomy incisions are particularly painful. Several methods of analgesia are available to provide adequate postoperative pain control. One of three techniques may be used to administer opioid analgesic agents: (1) epidural infusion, (2) patient-controlled intravenous dosing, or (3) conventional intermittent parenteral dosing. Often the patient is given the option of choosing preoperatively the technique of postoperative analgesia.

Provision of psychological support is an integral part of nursing care during the immediate preoperative period. Almost all patients experience some fear and anxiety during this time. In fact, moderate anxiety is considered indicative that a patient is emotionally ready for an operation and may help the patient cope with postoperative stress and discomfort (Gregersen & McGregor, 1989). Manifestations of anxiety in preoperative patients include a variety of psychophysiologic symptoms, such as increased tension, a sense of helplessness, decreased self-assurance, and focusing on the perceived object of fear (Carty, 1991).

Effective interventions for preoperative anxiety include (1) allowing the patient to verbalize concerns, (2) providing factual information to reduce fear that is based on distorted perceptions, and (3) providing reassurance about the nurses' and physicians' commitment to the patient's well-being. Sometimes, patients are severely anxious about an impending thoracic operation. If the patient's need for support exceeds what the nurse can realistically provide, psychiatric consultation may be necessary. Principles used to guide preoperative education and psychologic support are discussed more fully in Chapter 10, Education and Psychological Support for the Patient and Family.

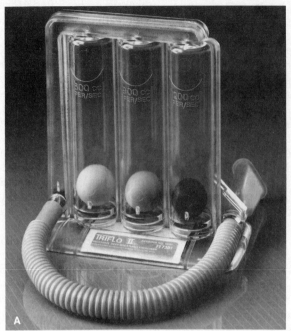 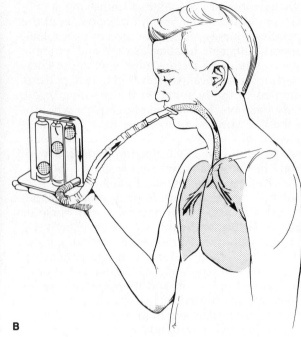

FIGURE 37-1. **(A)** An incentive spirometry device such as the Triflo II is used to promote lung expansion in the postoperative period. **(B)** Preoperative instruction typically includes allowing the patient to practice using the device. (Courtesy of Sherwood Medical Co., St. Louis, MO)

REFERENCES

Carty JL, 1991: Psychosocial aspects. In Alspach JG (ed): Core Curriculum for Critical Care Nursing, ed. 4. Philadelphia, WB Saunders

Cohen AJ, Thompson L, Edwards FH, Bellamy RF, 1991: Primary cysts and tumors of the mediastinum. Ann Thorac Surg 51:378

Davis RD, Oldham HN Jr, Sabiston DC Jr, 1990: The mediastinum. In Sabiston DC Jr, Spencer FC (eds): Surgery of the Chest, ed. 5. Philadelphia, WB Saunders

Doebbeling BN, Pfaller MA, Kuhns KR, et al., 1990: Cardiovascular surgery prophylaxis. J Thorac Cardiovasc Surg 99:981

Enright PL, Hodgkin JE, 1991: Pulmonary function tests. In Respiratory Care, ed. 3. Philadelphia, JB Lippincott

Gotch PM, 1991: The endocrine system. In Alspach JG (ed): Core Curriculum for Critical Care Nursing, ed. 4. Philadelphia, WB Saunders

Gregersen RA, McGregor MS, 1989: Cardiac surgery. In Underhill SL, Woods SL, Froelicher ES, Halpenny CJ (eds): Cardiac Nursing, ed. 2. Philadelphia, JB Lippincott

Hillis LD, Lange RA, Wells PJ, Winniford MD, 1992: Noncardiac surgery in patients with coronary artery disease. In Manual of Clinical Problems in Cardiology, ed. 4. Boston, Little, Brown

Kaiser AB, 1990: Use of antibiotics in cardiac and thoracic surgery. In Sabiston DC Jr, Spencer FC (eds): Surgery of the Chest, ed. 5. Philadelphia, WB Saunders

Kanarek DJ, 1989: Evaluation for pulmonary resection. In Grillo HC, Austen WG, Wilkins EW, et al. (eds): Current Therapy in Cardiothoracic Surgery. Toronto, BC Decker

Lumb PD, 1990: Perioperative pulmonary physiology. In Sabiston DC Jr, Spencer FC (eds): Surgery of the Chest, ed. 5. Philadelphia, WB Saunders

Mathisen DJ, 1991: Thymectomy: Avoidance and management of complications. In Waldhausen JA, Orringer MB (eds): Complications in Cardiothoracic Surgery. St. Louis, Mosby–Year Book

Metzler MH, 1989: Pre- and postoperative respiratory care. In Braun SR (ed): Concise Textbook of Pulmonary Medicine. New York, Elsevier

Pairolero PC, Payne WS, 1991: Postoperative care and complications in the thoracic surgery patient. In Baue AE, Geha AS, Hammond GL, et al. (eds): Glenn's Thoracic and Cardiovascular Surgery, ed 5. Norwalk, CT, Appleton & Lange

Reves JG, Greeley WJ, Leslie J, 1990: Anesthesia and supportive care for cardiothoracic surgery. In Sabiston DC Jr, Spencer FC (eds): Surgery of the Chest, ed. 5. Philadelphia, WB Saunders

Scalzi CC, Burke LE, 1989: Education of the patient and family: In-hospital phase. In Underhill SL, Woods SL, Froelicher ES, Halpenny CJ (eds): Cardiac Nursing, ed. 2. Philadelphia, JB Lippincott

Scott WJ, Kessler R, Wernly JA, 1990: Blood conservation in cardiac surgery. Ann Thorac Surg 50:843

Shields TW, 1989: Carcinoma of the lung. In Shields TW (ed): General Thoracic Surgery, ed. 3. Philadelphia, Lea & Febiger

Shields TW, 1994: General features and complications of pulmonary resections. In Shields TW (ed): General Thoracic Surgery, ed. 4. Baltimore, Williams & Wilkins

Shields TW, 1991: Lung cancer: Diagnosis and staging. In Baue AE, Geha AS, Hammond GL, et al. (eds): Glenn's Thoracic and Cardiovascular Surgery, ed. 5. Norwalk, CT, Appleton & Lange

Stein HJ, DeMeester TR, Hinder RA, 1992: Evaluation and surgical management of motor disorders of the esophageal body and lower esophageal sphincter. Curr Probl Surg 24:447

Wilson RS, 1991: Anesthesia for thoracic surgery. In Baue AE, Geha AS, Hammond GL, et al. (eds): Glenn's Thoracic and Cardiovascular Surgery, ed. 5. Norwalk, CT, Appleton & Lange

Wolfe WG, Smith PK, 1990: Preoperative assessment of pulmonary function: Quantitative evaluation of ventilation and blood gas exchange. In Sabiston DC Jr, Spencer FC (eds): Surgery of the Chest, ed. 5. Philadelphia, WB Saunders

Wong HY, Brunner EA, 1994: Preanesthetic evaluation and preparation. In Shields TW (ed): General Thoracic Surgery, ed. 4. Baltimore, Williams & Wilkins

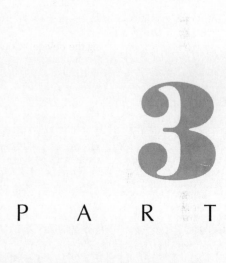

3

P A R T

THORACIC OPERATIONS

38

SURGICAL TREATMENT
OF PULMONARY DISEASE

CARCINOMA OF THE LUNG
   Indications for Surgical Treatment
   Preoperative Evaluation
   Types of Pulmonary Resections
   The Operative Procedure
   Results

OTHER PULMONARY DISEASES
   Metastatic Lung Tumors
   Benign Lung Disease

The pulmonary disease most commonly treated with surgery is carcinoma of the lung. Less often, pulmonary surgery is performed to remove a malignant tumor that has metastasized to the lung from outside the thorax or to treat benign forms of pulmonary disease.

CARCINOMA OF THE LUNG

By far the most common form of lung cancer is *bronchogenic carcinoma,* which arises from the epithelial lining of the bronchi. Bronchogenic lung cancer is further categorized according to histologic cell type as (1) adenocarcinoma, (2) squamous or epidermoid carcinoma, (3) small cell carcinoma, or (4) large cell carcinoma. Uncommon forms of lung cancer include *bronchoalveolar carcinoma,* which originates in the lung parenchyma, and *mesothelioma,* which arises in the pleura.

Bronchogenic lung cancer generally occurs in the form of a solitary tumor. Lesions that involve the mainstem, lobar, or segmental bronchi are considered *central*, and those that originate in distal bronchi, bronchioles, or lung parenchyma are termed *peripheral*. Most squamous cell tumors are located centrally in major bronchi; adenocarcinoma, on the other

hand, usually originates in the lung periphery. Malignant lung tumors occur more commonly in the right lung and usually in the upper lobes (Shields, 1994a). A *Pancoast,* or *superior sulcus tumor,* is a bronchogenic carcinoma that arises in the superior pulmonary sulcus or thoracic inlet and invades lymphatic tissue in the endothoracic fascia (Urschel, 1993) (Fig. 38-1).

Malignant lung tumors can spread by any of three routes. First, they may directly invade contiguous pulmonary parenchyma (tissue) and adjacent structures, such as the pleura, diaphragm, chest wall, or mediastinal organs. Second, lung tumors often spread to lymph nodes in the pulmonary hilum or mediastinum and are disseminated through the lymphatic system. Third, tumor cells can invade pulmonary veins in the lungs and spread to distant organs through the vascular system.

INDICATIONS FOR SURGICAL TREATMENT

For non–small cell bronchogenic lung cancer, the treatment of choice is surgical resection of the tumor and surrounding lymphatic tissue. However, the ability to surgically remove a lung tumor depends on the location and size of the tumor, presence of tumor cells in regional lymph nodes, and whether tumor has invaded nearby structures, such as the great ves-

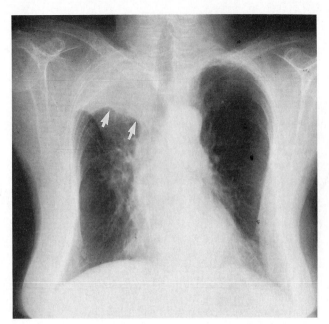

FIGURE 38-1. Chest radiograph demonstrating right Pancoast tumor (*arrows*). (Courtesy of Robert M. Vanecko, M.D.)

sels or trachea. Incomplete resection of a malignant tumor does not enhance survival and has little or no palliative benefit (Shields, 1993).

To determine a tumor's suitability for resection before surgical treatment, a clinical determination is made of the patient's anatomic stage of disease. The *International Staging System* provides standard nomenclature for categorizing the extent of disease in patients with lung cancer (Mountain, 1986). It consists of a three-letter code, with the first letter, "T," designating tumor size; the second, "N," the presence and extent of lymph node involvement; and the third, "M," the presence of distant metastasis.

Once TNM status is determined, the anatomic stage of disease is categorized as stage I, II, IIIA, IIIB, or IV. Staging of the disease enables the physician to select the most appropriate therapy and provide prognostic information. Stage I lung cancer is considered early disease, stage II cancer is intermediate, and stages III and IV represent advanced disease (Martini et al., 1992). TNM definitions and staging of lung cancer are described in more detail in Chapter 33, Pulmonary, Tracheal, and Pleural Diseases.

A lung tumor is assessed initially by its appearance on the chest roentgenogram. The roentgenogram demonstrates tumor size, location, and involvement of contiguous structures, such as the chest wall. The roentgenogram may also provide suggestive evidence of tumor involvement of mediastinal lymph nodes. If the mediastinal shadow is abnormal in appearance, computed tomography is usually performed to more clearly demonstrate the presence of mediastinal adenopathy (i.e., lymph node enlargement).

If lymph nodes 1 cm or larger are evident on the chest roentgenogram or computed tomogram, mediastinal exploration by mediastinoscopy or mediastinotomy is recommended before thoracotomy. Mediastinal lymph node involvement represents N2 as opposed to N1 disease, in which only pulmonary lymph nodes contain tumor (Fig. 38-2). Surgical resection is usually not recommended once tumor cells have spread to mediastinal lymphatic tissue. Surgical treatment of lung cancer is also contraindicated in the presence of distant metastasis. Consequently, any patient with signs or symptoms of distant metastasis undergoes scans of all potential metastatic sites (e.g., brain, upper abdomen, and bones) (Shields, 1993).

Surgical candidates are generally those patients with stage I or stage II disease (Table 38-1). Selected

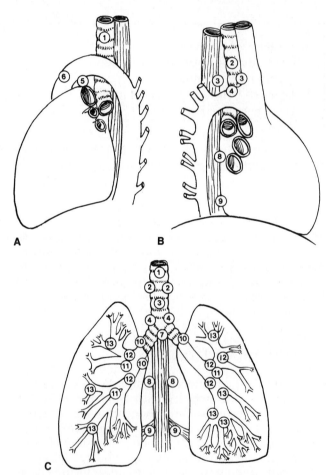

FIGURE 38-2. Left lateral **(A),** right lateral **(B),** and anterior **(C)** views demonstrating sites of lymph node metastasis in carcinoma of the lung. N2 nodes: *1,* highest mediastinal; *2,* upper paratracheal; *3,* pretracheal and retrotracheal; *4,* lower paratracheal; *5,* subaortic; *6,* para-aortic; *7,* subcarinal; *8,* paraesophageal; *9,* pulmonary ligament. N1 nodes: *10,* hilar; *11,* interlobar; *12,* lobar; *13,* segmental. (Beahrs OH, Myers MH [eds], 1992: American Joint Committee on Cancer: Manual for Staging of Cancer, ed. 4, p. 122. Philadelphia, JB Lippincott)

TABLE 38-1. MALIGNANT LUNG TUMORS TREATED WITH SURGICAL RESECTION

Non–Small Cell

Stage I

Proximal extent of tumor within lobar bronchus or at least 2 cm distal to carina

Associated atelectasis or obstructive pneumonitis involves less than entire lung

No demonstrable metastasis to regional lymph nodes

No distant metastasis

Stage II

Proximal extent of tumor within lobar bronchus or at least 2 cm distal to carina

Associated atelectasis or obstructive pneumonitis involves less than entire lung

Metastasis to peribronchial or ipsilateral hilar region present

No distant metastasis

Stage IIIA*

Tumor extends into chest wall, diaphragm, or mediastinal pleura or pericardium without involving heart, great vessels, trachea, esophagus, or vertebral body, or tumor in main bronchus within 2 cm of the carina without involving carina

or

Metastasis to ipsilateral mediastinal and subcarinal lymph nodes

Small Cell†

Isolated tumor and limited regional disease

---

* In selected patients only.

† As adjuvant to combination chemotherapy.

---

patients with stage IIIA lung tumors may be treated with surgical resection (e.g., those with peripheral tumors that have invaded the parietal pleura, diaphragm, or chest wall). Tumors categorized as stage IIIA because of confirmed N2 disease (i.e., tumor invasion of ipsilateral mediastinal or subcarinal lymph nodes) are generally not treated surgically. Surgical resection is contraindicated in patients with stage IIIB or stage IV lung cancer.

Unfortunately, surgical resection is possible in only 20% to 25% of patients with non–small cell lung tumors (Shields, 1993). Approximately 50% of patients diagnosed with lung cancer have evidence of distant metastasis; of the remaining potential operative candidates, approximately one half have intrathoracic spread that precludes surgical resection (Sabiston, 1990). Pulmonary resection may also be prohibited by the patient's general medical condition, particularly in the presence of severe underlying pulmonary impairment or cardiovascular disease. Table 38-2 displays potential contraindications to pulmonary resection in patients with lung cancer.

Small cell lung tumors are seldom treated with surgical resection. Small cell lung cancer has distinct biologic and clinical characteristics that distinguish it from other types of lung cancer (Mentzer et al., 1993b). Most important from a surgical perspective is a rapid doubling time that results in early tumor dissemination. Consequently, only a limited number of patients with small cell lung cancer have a single tumor and no evident metastases. Surgical resection may be appropriate in selected patients with small cell lung cancer as an adjunct to combination chemotherapy for removal of residual disease. Appropriate candidates for adjuvant surgical resection are those patients with an isolated tumor nodule and limited regional disease (Mentzer et al., 1993b).

PREOPERATIVE EVALUATION

The objective of pulmonary resection for lung cancer is to completely remove all visible tumor with regional lymph nodes that may contain malignant cells. In planning the resection, consideration is given to whether the tumor has spread to lymph nodes or invaded extraparenchymal structures, such as the chest wall, diaphragm, or pericardium. The pulmonary resection should be as conservative as possible without compromising the complete removal of local and regional disease within the thorax (Shields, 1993).

Preoperative pulmonary function testing and assessment of the patient's current functional status are performed to predict how much lung tissue can safely be removed. Patient age and presence of associated medical conditions, particularly cardiovascular disease, also influence a patient's ability to withstand a pulmonary resection. The planned pulmonary resection is based on an assessment of (1) the amount of lung tissue that must be removed to completely eradicate visible tumor, (2) the impairment that may be anticipated due to the loss of lung tissue, and (3) any associated medical problems that may impact on the patient's perioperative course (Kanarek, 1989).

Because of the association between smoking and lung cancer, many patients who require pulmonary

TABLE 38-2. POTENTIAL CONTRAINDICATIONS TO PULMONARY RESECTION FOR LUNG CANCER

Evidence of extrapulmonary spread
  Paralysis of recurrent laryngeal nerve
  Superior vena cava syndrome
  Phrenic nerve paralysis
  Pleural effesion with malignant cells
Technical considerations
  Involvement of the main pulmonary artery
  Involvement of the tracheal carina
Medical conditions
  Marginal pulmonary function
  Unstable angina or recent myocardial infarction
  Congestive heart failure
Distant metastases

resection have underlying obstructive pulmonary disease. In patients with severe pulmonary impairment, preoperative interventions, such as smoking cessation, intensive pulmonary hygiene, antibiotics (for existing infection), bronchodilator therapy, and pulmonary rehabilitation, are performed before surgical treatment to reduce perioperative risk (Reilly et al., 1993). Often these interventions can markedly improve pulmonary function.

Depending on tumor location, either a lobectomy or pneumonectomy is generally performed. A lesser pulmonary resection may be necessary in patients with marginal pulmonary function to ensure sufficient residual lung parenchyma for adequate ventilation. If pulmonary function is so marginal that the necessary surgical resection would not be tolerated, operative therapy is precluded. An alternative treatment modality (e.g., irradiation) may be performed for palliation of symptoms.

TYPES OF PULMONARY RESECTIONS

The various types of pulmonary resection operations are named according to the amount of lung tissue that is removed. The lungs are divided by fissures into lobes: three on the right and two on the left. The lobes are subdivided into bronchopulmonary segments: 10 in the right lung and 8 in the left lung (Shields, 1994b).

Lobectomy is the most commonly performed pulmonary resection for lung cancer. It is the procedure of choice when a tumor is confined to a lobe and neither N1 (lobar or hilar) nor N2 (mediastinal) lymph node metastasis is present that would preclude complete removal of all diseased tissue (Shields, 1993). A *bilobectomy* (i.e., removal of the right middle lobe along with either the upper or lower lobe) may be performed if a right-sided tumor extends across an interlobar fissure or if a fissure is absent. Because the right lung has three anatomic lobes, a bilobectomy allows preservation of one remaining lobe.

If the tumor can be removed completely without resecting an entire lobe of a lung, a wedge resection or segmentectomy may be performed. A *wedge resection* is the removal of a peripheral piece of lung tissue containing the tumor. It sacrifices the least amount of normal lung parenchyma. A *segmentectomy* is removal of an anatomic segment of a lobe, including the bronchus, and pulmonary artery and vein of the segment (Faber & Jensik, 1991). Although any segment can be resected, segmentectomy of the upper lobes is most commonly performed (Shields, 1993). When a wedge resection or segmentectomy is performed, it is not technically possible to remove all adjacent lobar lymph nodes (Faber & Jensik, 1991).

Wedge resection and segmentectomy are considered *limited pulmonary resections*. Although long-term survival after limited resection is similar to that for lobectomy in patients with stage I lung cancer, those who undergo limited resection are more likely to develop local recurrence of disease (Mentzer et al., 1993a). As a result, limited pulmonary resection is considered by many to be an inadequate operation for treatment of bronchogenic carcinoma if the patient can tolerate lobectomy. Limited resections are thus generally reserved for elderly patients or those with marginal cardiopulmonary status who have a stage I tumor that is less than 3 cm.

A *pneumonectomy,* or removal of an entire lung, is required for complete removal of lesions that involve the left or right main bronchus or that have spread or are fixed to the hilum (Sabiston, 1990). Most patients with good pulmonary function are able to withstand loss of an entire lung. However, operative mortality with pneumonectomy is higher than that associated with lobectomy. Also, in patients with a long smoking history, pulmonary or cardiac function may be impaired to the degree that removal of an entire lung is contraindicated. Preoperative studies that may be performed to assist in determining a patient's ability to tolerate pneumonectomy include (1) split-function studies that measure individual lung function, (2) radioisotope measurement of pulmonary ventilation and perfusion, (3) measurement of unilateral pulmonary artery pressure and pulmonary vascular resistance using balloon occlusion of the ipsilateral pulmonary artery, and (4) exercise testing with measurement of maximal oxygen consumption (Filderman & Matthay, 1989).

Five to 8% of patients have tumors that can be resected with *lobectomy and sleeve resection* (Lowe & Sabiston, 1990). A sleeve resection (also called a *bronchoplastic procedure*) enables the surgeon to avoid performing a pneumonectomy when tumor extends into a lobar bronchus. Candidates for sleeve resection lobectomy are patients with (1) a tumor that is centrally located, (2) metastatic lymph nodes near a main bronchus, or (3) compromised pulmonary function that precludes pneumonectomy (Van Schil et al., 1991).

A sleeve resection lobectomy consists of resecting the lobe en bloc (i.e., as a whole) with a portion of the common airway; the transected airway is then reconstructed to restore lung continuity (Mentzer et al., 1993a) (Fig. 38-3). Bronchoplastic techniques may be performed for resection of tumors of the upper and lower lobes on both the right and left sides but are most applicable for localized tumors originating in the right upper lobe orifice (Tedder & Lowe, 1992). Survival rates after sleeve resection are comparable with those achieved with conventional lobectomy or pneumonectomy (Lowe & Sabiston, 1990).

Sometimes tumor invasion necessitates surgical resection of structures contiguous to the lungs and bronchi. Any of the pulmonary resection procedures can be combined with en bloc removal of structures beyond the visceral pleura into which the tumor has extended (Shields, 1993). An *extrapleural pneumonectomy* is the removal of not only an entire lung but also the parietal pleura surrounding the lung, as well as portions of the diaphragm and pericardium. If tumor

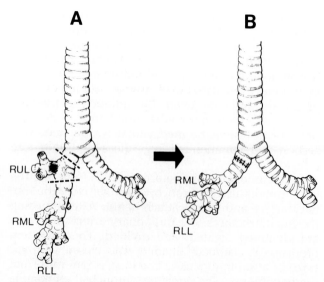

A   **B**

RUL

RML

RLL

RML

RLL

FIGURE 38-3. Schematic representation of bronchoplastic technique during sleeve lobectomy. **(A)** Tracheobronchial tree with tumor in orifice of right upper lobe (*RUL*) bronchus; right mainstream bronchus is divided (*dotted lines*), and RUL is removed en bloc. **(B)** Bronchial continuity is restored by reconstructing right mainstem bronchus. *RML*, right middle lobe; *RLL*, right lower lobe. (Mentzer SJ, Myers DW, Sugarbaker DJ, 1993: Sleeve lobectomy, segmentectomy, and thoracoscopy in the management of carcinoma of the lung. Chest 103:416S)

has invaded the chest wall, an *en bloc chest wall resection* may be performed along with the pulmonary resection. Some surgeons with extensive experience with tracheal surgery recommend *tracheal resection* in combination with pulmonary resection, if a lung tumor that is otherwise resectable encroaches on the carina of the mainstem trachea (Mathisen & Grillo, 1991).

Completion pneumonectomy is the name given to resection of a remaining lobe or lobes after a prior lobectomy or bilobectomy of the lung. Completion pneumonectomy is performed uncommonly. It is technically complex because adhesions from the prior pulmonary resection in the same hemithorax make mobilization of the residual lung difficult and blood loss greater (Gregoire et al., 1993). Accordingly, completion pneumonectomy is recommended only if there is sufficient pulmonary reserve in the contralateral lung to tolerate loss of the remaining ipsilateral lung, the patient's general condition is adequate to tolerate the procedure, and the risks of the procedure are balanced by the expected improvement in prognosis (McGovern et al., 1988).

THE OPERATIVE PROCEDURE

On arrival in the operating room, a preoperative dose of intravenous antibiotics is generally administered to reduce the likelihood of perioperative wound infec-

tion. Often an epidural catheter is placed to be used for postoperative infusion of opioid analgesic agents. Bronchoscopy is usually performed before thoracotomy to identify any previously undetected endobronchial abnormalities. A fiberoptic bronchoscope is inserted into the tracheobronchial tree after induction of general anesthesia and used to thoroughly examine segmental and subsegmental bronchi. Bronchoscopic visualization may reveal the tumor itself exposed in bronchial mucosa or abnormalities in the bronchial wall or lumen size produced by tumor infiltration or external compression (Shields, 1991).

Pulmonary resection operations are most commonly performed through a thoracotomy incision. After positioning the patient in a lateral decubitus position with the operative lung up, the skin of the operative field is prepared with an antibiotic solution to reduce skin flora. Typically, a posterolateral incision is performed (Fig. 38-4). Subcutaneous tissue along the course of the incision is divided, as well as the latissimus dorsi and serratus anterior muscles (Crawford & Kratz, 1990). The fifth or sixth interspace is incised for upper lobe or lower lobe resection, respectively. One or more ribs may be surgically divided or a small segment of rib is removed (i.e., the rib is "shingled") to facilitate spreading the chest wall for adequate exposure.

In patients with limited pulmonary reserve, a muscle-sparing incision may be performed alternatively. The term *muscle-sparing* denotes that the serratus anterior and latissimus dorsi muscles are retracted without being surgically divided when the chest wall is opened. A muscle-sparing thoracotomy incision appears to decrease pain and reduce shoulder girdle disability in the early postoperative period (Hazelrigg et al., 1991). Splinting and hypoventilation secondary to pain may therefore be less pronounced than after a standard thoracotomy incision in which major chest wall muscles are divided.

Initially, the pleural space is entered and the lung is freed from the chest wall in areas where it is tethered by adhesions. *Single lung ventilation* is used for pulmonary resection operations, as well as for most other types of thoracic operations. A double-lumen endotracheal tube is positioned in the right or left mainstem bronchus, on the same side as the operative lung (Fig. 38-5). Inflation of the cuff at the distal end of the tube occludes the bronchus, allowing ventilation of the contralateral lung only while the lung on the operative side is allowed to collapse. The lung to be resected is thus nonventilated, collapsed, and atelectatic during the procedure (Reves et al., 1990).

The final determination of resectability is made when the pleura is entered. Despite preoperative clinical staging, factors that preclude curative resection are occasionally identified after opening the thorax, such as (1) undetected pleural seeding; (2) extensive, fixed mediastinal lymph node involvement; (3) nonresectable direct extension of the tumor beyond the lung; or (4) inability to safely control the blood

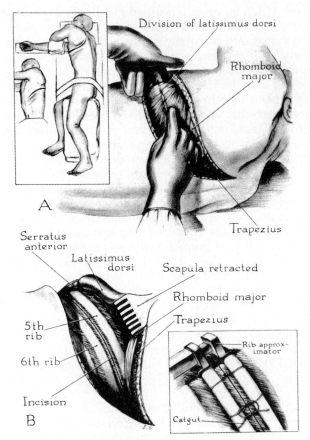

FIGURE 38-4. Posterolateral thoracotomy incision. **(A)** Skin incision extends from just below the nipple posteriorly to 1 inch below the tip of the scapula and then upward between the scapula and spine; when latissimus dorsi and serratus anterior muscles are divided, shoulder girdle glides upward and scapula retracts to expose rib cage. **(B)** Closure of the incision is begun by approximating ribs with rib approximator and securing them with heavy sutures. (Crawford FA, Jr, Kratz J, 1990: Thoracic incisions. In Sabiston DC Jr, Spencer FC [eds]: Surgery of the Chest, ed. 5, p. 191. Philadelphia, WB Saunders)

supply to the lung (Shields, 1993). If a histologic diagnosis has not been established before the operation, a biopsy specimen may be obtained for *frozen section examination* before the pulmonary resection is performed. Guided by digital palpation of the lung, the surgeon directs a biopsy needle device through the lung parenchyma into the lesion. Four or five samples of tissue are plucked from different sites within the lesion. Tissue specimens may also be submitted to be tested for tuberculosis or other bacterial or fungal infection.

If a lobectomy is to be performed, the fissure separating the involved lobe from the other lobe or lobes is carefully divided. All pulmonary artery and vein branches supplying the lobe to be resected are located, ligated, and divided. The lobar bronchus is then isolated, clamped, and divided. The remaining proximal bronchus is closed with sutures or staples. Removal of the lobe is completed by dividing any remaining connections to the other lobe or lobes.

A careful inspection of ipsilateral mediastinal lymph node stations is performed. Lymphatic spread may occur even with small tumors and affects both prognosis and the need for adjunctive therapy. Therefore, a thorough mediastinal lymph node sampling or a systematic mediastinal lymph node dissection is recommended regardless of tumor size (Shields, 1990).

A pneumonectomy is performed by severing the lung from its airway (bronchus) and vascular (pulmonary artery and veins) attachments. After exposing the hilar structures, the pulmonary artery and veins are identified, ligated, and divided. The mainstem bronchus is clamped, divided, and closed with sutures or a stapling device. The lung is removed from the hemithorax. The remaining bronchial segment is covered with adjacent tissue (e.g., pleura, pericardial fat, or pericardium) to help prevent disruption of the closure (Shields, 1994c). As during lobectomy, mediastinal lymph nodes are inspected and sampled. Hemostasis is achieved and the chest wall is closed.

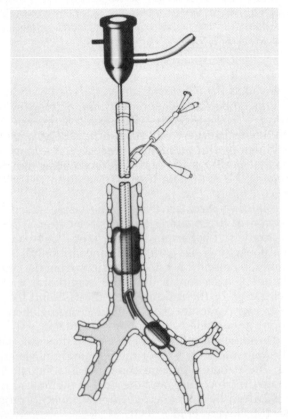

FIGURE 38-5. Double-lumen endotracheal tube positioned using pediatric flexible bronchoscope. (Lewis RJ, Caccavale JR, Sisler GE, Mackenzie JW, 1992: One hundred consecutive patients undergoing video-assisted thoracic operations. Ann Thorac Surg 54:422. Reprinted with permission of the Society of Thoracic Surgeons)

A segmentectomy is performed by identifying, ligating, and dividing the segmental arteries, veins, and bronchus. The segment is then bluntly dissected from surrounding segments of the lobe. Vascular and small airway connections to other segments are clamped, ligated, and divided, and the segment is removed. A wedge resection is performed by excising only the portion of lung containing the tumor and closing the remaining lung edge with staples or sutures (Fig. 38-6).

After lobectomy, segmentectomy, or wedge resection, two chest tubes are inserted into the pleural space through separate incisions. Pleural chest tubes are important to fully reexpand the operative lung and to evacuate blood and air from the pleural space. Negative suction is applied to facilitate lung expansion. The apposition of parietal and visceral pleural surfaces that occurs when the lung is fully expanded enhances cessation of bleeding and air leakage from the operative lung.

A chest tube is generally not placed after pneumonectomy unless excessive bleeding is anticipated. At the conclusion of the operation, pressure within the operative hemithorax is adjusted by thoracentesis to maintain the mediastinum in a midline position. Avoidance of a chest tube after pneumonectomy lessens the risk of empyema (i.e., infection of the pleural space). Infection is more likely after pneumonectomy because of the residual empty space in the

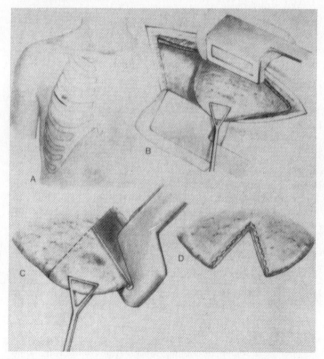

FIGURE 38-6. Wedge resection of peripheral lung parenchyma. Mechanical stapling device is used to excise wedge and close lung edges. (Hood RM, 1984: Stapling techniques involving lung parenchyma. Surg Clin North Am 3:474)

hemithorax after removal of the lung. This is in contrast to lesser pulmonary resection procedures in which the remaining ipsilateral lung almost always expands to fill the hemithorax.

Patients in whom N2 disease (mediastinal lymph node invasion) is confirmed during surgical resection are generally treated adjunctively with radiation therapy in the postoperative period. Radiation therapy may also be used in postoperative patients who develop local recurrence after pulmonary resection. Adjuvant chemotherapy has not proven beneficial in patients with non–small cell cancer.

RESULTS

The risk of operative death is generally less than 5% after pneumonectomy and approximately 2% after lobectomy (Sabiston, 1990). Limited pulmonary resections are associated with an operative risk of less than 1%. Postoperative complications are infrequent after pulmonary resection. Most common are respiratory complications (e.g., atelectasis, pneumonia, or respiratory failure). Other complications of pulmonary resection include cardiac arrhythmias, prolonged air leak, bronchopleural fistula, persistent air space, and empyema (Piccione & Faber, 1991). These complications are discussed in detail in Chapter 43, Complications of Thoracic Operations.

Despite curative resection, many patients die of recurrent carcinoma. Even in patients with stage I disease, who are presumed to have no lymph node or distant metastasis, local or distant disease sometimes recurs (Deschamps et al., 1990). Most deaths occur within the first 12 to 24 months after resection; patients rarely die of the original disease more than 5 years after operation (Shields, 1994d). Postoperative adjuvant therapy (irradiation or chemotherapy) has not been demonstrated to increase the number of long-term survivors; although it may control local recurrence, almost all patients who die of their disease do so with the presence of distant metastasis (Shields, 1993). Patients with lung cancer also have an increased risk for development of a second primary lung cancer.

Long-term results of surgical treatment vary primarily according to the TNM stage of the patient's disease at the time of operation. Cure of disease is most likely in patients with stage I lung cancer, that is, those with smaller, more peripheral tumors without nodal involvement or distant metastases (T1,N0,M0 or T2,N0,M0). Approximately 70% of patients with stage I tumors survive 5 years after surgical resection (Flehinger et al., 1992). Stage II lung tumors (T1,N1,M0 or T2,N1,M0), which are larger and more invasive, are associated with a 49% 5-year survival after surgical resection (Burt & Martini, 1991). Curative surgical resection is possible in only a small percentage of stage IIIA lung tumors. In those patients who do undergo surgical treatment, long-term survival is variable, depending on the presence and location of lymph node metastasis and the size of the tumor.

OTHER PULMONARY DISEASES

METASTATIC LUNG TUMORS

In some instances, pulmonary resection is performed for resection of a *pulmonary metastasis* from a primary tumor located elsewhere in the body. Surgery for pulmonary metastases is local therapy for systemic disease; its purpose is to remove macroscopic disease in preparation for further therapy to eradicate microscopic disease (Kodama et al., 1991). If isolated lesions are present in both lungs, a median sternotomy approach may be used. Through this midline incision, both pleural spaces can be entered and bilateral wedge resections of the lesions performed.

Surgical removal of metastatic lesions is associated with prolonged survival in patients with selected histologic types of tumors. For example, greater than 30% 3-year survival has been reported after removal of metastatic pulmonary tumors in patients with primary osteogenic sarcoma, soft tissue sarcoma, and urinary tract cancers; histologic cell types associated with less favorable or unfavorable results include colorectal, breast, uterine or cervical cancer, and melanoma (Pogrebniak et al., 1988). Other factors taken into consideration when selecting candidates for resection of metastatic pulmonary disease include (1) presence of any other metastatic lesions, (2) tumor-doubling time, (3) availability of adjuvant therapy (i.e., irradiation or chemotherapy), and (4) the disease-free interval.

BENIGN LUNG DISEASE

Benign lung tumors, such as hamartoma or fibroma, are frequently surgically removed because of an inability to definitively determine benignity without thoracotomy and removal of the tumor for histologic evaluation. Less commonly, a benign tumor is removed because it produces pneumonia or atelectasis secondary to bronchial compression.

Pulmonary resection is occasionally performed for benign pulmonary diseases, such as bronchiectasis, hemoptysis, radiation necrosis, or lung abscess. *Bronchiectasis* is a disease characterized by localized or diffuse dilatation and destruction of bronchi. Surgical removal of bronchiectatic lung segments may become necessary in patients with complications of the condition, such as recurrent pneumonia, hemoptysis, or copious sputum production. Pulmonary resection may also be necessary to remove lung tissue destroyed by *infection* (e.g., lung abscess, tuberculosis, or empyema) or *radiation necrosis.*

Infrequently, pulmonary resection is performed for treatment of a congenital abnormality, such as pulmonary sequestration or a pulmonary arteriove-nous malformation. *Pulmonary sequestration* is an abnormality in which a segment or lobe has no communication with the normal tracheobronchial tree and the arterial blood supply is from a systemic vessel (Reynolds, 1994). The anomaly can cause recurrent pulmonary infection or hemoptysis. Definitive treatment of pulmonary sequestration is removal of the involved segment or lobe with its anomalous blood supply. *Pulmonary arteriovenous malformation* describes an anomalous communication between a pulmonary artery and vein that can lead to hemoptysis, hemothorax, or systemic embolization. Surgical excision of the fistula and surrounding tissue is recommended.

Occasionally, *emphysematous bullae* (i.e., nonfunctioning, distended air sacs) are surgically resected. The operative procedure, termed a *bullectomy,* may be necessary for bullae that markedly impair pulmonary function or cause complications, such as pneumothorax, infection, or hemoptysis. Surgical treatment of pneumothorax and diseases of the pleura and trachea are discussed in Chapter 40, Surgery of the Pleura, Trachea, Chest Wall, and Mediastinum.

REFERENCES

Burt M, Martini N, 1991: Surgical treatment of lung carcinoma. In Baue AE, Geha AS, Hammond GL, et al. (eds): Glenn's Thoracic and Cardiovascular Surgery, ed. 5. Norwalk, CT, Appleton & Lange

Crawford FA Jr, Kratz JM, 1990: Thoracic incisions. In Sabiston DC Jr, Spencer FC (eds): Surgery of the Chest, ed. 5. Philadelphia, WB Saunders

Deschamps C, Pairolero PC, Trastek VF, Payne WS, 1990: Multiple primary lung cancers. J Thorac Cardiovasc Surg 99:769

Faber LP, Jensik RJ, 1991: Limited pulmonary resection. In Baue AE, Geha AS, Hammond GL, et al. (eds): Glenn's Thoracic and Cardiovascular Surgery, ed. 5. Norwalk, CT, Appleton & Lange

Filderman AE, Matthay RA, 1989: Preoperative pulmonary evaluation. In Shields TW (ed): General Thoracic Surgery, ed. 3. Philadelphia, Lea & Febiger

Flehinger BJ, Kimmel M, Melamed MR, 1992: The effect of surgical treatment on survival from early lung cancer. Chest 101:1013

Gregoire J, Deslauriers J, Guojin L, Rouleau J, 1993: Indications, risks, and results of completion pneumonectomy. J Thorac Cardiovasc Surg 105:918

Hazelrigg SR, Landreneau RJ, Boley TM, et al., 1991: The effect of muscle-sparing versus standard posterolateral thoracotomy on pulmonary function, muscle strength, and postoperative pain. J Thorac Cardiovasc Surg 101:394

Kanarek DJ, 1989: Evaluation for pulmonary resection. In Grillo HC, Austen WG, Wilkins EW Jr, et al. (eds): Current Therapy in Cardiothoracic Surgery. Toronto, BC Decker

Kodama K, Doi O, Higashiyama M, et al., 1991: Surgical management of lung metastases. J Thorac Cardiovasc Surg 101:901

Lowe JE, Sabiston DC Jr, 1990: Bronchoplastic techniques in the surgical management of benign and malignant pulmonary lesions. In Sabiston DC Jr, Spencer FC (eds): Surgery of the Chest, ed. 5. Philadelphia, WB Saunders

Martini N, Burt ME, Bains MS, et al., 1992: Survival after resection of stage II non-small cell lung cancer. Ann Thorac Surg 54:460

Mathisen DJ, Grillo HC, 1991: Carinal resection for bronchogenic carcinoma. J Thorac Cardiovasc Surg 102:16

McGovern EM, Trastek VF, Pairolero PC, Payne WS, 1988: Completion pneumonectomy: Indications, complications, and results. Ann Thorac Surg 46:141

Mentzer SJ, Myers DW, Sugarbaker DJ, 1993a: Sleeve lobectomy, segmentectomy, and thoracoscopy in the management of carcinoma of the lung. Chest 103:415S

Mentzer SJ, Reilly JJ, Sugarbaker DJ, 1993b: Surgical resection in the management of small-cell carcinoma of the lung. Chest 103:349S

Mountain CF, 1986: A new international staging system for lung cancer. Chest 89:2255

Piccione W Jr, Faber LP, 1991: Management of complications related to pulmonary resection. In Waldhausen JA, Orringer MB (eds): Complications in Cardiothoracic Surgery. St. Louis, Mosby–Year Book

Pogrebniak HW, Stovroff M, Roth JA, Pass HI, 1988: Resection of pulmonary metastases from malignant melanoma: Results of a 16-year experience. Ann Thorac Surg 46:20

Reilly JJ Jr, Mentzer SJ, Sugarbaker DJ, 1993: Preoperative assessment of patients undergoing pulmonary resection. Chest 103:342S

Reves, JG, Greeley WJ, Leslie J, 1990: Anesthesia and supportive care for cardiothoracic surgery. In Sabiston DC Jr, Spencer FC (eds): Surgery of the Chest, ed. 5. Philadelphia, WB Saunders

Reynolds M, 1994: Congenital lesions of the lung. In Shields TW (ed): General Thoracic Surgery, ed. 4. Baltimore, Williams & Wilkins

Sabiston DC Jr, 1990: Carcinoma of the lung. In Sabiston DC Jr, Spencer FC (eds): Surgery of the Chest, ed. 5. Philadelphia, WB Saunders

Shields TW, 1990: Behavior of small bronchial carcinomas. Ann Thorac Surg 50:691

Shields TW, 1994a: Lung cancer: Etiology, carcinogenesis, molecular biology, and pathology. In Shields TW (ed): General Thoracic Surgery, ed. 4. Baltimore, Williams & Wilkins

Shields TW, 1994b: Surgical anatomy of the lungs. In Shields TW (ed): General Thoracic Surgery, ed. 4. Baltimore, Williams & Wilkins

Shields TW, 1994c: General features and complications of pulmonary resections. In Shields TW (ed): General Thoracic Surgery, ed. 4. Baltimore, Williams & Wilkins

Shields TW, 1994d: Surgical treatment of non–small cell bronchial carcinoma. In Shields TW (ed): General Thoracic Surgery, ed. 4. Baltimore, Williams & Wilkins

Shields TW, 1991: Lung cancer: Diagnosis and staging. In Baue AE, Geha AS, Hammond GL, et al. (eds): Glenn's Thoracic and Cardiovascular Surgery, ed. 5. Norwalk, CT, Appleton & Lange

Shields TW, 1993: Surgical therapy for carcinoma of the lung. Clin Chest Med 14:121

Tedder M, Lowe JE, 1992: Complications following bronchoplastic procedures. In Wolfe WG (ed): Complications in Thoracic Surgery. St. Louis, Mosby–Year Book

Urschel HC, 1993: New approaches to Pancoast and chest wall tumors. Chest 103:360S

Van Schil PE, de la Riviere AB, Knaepen PJ, et al., 1991: TNM staging and long-term follow-up after sleeve resection for bronchogenic tumors. Ann Thorac Surg 52:1096

CHAPTER 39

SURGICAL TREATMENT OF ESOPHAGEAL DISEASE

GASTROESOPHAGEAL REFLUX
MOTILITY DISORDERS
  Achalasia
  Diffuse Esophageal Spasm
ESOPHAGEAL DIVERTICULUM

ESOPHAGEAL CANCER
  Esophageal Resection
  Palliative Surgical Interventions
OTHER ESOPHAGEAL DISORDERS
  Esophageal Perforation
  Benign Disease Requiring Esophagectomy

A variety of diseases can affect the esophagus and impair normal physiologic function. Those that may require surgical intervention are the focus of this chapter and include gastroesophageal reflux, motility disorders, esophageal diverticula, cancer of the esophagus, and esophageal perforation.

GASTROESOPHAGEAL REFLUX

Gastroesophageal reflux is the most common functional abnormality of the esophagus requiring surgical intervention. It is estimated to account for 75% of esophageal pathology (Stein et al., 1992a). Although some degree of gastroesophageal reflux is considered physiologic, pathologic reflux is said to exist when symptoms or esophageal injury develop because of an increase in frequency or amount of reflux or because of delayed clearing of refluxed material. The precise mechanism for pathologic reflux is unknown. It occurs commonly with conditions such as hiatal hernia or scleroderma.

Continued reflux of gastric contents eventually produces esophageal tissue ulceration and can lead to bleeding, perforation, or stricture formation. In addition, gastroesophageal reflux can cause destruction of the normal squamous cell lining of the lower esophageal sphincter (LES), which is then replaced with columnar epithelium. This phenomenon, termed *Barrett's esophagus*, predisposes the patient to development of adenocarcinoma of the distal esophagus. Other abnormalities of the distal esophagus have also been linked to Barrett's esophagus, including Barrett's stricture and Barrett's ulcer (Pera et al., 1992).

Medical therapy for gastroesophageal reflux includes antacids, hydrogen ion antagonists (e.g., cimetidine or ranitidine), dietary modifications, and elevation of the head of the patient's bed (Backer & LoCicero, 1986). Surgical treatment is indicated in patients who have intractable symptoms despite medical therapy or in those who develop complications of reflux, such as ulcerative esophagitis or stricture. Diagnostic studies used to evaluate gastroesophageal reflux and the need for surgical intervention include esophageal manometry and pH monitoring to document and quantify reflux and esophagoscopy to ascertain the degree of esophagitis.

Antireflux operations comprise a number of surgical procedures that have been developed and modified over the years. They may be performed as primary treatment for gastroesophageal reflux or concomitantly with surgical procedures that may be complicated by postoperative gastroesophageal reflux (e.g., esophagomyotomy). The primary goal of all antireflux procedures is to eliminate reflux of gastric contents while maintaining the patient's ability to swallow normally, belch to relieve gastric distention, and vomit when necessary (Stein et al., 1992a).

The three most commonly performed antireflux procedures are the Nissen fundoplication, Belsey Mark IV operation, and Hill posterior gastropexy. All are designed to restore the factors that normally are important in controlling reflux, that is, an intra-abdominal segment of distal esophagus and distal esophagus at a narrow diameter as it enters the gastric pouch (Skinner, 1994). Restoration of distal esophagus to the abdominal compartment reduces reflux of gastric contents upward into the esophagus because pressure in the abdominal compartment is positive and that in the thorax is negative. Maintaining a narrowed diameter of distal esophagus is accomplished by plication, or folding stomach tissue around a portion or all of the circumference of the distal esophagus. Factors that influence the choice of antireflux procedure include (1) whether a thoracic or abdominal incision is preferable, (2) whether the patient has had a prior antireflux procedure, (3) whether concomitant esophageal resection or esophagomyotomy is likely to be necessary, and (4) the patient's body habitus (Skinner, 1990).

A *Nissen fundoplication* is usually performed through an abdominal incision, although a thoracotomy is sometimes used. After mobilizing the distal esophagus and proximal stomach, the fundus of the stomach is wrapped around the entire circumference of the distal esophagus (Fig. 39-1). Complications specifically associated with Nissen fundoplication include (1) splenic injury, leading to postoperative hemorrhage and the possible need for splenectomy; (2) "slipped Nissen," in which the gastric wrap slips distally, creating a two-chambered stomach: and (3) gas-bloat syndrome, characterized by an inability to belch (Backer & LoCicero, 1986).

A *Belsey Mark IV operation* is performed using a left lateral thoracotomy incision. In this procedure, the gastric fundus is wrapped around approximately two thirds of the circumference of the distal esophagus and the wrapped segment is placed beneath the diaphragm. The *Hill gastropexy*, performed through an abdominal incision, consists of securing the posterior aspect of the gastroesophageal junction within the abdominal compartment and partially wrapping stomach around the distal esophagus. Complications of the latter two procedures are primarily those associated with a thoracotomy incision (Belsey Mark IV) or a laparotomy incision (Hill gastropexy).

MOTILITY DISORDERS

Motility disorders are pathologic abnormalities of the esophagus characterized by abnormal peristalsis, sphincter dysfunction, or a combination of the two. They may affect the upper esophageal sphincter (UES), the body of the esophagus, or the LES.

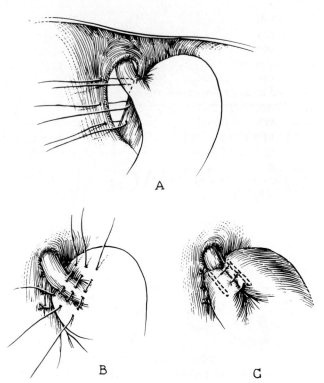

FIGURE 39-1. Nissen fundoplication performed through an abdominal incision. **(A)** Sutures are placed in the crura posteriorly to narrow the hiatus. **(B)** After full mobilization of the fundus, the stomach is passed behind the esophagus and a series of sutures is placed through the stomach and esophagus. **(C)** When these are tied, approximately a 4-cm segment of esophagus is restored within the abdomen. (Zuidema GD, 1972: Surgical treatment: Abdominal approach. In Skinner DB [ed]: Gastroesophageal Reflux and Hiatal Hernia, p. 154. Boston, Little, Brown)

ACHALASIA

The motility disorder most commonly treated with surgical therapy is *achalasia*, an impairment that primarily involves the smooth muscle of the body of the esophagus. Achalasia is characterized by absent peristalsis in the body of the esophagus, excessive pressure in the LES, and a failure of the LES to relax in response to swallowing (Ellis, 1990). The neurologic defect responsible for its development remains poorly understood (Ferguson, 1991a). Achalasia almost always causes dysphagia and may also be associated with regurgitation of solid foods, epigastric discomfort, and weight loss. Nonsurgical therapy consists of forceful dilatation of the esophageal lumen at the level of the LES, using a hydrostatic or pneumatic dilator.

Alternatively, achalasia may be treated with *esophagomyotomy*, a surgical procedure designed to improve the transport of a swallowed bolus through the esophagus (Stein et al., 1992b). The operation consists of making a partial-thickness incision in the outer, muscular layer of the gastroesophageal junction to diminish LES pressure (Fig. 39-2). Esophagomyotomy is most commonly performed through a thoracotomy incision. A nasogastric tube is passed to decompress the stomach and single lung ventilation (i.e., sustained deflation of the ipsilateral lung) is performed to improve exposure. The esophagus is mobilized carefully, avoiding damage to the vagus nerve that passes along the esophageal wall.

A longitudinal incision is made in the esophagus, dividing the circular muscle layer to the level of the mucosa. The length of the incision depends on anatomic circumstances, but it is usually 5 to 7 cm (Ellis, 1990). Opinion varies among surgeons concerning

the appropriate proximal and distal extent of the incision. In general, it begins proximally a short distance above the gastroesophageal junction and usually extends distally 1 to 5 cm onto the stomach. The muscular layer is also dissected laterally to permit outward bulging of the mucosa and prevent subsequent fibrotic closure of the muscular layer (Wilkins, 1994). The most commonly performed operative technique is called a *modified Heller esophagomyotomy*. Controversy exists concerning the need for performing a concomitant antireflux procedure to prevent postoperative gastroesophageal reflux that may result from surgical alteration of LES anatomy (Ferguson, 1991a).

DIFFUSE ESOPHAGEAL SPASM

Another form of motility disorder, *diffuse esophageal spasm*, may also be treated with esophagomyotomy. In this disorder, LES relaxation occurs appropriately, but nonperistaltic, repetitive contractions occur in the body of the esophagus, producing chest pain, dysphagia, and regurgitation. Pharmacologic treatment is the mainstay of therapy for diffuse esophageal spasm and successfully relieves symptoms in a majority of patients. Surgical treatment is generally reserved for patients with severe symptoms not relieved with medical therapy (Naunheim & Baue, 1991).

Esophagomyotomy for diffuse esophageal spasm is similar to that for achalasia except that the incision is extended proximally to the apex of the intrathoracic esophagus (Wilkins, 1994). Because myotomy of the distal esophageal body markedly reduces contraction amplitude, the incision is extended distally across the gastroesophageal junction to reduce resistance to emptying of the surgically altered esophagus (Stein, 1992b). An antireflux procedure may be necessary to prevent postoperative gastroesophageal reflux.

ESOPHAGEAL DIVERTICULUM

An esophageal diverticulum is an epithelial-lined blind pouch leading from the main lumen of the esophagus (Trastek, 1994). It is formed by localized herniation of esophageal mucosa through the outer muscular layer. Esophageal motility disorders are thought to contribute to diverticulum development. Esophageal diverticula are categorized according to location and etiology: (1) pharyngoesophageal pulsion, (2) epiphrenic pulsion, or (3) parabronchial traction. *Pulsion diverticula* develop as a result of forces within the esophageal mucosa acting against an area of resistance, and *traction diverticula* are caused by forces exerted from outside the esophagus, such as inflammatory adhesions (Ferguson, 1991b).

Most common is a *pharyngoesophageal pulsion*, or *Zenker's diverticulum*, which extends from the main lumen of the esophagus at or just below the cricopharyngeus muscle (primary component of the

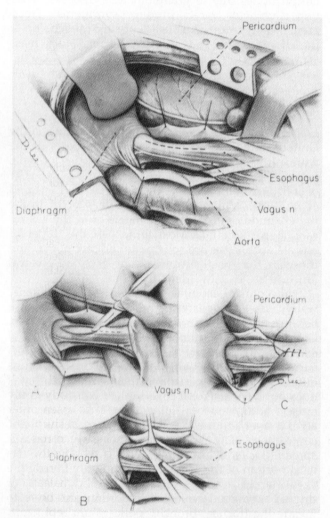

FIGURE 39-2. Esophagomyotomy. **(Top)** Transthoracic exposure of distal esophagus. The left lung has been retracted cephalad, and the mediastinal pleura has been opened. **(Bottom)** Technique of esophagomyotomy. **(A)** Beginning the incision. **(B)** Dissection of the mucosa from the muscularis. **(C)** Restoration of esophagogastric junction to intra-abdominal position with sutures to narrow esophageal hiatus, if necessary. (Ellis FH Jr, Kiser JC, Schlegel JF, et al., 1967: Esophagomyotomy for esophageal achalasia: Experimental, clinical, and manometric aspects. Ann Surg 166:646)

UES). Once the diverticulum forms, it enlarges and descends dependently owing to constant distention with ingested food (Trastek, 1994). Progressive symptoms of dysphagia, foul breath, noisy swallowing, and regurgitation are typical.

For small Zenker's diverticula, *cricopharyngeal esophagomyotomy* is usually recommended to prevent continued filling of the diverticulum with ingested material. Cricopharyngeal esophagomyotomy is performed through an incision in the neck. The pharynx and cervical esophagus are exposed by retracting the sternocleidomastoid muscle and carotid sheath laterally and the trachea and larynx medially (Stein et al., 1992c). A vertical, partial-thickness incision is made in the cricopharyngeus muscle, dividing the muscle fibers down to the mucosal layer of the esophageal wall. Typically, the incision begins at the neck of the diverticulum and extends distally onto the esophagus. As with any esophagomyotomy, complete division and lateral dissection of the muscular layer is performed so that the mucosa bulges diffusely through the divided muscle layer.

For larger diverticula, either pharyngoesophageal diverticulopexy or diverticulectomy may be performed. *Diverticulopexy* consists of suturing the diverticulum in an inverted position to prevent its distention with food and allow its contents to drain freely into the esophagus. The procedure uses the same surgical exposure as for cricopharyngeal esophagomyotomy. If a diverticulum is so large that it would be redundant if suspended or if its walls are thickened, *diverticulectomy* is performed instead (Stein et al., 1992c). A diverticulectomy consists of amputating the diverticulum from the esophagus (Fig. 39-3). Esophagomyotomy is concomitantly performed.

Less common than Zenker's diverticulum is an *epiphrenic pulsion diverticulum* (i.e., a herniation of esophageal mucosa through muscular fibers just above the level of the diaphragm). Surgical therapy (diverticulectomy) is sometimes necessary for an epiphrenic diverticulum if it is associated with progressive symptoms or enlargement. The diverticulum is exposed through a thoracotomy incision and amputated from the esophagus. An extended esophagomyotomy is also performed. This type of diverticulum is frequently associated with a *sliding hiatal hernia,* which is concomitantly repaired along with performance of an antireflux procedure (Trastek, 1994).

The third type of esophageal diverticulum, *parabronchial traction diverticulum,* may develop from inflammation and scarring of adjacent tracheobronchial lymph nodes due to granulomatous diseases. Traction diverticula rarely produce symptoms. Treatment, when required, consists of surgical excision of the diverticulum and adjacent inflammatory mass (Trastek, 1994).

ESOPHAGEAL CANCER

Esophageal cancer is a relatively unusual disease in the United States but is common in other parts of the world. It is a devastating illness that carries a dismal prognosis regardless of treatment modality. The overall survival rate at 5 years is only 3% to 4% (Lund et al., 1990). Malignant neoplasms may occur in the upper, middle, or lower esophagus or in the gastroesophageal junction. Most tumors of the upper or middle esophagus are squamous cell carcinoma, and those in the distal esophagus or gastroesophageal junction are usually adenocarcinoma.

Symptoms of esophageal cancer (e.g., dysphagia, weight loss) occur late in the course of the disease because the esophagus distends easily (Steiger, 1991). Consequently, the tumor may not be detected until extensive local, regional, or distant spread has occurred (Naunheim et al., 1992). Also, the esophagus differs from other gastrointestinal viscera in that it does not have a serosal covering but consists of only muscle and a mucosal lining. The lack of an outer serosal layer and the extensive submucosal lymphatic connections of the esophagus favor early metastatic spread (Backer & LoCicero, 1986). Tumors in the cervical portion of the esophagus commonly invade the vagal nerves, trachea, vertebrae, carotid vessels, or thyroid; those in the thoracic portion are likely to invade the trachea, bronchi, pericardium and heart, pulmonary vessels, vertebrae, or aorta (Steiger, 1991).

Treatment of esophageal cancer is somewhat controversial because no single or combination therapy has significantly improved long-term survival. Surgical therapy includes a number of procedures designed to remove malignant disease or palliate symptoms (Table 39-1). Operative intervention is appropriate only in carefully selected patients. It can impose significant morbidity and yet, if successful,

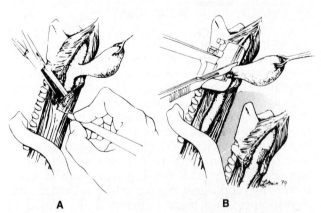

A   **B**

FIGURE 39-3. Cervical esophagomyotomy and concomitant resection of Zenker's diverticulum. **(A)** After mobilization of the diverticulum, the esophagomyotomy is performed. **(B)** The base of the diverticulum is then stapled and amputated. (Orringer MB, 1980: Extended cervical esophagomyotomy for cricopharyngeal dysfunction. J Thorac Cardiovasc Surg 80:672)

TABLE 39-1. SURGICAL PROCEDURES FOR TREATMENT OF ESOPHAGEAL CANCER

Esophagectomy with esophagogastrostomy
Esophagectomy with colon interposition
Proximal esophagostomy with gastrostomy and jejunostomy
Intraluminal intubation
Laser therapy
Brachytherapy

may alleviate the severe dysphagia that accompanies advanced disease and can ultimately preclude even the swallowing of saliva.

The morbidity associated with surgical therapy in patients with esophageal cancer is related to several factors. First, an operation on the esophagus is a major surgical procedure, necessitating a thoracotomy, abdominal incision, or both. Second, patients are frequently nutritionally compromised at the time of operation because of the dysphagia produced by esophageal obstruction. Wound healing, specifically that of the esophageal anastomosis, may be impaired. Third, many patients with esophageal tumors have abused alcohol or cigarettes, both of which are independent risk factors for esophageal cancer. Associated cardiovascular, pulmonary, or hepatic disease is frequently present.

ESOPHAGEAL RESECTION

Esophageal resection has historically been associated with disappointing results; because of the tendency for early lymphatic and hematogenous metastasis, tumor resection may not significantly increase long-term survival. Many surgeons believe that all surgical therapy for esophageal cancer is palliative. Still, when esophageal resection is performed in the early stage of the disease, cure is sometimes achieved. Attempts to improve the ability to achieve cure with surgical resection have focused in three areas: (1) subtotal esophagectomy (i.e., removing almost all of the esophagus), (2) en bloc resection (i.e., removing all tumor in a resected block of tissue, surrounded by normal tissue on all sides), and (3) more complete lymphadenectomy (lymph node removal) (Ribet et al., 1992). Also, some surgeons advocate a combined treatment approach, including chemotherapy and radiation therapy before operation (Naunheim et al., 1992). Others favor surgical resection without preoperative adjuvant therapy.

Resection of an esophageal tumor is undertaken if there is no lymphatic or hematologic evidence of distant spread and the patient is medically able to withstand a major operation. The size and extent of the primary lesion and potential involvement of contiguous structures also influence the ability to perform operative resection. Before surgical treatment, patients often undergo "triple endoscopy": esopha-goscopy, bronchoscopy, and direct laryngoscopy. Esophagoscopy is essential to obtain tissue samples for histologic confirmation of the diagnosis. Bronchoscopy allows detection of direct invasion of the tracheobronchial tree, and laryngoscopy allows inspection of vocal cord motion to detect involvement of the recurrent laryngeal nerve (Steiger, 1991).

Surgical resection of esophageal tumors consists of removal of the tumor plus an adequate margin of tumor-free tissue above and below the tumor. Depending on the operative technique, adjacent lymph nodes may also be removed. For tumors in the upper or middle third of the esophagus, only esophagus is resected; for tumors of the lower third or gastric cardia, a portion of stomach is resected in addition to esophagus (DeMeester & Barlow, 1988). Because of the poor prognosis associated with tumors in the upper one third of the esophagus, surgical resection is seldom performed except in patients who demonstrate a favorable response to preoperative chemotherapy.

Nearly all of the esophagus is generally removed during resection because of the tendency for tumors to spread in both directions along the length of the esophagus. The remaining proximal and distal esophagus provides insufficient length for direct reattachment without excessive tension on the anastomosis, and a replacement conduit is necessary to bridge the defect. One of three visceral structures can be used to replace the resected segment of esophagus: (1) stomach, (2) colon, or (3) jejunum. Each is associated with particular advantages in specific clinical situations (Table 39-2). The determination of which to use as a substitute conduit is based on the location and length of esophagus that must be replaced and the blood supply and freedom from disease of the replacement viscera.

TABLE 39-2. CHOICES FOR ESOPHAGEAL REPLACEMENT CONDUIT

Stomach

Requires only one anastomosis
Gastric esophagitis more common
Postoperative dysphagia common
Adynamic conduit

Colon

Durable
Longest graft
Dysphagia, gastric esophagitis less common
Adynamic conduit
Requires three anastomoses

Jejunum

Dynamic conduit
Shortest graft
Requires three anastomoses

The most convenient and widely used visceral structure for esophageal replacement is the stomach (Hiebert, 1991; Huang, 1994). Advantages of using stomach as the replacement viscera include the following: (1) it has a rich blood supply and submucosal collateral circulation, (2) it has a thick, resilient muscular wall, and (3) it can be mobilized to reach superiorly to any level of the chest or neck for esophageal substitution (Orringer, 1991).

Sometimes, it is not possible to use the stomach to replace resected esophagus. It may be damaged due to caustic burn, scar, ulceration, or previous operation (Hiebert, 1991). Alternatively, a segment of colon or jejunum may be used as a conduit to replace resected esophagus. Colon is a more durable substitute, and jejunum is a dynamic graft that contributes to bolus transport (Stein et al., 1992b). However, colon or jejunum interposition requires three anastomoses, increasing the likelihood of anastomotic complications. Colon is most often selected when stomach cannot be used. Jejunum interposition is performed rarely. The primary indication for using jejunum is reconstruction of the cervical esophagus after radical resection (Paletta & Jurkiewicz, 1991).

Esophagectomy With Esophagogastrostomy

An operation to remove esophagus and replace it with stomach is called *esophagectomy* (removal of the esophagus) with *esophagogastrostomy* (reattachment of the fundus of the stomach to the remaining proximal esophageal remnant) (Fig. 39-4). Although the cardia is the stomach's most proximal anatomic component, the fundus of the stomach actually lies superior to the

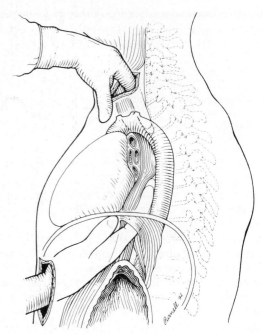

FIGURE 39-5. Technique of transhiatal esophagectomy; working through incisions in the upper abdomen and neck, the surgeon uses his or her fingers to bluntly free the esophagus from surrounding mediastinal attachments. (Shriver CD, Burt M, 1992: Transhiatal esophagectomy. Semin Thorac Cardiovasc Surg 4:309)

cardia and can be more easily extended upward for anastomosis to the proximal esophageal segment. Also, in tumors of the lower esophagus or gastroesophageal junction, the cardia often must be sacrificed to obtain an adequate distal tumor-free margin.

Esophagectomy with esophagogastrostomy may be performed by one of two approaches: a transhiatal approach or a transthoracic approach. In a *transhiatal approach* the upper abdomen is explored through a midline abdominal incision to detect visible local metastatic disease. If none is apparent, the stomach is mobilized widely (i.e., freed from tethering attachments) with care to preserve its blood supply. Through a separate incision in the left side of the neck, the cervical esophagus is exposed. Working primarily through the abdominal incision, the surgeon inserts his or her hand through the diaphragmatic hiatus (paraesophageal opening in the diaphragm) into the mediastinum (Fig. 39-5). The surgeon uses blunt dissection, (fingers or blunt instruments) to blindly (with limited visualization) free the esophagus from surrounding tissue. This technique is possible because only small blood vessels and tissue attach the esophagus to surrounding structures in the mediastinum.

When the esophagus is entirely mobilized, the cervical esophagus is stapled and divided. The esophagus is pulled downward and out through the abdominal incision. The proximal stomach is stapled and

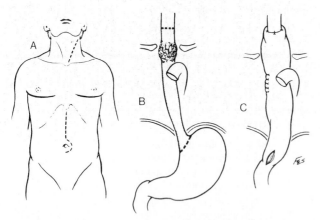

FIGURE 39-4. Esophagectomy and esophagogastrostomy using transhiatal approach. **(A)** Incisions. **(B)** Extent of esophageal resection (*shaded area*). **(C)** The stomach has been pulled upward into the mediastinum, and the gastric fundus has been anastomosed to the remaining cervical esophageal segment; a pyloromyotomy has been performed to facilitate gastric emptying. (Ellis FH Jr, 1980: Esophagogastrectomy for carcinoma: Technical considerations based on anatomic location of lesion. Surg Clin North Am 60:275)

divided, and the diseased esophageal segment is removed. Next, the gastric fundus is maneuvered upward through the diaphragmatic hiatus and mediastinum to the open neck incision, where the anastomosis between gastric fundus and the remaining cervical esophageal segment is performed. Because the stomach can be elongated to reach the upper chest without disrupting its distal continuity with the duodenum, only a single visceral anastomosis (i.e., proximal stomach to esophageal remnant) is necessary to restore continuity of the alimentary tract. Once the stomach is positioned and sutured to proximal esophagus, most of it lies within the thorax. It is preferably positioned in the usual anatomic location of the esophagus (i.e., in the posterior mediastinum). If the posterior mediastinum is fibrotic from prior radiation therapy or a surgical procedure, the stomach may alternatively be positioned behind the sternum in the anterior mediastinum (Orringer, 1991).

A transhiatal approach avoids a thoracotomy incision and its potential pulmonary complications and associated postoperative pain. In addition, the esophageal anastomosis is in the neck rather than the thorax. Cervical anastomotic leaks (i.e., those that occur in the neck) have less severe consequences and are more easily managed (Daniel et al., 1992). Manipulation within the neck occasionally injures the recurrent laryngeal nerve.

A *transthoracic approach,* like a transhiatal approach, includes an upper abdominal incision through which the stomach is mobilized. However, instead of a neck incision, a right or left thoracotomy is performed. Through the thoracotomy incision, the entire esophagus is exposed and under direct visualization is freed from its mediastinal attachments along with surrounding lymph and fatty tissue. A transthoracic approach provides better exposure, allowing easier mobilization of viscera. Hemorrhage, pneumothorax, or injuries to intrathoracic structures may be less likely than with the limited exposure provided by a transhiatal approach (Backer & LoCicero, 1986). A transthoracic approach also allows an en bloc esophagectomy (i.e., radical excision of regional mediastinal lymph nodes and other tissue surrounding the esophagus).

Regardless of operative approach, the vagus nerves are divided in the process of performing esophagectomy with esophagogastrostomy. Because vagotomy impairs gastric emptying, many surgeons routinely revise the gastric pylorus to facilitate gastric outflow. A *pyloromyotomy* (division of serosa and muscle layers of the pylorus) or *pyloroplasty* (full-thickness division of pylorus and suture reclosure) is usually performed. However, the advisability of performing concomitant revision of the pylorus remains controversial because it sometimes results in duodenogastric reflux and the development of gastroesophagitis.

A jejunostomy tube is almost always placed concomitantly with esophagectomy to provide an alter-native means for providing alimentation to the patient during the postoperative period. Esophageal contents must be diverted and oral nourishment withheld for approximately 1 week to allow adequate healing of the esophageal anastomosis. During this period, adequate nutrition is important to ensure recovery from operation and wound healing in these patients who are usually malnourished and debilitated because of the underlying disease. Jejunostomy feedings avoid infectious complications associated with intravenous hyperalimentation and potential gastroesophageal reflux from tube feedings delivered by means of gastrostomy. A nasogastric tube is also placed to divert secretions from the esophagus and prevent distention of the anastomotic site. A contrast swallow study is generally performed 7 or 8 days after surgery to confirm the integrity of the anastomosis. If no leak is present and bowel function has resumed, oral feedings are gradually reinstituted.

Esophagectomy With Colon Interposition

The surgical procedure to substitute colon for resected esophagus is called *esophagectomy with colon interposition* (Fig. 39-6). If colon is to be used as the replacement viscera, a number of preoperative inter-

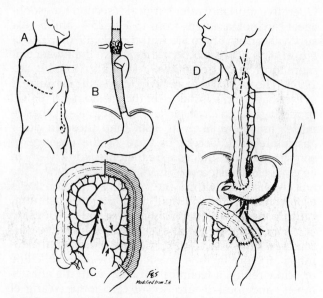

FIGURE 39-6. Esophagectomy with colon interposition using transthoracic approach. **(A)** Incisions. **(B)** Extent of esophageal resection (*shaded area*). **(C)** Segment of left colon to be used for interposition (*shaded area*). **(D)** Colon segment has been anastomosed to the esophagus proximally and stomach distally; remaining bowel segments have been anastomosed to restore bowel continuity; a pyloromyotomy has been performed to facilitate gastric emptying. (Ellis FH Jr, 1980: Esophagogastrectomy for carcinoma: Technical considerations based on anatomic location of lesion. Surg Clin North Amer 60:277)

ventions are performed. The patient is restricted to a clear liquid diet to cleanse the bowel of fecal material, and oral antibiotics are administered to reduce bacterial flora in the bowel. A colonoscopy may be performed to visually inspect the colon. In addition, a barium enema may be performed to assess anatomic configuration of the colon and to detect any pathology. Because the location of arterial blood vessels to the colon is occasionally anomalous, an angiogram may be performed as well to define vascular anatomy.

As with esophagogastrostomy, colon interposition may be performed through a transhiatal or a transthoracic approach. Either the right (proximal) or left (distal) colon may be used to replace the esophagus. The right colon is the easiest to mobilize but has a variable blood supply and shorter vascular pedicle; the left colon can span longer defects and is thicker, making it easier to suture (Hiebert, 1991). Through the laparotomy incision, the necessary length of colon is harvested, making sure that blood supply to both the resected portion and remaining bowel is adequate. The segment of colon is anastomosed to the esophagus proximally and the stomach distally. The two remaining bowel segments in the abdomen are anastomosed to restore bowel continuity.

Results

Operative mortality after surgical resection for esophageal carcinoma ranges from 15% to 25%, and 5-year survival is from 6% to 9% (Lund et al., 1990). *Respiratory* and *cardiovascular complications* are the most common form of perioperative morbidity (Law et al., 1992). The primary complication specifically related to esophagectomy is failure of the anastomosis to heal properly (i.e., an *anastomotic leak*). Esophageal anastomoses are more likely to leak than those in other gastrointestinal viscera because of the absence of serosa covering the esophagus. Breakdown of an esophageal anastomosis is most serious when the anastomosis is within the thorax. The nonsterile esophageal secretions spill into the mediastinum, causing mediastinitis. *Esophageal stricture* can develop at the anastomotic site and lead to postoperative dysphagia (Lam et al., 1992). Possible causes of anastomotic stricture include anastomotic leakage, alkaline or acidic reflux, a technical problem with the anastomosis, and local recurrence of carcinoma (Wang et al., 1992).

None of the substitute viscera functions as well as the native esophagus in which peristalsis propels food into the stomach (Collard et al., 1992). Although most patients are able to achieve adequate oral alimentation, modifications in the amount and type of food ingested may be necessary to avoid uncomfortable postprandial symptoms. After esophagogastrostomy, maintaining an upright position during and after meals may be necessary to avoid postprandial regurgitation (Morton et al., 1991). The complications of esophageal operations are discussed further in Chapter 43, Complications of Thoracic Operations.

PALLIATIVE SURGICAL INTERVENTIONS

Palliative surgical therapy is sometimes performed to alleviate the disabling and unpleasant symptoms that eventually develop in patients with incurable esophageal cancer. Objectives of palliative procedures include (1) relief of dysphagia, (2) diversion of saliva and prevention of aspiration, (3) prevention of tumor ulceration (with resulting hemorrhage) or infection (with resulting sepsis), and (4) provision of a route for enteral alimentation. Procedures designed to achieve these objectives may necessitate lengthy hospitalization and cause untoward complications.

Average patient survival in patients receiving palliative therapy is only 4 months (Ellis, 1990). Therefore, interventions must be carefully planned to enhance rather than detract from the patient's quality of life during this short interval. The most reasonable goal is maximizing the number of days that a patient is able to both swallow and be at home with family (Pagliero, 1991). Esophagectomy with esophagogastrostomy is sometimes performed as a palliative procedure to relieve dysphagia in severely symptomatic patients with minimal local spread to regional lymphatic tissue. However, many surgeons consider the significant operative risk unacceptable given the short life expectancy (Lund et al., 1990).

In patients unable to swallow saliva, a *proximal esophagostomy and gastrostomy* or *jejunostomy* may be performed. In this procedure, the esophagus is stapled and divided above the tumor and a fistula is surgically created between the proximal esophageal remnant and the skin, allowing saliva to drain into an external esophagostomy pouch. A gastrostomy or jejunostomy feeding tube is placed concomitantly for alimentation. Alternatively, *esophageal dilatation* (i.e., *bougienage*) may be performed to dilate the obstructed esophageal segment or the obstructed segment may be intubated with a prosthetic stent (*esophageal intubation*). Either *laser therapy* or *brachytherapy* (implantation of radioactive isotopes in the tumor) may be performed through esophagoscopy to destroy tumor that is occluding the esophageal lumen. Unfortunately, only modest success is achieved with any of these measures.

OTHER ESOPHAGEAL DISORDERS

ESOPHAGEAL PERFORATION

Esophageal perforation may occur as a consequence of severe vomiting, penetrating trauma, instrumentation, or foreign body ingestion. The resultant leakage of digestive fluids, food, and bacteria into the periesophageal spaces causes diffuse cellulitis and leads to localized or extensive suppuration (Ellis, 1990).

The diagnosis of esophageal perforation is suggested by severe chest pain, fever, and radiographic evidence of mediastinal or subcutaneous air, particularly when these findings are associated with a clinical history of instrumentation, trauma, or vomiting. Definitive diagnosis is achieved by contrast swallow study or esophagoscopy.

Treatment of esophageal perforation includes intravenous antibiotic therapy and prompt surgical exploration to drain the infected area and repair the esophageal wall. If surgical treatment is delayed or infection is extensive, primary repair of the esophagus may not be possible. Instead, *esophageal diversion* is performed; the upper esophagus is divided and the proximal esophageal segment is brought out through the skin of the neck as a fistula to drain saliva (Fig. 39-7). The distal esophageal segment is sutured closed, and its upper end is attached to the back of the newly created esophageal stoma. Gastric drainage and enteral feeding tubes are placed to decompress the stomach and provide alimentation. Esophageal reconstruction is performed after the infection resolves. Esophageal perforation is discussed further in Chapter 32, Cardiac and Thoracic Trauma, and Chapter 34, Esophageal Diseases.

BENIGN DISEASE REQUIRING ESOPHAGECTOMY

Esophagectomy is sometimes performed for treatment of benign diseases, such as esophageal motility disorders, caustic injury, or connective tissue disorders (e.g., scleroderma). It is indicated in patients whose esophageal function has been destroyed by the underlying disease process or who have already undergone multiple surgical procedures on the esophagus (Stein et al., 1992b). Esophagectomy may also be considered for patients with Barrett's esophagus and high-grade dysplasia (i.e., markedly abnormal cells) (Pera et al., 1992). These patients have a high incidence of early invasive carcinoma that might not otherwise be detected and treated while the possibility for cure exists.

Proper patient selection for complex reconstructive operations is difficult and controversial; analysis and comparison of results of the various reconstructive procedures is limited by the highly variable clinical and anatomic features among individual patients (Ellis & Gibb, 1990). Some surgeons consider colon to be the replacement conduit of choice in patients with benign disease. Although colon interposition is technically a more difficult procedure, the colon may be a preferable long-term replacement viscera. It is more durable over time and provides a better quality of deglutition (swallowing) than stomach (Stein et al., 1992b).

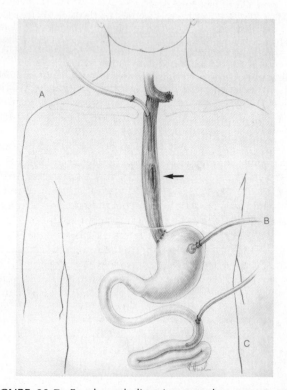

FIGURE 39-7. Esophageal diversion may be necessary for treatment of esophageal rupture (*arrow*) if diagnosis is delayed and infection well established. (**A**) The esophagus is divided at the level of the sternal manubrium, bringing the proximal end out to the skin. The distal esophagus is closed and attached to the back of the esophageal stoma. Distal to this closure line, a drainage catheter is inserted through a pursestring suture in the side of the esophagus and brought out through a small incision on the opposite side of the neck. (**B**) Through a laparotomy incision, the cardia is closed and a gastrotomy tube is inserted. (**C**) A jejunostomy tube is inserted for enteral feeding. (Skinner DB, 1991: Esophageal rupture. In Atlas of Esophageal Surgery, p. 181. New York, Churchill Livingstone)

REFERENCES

Backer CL, LoCicero J III, 1986: Surgical management of esophageal disorders. Crit Care Q 9:12

Collard JM, Otte JB, Reynaert M, Kestens PJ, 1992: Quality of life three years or more after esophagectomy for cancer. J Thorac Cardiovasc Surg 104:391

Daniel TM, Fleisher KJ, Flanagan TL, et al., 1992: Transhiatal esophagectomy: A safe alternative for selected patients. Ann Thorac Surg 54:686

DeMeester TR, Barlow AP, 1988: Surgical management for carcinoma of the thoracic esophagus and cardia. Curr Probl Surg 25:559

Ellis FH Jr, 1990: Disorders of the esophagus in the adult. In Sabiston DC Jr, Spencer FC (eds): Surgery of the Chest, ed. 5. Philadelphia, WB Saunders

Ellis FH Jr, Gibb SP, 1990: Esophageal reconstruction for complex benign esophageal disease. J Thorac Cardiovasc Surg 99:192

Ferguson MK, 1991a: Achalasia: Current evaluation and therapy. Ann Thorac Surg 52:336

Ferguson MK, 1991b: Evolution of therapy for pharyngoesophageal (Zenker's) diverticulum. Ann Thorac Surg 51:848

Hiebert CA, 1991: Surgical options for esophageal excision replacement: Colon interposition. In Baue AE, Geha AS, Hammond GL, et al. (eds): Glenn's Thoracic and Cardiovascular Surgery, ed. 5. Norwalk, CT, Appleton & Lange

Huang GJ, 1994: Replacement of the esophagus with the stomach. In Shields TW (ed): General Thoracic Surgery, ed. 4. Baltimore, Williams & Wilkins

Lam TC, Fok M, Cheng SW, Wong J, 1992: Anastomotic complications after esophagectomy for cancer. J Thorac Cardiovasc Surg 104:395

Law SY, Fok M, Cheng SW, Wong J, 1992: A comparison of outcome after resection for squamous cell carcinomas and adenocarcinomas of the esophagus and cardia. Surg Gynecol Obstet 175:107

Lund O, Kimose HH, Aagaard MT, et al., 1990: Risk stratification and long-term results after surgical treatment of carcinomas of the thoracic esophagus and cardia. J Thorac Cardiovasc Surg 99:200

Morton KA, Karwande SV, Davis RK, et al., 1991: Gastric emptying after gastric interposition for cancer of the esophagus or hypopharynx. Ann Thorac Surg 51:759

Naunheim KS, Baue AE, 1991: Esophageal dysmotility. In Baue AE, Geha AS, Hammond GL, et al. (eds): Glenn's Thoracic and Cardiovascular Surgery, ed. 5. Norwalk, CT, Appleton & Lange

Naunheim KS, Petruska PJ, Roy TS, et al., 1992: Preoperative chemotherapy and radiotherapy for esophageal carcinoma. J Thorac Cardiovasc Surg 103:887

Orringer MB, 1991: Surgical options for esophageal resection and reconstruction with stomach. In Baue AE, Geha AS, Hammond GL, et al. (eds): Glenn's Thoracic and Cardiovascular Surgery, ed. 5. Norwalk, CT, Appleton & Lange

Pagliero KM, 1991: Palliative treatment for carcinoma of the esophagus. In Baue AE, Geha AS, Hammond GL, et al. (eds): Glenn's Thoracic and Cardiovascular Surgery, ed. 5. Norwalk, CT, Appleton & Lange

Paletta CE, Jurkiewicz MJ, 1991: Esophageal replacement: Microvascular jejunal transplantation. In Baue AE, Geha AS, Hammond GL, et al. (eds): Glenn's Thoracic and Cardiovascular Surgery, ed. 5. Norwalk, CT, Appleton & Lange

Pera M, Trastek VF, Carpenter HA, et al., 1992: Barrett's esophagus with high-grade dysplasia: An indication for esophagectomy. Ann Thorac Surg 54:199

Ribet M, Debrueres B, Lecomte-Houcke M, 1992: Resection for advanced cancer of the thoracic esophagus: Cervical or thoracic anastomosis. J Thorac Cardiovasc Surg 103:784

Skinner DB, 1994: Gastroesophageal reflux. In Shields TW (ed): General Thoracic Surgery, ed. 4. Baltimore, Williams & Wilkins

Skinner DB, 1990: The Belsey Mark IV antireflux repair. In Sabiston DC Jr, Spencer FC (eds): Surgery of the Chest, ed. 5. Philadelphia, WB Saunders

Steiger Z, 1991: Esophageal cancer. In Baue AE, Geha AS, Hammond GL, et al. (eds): Glenn's Thoracic and Cardiovascular Surgery, ed. 5. Norwalk, CT, Appleton & Lange

Stein HJ, DeMeester TR, Hinder RA, 1992a: Evaluation and surgical management of the gastroesophageal reflux disease. Curr Probl Surg 24:482

Stein HJ, DeMeester TR, Hinder RA, 1992b: Evaluation and surgical management of motor disorders of the esophageal body and lower esophageal sphincter. Curr Probl Surg 24:447

Stein HJ, DeMeester TR, Hinder RA, 1992c: Evaluation and surgical management of pharyngoesophageal swallowing disorders. Curr Probl Surg 24:429

Trastek VF, 1994: Esophageal diverticula. In Shields TW (ed): General Thoracic Surgery, ed. 4. Baltimore, Williams & Wilkins

Wang LS, Huang MH, Huang BS, Chien KY, 1992: Gastric substitution for resectable carcinoma of the esophagus: An analysis of 368 cases. Ann Thorac Surg 53:289

Wilkins EW, 1994: Motor disturbances of deglutition. In Shields TW (ed): General Thoracic Surgery, ed. 4. Baltimore, Williams & Wilkins

40

SURGERY OF THE PLEURA, TRACHEA, CHEST WALL, AND MEDIASTINUM

OPERATIONS ON THE PLEURA
  Pleural Abrasion
  Pleurectomy
  Decortication
OPERATIONS ON THE TRACHEA
  Tracheal Resection and Reconstruction
  Tracheostomy
OPERATIONS ON THE CHEST WALL
  Resection of Primary Chest Wall
    Neoplasms
  Thoracoplasty

OPERATIONS INVOLVING MEDIASTINAL
    STRUCTURES
  Thymectomy for Myasthenia Gravis
  Resection of Primary Mediastinal
    Neoplasms and Cysts
  Surgical Bypass of the Superior Vena
    Cava

By far, the majority of thoracic operations are performed for treatment of pulmonary or esophageal diseases, as discussed in Chapter 38, Surgical Treatment of Pulmonary Disease, and Chapter 39, Surgical Treatment of Esophageal Disease. In this chapter the focus is on less commonly performed types of thoracic surgery—operations that involve the pleura, trachea, chest wall, or specific structures within the mediastinum.

OPERATIONS ON THE PLEURA

PLEURAL ABRASION

Pleural abrasion, also called *pleurodesis* or *pleural scarification*, is an operation in which the visceral and parietal pleural surfaces are mechanically abraded. The most common reason for performing pleural abrasion is to prevent recurrent pneumothorax and lung col-

lapse in patients with a predilection for *spontaneous pneumothoraces*. These patients, who are typically slender, young adults with otherwise normal lungs, have a propensity for developing pneumothoraces owing to idiopathic rupture of air-filled blebs on the lung's surface. Patients who have experienced an initial episode of spontaneous pneumothorax have a 20% risk of recurrence after the first episode and a 60% to 80% risk after the second episode; most recurrences are on the ipsilateral side (Deslauriers et al., 1989).

An initial episode of spontaneous pneumothorax is most commonly treated with thoracostomy drainage of the pleural space. Pleural abrasion is generally reserved for patients who experience a second or third spontaneous pneumothorax. Certain situations, however, dictate pleural abrasion after a single episode of spontaneous pneumothorax. For example, surgical therapy is performed after the first pneumothorax in patients in whom a recurrent episode could be life threatening, such as airline pilots, scuba divers, and individuals who spend time in an area remote from available medical care. Sometimes, surgical therapy becomes necessary after an initial pneumothorax because the visceral pleura fails to seal and an air leak persists beyond 7 to 10 days. An operation is also recommended in patients who experience spontaneous pneumothorax after a previous pneumothorax on the contralateral side or in the rare circumstance of simultaneous bilateral pneumothoraces.

Pleural abrasion is frequently performed through video-assisted thoracoscopy. Alternatively, a small axillary thoracotomy incision may be used. With a dry gauze sponge, the visceral pleura is mildly abraded and the parietal pleura is rubbed to cause erythema and mild capillary bleeding (DeMeester & LaFontaine, 1990). The resulting pleural inflammation causes adhesion formation and pleural symphysis (i.e., a fusing together of the pleural surfaces). Sometimes, a bleb at the apex of the lung is identified during the operation. If so, it is resected using a stapling device. Pleural abrasion is highly successful in preventing recurrent pneumothoraces. In the event of subsequent bleb rupture, the pleural symphysis prevents accumulation of air in the pleural space and collapse of the lung. Rarely, pleural abrasion is inadequate to prevent portions of the lung from collapsing. A reoperation may be necessary to further abrade the pleural surface and staple the portion of lung tissue from which air is leaking.

Occasionally, pleural abrasion is performed for treatment of *malignant pleural effusion.* It is an effective method of preventing fluid reaccumulation if more conservative therapy fails. However, few patients with malignant pleural effusion survive longer than 6 months (Lynch, 1992). Given the limited life-expectancy in this group of patients, the morbidity of the operation is generally thought to outweigh the benefit. For similar reasons, pleural abrasion is usually not recommended for pneumothorax secondary to *Pneumocystis carinii* pneumonia in patients with acquired immunodeficiency syndrome.

PLEURECTOMY

A *pleurectomy*, or removal of the parietal pleura, is another surgical technique for causing adhesion formation and pleural symphysis. A small thoracotomy incision is made through which the intercostal muscles are divided and the pleural space is entered. When treating pneumothorax, the parietal pleura is stripped from the endothoracic fascia in the area over the apex of the lung (Deslauriers et al., 1991). As during pleural abrasion, identified apical blebs are excised with a stapling instrument.

Pleurectomy is performed less commonly than pleural abrasion for treatment of spontaneous pneumothorax. It is associated with a higher incidence of morbidity than pleurodesis, and it makes subsequent thoracotomy for unrelated disease more difficult (DeMeester & LaFontaine, 1990). A more extensive pleurectomy can be an effective operation for preventing recurring malignant pleural effusions. As with pleural abrasion, however, the palliative benefits of pleurectomy are seldom thought to outweigh the associated morbidity of the operation in patients with limited life expectancy due to a terminal illness.

Pleurectomy is occasionally performed for treatment of *mesothelioma,* a type of cancer that arises in the pleura. The most common form of mesothelioma is a diffuse, malignant variety that is often associated with asbestos exposure. Malignant mesothelioma is usually a fatal disease. Survival time after diagnosis averages only 6 to 14 months (Deslauriers et al., 1991). No presently available form of therapy has proven effective, and the role of surgical therapy is controversial. Pleurectomy may be performed in selected patients. In others, pleural resection is combined with removal of the ipsilateral lung, an operation known as *extrapleural pneumonectomy.* Neither pleurectomy nor extrapleural pneumonectomy has been shown to definitively increase survival time (Rusch et al., 1991). Consequently, many physicians advocate only supportive therapy for patients with malignant mesothelioma.

DECORTICATION

Decortication is the surgical removal of a restrictive, fibrous membrane or layer of tissue from the pleural surface of the lung and, if necessary, from the chest wall and diaphragm (Shields, 1994a). The purpose of the operation is to free lung that has become entrapped by the abnormal fibrous tissue, sometimes called a "fibrous peel." Most commonly, decortication is performed to remove a fibrous peel that has developed secondary to an inadequately drained hemothorax or as a result of empyema.

Both hemothorax and empyema are initially treated with chest tube thoracostomy drainage. If a significant hemothorax is undetected or inadequately drained, the blood remaining in the pleural space eventually becomes organized and cannot be evacuated with tube drainage. When this occurs, operative evacuation of the blood and decortication of the fibrous peel overlying the lung becomes necessary to achieve lung reexpansion. Similarly, decortication may become necessary in patients with empyema if the cavity is unusually thick walled and does not decrease in size over time (DeMeester & LaFontaine, 1990). Decortication is typically performed through a posterolateral thoracotomy incision in the fifth or sixth intercostal space. A rib may be resected to provide better exposure of the pleural space. A small incision is made in the visceral pleura. By using primarily blunt dissection, and sharp dissection as necessary, the visceral peel covering the lung is removed, allowing underlying lung to expand (Fig. 40-1). When decortication includes removal of both

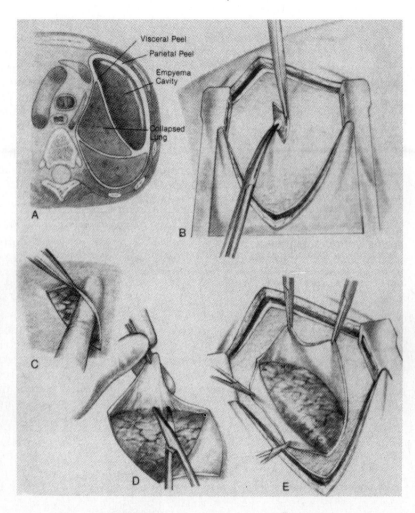

FIGURE 40-1. Decortication of the pleura. **(A)** Cross-sectional diagram of thorax demonstrating the relationship of the empyema cavity and its walls to the chest wall and underlying lung. **(B)** The chest has been opened and the empyema space entered; the thick parietal peel has been incised and retracted; dissection of the visceral peel from underlying lung is begun through a small incision in the visceral peel. **(C)** Sometimes the peel can be separated from the lung with gentle blunt dissection. **(D)** Sharp dissection may be necessary. **(E)** The area of decorticated lung is now able to expand from its partially collapsed state. (Hood MR, 1993: Operations for trauma. In Techniques in General Thoracic Surgery, ed. 2, p. 54. Philadelphia, Lea & Febiger)

the visceral and parietal peels that form an empyema sac, the operation is called an *empyemectomy*. The primary postoperative problems associated with decortication are sepsis, persistent air leak, and bleeding (Shields, 1994a).

OPERATIONS ON THE TRACHEA

TRACHEAL RESECTION AND RECONSTRUCTION

Resection and reconstruction of the trachea may be indicated in the treatment of various pathologic conditions affecting the trachea, including tracheal tumors, damage to the trachea from intubation or trauma, and tracheoesophageal fistulae. Surgery of the trachea has evolved more slowly than other types of thoracic surgery owing to the rarity of tracheal tumors, the anatomic complexities of reconstruction of the trachea, and the biologic incompatibilities that have occurred with prosthetic materials used for tracheal replacement (Grillo, 1989a).

Primary tumors of the trachea are rare. Most are malignant and are either squamous cell carcinoma or adenoid cystic carcinoma. Because tracheal tumors are not easily visible on a chest roentgenogram, they are usually not diagnosed until the patient develops symptoms of progressive airway obstruction (Grillo, 1989b). *Traumatic damage* to the trachea may result from prolonged or traumatic intubation, traumatic laceration, radiation therapy, tracheal burns, aspiration of a caustic substance, or infection. The most common etiology of tracheal damage is injury caused by intubation of the trachea with an endotracheal or tracheostomy tube.

Damage to the trachea may result in stricture formation, tracheal malacia, or development of an tracheoesophageal fistula. *Tracheal stricture* is often the result of intubation injury. Two principal types of stricture can develop after intubation: (1) stricture at the level of a tracheostomy stoma or (2) stricture at the level of a tracheostomy or endotracheal tube cuff (Grillo & Mathisen, 1991). *Tracheal malacia,* or collapse of a segment of tracheal wall, may be caused by endotracheal tube cuff injury or may develop secondary to chronic compression from a lesion external to the trachea (Grillo & Mathisen, 1991). *Tracheoesophageal fistula* can occur as a complication of prolonged intubation of the trachea or secondary to esophageal perforation and resultant infection.

Diseased or damaged segments of trachea are surgically removed with circumferential resection of the involved portion of trachea. To date, no prosthetic graft has proved successful for replacement of resected trachea. Inflammation with resultant granulation tissue and stricture formation typically develops after prosthesis implantation in the trachea. Consequently, tracheal reconstruction is generally performed by direct anastomosis of the tracheal segments above and below the area of circumferential resection. In the average adult, it is usually possible to remove up to one half of the length of the trachea and successfully reconstruct it with primary anastomosis of the remaining segments.

Depending on the area of tracheal pathology, operations to resect and reconstruct the trachea may be performed through a cervical incision, a median sternotomy, or a posterolateral thoracotomy. The various surgical approaches are based on a knowledge of the trachea's anatomic position in the thorax. When viewed laterally, the trachea in an erect individual courses downward and backward from a nearly subcutaneous position at the infracricoid level to rest against the esophagus and vertebral column at the level of the carina (Grillo, 1989a). Consequently, resection of a lesion in the upper trachea is best performed through an anterior cervical incision with or without a vertical partial sternal division (Grillo, 1990). A posterolateral thoracotomy incision is more suitable for a lesion in the lower trachea.

Operations on the trachea necessitate special techniques to ensure adequate ventilation. Principles of airway management during tracheal resection and reconstruction include (1) full control of the airway at all times, (2) bronchoscopic examination of the airway by both the surgeon and anesthesiologist, (3) slow and gentle induction of anesthesia, and (4) spontaneous ventilation during and after the operation (Grillo, 1989a).

Initially, the patient is intubated in a normal fashion. The trachea is exposed and mobilized carefully to preserve adequate blood supply. Traction sutures are placed in the trachea above and below the lesion. After making an incision in the anterior surface of the trachea distal to the lesion, the endotracheal tube is withdrawn so that its tip is above the incision. A sterile, specially designed, flexible endotracheal tube is inserted through the incision into the distal trachea to continue ventilation while tracheal integrity is disrupted. After resecting the diseased or damaged section, the traction sutures are used to approximate the remaining proximal and distal tracheal segments and a primary anastomosis is performed (Fig. 40-2).

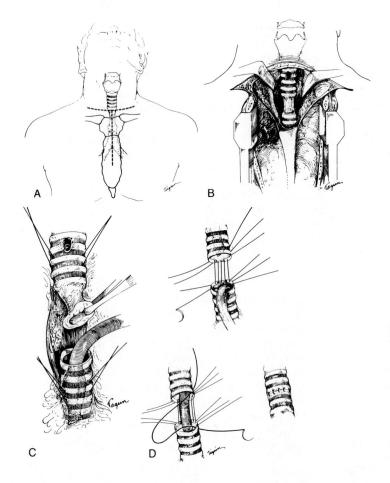

FIGURE 40-2. Resection and reconstruction of the upper trachea. **(A)** Collar incision is often sufficient, but median sternotomy improves access to mediastinum. **(B)** Retraction of innominate vein and artery to adequately expose trachea. **(C)** Division of trachea and intubation of distal trachea across operative field. **(D)** Tracheal segment has been resected; posterolateral sutures are placed to begin anastomosis of proximal and distal trachea (*top*). Proximal endotracheal tube is advanced into distal trachea (*bottom left*) and anterior sutures are placed (*bottom right*). (Grillo HC, 1972: Tracheal reconstruction: Indications and techniques. Arch Otolaryngol 96:37. Copyright 1972, American Medical Association)

To achieve a satisfactory result with tracheal resection and reconstruction, it is important to avoid undue tension at the anastomotic site. At the conclusion of the operation, sutures may be placed between the patient's chin and chest to maintain the head in a forward position. These so-called guardian sutures prevent tension on the tracheal anastomosis that would occur with hyperextension of the neck. The sutures are left in place for approximately 7 days (La-Muraglia et al., 1991).

Patients are usually extubated shortly after tracheal surgery to avoid injury to the anastomosis from an endotracheal tube. Providing adequate postoperative pulmonary hygiene necessitates special considerations. Coughing and deep breathing regimens are essential to prevent atelectasis. Endotracheal suctioning and reintubation are avoided, if at all possible, because of potential injury to or disruption of the tracheal anastomosis. If endotracheal suctioning does become necessary, it is performed by the surgeon, using a bronchoscope to provide visual guidance. Potential complications of tracheal operations include anastomotic dehiscence, infection, and tracheal stenosis at the anastomotic site. Anastomotic dehiscence is usually a fatal complication.

TRACHEOSTOMY

Tracheostomy, also called *tracheotomy*, is performed in two situations: (1) to overcome upper airway obstruction or (2) for long-term airway management in patients who have required prolonged endotracheal intubation (Astrachan & Sasaki, 1991). Most commonly, it is performed for the latter indication, typically in critically ill patients who require mechanical ventilation for more than 10 to 14 days. Tracheostomy reduces the likelihood of complications associated with prolonged intubation with an endotracheal tube. It also frees the patient's nose or mouth of the tube and allows resumption of oral feedings if the patient's level of consciousness and swallowing mechanism are not impaired.

Tracheostomy is preferably performed as a planned procedure in an operating room with a nasal or oral endotracheal tube in place and with the assistance of an anesthesiologist (Boyd et al., 1990). Either general or local anesthesia may be used. The patient's head is extended to place a maximal amount of trachea above the sternal notch (Mathisen, 1989). A short horizontal skin incision is made 1 to 2 cm below the cricoid cartilage. The strap muscles are separated, and the thyroid isthmus is divided or retracted to expose the trachea. A vertical incision is created in the anterior surface of the trachea in the area of the third tracheal ring (Fig. 40-3). A tracheostomy tube with a high-volume, low-pressure cuff is inserted through the opening and secured with skin sutures or tapes passed through the flanges of the tube. Generally, it is not necessary to close the incision; instead, a dry, sterile gauze dressing is applied (Boyd et al., 1990).

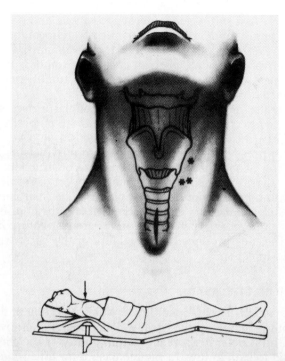

FIGURE 40-3. Tracheostomy. **(Top)** A 2- to 3-cm vertical incision is made in the anterior surface of the trachea in the area of the third tracheal ring. **(Bottom)** Proper positioning of the patient during tracheostomy to extend the head and improve exposure. (Astrachan DI, Sasaki CT, 1991. Tracheotomy. In Baue AE, Geha AS, Hammond GL, et al. [eds]: Glenn's Thoracic and Cardiovascular Surgery, ed. 5, p. 605. Norwalk, CT, Appleton & Lange)

OPERATIONS ON THE CHEST WALL

RESECTION OF PRIMARY CHEST WALL NEOPLASMS

Chest wall resection is most often performed to treat primary neoplasms of the chest wall. *Chest wall tumors* may arise from any of a variety of cell types and may involve the soft tissues of the thorax, the bony structures, or both. They generally occur as slowly enlarging masses that are asymptomatic; with continued growth, nearly all malignant tumors and two thirds of benign tumors become painful (Pairolero, 1990). In contrast to masses in other locations, an excisional biopsy (i.e., excision of the entire mass) instead of needle aspiration or incisional biopsy is recommended to achieve accurate histologic diagnosis of a primary chest wall tumor.

The treatment of choice for both benign and malignant chest wall tumors is generally surgical resection. Benign tumors often become painful if not resected, and some benign tumors undergo malignant degeneration. Malignant tumors of the chest wall are treated with wide surgical resection; the tumor is removed en bloc (as a whole) along with any contiguous structures invaded by the tumor. To allow adequate tumor-free margins, several centimeters of tumor-free soft tissue, a normal rib above and below the tumor, and 5 cm of tumor-free rib are included in the resection (McCormick, 1991). Occasionally palliative resection of a malignant chest wall tumor is performed to reduce pain or to remove a tumor that is infected, ulcerated, or bleeding.

If the removal of a chest wall neoplasm necessitates resection of a significant amount of rib segments, the resulting defect may need to be covered with prosthetic material or muscle to provide stabilization of the chest wall. Adequate reconstruction of the thorax is important to ensure support of respiration and protection of underlying organs (Pairolero, 1990). The primary complications of chest wall resection and reconstruction operations are respiratory insufficiency produced by instability of the chest wall and infection.

THORACOPLASTY

Thoracoplasty is an operation in which a portion of the bony structure of the chest wall is resected. Removal of the skeletal support allows that portion of the chest wall to sink in toward the mediastinum, thus reducing the size of the hemithorax and partially collapsing underlying lung (Shields, 1994b). The operation is performed infrequently for treatment of chronic empyema when more conservative therapy has failed to obliterate the infected cavity. Thoracoplasty may be considered when an empyema cavity fails to close with chronic drainage alone, when muscle flaps are unavailable or inadequate to fill the space, or if the lung cannot expand (Deslauriers et al., 1991). The operation is cosmetically disfiguring and can lead to chronic spine and shoulder problems (Ali & Unouh, 1990).

OPERATIONS INVOLVING MEDIASTINAL STRUCTURES

THYMECTOMY FOR MYASTHENIA GRAVIS

Thymectomy, or removal of the thymus gland, is most often performed for the treatment of *myasthenia gravis*, a disease characterized by impaired neuromuscular transmission in voluntary muscles. Patients with myasthenia gravis develop progressive weakness and easy fatigability of voluntary muscles. Ocular, shoulder, and upper extremity muscles are most often affected (Ewing & Hardy, 1991). For reasons that are incompletely understood, surgical resection of the thymus gland sometimes produces significant clinical improvement in patients with myasthenia gravis. Sixty to 85% of patients demonstrate clinical improvement after thymectomy, and complete remission of disease is reported in 20% to 35% (Ewing & Hardy, 1991).

Precise indications and timing for thymectomy in patients with myasthenia gravis are somewhat con-

troversial. Surgical resection is recommended in all patients with myasthenia gravis and a thymoma (tumor of the thymus gland). Ten to 15% of patients with myasthenia gravis have a thymoma and 30% to 50% of patients with thymoma have associated myasthenia gravis (Kirschner, 1991). In patients without thymoma, surgical therapy is typically performed in patients with generalized symptoms of myasthenia gravis, including ptosis, dysarthria, dysphagia, and weakness of respiratory muscles.

The thymus gland is a bilobular structure with an H-shaped configuration. Most of the thymus is in the anterior mediastinum, overlying the pericardium and great vessels at the base of the heart; the upper poles of each lobe extend into the neck and are attached to the thyroid gland (Trastek & Shields, 1994). Thymectomy may be performed through one of several incisions, including a partial upper sternal-splitting incision, a transverse cervical incision, or a median sternotomy incision with cervical extension (Trastek & Pairolero, 1991). After entering the mediastinal cavity, the thymus is carefully freed from attaching tissue (Fig. 40-4). Both pleural cavities may be opened to adequately expose the phrenic nerves and avoid injury during the dissection.

Patients who undergo thymectomy for myasthenia gravis require careful monitoring of postoperative respiratory status. In patients with disease of relatively short duration, extubation is considered several hours after operation; patients with more severe myasthenia gravis may require intubation for longer periods (Olanow & Wechsler, 1990).

RESECTION OF PRIMARY MEDIASTINAL NEOPLASMS AND CYSTS

The majority of *mediastinal masses* represent metastatic spread of malignant disease and are not treated surgically. However, a variety of primary neoplasms or cysts can originate in the mediastinum. Most common are cysts, neurogenic tumors, thymomas, lymphomas, and germ cell tumors (Davis et al., 1990). A mediastinal mass is generally detected by its appearance on a chest roentgenogram. A presumptive diagnosis can often be established because most mediastinal masses have a predilection for specific age groups and anatomic locations within the mediastinum (Pearson, 1992). Masses in the anterosuperior mediastinum are most common and include thymoma, lymphoma, and germ cell tumors. Masses in the middle mediastinal subdivision are most often lymphomas or cysts, and those in the posterior mediastinum usually are neurogenic tumors. These neoplasms are discussed in greater detail in Chapter 35, Diseases of the Mediastinum and Chest Wall.

Symptoms are present in more than half of adults diagnosed with mediastinal lesions (Cohen et al., 1991). Malignant masses are more likely to cause symptoms of compression or obstruction because malignant disease is often accompanied by distortion

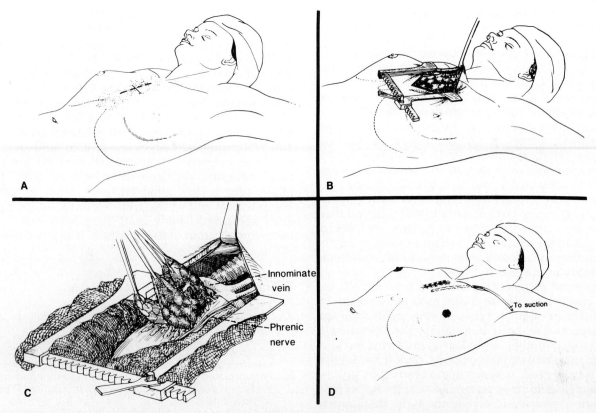

FIGURE 40-4. Thymectomy. **(A)** A short midline incision is made. **(B)** Manubrium and sternum are divided, and mediastinum is exposed by spreading sternum and retracting incision cephalad. **(C)** After ligation and division of its blood supply, the entire thymus is freed from adjacent pericardium and mediastinal pleura by blunt and sharp dissection. Care is taken to remove all thymic tissue, including cervical extensions, while carefully preserving phrenic nerves. **(D)** Incision has been closed. A small catheter is placed for suction drainage if pleural spaces have not been violated. A chest tube is necessary if pleura has been entered. (Trastek VF, Payne WS, 1989: Surgery of the thymus gland. In Shields TW [ed]: General Thoracic Surgery, ed. 3, p. 1129. Philadelphia, Lea & Febiger)

and fixation of vital structures that are otherwise mobile enough to conform to distortion from pressure (Shields, 1991).

Definitive diagnosis of a mediastinal mass before surgical exploration is important. Although many benign and malignant mediastinal masses are best treated with surgical resection, other modalities may be preferable for specific tumors. For example, primary mediastinal seminoma is highly curable with radiation therapy, and surgical resection is no longer performed as definitive treatment of this tumor (Ginsberg, 1992). Tissue for histologic examination may be obtained through mediastinoscopy, mediastinotomy, or, less commonly, thoracoscopy or thoracotomy. In some instances, a cytologic diagnosis can be made from fluid obtained with fine-needle aspiration of a mediastinal mass.

Depending on the location and extent of a mediastinal tumor, surgical resection may be performed using a median sternotomy or right or left posterolateral thoracotomy incision. Neurogenic tumors with intraspinal extension may be approached using a thoracotomy incision that is extended vertically upward along the vertebrae. After entering the mediastinal cavity and exposing the lesion, the surgeon excises all of the mass or as much as is technically possible without injuring nearby vital structures. Even if all malignant disease cannot be totally excised, surgical "debulking" of a mediastinal tumor may be an important component of multimodal therapy. In other cases, such as with nonseminomatous mediastinal germ cell tumors, adjunctive surgical excision may be performed to remove vestiges of residual disease after induction chemotherapy (Ginsberg, 1992).

Postoperative care after removal of a mediastinal mass is similar to that of patients who undergo other noncardiac thoracic operations. If a median sternotomy incision has been used, patients typically experience less postoperative pain and pulmonary morbidity than after thoracotomy in which major chest wall muscles are divided. Mediastinal tube drainage is usually necessary for 24 to 48 hours.

SURGICAL BYPASS OF THE SUPERIOR VENA CAVA

An operation to bypass the superior vena cava (SVC) may be performed in selected patients for treatment of the clinical entity known as *SVC syndrome*. The syndrome is characterized by venous hypertension in the upper body that develops when the SVC is (1) occluded with intraluminal thrombus, (2) obstructed by invasive tumor, or (3) compressed by extrinsic pressure (Hartz & Shields, 1991). Candidates for bypass of the SVC include patients with nearly complete SVC obstruction and reversed flow through the azygous vein. Pronounced cerebral or airway symptoms are typically present (Little, 1989). Surgical therapy is most often performed in patients with severe SVC syndrome caused by a benign process. It may be appropriate for selected patients with SVC syndrome secondary to malignant disease.

The most commonly performed type of SVC bypass consists of placing a vein graft between the innominate or jugular vein and the right atrial appendage of the heart (Fig. 40-5). The operation is performed through a median sternotomy incision, which may be extended onto the neck if the jugular vein is to be used. A biopsy of the obstructing process in the mediastinum is performed, and the upper pericardium is opened to expose the right atrial appendage. The innominate or jugular vein is exposed and mobilized.

Although a number of conduits have been used to bypass the SVC, autologous vein is most likely to remain patent (Doty & Jones, 1991). A *composite*, or *spiral vein*, *graft* is often created to avoid potential venous drainage problems associated with harvesting a vein of similar size to the SVC. The composite graft is fashioned from a segment of autologous saphenous vein harvested from the leg. The vein segment is divided longitudinally and wrapped in spiral fashion around a plastic thoracostomy tube similar in diameter to the vein to which the graft will be anastomosed. The saphenous vein edges are sutured, and an end-to-end anastomosis is created between the innominate or jugular vein and the composite graft. The plastic tube is then removed from within the graft. The proximal end of the graft is sutured to the right atrial appendage. Early graft thrombosis is the primary complication of the operation (Hartz & Shields, 1991).

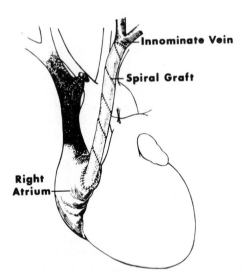

FIGURE 40-5. Venous bypass for superior vena cava syndrome. The innominate vein (at the junction of the left internal jugular and subclavian veins) is anastomosed to the spiral vein graft. Anastomosis of the spiral vein graft to the right atrium completes bypass of the obstructed superior vena cava. (Doty DB, Baker WH, 1976: Bypass of SVC with spiral vein graft. Ann Thorac Surg 22:492. Reprinted with permission of the Society of Thoracic Surgeons)

REFERENCES

Ali I, Unouh H, 1990: Management of empyema thoracis. Ann Thorac Surg 50:355

Astrachan DI, Sasaki CT, 1991: Tracheotomy. In Baue AE, Geha AS, Hammond GL, et al. (eds): Glenn's Thoracic and Cardiovascular Surgery, ed. 5. Norwalk, CT, Appleton & Lange

Boyd AD, Bernhard WN, Sparaco RJ, 1990: Tracheal intubation and mechanical ventilation. In Sabiston DC Jr, Spencer FC (eds): Surgery of the Chest, ed. 5. Philadelphia, WB Saunders

Cohen AH, Thompson L, Edwards FH, Bellamy RF, 1991: Primary cysts and tumors of the mediastinum. Ann Thorac Surg 51:378

Davis RD, Oldham HN Jr, Sabiston DC Jr, 1990: The mediastinum. In Sabiston DC Jr, Spencer FC (eds): Surgery of the Chest, ed. 5. Philadelphia, WB Saunders

DeMeester TR, Lafontaine E, 1990: The pleura. In Sabiston DC Jr, Spencer FC (eds): Surgery of the Chest, ed. 5. Philadelphia, WB Saunders

Deslauriers J, Leblanc P, McClish A, 1989: Bullous and bleb diseases of the lung. In Shields TW (ed): General Thoracic Surgery, ed. 3. Philadelphia, Lea & Febiger

Deslauriers J, Beauchamp G, Desmeules M, 1991: Benign and malignant disorders of the pleura. In Baue AE, Geha AS, Hammond GL, et al. (eds): Glenn's Thoracic and Cardiovascular Surgery, ed. 5. Norwalk, CT, Appleton & Lange

Doty DB, Jones KW, 1991: Superior vena cava syndrome. In Baue AE, Geha AS, Hammond GL, et al. (eds): Glenn's Thoracic and Cardiovascular Surgery, ed. 5. Norwalk, CT, Appleton & Lange

Ewing HP, Hardy JD, 1991: The mediastinum. In Baue AE, Geha AS, Hammond GL, et al. (eds): Glenn's Thoracic and Cardiovascular Surgery, ed. 5. Norwalk, CT, Appleton & Lange

Ginsberg RJ, 1992: Mediastinal germ cell tumors: The role of surgery. Semin Thorac Cardiovasc Surg 4:51

Grillo HC, 1989a: Tracheal anatomy and surgical approaches. In Shields TW (ed): General Thoracic Surgery, ed. 3. Philadelphia, Lea & Febiger

Grillo HC, 1989b: Benign and malignant diseases of the trachea. In Shields TW (ed): General Thoracic Surgery, ed. 3. Philadelphia, Lea & Febiger

Grillo HC, 1990: Congenital lesions, neoplasms, and injuries of the trachea. In Sabiston DC Jr, Spencer FC (eds): Surgery of the Chest, ed. 5. Philadelphia, WB Saunders

Grillo HC, Mathisen DJ, 1991: The trachea: Tumors, strictures, and tracheal collapse. In Baue AE, Geha AS, Hammond GL, et al. (eds): Glenn's Thoracic and Cardiovascular Surgery, ed. 5. Norwalk, CT, Appleton & Lange

Hartz RS, Shields TW, 1991: Vein grafts and prosthetic grafts for replacement of the superior vena cava. In Shields TW (ed): The Mediastinum. Philadelphia, Lea & Febiger

Kirschner PA, 1991: Myasthenia gravis. In Shields TW (ed): The Mediastinum. Philadelphia, Lea & Febiger

LaMuraglia MV, Meister M, DiBona N, 1991: Tracheal resection and reconstruction: Indications, surgical procedure, and postoperative care. Heart Lung 20:245

Little AG, 1989: Superior vena cava syndrome. In Grillo HC, Austen WG, Wilkins EW, et al. (eds): Current Therapy in Cardiothoracic Surgery. Toronto, BC Decker

Lynch TJ, 1992: Management of malignant pleural effusion. Chest 103:385S

Mathisen DJ, 1989: Tracheostomy. In Grillo HC, Austen WG, Wilkins EW, et al. (eds): Current Therapy in Cardiothoracic Surgery. Toronto, BC Decker

McCormick P, 1991: Chest wall tumors. In Baue AE, Geha AS, Hammond GL, et al. (eds): Glenn's Thoracic and Cardiovascular Surgery, ed. 5. Norwalk, CT, Appleton & Lange

Olanow CW, Wechsler AS, 1990: Surgical management of myasthenia gravis. In Sabiston DC Jr, Spencer FC (eds): Surgery of the Chest, ed. 5. Philadelphia, WB Saunders

Pairolero PC, 1990: Surgical management of neoplasms of the chest wall. In Sabiston DC Jr, Spencer FC (eds): Surgery of the Chest, ed. 5. Philadelphia, WB Saunders

Pearson FG, 1992: Mediastinal tumors. Semin Thorac Cardiovasc Surg 4:1

Rusch VW, Piantadosi S, Holmes EC, 1991: The role of extrapleural pneumonectomy in malignant mesothelioma. J Thorac Cardiovasc Surg 102:1

Shields TW, 1994a: Decortication of the lung. In Shields TW (ed): General Thoracic Surgery, ed. 4. Baltimore, Williams & Wilkins

Shields TW, 1994b: Thoracoplasty. In Shields TW (ed): General Thoracic Surgery, ed. 4. Baltimore, Williams & Wilkins

Shields TW, 1991: Primary mediastinal tumors and cysts and their diagnostic investigation. In Shields TW (ed): The Mediastinum. Philadelphia, Lea & Febiger

Trastek VF, Shields TW, 1994: Surgery of the thymus gland. In Shields TW (ed): General Thoracic Surgery, ed. 4. Baltimore, Williams & Wilkins

Trastek VF, Pairolero PC, 1991: Standard thymectomy. In Shields TW (ed): The Mediastinum. Philadelphia, Lea & Febiger

4

P A R T

POSTOPERATIVE
MANAGEMENT

POSTOPERATIVE MANAGEMENT OF THORACIC SURGICAL PATIENTS

THE POSTOPERATIVE REGIMEN
  Early Management
  Continued Management
PULMONARY HYGIENE INTERVENTIONS
DRAINAGE AND OBLITERATION OF THE
    PLEURAL SPACE
CONTROL OF POSTOPERATIVE PAIN

POTENTIAL POSTOPERATIVE PROBLEMS
SPECIAL CONSIDERATIONS
  Considerations After Esophageal Surgery
  Considerations in Patients With
    Malignant Disease
DISCHARGE PREPARATION

Thoracic surgery may be performed as treatment for diseases of the lungs, esophagus, or mediastinum. Pulmonary resection is the most frequently performed thoracic operation, usually in patients with carcinoma of the lung. Although the postoperative regimen varies somewhat depending on the specific pathology and type of operation, many components of postoperative care are similar for all types of noncardiac thoracic surgery. Most patients follow a predictable course of recovery. Typically, they remain in an intensive or intermediate care unit for 24 hours after surgery and then continue their convalescence on a general postoperative unit. Many patients can be discharged after 5 to 7 days.

THE POSTOPERATIVE REGIMEN

EARLY MANAGEMENT

Transfer from the operating room to the recovery room or intensive care unit is performed when the operation is concluded and the patient's vital signs demonstrate hemodynamic stability. The anesthesiologist or surgeon accompanies the patient and communicates information to the nurse regarding (1) the operation performed and type of anesthesia used, (2)

any significant intraoperative findings or complications, (3) the amount of blood products and fluids administered intraoperatively, and (4) any current medication or fluid infusions.

The nurse's first priority on patient arrival is reestablishment of monitoring capabilities, chest tube suction, and, if the patient is still intubated, mechanical ventilation. Vital signs are measured to confirm hemodynamic stability, and an overall assessment of the patient's condition is performed. Intravenous catheters are assessed for patency and proper infusion rates. The arterial catheter, chest tubes, urethral catheter, and nasogastric tube are examined for proper functioning.

Continuous electrocardiographic, arterial pressure, and pulse oximetry monitoring are generally performed during the period that the patient is in the recovery room or intensive care unit. Vital signs, including heart rate, respiratory rate, blood pressure, and temperature are recorded every 1 to 2 hours, or more frequently if the patient's condition is unstable (Table 41-1).

Breath sounds are auscultated every 2 to 4 hours, and the presence of diminished or adventitious sounds is noted. Many patients can be extubated in the operating room or shortly after admission to the recovery area. If so, supplemental oxygen using a

TABLE 41-1. DESIRABLE PARAMETERS IN POSTOPERATIVE THORACIC SURGICAL PATIENTS

Parameter	Desired Values
Heart rate	60–100 beats per minute
Blood pressure	100–140 mm Hg (systolic)
Respiratory rate	16–24 breaths per minute
Oxygen saturation	>90%
Temperature	37.0°C
Urine output	>30 mL/h
Chest tube output	<100 mL/h

high humidity delivery system is administered for several days. In patients who have undergone airway or lung surgery, early extubation is particularly desirable since extended mechanical ventilation may cause barotrauma and contribute to bronchopleural fistula development (Quill, 1992).

If mechanical ventilation is required, an intermittent mandatory ventilation mode is generally used and the patient is weaned during the first 24 hours. Pulse oximetry monitoring is performed and arterial blood gases are measured after changes are made in ventilatory parameters or as warranted by changes in the patient's condition. While the patient is ventilated, a nasogastric tube is usually in place to prevent gastric distention from swallowed air. Weaning and extubation are performed when the patient demonstrates adequate respiratory parameters for self-ventilation (e.g., arterial oxygen tension more than 60 mm Hg, arterial carbon dioxide tension less than 50 mm Hg, respiratory rate less than 30 breaths per minute, and vital capacity more than 10 mL/kg (Deschamps et al., 1992a). Other factors that influence the timing of weaning include the patient's level of mentation and respiratory muscle strength as assessed by negative inspiratory force measurements.

Patients are generally normovolemic with electrolytes in balance when leaving the operating room (Deschamps et al., 1992a). Maintenance intravenous fluids are administered until the patient is alert enough to take liquids orally. Patients who have undergone pneumonectomy are particularly sensitive to volume overload because one half of the pulmonary vascular bed has been removed (Hawthorne, 1992). Consequently, after pneumonectomy fluid status is carefully monitored, maintenance fluid repletion is reduced, and blood transfusion is avoided if possible (Deschamps et al., 1992b). In patients with a history of cardiac disease, a central venous or pulmonary artery catheter may be in place to guide perioperative fluid administration. Intake and output from the urinary drainage catheter are recorded hourly.

Chest tubes are assessed frequently during the early postoperative hours to ensure patency and to record blood loss. The rate of bleeding is generally 100 mL/h or less and decreases over the first few postoperative hours. Some thoracic surgeons advocate routine "milking" or "stripping" of tubes to maintain patency. More commonly, milking of chest tubes is performed only to restore patency when a tube is occluded. Milking the tube mechanically dislodges clot or fibrin in the tubing and creates a brief pulse of increased suction (Erickson, 1989). In addition to monitoring chest tube output, postoperative bleeding is assessed by serial hematocrit evaluations, examination of a postoperative chest roentgenogram for detection of hemothorax, and observation of the patient for clinical manifestations of hypovolemia.

A chest roentgenogram, complete blood cell count, and blood chemistry survey are obtained shortly after patient arrival in the recovery area. The chest roentgenogram demonstrates the position of intrathoracic tubes and catheters and allows early detection of pathophysiologic events, such as pneumothorax, hemothorax, atelectasis, or mediastinal shift. It also provides a baseline for comparison with subsequent roentgenograms when evaluating clinical problems that arise during the postoperative period. Ideally, the initial postoperative chest roentgenogram demonstrates full lung expansion (i.e., no pneumothorax) and minimal or no hemothorax. The roentgenogram in a patient who has undergone pneumonectomy demonstrates an empty hemithorax on the operative side with only a small amount of fluid in the space.

While the patient is on bed rest, repositioning is performed every 2 hours. Repositioning the patient at regular intervals lessens ventilation–perfusion mismatching that occurs because pulmonary arterial blood flow is directed preferentially to dependent portions of lung and remaining segments are better ventilated. Intermittent repositioning also lessens retention of bronchial secretions in dependent portions of the lungs and facilitates drainage of accumulated blood from the pleural space.

Generally, the head of the bed is maintained in a slightly elevated position (45 degrees) to enhance effectiveness of deep breathing and clearing of secretions. Particularly in obese patients, elevating the head of the bed avoids impingement of abdominal viscera on diaphragmatic movement. After pneumonectomy, the patient is positioned either on the back or with the operative side down to avoid retention of secretions and hypoventilation in the remaining lung.

CONTINUED MANAGEMENT

In patients who have undergone pulmonary resection, an oral diet is generally resumed on the first postoperative day and gradually advanced. Medications that the patient has been taking preoperatively are reinstituted with the diet. An NPO status is maintained for longer periods after esophageal resection or repair procedures, as discussed later in the chapter. Daily weights are obtained throughout the postoperative period to assist in evaluation of the patient's fluid status.

The patient can usually ambulate to the bathroom and sit in a chair on the first postoperative day, unless prolonged mechanical ventilation is necessary. Getting the patient out of bed is one of the most important postoperative lung expansion maneuvers; it increases functional residual capacity as much as 10% to 20% (Ronan & Murray, 1992). Ambulation in the corridor at least two to three times per day begins on the second postoperative day if the hemodynamic and ventilatory status are stable. Activity should progress so that each day walking is performed more frequently and for longer periods. By the fourth or fifth postoperative day, the patient is usually spending most of the day out of bed and ambulating in the corridor three to four times daily. The patient is also encouraged to gradually increase range of motion to the arm on the operative side.

After the first 24 hours, the sterile dressing covering the surgical incision is removed and the incision remains uncovered. The incision is cleansed daily and inspected for drainage or erythema of surrounding tissue. The need for perioperative antibiotic prophylaxis in patients who undergo thoracic operations remains controversial. A preoperative dose is almost always given, and many surgeons administer one or two doses during the postoperative period. A cephalosporin (vancomycin in penicillin-allergic patients) is typically chosen for prophylaxis against infection because of its broad antibiotic spectrum and low incidence of associated toxicity and side effects (Kaiser, 1990).

PULMONARY HYGIENE INTERVENTIONS

Attention to the patient's pulmonary status is one of the most important components of postoperative nursing management in thoracic surgical patients. Observation of the patient's respirations and careful auscultation may reveal early evidence of atelectasis, pneumothorax, or pulmonary edema before clinical deterioration of the patient (Table 41-2).

A number of factors associated with thoracic operations impair the efficiency of respiratory gas exchange and ventilation during the postoperative period. Some degree of atelectasis is always present due to the decrease in functional residual capacity that accompanies a thoracotomy (Joob & Hartz, 1994). Incisional discomfort, immobility, and pain medications contribute to continued atelectasis. In addition, many operations on the thorax are performed using single lung anesthesia, in which one lung is maintained in a deflated state for the duration of the operation. After operations on the esophagus, a nasogas-

TABLE 41-2. CLINICAL INDICATORS OF RESPIRATORY INSUFFICIENCY

Patient Appearance

Agitation
Confusion
Anxiety
Somnolence
Ashen color
Diaphoresis

Vital Signs

Tachypnea
Tachycardia
Elevated temperature

Arterial Blood Gas Measurements

Decreasing Pao_2
Decreasing oxygen saturation
Increasing $PaCo_2$

Pulmonary Auscultation

Diminished breath sounds
Rhonchi
Rales

tric tube remains in place for several postoperative days and impairs effective coughing and clearing of secretions.

The postoperative changes in pulmonary function are present immediately after a thoracic operation, slowly worsen during the next 1 to 2 days and, in most patients, then return to normal (Anderson & Bartlett, 1991). Patients who undergo pulmonary resection are at particular risk for respiratory complications because the loss of functional lung tissue is often superimposed on underlying obstructive pulmonary disease. Consistent pulmonary hygiene interventions are necessary to evacuate retained pulmonary secretions and eliminate atelectasis. Although pneumonia after thoracotomy is less common than in the past, it remains an important source of perioperative morbidity and mortality (Nelson & Moran, 1992).

Respiratory maneuvers that facilitate maximal lung inflation are important since shallow breathing, the lack of spontaneous deep breaths, and alveolar collapse are the steps that lead to postoperative deterioration of pulmonary function (Anderson & Bartlett, 1991). As soon as consciousness is regained, the patient is assisted in *deep breathing and coughing maneuvers* every 1 to 2 hours to ensure that pulmonary secretions are cleared and atelectatic segments are reexpanded. Typically, the patient uses an incentive spirometry device to intermittently take and sustain a series of deep inspirations. After several cycles of deep breathing, the patient coughs forcefully. A pillow or blanket is usually placed against the incisional area to brace the chest wall and reduce discomfort.

Some thoracic surgeons also advocate routine chest physiotherapy (e.g., postural drainage, chest percussion, and vibration). However, these procedures produce a fair amount of discomfort in the presence of a thoracotomy incision. Unless significant underlying pulmonary impairment is present, many patients can effectively clear secretions and maintain full lung expansion with incentive spirometry, coughing, and early ambulation alone. More aggressive interventions, including chest physiotherapy or aerosolized bronchodilator treatments, are promptly instituted in (1) patients with tenacious secretions or marginal pulmonary function or (2) those with fever and auscultatory or radiographic evidence of atelectasis.

Nasotracheal suctioning is performed in patients who are unable to clear secretions with coughing. With the patient in an upright position, a catheter is inserted through the nose until it reaches the pharynx, where a gagging reflex is produced. As the patient takes slow, deep breaths, the catheter is advanced at the beginning of a deep inspiration through the vocal cords and into the trachea (Pairolero & Payne, 1991). Once the catheter is in the trachea, it can be intermittently attached to low suction for 5 to 10 seconds at a time. A small amount of saline may be instilled through the catheter to induce coughing and loosen tenacious secretions.

A high concentration of oxygen is administered throughout the suctioning procedure and the patient is closely observed for evidence of cardiac arrhythmias or profound hypoxemia. Nasotracheal suctioning is generally quite discomforting for the patient. It is made easier if patient cooperation is elicited at the beginning of the procedure and the catheter is well lubricated and inserted gently.

Infrequently, a patient retains copious amounts of secretions that cannot be evacuated with nasotracheal suctioning. *Serial bronchoscopy* with deep lavage and suctioning may be required to prevent respiratory failure and the need for intubation and mechanical ventilation. In patients receiving aggressive pulmonary hygiene therapy, adequate rest periods must be provided between treatments. Otherwise, fatigue and increased oxygen consumption associated with the interventions can worsen hypoinflation or hypoxemia (Hawthorne, 1992).

Prolonged mechanical ventilation may be required in the postoperative period for a number of reasons, including prolonged anesthesia, fluid overload, potential space problems after pulmonary resection (i.e., when spontaneous ventilation does not result in expansion of the operative lung to fill the entire hemithorax), hemodynamic instability, myocardial ischemia or infarction, or acute respiratory failure (Todd, 1989). Underlying chronic obstructive pulmonary disease and chest wall splinting secondary to inadequate pain control may also contribute to the need for prolonged ventilatory support.

DRAINAGE AND OBLITERATION OF THE PLEURAL SPACE

Most noncardiac thoracic operations are performed through a thoracotomy incision. At the conclusion of the operation, chest drainage tubes are placed in the pleural space for postoperative evacuation of blood and air from the thorax. Usually two large-bore chest tubes are placed in the operative hemithorax. The tubes are inserted through separate small skin incisions in the anterolateral chest wall so that the patient can lie comfortably in a supine position without compressing the chest tubes (Deschamps et al., 1992a). Generally, one chest tube is directed anteriorly toward the apex to evacuate air that rises to the top of the pleural space; the other tube is directed posteriorly to drain fluid that collects in dependent areas.

Postoperative drainage of the pleural space is unique because of the negative pressure that normally exists within the thorax. Chest tubes are connected to a sterile drainage system with the capability of underwater seal and suction drainage. A controlled amount of continuous suction (-20 cm H_2O is the conventional amount) is commonly applied to the pleural space during the early postoperative period. Applying suction helps achieve full expansion of the lung so that visceral and parietal pleural surfaces appose; cessation of both air leakage and bleeding is enhanced by apposition of the two pleural surfaces. Except when excessive amounts of lung tissue have been removed, the remaining lung tissue usually expands to fill the entire hemithorax. Once the lung is fully expanded, the chest drainage system is often converted to water seal drainage without suction.

The surgeon achieves hemostasis and seals leaking alveolar surfaces of the lung before closing a thoracotomy incision. Nevertheless, some degree of bleeding and (after pulmonary resection operations) air leakage can be anticipated in the postoperative period. Bleeding usually originates from oozing surfaces of incised pulmonary parenchyma or from areas where pleural adhesions have been divided. Adequate chest tube drainage prevents accumulation of blood in the pleural space. A hemothorax prevents full expansion of the ipsilateral lung. It also provides an excellent medium for growth of bacteria and may lead to empyema and possible entrapment of the lung in a collapsed state. Sometimes blood pools in the pleural space while the patient is lying in one position for a prolonged period of time; if so, a large quantity of blood (400 to 500 mL) may drain rapidly into the chest tube drainage system when the patient is repositioned.

Chest drainage is also important to evacuate air from the pleural space. Patients who have had removal of a portion of a lung normally have air leakage that persists for several days. Air leakage after lobectomy usually originates from areas where incomplete fissures have been divided (Pairolero & Payne, 1991).

Air leaks after wedge resection or segmentectomy arise from raw parenchymal surfaces produced through creation of intersegmental planes (Duhay-longsod & Wolfe, 1992). Air may also leak from de-nuded parenchyma in areas where the lung was adherent to the undersurface of the chest wall.

Occasionally, an air leak persists for more than a week. In most instances, such prolonged air leaks represent inadequate healing or closure of distal bronchioles or alveoli (i.e., an bronchoalveolar-pleural fistula) (Rice & Kirby, 1992). If a vigorous air leak is present, it is advisable to maintain negative suction to the chest tubes at all times. Extension tubing may be added to the suction source to allow the patient to ambulate freely in the room. Once the lung is fully expanded and the air leak is small, suction is often discontinued and the tubes are maintained with underwater seal drainage. This allows the patient to ambulate more freely. Most persistent air leaks eventually seal with continued thoracostomy drainage.

Sometimes, an air leak persists that is slight enough so that it produces only intermittent bubbling in the water seal chamber and thus remains undetected. If there is any uncertainty about whether a slight air leak remains, the surgeon may choose to obtain a chest roentgenogram while the chest tube is clamped. If the chest roentgenogram reveals a pneumothorax or the patient develops symptoms, the tube is promptly unclamped. This maneuver, which is the only indication for clamping a chest tube, reveals the need for continued pleural drainage and spares the patient the discomfort of having a tube removed only to require insertion of another tube several hours later.

While chest tubes are in place, chest roentgenograms are generally obtained on a daily basis to evaluate lung expansion and the presence of pleural air or fluid. Chest tubes are removed when there is no leakage of air and when bleeding has ceased or is less than 100 to 150 mL per 24 hours. In patients in whom an esophageal resection has been performed, chest tubes usually remain until the absence of leakage from the esophageal anastomosis is confirmed by contrast esophagography. Chest tubes may also remain in place in patients requiring prolonged mechanical ventilation with high levels of positive end-expiratory pressure because of the likelihood of barotrauma with resultant tension pneumothorax.

Removal of a pleural chest tube requires careful adherence to technique to prevent iatrogenic pneumothorax. In mechanically ventilated patients, one person delivers and sustains a deep inspiration with a self-inflating bag while a second person removes the chest tube and applies an occlusive dressing. In self-ventilating patients, one of two techniques is generally advocated by thoracic surgeons. The rationale guiding both techniques is to minimize the likelihood of the patient gasping as the tube is removed and thereby drawing air into the pleural space through the subcutaneous tube tract. The tube is removed quickly from the chest either (1) while the patient is performing a Valsalva maneuver after a deep inspiration or (2) during a full exhalation. With either technique, an occlusive dressing is applied to the chest tube site as the tube is withdrawn.

Operations performed through median sternotomy incisions (e.g., mediastinal tumor resection) necessitate tube thoracostomy drainage of blood from the mediastinum. Mediastinal tubes are inserted through small incisions below the xiphoid process. Patients who have undergone pneumonectomy generally have no chest tube placed. During a pneumonectomy, the entire lung is removed from the hemithorax and the remaining bronchial segment is securely closed with suture. Application of continuous negative suction to the empty hemithorax could produce undesirable shifting of the mediastinum toward the operative side. If no chest tube is placed, pressure within the operative hemithorax is adjusted at the conclusion of the operation to approximate a negative pressure of 2 to 4 cm H_2O during inspiration and a positive pressure of 2 to 4 cm H_2O during expiration (Shields, 1994). Adjusting pressure in the empty hemithorax maintains the mediastinum in a midline position. It is generally accomplished after closing the thoracic incision by aspiration of air through thoracentesis.

A chest tube may be inserted at the time of pneumonectomy if the pleural space is infected or unusual bleeding is anticipated; some surgeons routinely place chest tubes when performing a pneumonectomy. A chest tube placed in a patient who has undergone pneumonectomy is connected to water seal drainage *without* suction. Management of chest tubes is discussed in more detail in Chapter 42, Pleural Thoracostomy Drainage.

CONTROL OF POSTOPERATIVE PAIN

Pain control is a major consideration in the postoperative period. A thoracotomy incision usually necessitates division of major chest wall muscles, retraction of the chest wall, and surgical fracture or resection of one or more rib segments. It is normal for the patient to have a fair amount of postoperative discomfort, particularly when moving about and when performing deep breathing and coughing exercises. Excessive pain and splinting can result in a decrease in vital capacity, retention of secretions, atelectasis, ventilation–perfusion mismatch, and deterioration of arterial blood oxygenation (Deschamps et al., 1992a). Postoperative pain has several other detrimental effects, including (1) an increase in cardiac work that may provoke cardiac arrhythmias or myocardial ischemia; (2) an increase in vagal tone, resulting in a propensity for nausea and vomiting; and (3) elevated hormonal tone leading to water retention and hyperglycemia (Joob & Hartz, 1994).

One of the most common methods of pain management in thoracic surgical patients is *epidural anesthesia* (i.e., delivery of analgesic agents through a catheter positioned in the epidural space) (Fig. 41-1). The catheter may be inserted in the operating or recovery room and usually remains in place for 3 to 4 days. The direct application of narcotics into the epidural space produces effective pain relief without the heavy sedation and respiratory depression associated with intravenous or intramuscular narcotics (Bragg, 1989). As a result, patients arrive in the recovery area alert and relatively pain free, thus reducing the likelihood of hypoventilation (Hawthorne, 1992).

Agents commonly used for epidural analgesia include the opioids fentanyl, morphine, methadone, and meperidine and the local anesthetic bupivacaine (Marcaine) (Piccione & Faber, 1991). Dosage and catheter care are generally managed by an anesthesiologist, but the nurse must be aware of the desired and adverse effects of the medications being given. The level of analgesia and degree of respiratory depression or somnolence must be continuously assessed so that adjustments can be made to maintain an adequate level of pain control without excessive sedation (Bojar et al., 1989).

A disadvantage of epidural analgesia is that an infusion pump is necessary for dosage titration. A urethral catheter usually remains in place as well because of possible associated urinary retention. Patient mobility is somewhat curtailed by these attachments,

and assistance must be given to the patient to ensure progressive mobility. Common side effects of epidural analgesia include pruritus, nausea and vomiting, and urinary retention (Bragg, 1989). Epidural analgesia may also be complicated by dural puncture and spinal headache, total spinal blockade, hypotension, and tachyphylaxis (Bragg, 1991).

Postoperative pain control may alternatively be achieved with parenteral administration of opioids. Morphine sulfate is commonly used. During the early postoperative period, opioids are generally administered intravenously if the patient is mechanically ventilated or under continuous observation in an intensive care unit. When the patient is moved to a general nursing unit, an intramuscular route is used for narcotic administration. A disadvantage of intramuscular narcotics is the varying level of analgesia, with excessive pain at low narcotic levels and possible respiratory depression or confusion at high levels.

Alternatively, intravenous narcotics may be administered on the general nursing unit using a patient-controlled system (i.e, *patient-controlled analgesia*). Commercially designed pump systems allow the patient to self-administer predetermined doses of pain medication intravenously. A lockout interval prevents the patient from administering medication too frequently. Newer devices allow delivery of a continuous infusion of medication that can be supplemented with patient-controlled boluses; the new devices also record a profile of the drug administration (Lubenow & Faber, 1992). Morphine or meperidine is commonly used.

An infrequently used method of postoperative pain management is *interpleural regional analgesia*. A catheter is placed percutaneously through the chest wall directly into the pleural space. Pain medication is then infused continuously or intermittently into the space between the visceral and parietal pleura. Local anesthetics infused into the pleural space diffuse through the parietal pleura to the intercostal neurovascular bundle, producing a unilateral nerve block at multiple levels (Lubenow & Faber, 1992). If more than one chest tube is in place, the physician may order clamping of the posterior tube for 15 to 20 minutes after medication administration to enhance its absorption. It is important that the remaining chest tube not be clamped if an air leak is present.

In patients with persistent chest wall pain, the surgeon may perform *intercostal nerve blockade*. Bupivacaine solution is injected percutaneously into the area of the intercostal nerve (subcostal groove on the undersurface of the rib) of several subsequent rib segments. If successful pain relief is achieved, the procedure may be repeated.

Regardless of the system used for pain control, it is necessary to medicate the patient adequately so that deep breathing, coughing, and ambulation can be performed without a great deal of discomfort. However, toxic effects may result from overzealous pain control. Probably the most commonly seen deleteri-

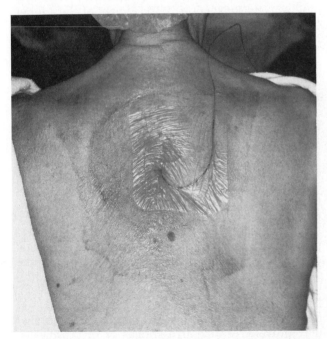

FIGURE 41-1. Epidural catheter has been placed just before anesthesia induction in this patient who is about to undergo a thoracotomy for pulmonary resection.

ous effects are oversedation, confusion, and psychosis. Development of any neurologic changes should prompt reassessment and reduction of medication dosing.

Because patients tend to require prolonged use of narcotics during the first week after thoracotomy, constipation is almost routine and ileus can occur. Daily assessment of bowel function is important, and administration of laxatives may be necessary. Signs of developing ileus include abdominal distention, absence of bowel sounds, and lack of bowel movements or flatus. In the late postoperative period and by the time of discharge, the patient is generally taking only oral analgesics. Acetaminophen (Tylenol) with codeine or hydrocodone bitartrate (Vicodin) may be prescribed when the patient is discharged.

POTENTIAL POSTOPERATIVE PROBLEMS

The major problems that can arise in the postoperative period are arrhythmias, myocardial infarction, respiratory insufficiency, and hemorrhage. *Postoperative arrhythmias* occur in 3% to 30% of patients who undergo thoracic operations (Duhaylongsod & Wolfe, 1992). Despite extensive experimental and clinical investigation, the etiology of most arrhythmias that occur after thoracotomy is multifactorial and incompletely understood (Ferguson, 1992). At greatest risk for cardiac arrhythmias are older patients and those who have undergone pneumonectomy.

Supraventricular tachycardia, especially atrial fibrillation or atrial flutter, is particularly common in postoperative patients (Fig. 41-2). Digoxin is generally used for treatment of supraventricular tachycardia; it may also be given prophylactically to patients with increased risk for postoperative supraventricular arrhythmias. Other antiarrhythmic agents used to treat postoperative supraventricular tachycardia include quinidine, procainamide, and calcium-channel antagonists, such as verapamil. Beta-blocking medications are used infrequently because of the prevalence of underlying obstructive pulmonary disease in

thoracic surgical patients and the potential for bronchospasm.

Postoperative ventricular arrhythmias are less common and almost always occur transiently. They are often the result of a precipitating factor, such as hypoxemia or hypokalemia. Intravenous lidocaine is administered while the causative factor is corrected if premature ventricular contractions are multifocal, occur in couplets or at a frequency greater than six per minute, or fall on the T wave of the preceding complex. Less commonly, ventricular arrhythmias occur secondary to acute myocardial ischemia or infarction.

Perioperative *myocardial infarction* occurs in a small number of patients who undergo thoracic operations. Patients at greatest risk are those with underlying coronary artery disease and unstable angina, recent myocardial infarction, congestive heart failure, uncontrolled hypertension, or severe aortic stenosis (Hillis et al., 1992). Perioperative myocardial ischemia is most likely during the first 48 hours when major alterations occur in adrenergic activity, plasma catecholamine levels, body temperature, pulmonary function, fluid balance, and pain (Mathisen & Wain, 1992).

Respiratory insufficiency occurs occasionally during the postoperative period. Patients at greatest risk are those with marginal pulmonary function who undergo lobectomy or pneumonectomy and debilitated patients who undergo esophageal resection. Respiratory failure almost always necessitates prolonged intubation and mechanical ventilation, which can lead to a number of deleterious consequences. The presence of an indwelling endotracheal tube provides a route for tracheobronchial contamination that can lead to pneumonia. Also, mechanical ventilation can produce barotrauma, possible rupture of bronchial anastomoses, and continuation of parenchymal air leaks.

Excessive bleeding is uncommon after noncardiac thoracic operations. It can originate from oozing blood vessels in the parenchyma or chest wall muscles or occur secondary to a coagulation abnormality. Rarely, disruption of a pulmonary artery or vein ligature causes massive hemorrhage. Sustained blood

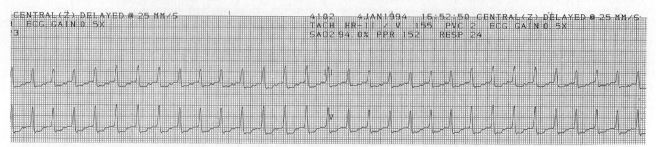

FIGURE 41-2. Supraventricular tachyarrhythmias sometimes develop in the early postoperative period after major thoracic operations. This patient underwent lobectomy 2 days earlier; electrocardiogram demonstrates atrial flutter with a ventricular rate of 152 beats per minute.

loss greater than 150 mL/h in the absence of abnormal coagulation usually necessitates reexploration of the thorax. Manifestations of excessive bleeding are less obvious in patients who have undergone pneumonectomy without chest tube placement. Because blood accumulates in the empty hemithorax, other indicators of bleeding, such as hematocrit level, radiographic evidence of an increasing fluid level in the operative hemithorax, and clinical signs of hypovolemia, are used to detect significant blood loss. Complications are discussed in more detail in Chapter 43, Complications of Thoracic Operations.

SPECIAL CONSIDERATIONS

CONSIDERATIONS AFTER ESOPHAGEAL SURGERY

Patients who have undergone an esophageal surgical procedure almost always have a nasogastric tube placed at the time of operation. Maintaining proper function of the nasogastric tube is particularly important in the early period after general anesthesia when the patient has not yet regained the cough reflex; regurgitation and aspiration can occur if the tube is not functioning properly (Orringer, 1991a). Also, because the nasogastric tube interferes with the patient's ability to cough and clear secretions effectively, pulmonary hygiene interventions are essential to avoid retention of secretions and atelectasis.

The length of time that a nasogastric tube remains in place depends on two factors: (1) the return of normal bowel function and (2) the likelihood of postoperative esophageal disruption. Operations that require only a partial-thickness incision or the placement of sutures in the esophagus are less often associated with esophageal disruption than are procedures that necessitate surgical division and anastomosis of the esophagus (Table 41-3). However, esophageal perforation can occur after any operation on the esophagus. For example, during antireflux operations, the esophagus may be perforated during intraoperative esophagoscopy, secondary to stricture disruption during esophageal dilatation, or at the site of gastric or esophageal sutures placed during the repair (Orringer, 1991b). Consequently, esophageal integrity is generally evaluated by contrast esophagogram before beginning postoperative oral nourishment; an esophagogram is repeated if the patient develops unexplained fever or chest pain after a diet is resumed.

After operations in which esophageal disruption is unlikely, the nasogastric tube remains in place for 24 to 48 hours and oral feedings can generally be resumed when the patient begins passing flatus or has a bowel movement. After operations in which the esophagus has been surgically divided, nasogastric suction is continued for approximately 5 days. The nasogastric tube is secured with tape and the patient

TABLE 41-3. RISK OF ESOPHAGEAL DISRUPTION AFTER ESOPHAGEAL OPERATIONS

Operations with Less Risk*

Esophagomyotomy
Antireflux procedures
 Nissen fundoplication
 Belsey Mark IV operation
 Hill posterior gastropexy

Operations with Greater Risk†

Esophagectomy or esophagogastrectomy
 With esophagogastrostomy
 With colon interposition
 Repair of esophageal perforation

* Procedures include partial-thickness incision or placement of sutures in esophagus.

† Procedures include surgical division and anastomosis of the esophagus.

restrained, if necessary, to prevent tube dislodgment. Reinsertion or manipulation of a nasogastric tube after esophageal resection is performed by the surgeon. If a proximal esophageal anastomosis is present, endotracheal suctioning is avoided or performed with caution because of the potential for disrupting the anastomosis if the catheter is introduced into the esophagus.

Malnourishment is a common problem in patients who require esophageal resection. The underlying disease is usually esophageal cancer with associated dysphagia and a compromised nutritional status. A feeding jejunostomy is generally placed intraoperatively so that adequate nutrition can be maintained throughout the postoperative period. If the gastrointestinal tract is functional, enteral feedings are preferable because of the risk of sepsis associated with central venous hyperalimentation.

Enteral alimentation through a feeding jejunostomy is initiated when bowel sounds are present and the patient is passing flatus. A number of commercial enteral feedings are available. Typically, a feeding solution is selected that (1) is isotonic, (2) provides at least one calorie per milliliter so that large volumes need not be infused, and (3) is unlikely to produce diarrhea. If persistent diarrhea occurs with enteral feedings or if the patient develops a postoperative ileus, enteral feedings are temporarily discontinued. Intravenous hyperalimentation may be instituted alternatively.

A contrast esophagogram is performed 5 to 7 days after surgery to assess integrity of the esophageal wall. If no leak is demonstrated (i.e., no contrast medium leaks into the mediastinum), feedings are resumed gradually, beginning with clear liquids and progressing according to the patient's tolerance. If a leak is present, an NPO status is maintained and enteral or intravenous alimentation is continued. Unless residual tumor or infection remains in the area of the anastomosis, a postoperative anastomotic leak usually heals spontaneously, although it may take several weeks. Oral nourishment is resumed when an intact esophagus is demonstrated by esophagogram.

Esophageal resection for cancer generally necessitates removal of most of the esophagus and substitution of the stomach or a segment of colon in its place. After esophagectomy, gastric emptying may be delayed and patients may experience some difficulty in resuming oral feedings. Neither of the substitute viscera (i.e., stomach or colon) functions as well as native esophagus in which peristalsis propels food into the stomach (Collard et al., 1992). An H_2-receptor antagonist (e.g., cimetidine) agent and metoclopramide may be prescribed (Wolfe & Sebastian, 1992). Several other interventions may also be helpful. First, the patient is maintained on a mechanically soft diet to enhance passage of the food through the replacement viscera. Second, the patient is instructed to take small bites and to chew food thoroughly. Often six small meals are tolerated better than three larger ones. Finally, the patient is instructed to maintain an upright position during and after meals. Generally, gastric emptying improves gradually.

CONSIDERATIONS IN PATIENTS WITH MALIGNANT DISEASE

The diagnosis of a malignancy is devastating news for both the patient and family. Both lung cancer and esophageal cancer, the two most common thoracic malignancies, are associated with a grim prognosis unless detected early in the disease. Sometimes the patient will have had some clinical manifestations of the neoplasm, but in other cases the patient may have had no warning symptoms that a tumor was present until the time of diagnosis. If the definitive diagnosis is made during an operative procedure, the nurse at the bedside may be confronted with the patient, on awakening from general anesthesia, requesting information about the diagnosis. The family may also seek assistance from the nurse in discussing operative findings with the patient during the initial postoperative visit. Their initial visit with the patient may be particularly stressful when an exploratory thoracotomy has been performed and plans for surgical resection abandoned due to tumor location or metastatic spread.

Provision of adequate emotional support to the patient and family during this period is dependent on the nurse and physician working together to provide appropriate information and counseling. Although it is the surgeon's responsibility and prerogative to determine when and what information about the diagnosis is communicated to the patient, it is somewhat unpredictable when the patient will awaken fully from general anesthesia and become alert enough to ask for and retain information. Consequently, the patient may request information when the surgeon is unavailable to come to the patient's bedside. If the patient is persistently asking for information, the surgeon may delegate another physician or a clinical nurse specialist to talk with the patient.

A nurse who assumes responsibility for providing a patient or family with preliminary information about a malignant diagnosis should (1) feel comfortable with the responsibility, (2) be knowledgeable enough about the disease and operative findings to impart the information accurately, (3) have a clear understanding of the precise information to be communicated, and (4) defer questions about the prognostic implications or projected therapy to the appropriate physician. This type of responsibility is generally reserved for a clinical nurse specialist or those clinical nurses with expert knowledge who have a close, collaborative working relationship with the thoracic surgeon and well-developed communication and interpersonal skills.

More frequently, it is the physician who provides information about a malignant diagnosis and the nurse who remains at the bedside and intervenes with the patient and family as they begin to cope with implications of the diagnosis. Several obstacles must be overcome for the nurse to provide adequate emotional support. First, the patient remains in the postoperative setting only during the acute phase of the illness. A limited amount of time is available before the patient is discharged or transferred to another setting. Second, cardiothoracic nurses spend the majority of their time developing acute or critical care nursing skills. Providing counseling for patients who face chronic illness due to malignancy calls on skills that the cardiothoracic surgical nurse uses less frequently. Finally, there are usually legitimate time constraints that preclude the nurse from either sitting down to spend time talking with the patient or ensuring that there will be a period of time to talk without multiple interruptions.

In view of these constraints, it is important to build into the plan of care interventions for meeting the patient's emotional needs. Staff nurses can play a crucial role in supporting the patient and family, even if they cannot realistically set aside blocks of time specifically for this purpose. There is a particular intimacy that develops between patient and nurse as a result of the physical care that the nurse provides. This helps to counteract the above constraints and fosters open communication, if the nurse actively observes and listens for cues from the patient. Frequently, all that is necessary to begin the process are such simple signals to the patient as sitting down in the room, maintaining eye contact, and asking questions in a manner that conveys an interest in more than a cursory answer. Whether or not the patient chooses to discuss the illness and its implications, these nursing interventions demonstrate to the patient that the nurse is available to discuss feelings and concerns. Appropriate consultations for supportive therapy are initiated before discharging the patient.

DISCHARGE PREPARATION

Anticipatory planning for discharge is begun before surgery or early in the postoperative course so that arrangements for special circumstances can be handled efficiently and without delaying discharge from the hospital. Discharge preparation of a postoperative thoracic surgical patient is generally straightforward. Some patients, however, have more complex discharge needs. If the patient goes home with enteral feedings, a tracheostomy, or an open wound, visits from a community-based nursing service may be indicated. Even if there are no skilled nursing needs, homemaker services for shopping, meal preparation, or assistance with bathing may be necessary if the patient is elderly, lives alone, or has other disabilities. The nurse at the bedside is usually in the best position to assess the patient's functional capacity and the need for special assistance at home.

By the day of discharge, most patients will be ambulatory and performing all self care activities. The amount and type of prescribed activity at discharge is somewhat variable, depending on the patient's underlying condition and the type of operative procedure performed. Patients are encouraged to remain out of bed for most of the day and to take short walks at least three times daily; stair climbing may be performed as well. Fatigue and mild dyspnea with exertion are common. Sexual activity can be resumed as soon as the patient is ambulating for several blocks and climbing stairs without dyspnea. The patient should be advised that normal sexual drive may be diminished because of the physical and emotional fatigue associated with a major operation.

The patient is generally the best judge of how much activity can be performed without excessive fatigue. Most patients who undergo major pulmonary resection procedures continue to experience some dyspnea with exertion for the first few postoperative weeks. However, shortness of breath that worsens after discharge from the hospital or that develops precipitously is not typical and should be promptly reported to the physician.

Lifting and vigorous upper extremity physical activities are generally prohibited for 1 to 2 months. Patients are instructed to avoid carrying heavy items, such as groceries, children, or laundry, and also activities such as golf or swimming during this period. Most surgeons recommend that the patient refrain from driving for a month after a major thoracic operation. However, the patient can ride in a car and usually can travel by train or plane. Long car trips should include intermittent opportunities for the patient to get out of the car and ambulate. Return to work depends on the type of work and the patient's stamina. If the job does not involve lifting or strenuous physical exertion, the patient can usually return within 4 to 6 weeks.

If the patient has a lateral thoracotomy incision, chest wall discomfort generally persists for 2 to 3 months. An oral pain medication, such as acetaminophen with codeine, is prescribed for the first few weeks at home. A heating pad or warm baths or showers may also be helpful. The patient may be reluctant to use the affected arm. Exercises such as brushing one's hair or "climbing" the affected hand up a wall are helpful in restoring the patient's range of motion to the shoulder.

Insomnia and anorexia are common complaints during the first few weeks at home. As the patient increasingly resumes normal activities of daily living, the sleeping pattern usually improves. Also, as the patient becomes more active, appetite begins to increase. The patient is encouraged to eat a diet that is high in protein and calories. Smaller, more frequent meals may be better tolerated than three large meals. The patient's weight may continue to drift downward several pounds during the first postoperative month. However, the physician should be notified if the weight loss is more than 5 pounds or if weight loss continues more than a month after surgery. This is particularly true in patients who have undergone surgical resection of a malignant tumor.

Medications that the patient was taking before the operation are generally continued. Digoxin may be prescribed for 4 to 6 weeks in patients who have had postoperative atrial fibrillation or other supraventricular arrhythmia. Generally, no other special medications are necessary after a thoracic operation. The patient is instructed to cleanse the incision daily while showering or bathing and to report any evidence of infection (e.g., incisional erythema or drainage or temperature more than 101°F [38.3°C]). If the patient was smoking before the operation, counseling is provided about smoking cessation. Smoking is harmful because of its vasoconstrictive effects on blood vessels and its irreversible damage to the lungs. Motivation to discontinue smoking is usually high after a thoracic operation, and the likelihood of success is enhanced by the patient's abstinence from smoking during the hospitalization.

If the patient has had surgical resection of a malignancy, adjunctive radiation or chemotherapy may be recommended. Usually, treatments are initiated several weeks after the operation, when the patient has recovered from the initial stress of the surgery. These treatments can often be performed during outpatient visits. Before discharge, the nurse ascertains that all necessary arrangements for adjuvant therapy have been made and that the patient understands the plan for therapy. Often multiple physicians have been involved in the patient's care, and the nurse can help clarify for the patient the plan for ongoing medical supervision.

REFERENCES

Anderson HL III, Bartlett RH, 1991: Respiratory care of the surgical patient. In Burton GG, Hodgkin JE, Ward JJ (eds): Respiratory

Care: A Guide to Clinical Practice, ed. 3. Philadelphia, JB Lippincott

Bojar RM, Murphy RE, Payne DD, Diehl JT, 1989: Postoperative care. In Manual of Perioperative Care in Cardiac and Thoracic Surgery. Boston, Blackwell Scientific Publications

Bragg CL, 1989: Practical aspects of epidural and intrathecal narcotic analgesia in the intensive care setting. Heart Lung 18:599

Bragg CL, 1991: Intrapleural analgesia. Heart Lung 20:30

Collard JM, Otte JB, Reynaert M, Kestens PJ, 1992: Quality of life three years or more after esophagectomy for cancer. J Thorac Cardiovasc Surg 104:391

Deschamps C, Allen MS, Trastek VF, Pairolero PC, 1992a: Postoperative management. Chest Surg Clin North Am 2:713

Deschamps C, Pairolero PC, Allen MS, Trastek VF, 1992b: Postpneumonectomy pulmonary edema. Chest Surg Clin North Am 2:785

Duhaylongsod FG, Wolfe WG, 1992: Complications of pulmonary resection. In Wolfe WG (ed): Complications in Thoracic Surgery. St. Louis, Mosby–Year Book

Erickson RS, 1989: Mastering the ins and outs of chest drainage. II. Nursing 89 19:47

Ferguson TB, 1992: Arrhythmias associated with thoracotomy. In Wolfe WG (ed): Complications in Thoracic Surgery. St. Louis, Mosby–Year Book

Hawthorne MH, 1992: Recognition of thoracic surgical complications: A nursing perspective. In Wolfe WG (ed): Complications in Thoracic Surgery. St. Louis, Mosby–Year Book

Hillis LD, Lange RA, Wells PJ, Winniford MD, 1992: Noncardiac surgery in patients with coronary artery disease. In Manual of Clinical Problems in Cardiology, ed. 4. Boston, Little, Brown

Joob AW, Hartz RS, 1994: General principles of postoperative care. In Shields TW (ed): General Thoracic Surgery, ed. 4. Baltimore, Williams & Wilkins

Kaiser AB, 1990: Use of antibiotics in cardiac and thoracic surgery. In Sabiston DC Jr, Spencer FC (eds): Surgery of the Chest, ed. 5. Philadelphia, WB Saunders

Lubenow TR, Faber LP, 1992: Post-thoracotomy analgesia. Chest Surg Clin North Am 2:721

Mathisen DJ, Wain JC Jr, 1992: Cardiac complications following pulmonary resection. Chest Surg Clin North Am 2:793

Nelson ME, Moran JF, 1992: Post-thoracotomy pneumonia. In Wolfe WG (ed): Complications in Thoracic Surgery. St. Louis, Mosby–Year Book

Orringer MB, 1991a: Complications of esophageal resection and reconstruction. In Waldhausen JA, Orringer MB (eds): Complications in Cardiothoracic Surgery. St. Louis, Mosby–Year Book

Orringer MB, 1991b: Complications of hiatus hernia surgery. In Waldhausen JA, Orringer MB (eds): Complications in Cardiothoracic Surgery. St. Louis, Mosby–Year Book

Pairolero PC, Payne WS, 1991: Postoperative care and complications in the thoracic surgery patient. In Baue AE, Geha AS, Hammond GL, et al. (eds): Glenn's Thoracic and Cardiovascular Surgery, ed. 5. Norwalk, CT, Appleton & Lange

Piccione W Jr, Faber LP, 1991: Management of complications related to pulmonary resection. In Waldhausen JA, Orringer MB (eds): Complications in Cardiothoracic Surgery. St. Louis, Mosby–Year Book

Quill TJ, 1992: Anesthetic complications in thoracic surgery. In Wolfe WG (ed): Complications in Thoracic Surgery. St. Louis, Mosby–Year Book

Rice TW, Kirby TJ, 1992: Prolonged air leak. Chest Surg Clin North Am 2:803

Ronan KP, Murray MJ, 1992: Perioperative assessment and mechanical ventilation. Chest Surg Clin North Am 2:745

Shields TW, 1994: General features and complications of pulmonary resections. In Shields TW (ed): General Thoracic Surgery, ed. 4. Baltimore, Williams & Wilkins

Todd TR, 1989: The respiratory intensive care unit. In Grillo HC, Austen WG, Wilkins EW, et al. (eds): Current Therapy in Cardiothoracic Surgery. Toronto, BC Decker

Wolfe WG, Sebastian MW, 1992: Complications following esophagectomy and esophagogastrostomy. In Wolfe WG (ed): Complications in Thoracic Surgery. St. Louis, Mosby–Year Book

42

PLEURAL THORACOSTOMY DRAINAGE

<table>
<tr>
<td>

INDICATIONS FOR PLEURAL DRAINAGE
  Postoperative Drainage
  Pleural Drainage in Nonsurgical Patients
PRINCIPLES OF PLEURAL DRAINAGE
  Chest Tube Insertion
  Maintenance of Pleural Drainage
  Chest Tube Removal

</td>
<td>

SPECIAL SITUATIONS
  Massive Air Leak
  Chronic Pleural Drainage
  Pleural Sclerosis
  Pneumothorax Associated With Acquired
    Immunodeficiency Syndrome

</td>
</tr>
</table>

Thoracostomy drainage is an integral component in the care of thoracic surgical patients. Chest tubes may be placed to drain fluid or air from any of the three distinct compartments that compose the thorax (i.e., the mediastinum and the right and left pleural spaces). Mediastinal chest tubes are routinely placed at the conclusion of cardiac operations or other procedures performed through a median sternotomy incision (e.g., mediastinal tumor resection). The discussion in this chapter focuses on thoracostomy drainage of the pleural spaces.

The pleural space in each hemithorax lies between the visceral pleura, a thin sheet of tissue that covers the surfaces of the lungs, and the parietal pleura, the tissue lining that covers the undersurfaces of the ribs, the diaphragm, and the structures of the mediastinum (Munnell, 1991). Under normal conditions, each lung is fully expanded and completely fills the hemithorax. Consequently, the visceral and parietal pleural surfaces are apposed and the so-called pleural space is a potential space only, containing no air and only 5 to 10 mL of fluid. Pressure within the space is slightly negative in comparison to atmospheric pressure. It varies from approximately -9 to -12 cm H_2O on inspiration and from -3 to -6 cm H_2O on expiration (Waldhausen & Pierce, 1985).

INDICATIONS FOR PLEURAL DRAINAGE

POSTOPERATIVE DRAINAGE

Most noncardiac thoracic operations are performed through a thoracotomy incision and thus necessitate opening one of the pleural spaces. At the conclusion of a thoracotomy, chest tubes are placed in the operative hemithorax to achieve two objectives: (1) evacuation of blood and air from the pleural space and (2) maintenance of lung expansion in the presence of visceral pleural disruption. Usually two large-bore tubes are inserted through separate incisions in the operative side of the thorax.

One tube is positioned posteriorly and toward the base of the lung for drainage of blood that collects in dependent areas. Bleeding can be expected during the first 12 to 18 hours after a thoracic operation. Generally, blood loss into the chest drainage system occurs at a rate of 75 to 100 mL/h for the first several postoperative hours and gradually subsides. Adequate postoperative evacuation of blood from the chest is important. Blood that accumulates in the pleural space impedes expansion of the ipsilateral lung. An undrained hemothorax may also lead to infection of the pleural space (empyema) and potential entrapment of the lung in a collapsed state.

The second chest tube placed at the time of thoracotomy is positioned anteriorly near the apex of the lung for drainage of air. In patients who have undergone partial lung resection (i.e., lobectomy, segmentectomy, or wedge resection), air usually leaks for several days from remaining parenchymal tissue in areas where incomplete fissures were divided or adhesions were freed. Evacuation of air from the pleural space is essential to allow full expansion of remaining lung tissue.

The portion of lung remaining after pulmonary resection (usually one or two lobes) almost always expands fully to obliterate the pleural space. Several compensatory mechanisms that occur after pulmonary resection facilitate postoperative pleural space obliteration, including shift of the mediastinum toward the operative side, narrowing of the ipsilateral intercostal spaces, and elevation of the ipsilateral hemidiaphragm (Joob & Hartz, 1994). Once the lung fills the hemithorax, apposition of the pleural surfaces results in cessation of air leakage in most patients within 24 to 48 hours (Duhaylongsod & Wolfe, 1992). Less frequently, persistent air leakage necessitates prolonged chest tube drainage or, in rare cases, surgical intervention. In other cases, air leakage stops but remaining lung fails to fully fill the hemithorax. If so, an air-filled space remains. Usually a persistent air space causes no clinical sequelae and gradually disappears over months (Shields, 1994a). Infrequently, a residual air space becomes infected.

In patients who undergo pneumonectomy, a chest tube is often not placed unless infection is present or excessive bleeding is suspected. Intrapleural pressure is adjusted at the conclusion of the operation by aspirating air from the pleural space with a syringe after the operative hemithorax is closed. Reducing pressure in the empty hemithorax prevents shifting of mediastinal contents to the nonoperative side with resultant respiratory impairment. The empty hemithorax eventually fills with gelatinous fluid. If a chest tube is placed at the time of pneumonectomy, it is connected to passive drainage *without suction* since the application of suction would cause undesirable mediastinal shifting toward the operative hemithorax.

PLEURAL DRAINAGE IN NONSURGICAL PATIENTS

Pneumothorax

Pneumothorax in nonsurgical patients most often results from rupture of a pseudocyst, or air-filled bleb, in the peripheral lung tissue. Primary spontaneous pneumothorax occurs as a result of rupture of subpleural blebs in lungs that are otherwise normal; secondary spontaneous pneumothorax usually occurs in older individuals with chronic obstructive lung disease or bullous emphysema (Deslauriers et al., 1989). Pneumothorax can also occur due to iatrogenic perforation of the lung during invasive procedures, such as subclavian vein catheter insertion or transthoracic needle biopsy. Pneumothorax associated with trauma is usually due to lung injury caused by fractured rib segments or a penetrating object (Symbas, 1989a). In patients receiving mechanical ventilation with high levels of positive end-expiratory pressure, pneumothorax can occur due to overdistention and rupture of alveoli (Ronan & Murray, 1992).

Pneumothorax causes a reduction in pulmonary volumes, pulmonary compliance, and diffusing capacity; the pathophysiologic consequences depend on its size, the condition of the underlying lung, and the presence of tension (DeMeester & Lafontaine, 1990). Because the chest wall is relatively noncompliant, air accumulating in the pleural space causes the ipsilateral lung to collapse. If air leakage continues without drainage of the pleural space, the increasing intrapleural pressure causes shifting of mediastinal contents toward the contralateral hemithorax, a condition known as *tension pneumothorax* (Fig. 42-1). If untreated, tension pneumothorax can cause severe respiratory distress or even death. Treatment of tension pneumothorax is emergent chest tube thoracostomy, which may be performed without a confirmatory chest roentgenogram if warranted by findings on a physical examination and by the patient's clinical condition (Fry & Paape, 1994).

Fluid Collections

Fluid in the pleural space may be blood (hemothorax), serous fluid (pleural effusion), pus (empyema),

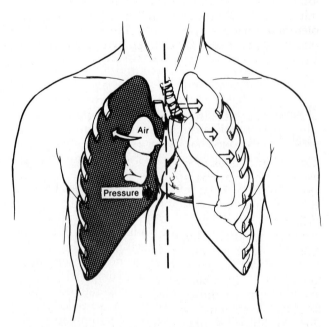

FIGURE 42-1. Diagrammatic representation of tension pneumothorax with total collapse of lung and shifting of mediastinum to contralateral side. (Hudak CM, Gallo BM, Benz JJ, 1990: Intervention alternatives: Respiratory system. In Critical Care Nursing, ed. 5, p. 337. Philadelphia, JB Lippincott)

or chyle (chylothorax). *Hemothorax* in nonsurgical patients is most often the result of chest trauma. Although some degree of bleeding occurs with almost all cases of chest trauma, significant hemothorax can result from injury to the heart, great vessels, or intercostal or pulmonary parenchymal blood vessels. Tube thoracostomy drainage in patients with traumatic hemothorax is used not only for evacuation of blood from the pleural space but also to salvage shed blood for autotransfusion.

Pleural effusion occurs when the equilibrium of fluid entering and leaving the pleural space is disturbed. Under normal conditions, 5 to 10 L of fluid flows from systemic capillaries in the parietal pleura into the pleural space each day (DeMeester & Lafontaine, 1990). The fluid is rapidly absorbed by pulmonary capillaries and lymphatics, leaving only a small amount of fluid in the pleural space. A variety of conditions can cause an imbalance in pleural fluid movement. Pleural effusion most commonly occurs secondary to malignant disease.

Empyema occurs when the normally sterile pleural space becomes infected. An empyema can develop as a complication of a prior thoracic procedure, chest trauma, or pulmonary infection. The infectious process causes accumulation of suppurative fluid in the pleural space and can lead to sepsis if the space is not adequately drained. *Chylothorax* occurs when chyle (lymph fluid originating in the intestinal tract) enters the pleural space as a result of disruption or obstruction of the thoracic duct, a large intrathoracic lymphatic channel located near the esophagus. Chylothorax is most often the result of intraoperative injury of the thoracic duct (Glinz, 1991). Chylous pleural drainage is distinguished from other types of pleural effusions by its characteristic milky appearance.

PRINCIPLES OF PLEURAL DRAINAGE

CHEST TUBE INSERTION

Clear plastic tubes of varying diameter are generally used for chest thoracostomy drainage. A smaller diameter tube (18 to 24 F) is adequate for evacuation of air or a transudative effusion. A larger bore tube (32 to 36 F) is advantageous for drainage of blood or suppurative material. Chest tubes have multiple drainage holes, distance markers, and a radiopaque stripe that outlines the proximal drainage hole (Miller & Sahn, 1987). The tubes are made of pliable material to avoid lung injury during insertion or while the tube is in place. They must be rigid enough, however, so that the lumen is not compromised by kinking or pressure (Hood, 1989).

Chest tubes are typically inserted through skin incisions located on the anterolateral aspect of the thorax (Deschamps et al., 1992). The specific site of insertion is determined by the nature of the material to be drained. Air, a low-density gas, tends to collect in the upper half of the pleural space and fluid, because of its higher density, accumulates inferiorly when the patient is upright and posteriorly when the patient is supine (Courad et al., 1990).

In most patients, a chest tube inserted into any location in the pleural space will effectively evacuate either air or fluid. However, specific placement of the tube makes drainage of the pleural space more efficient. A chest tube designed to evacuate pneumothorax is usually inserted in the third interspace in the midclavicular line of the anterior chest wall. This insertion site allows the tube to be directed so that its drainage holes lie between the apex of the lung and the anterior chest wall. A tube placed in this location is also less likely to injure great vessels, subclavian artery or vein, or pulmonary hilum during insertion (Elefteriades & Geha, 1985).

Conversely, a tube placed to drain fluid is inserted in the fifth or sixth intercostal space in the midaxillary line and directed posteriorly, because fluid can be expected to collect dependently in the costophrenic and costovertebral angles. Tubes are rarely placed in the posterior chest because of resultant inability of the patient to recline in a supine position without discomfort or occlusion of the tube. Chest tube insertion is a painful procedure; if time and the patient's condition permit, a parenteral dose of narcotic medication is administered 20 to 30 minutes before insertion of the tube. The skin in the area of the chosen insertion site is cleansed with an antiseptic solution (e.g., povidone-iodine) and a sterile drape is applied. Local anesthesia is achieved by infiltrating the skin, subcutaneous tissue, intercostal tissue, and parietal pleura with 1% lidocaine solution.

Using sterile technique, the surgeon makes a small transverse skin incision at the intercostal space below that selected for insertion of the tube (Symbas, 1989b). A hemostat is used to bluntly dissect subcutaneous tissue overlying the rib, thereby creating a tract before separating intercostal muscle on the superior margin of the rib and penetrating the parietal pleura (Fig. 42-2). Creation of a subcutaneous tract prevents air leakage at the tube insertion site while the tube is in place. It also provides a more occlusive soft tissue closure of the chest wall at the time of chest tube removal (Munnell, 1991).

Before inserting the tube into the pleural space, the surgeon inserts a fingertip to ensure that it is the pleural space that has been entered and that the lung is not adherent to parietal pleura. After digital exploration, the chest tube is clamped near its tip and advanced into the pleural space in the appropriate direction to maximize drainage. All drainage holes are positioned within the pleural space so that air evacuated from the pleural space does not enter the subcutaneous tissue (Munnell, 1991).

Typically, the chest tube is connected by 6 feet of latex tubing to a prepared drainage system placed below the level of the chest. This length of tubing

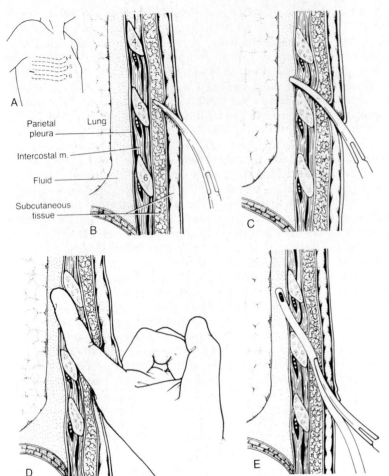

FIGURE 42-2. Schematic demonstrating steps of chest tube insertion. **(A)** Using local anesthesia, a small transverse skin incision is made in midaxillary line of fifth intercostal space. **(B)** Tract is developed through subcutaneous tissue using blunt dissection with hemostat. **(C)** The intercostal muscles are separated over the edge of the fifth rib, and the parietal pleura is gently penetrated. **(D)** Fingertip is inserted to confirm entry into the pleural space and ensure that lung is not adherent to the parietal pleura. **(E)** Tip of chest tube is inserted through subcutaneous tract and advanced into appropriate position so that all drainage holes are within pleural space. (Symbas PN, 1989: Contusion of the heart. In Cardiothoracic Trauma, p. 8. Philadelphia, WB Saunders)

allows the patient to turn and move about comfortably and minimizes the likelihood that drainage will be drawn back into the chest with deep inspirations (Erickson, 1989a). All connections are secured with tape to prevent disconnection. The tube is sutured to the skin at the insertion site to avoid dislodgement and a petrolatum gauze, occlusive dressing is applied to provide an airtight seal. A chest roentgenogram is obtained to confirm proper tube position and to ensure that the most proximal side hole, as identified by a short interruption in the radiopaque line on the tube, is clearly within the pleural space.

Because of the risk of infecting the pleural space and producing an empyema, most thoracic surgeons prefer not to advance or manipulate a chest tube once it is in place. Consequently, if the position of a tube is inadequate to evacuate pleural air or fluid effectively, placement of an additional tube through a separate incision may be necessary.

In some patients, air or fluid cannot move freely within the pleural space because of adhesions (i.e., areas in which visceral and parietal pleura are adherent to one another). In such cases, the air or fluid is said to be *loculated*. Loculated collections usually oc-

cur in patients who have had previous thoracic operations, radiation therapy, pulmonary infection, or inflammatory processes. In these patients, more precise tube placement is required for air or fluid to be evacuated. In certain cases, it may be necessary to place the tube under ultrasound or computed tomographic guidance. Alternatively, video-assisted thoracoscopy may be performed. During thoracoscopy, the pleural surfaces are visualized and adhesions can be mechanically disrupted to allow free drainage of fluid or air from the pleural space.

Chest tube insertion can be associated with major complications if intrathoracic or intra-abdominal structures are injured. The incidence of significant technical complications secondary to chest tube insertion is 1% to 2% (Douglas, 1992). If the tube is not inserted directly over the top of the chosen rib, the intercostal artery or vein that lies on the inferior surface of the rib can be lacerated (Keagy & Wilcox, 1989). Forceful insertion in an area where lung is adherent to the chest wall may lacerate pulmonary parenchyma. A chest tube that is placed too low can perforate the diaphragm and lacerate the liver, spleen, or stomach (Miller & Sahn, 1987). Rarely, the heart or one of the great vessels is lacerated by a chest tube, causing significant hemothorax. Injury to intra-thoracic or intra-abdominal structures is more likely when (1) a trocar is used during chest tube insertion or (2) a tube is inserted without digital exploration of the insertion site to ensure that the subcutaneous tract leads into the pleural space and to determine whether any tissue or organ is adherent to pleura at the insertion site (Symbas, 1989b).

MAINTENANCE OF PLEURAL DRAINAGE

The Drainage System

A variety of commercial chest drainage systems are available. All are designed using basic principles that provide a sterile system for passive or suction drainage of air and fluid, while at the same time preventing outside air from entering the thoracic cavity. The classic "three bottle" system was used for many years to provide thoracostomy drainage (Fig. 42-3). Today, these glass bottle systems have been largely replaced by disposable drainage systems, consisting of a single plastic circuit compartmentalized into three chambers. The design of disposable drainage systems varies according to the specific manufacturer. Most common are systems, such as the Pleur-evac (Deknatel, Fall River, MA), that incorporate the principles of the three glass bottle system. This type of chest drainage system is described below.

The first chamber of the drainage system (i.e., the chamber nearest the chest tube) is for collection of fluid. Graded labeling on the chamber allows quantification of the amount of fluid drainage. The second, or "water seal," chamber controls flow of air through the system so that it can move in one direction only, that is, out of the pleural space. A small amount (2 cm) of sterile water or saline is placed in the second chamber to create a water seal or one-way valve. When air trapped in the pleural space exceeds 2 cm H_2O pressure, it bubbles through the water in the second chamber and out through the atmospheric vent. However, outside air that enters the second chamber through the vent cannot penetrate the water seal to enter the first chamber.

The third, or "suction," chamber regulates the amount of negative suction applied to the pleural space. Generally, 20 cm of sterile water or saline is placed in the third chamber. To establish suction, tubing from the chamber is connected to a wall suction unit that creates negative pressure by removing air from the drainage system. Outside air can enter the third chamber through an atmospheric vent that is separated from the suction source by the column of water in the third chamber. Therefore, the degree of negative pressure within the drainage system is controlled by the amount of water in the chamber. When negative pressure reaches an amount equal to the height of the water column, outside air begins to bubble through the water, preventing negative pressure from exceeding this amount.

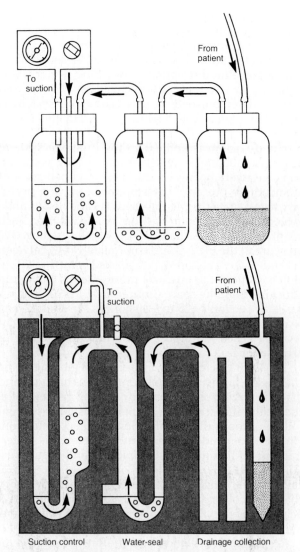

Suction control   Water-seal   Drainage collection

FIGURE 42-3. (Top) Classic "three bottle" chest drainage system. The first chamber (*right*) collects fluid evacuated from the pleural space. The second chamber, containing a small amount of sterile water or saline, provides a water seal that prevents atmospheric air from entering the pleural space through the chest tube. The third chamber, filled with 20 cm of sterile water or saline, allows regulation of the amount of suction. **(Bottom)** Disposable chest drainage system designed using principles of the three-bottle system. (Luce JM, Tyler ML, Pierson DJ, 1984: Drainage, obliteration, and decortication of the pleural space. In Intensive Respiratory Care, p. 166. Philadelphia, WB Saunders)

Assessment and Maintenance of the System

When a chest tube is in place, the chest drainage system to which it is attached must be viewed as an extension of the pleural space. Periodic assessment of the system for proper functioning is essential. The tubing and drainage chambers are always maintained in a position beneath the level of the chest to prevent siphoning of fluid from the drainage chamber into the pleural space (Bojar, 1989). If water seal drainage without suction is used, the tubing to the wall suction unit is disconnected since this segment of tubing serves as the atmospheric vent for the second chamber. Because fluid evaporates over time, water levels in the water seal and suction chambers are assessed daily and replenished as necessary. The system is inspected regularly to identify cracks in the plastic housing.

When suction is applied to the drainage system, vigorous bubbling is not necessary. As long as continuous, gentle bubbling occurs, the prescribed amount of suction is present. The amount of suction necessary to evacuate the pleural space is variable but must exceed the intrapleural vacuum created during each inspiration (Joob & Hartz, 1994). Recall that negative pressure in the pleural space normally varies between -3 and -12 cm H_2O pressure. Consequently, -20 cm H_2O is sufficient to evacuate most gaseous and liquid effusions from the space (Courad et al., 1990). Higher levels of suction (-25 to -40 cm H_2O pressure) may be required in selected situations, such as a persistent residual space, fibrinous hemothorax, empyema, or profuse air leak.

The tubing is regularly inspected, beginning at the chest wall, to ensure that all connections are tight and that the tubing is not kinked. Tubing between the chest tube and drainage system is adjusted to prevent coiling or loops that would allow fluid accumulation. Fluid in a dependent loop of tubing creates a "water-trap" effect that may inhibit drainage and negate suction (Hood, 1989). If a column of fluid greater than 20 cm (i.e., the height of the water column in the third chamber) collects in a dependent loop, no suction is being applied to the pleural space despite continuous bubbling in the third chamber.

Respiratory oscillation and the presence of an air leak are assessed by instructing the patient to inhale and exhale deeply while suction is momentarily disconnected. With passive water seal drainage, fluid in the water seal chamber rises and falls in synchrony with the patient's respirations as negative pressure in the thorax increases during inhalation and decreases during exhalation. In patients receiving positive-pressure mechanical ventilation, oscillatory variations are reversed; the water column falls during inhalation and rises during exhalation.

Bubbling in the water seal chamber indicates air leakage from the lung into the pleural space or a disrupted connection in the drainage system. If an air leak is small, bubbling will not occur continuously. The patient is instructed to take a deep breath and cough. If air is present in the pleural space, the positive pressure created by coughing will cause air to be expelled into the drainage system and through the water in the water seal chamber. Cessation of an air leak is manifested by an inability to evoke bubbling in the water seal chamber with suction disconnected and while the patient is coughing.

Infrequently, bubbling in the water seal chamber represents leakage of outside air into the system through a loose tubing connection or a defect in the drainage unit. If no intrathoracic problem accounts for an air leak or if an audible sucking sound is detected, the drainage system is assessed promptly. The dressing is removed to determine if air is being drawn in through the chest tube insertion site. Tape is removed from each of the connections to ensure that they are airtight.

The location of a leak in the drainage system is identified by applying a clamp on the tubing at progressively distal sites to the chest wall, beginning with the chest tube as it exits the chest and moving distally toward the drainage system (Munnell, 1991). If clamping the tubing results in cessation of air leakage (i.e., absence of bubbling in the water seal chamber), the leak is located proximal to the clamp. Air leakage that continues with a clamp applied to tubing just proximal to the drainage unit itself is indicative of a defect in the drainage unit; the unit should be replaced.

If fluid in the water seal chamber does not fluctuate when suction is momentarily disconnected, the tube is essentially nonfunctional. Absence of respiratory fluctuation may represent full lung expansion and occlusion of drainage holes by the surface of the lung. Alternatively, the tube may be kinked or occluded with fibrinous clot or debris. If the tube lumen is occluded and the patient has residual air or fluid in the pleural space, the tube may be "stripped" to restore patency.

Stripping (also called "milking") *a chest tube* consists of occluding the tube proximally with both hands and moving the distal hand in a sweeping motion along the length of the tube (Fig. 42-4). The proximal hand is then removed while the tube is still occluded distally. Stripping a chest tube mechanically dislodges clots or fibrin in the tubing and creates a brief pulse of increased suction (Erickson, 1989b). If chest tube patency is not restored by stripping a nonfunctional tube and pleural drainage is still required, the tube is removed and replaced with another tube (Hood, 1989).

Protocols for performance of chest tube stripping vary because the procedure is known to create excessive negative suction. While some thoracic surgeons advocate routine stripping of chest tubes, others believe it should be reserved for restoring patency to tubes that are nonfunctional. The effects of briefly increased suction within the pleural space are unknown, but it is postulated that stripping could injure lung tissue or exacerbate blood loss in patients with active bleeding. Furthermore, in most instances routine stripping does not appear to be necessary to maintain tube patency (Lim-Levy et al., 1986).

Clamps are almost never applied to chest tubes. During patient transport or ambulation, suction is disconnected, converting the system to passive water

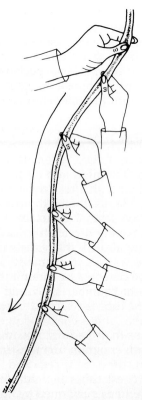

FIGURE 42-4. Stripping a chest tube. The tube is occluded proximally with both hands; one hand is held stationary while the other (still maintaining compression) is moved in a sweeping motion along the tube several times. While the tube is still occluded at the distal location, the proximal hand is released, creating a brief pulse of increased negative suction. The procedure is facilitated by putting lubricant on the hand used to strip the tube. (Courtesy of Deknatel, Inc., Fall River, MA)

seal drainage. If a chest tube becomes accidentally disconnected, it is promptly reconnected to the chest drainage system with suction. The physician is notified and a chest roentgenogram is obtained to ensure that the lung remains expanded. If there is evidence of an active air leak, the disconnected tube should not be clamped before reconnecting the chest drainage system. Any tipping that causes spillage of contents of the drainage system from one chamber to another requires replacement of the drainage system.

Replacement of the system may also be required if the collection chamber becomes filled. After preparing a new system for use, tape securing the chest tube to the connecting tubing is removed carefully. The chest tube is momentarily clamped while the connecting tubing of the system in use is disconnected and that of the new drainage system is connected to the chest tube. The clamp is then removed and tape is reapplied at the connection site. Replacing the drainage system in a patient with a profuse air leak should be performed with a physician in attendance and is discussed later in the chapter.

Cytologic, microbiologic, or cellular analysis of pleural fluid may be important to establish etiology of a pleural effusion. Pleural fluid for analysis is best obtained by the physician at the time of chest tube insertion. Although most chest drainage systems have a self-sealing diaphragm on the drainage chamber for pleural fluid aspiration, laboratory analysis of fluid that has accumulated in the drainage chamber over a period of days is usually not helpful in making critical clinical decisions. For example, fluid in the drainage chamber is not useful for microbiologic analysis if infection is suspected because it is likely to be colonized with bacteria even if fluid within the pleural space is not infected. Because the chest tube and latex connecting tubing are not self-sealing, it is not advisable to obtain fluid through needle aspiration of the tubing. Consequently, if pleural fluid for microbiologic analysis is required after a chest tube has been inserted, the physician usually clamps the chest tube, disconnects it from the latex tubing, and carefully swabs the inside of the tube distal to the clamp with a sterile applicator.

Patient Management

With properly positioned chest tubes, the pleural space can almost always be effectively drained. Failure to achieve drainage or lung reexpansion with an appropriately positioned tube represents either (1) air or fluid accumulation at a rate greater than can be drained by the chest tube or (2) underlying lung that is incapable of expanding (Bolling, 1991).

Suction drainage is usually maintained in patients with hemothorax or moderate to large pleural effusions. The amount of fluid drainage is measured hourly in patients with active bleeding and at least every 8 to 12 hours in patients with lesser amounts of drainage. The character of the drainage is documented. Terms used to characterize pleural fluid include active (bright red) bleeding, old (dark) blood, and the adjectives serosanguineous, straw-colored, purulent, and chylous.

Large, chronic pleural effusions are drained gradually to avoid complications that can result from rapid evacuation of pleural fluid. Unilateral pulmonary edema or sudden hypotension secondary to a vasovagal reaction may occur and appear to be related to the rapidity with which fluid is drained from the pleural space (Douglas, 1992). Typically, a clamp is applied if a liter of fluid drains within 30 minutes after tube insertion. The clamp is removed several hours later to allow continued drainage. If the collection chamber becomes filled, the drainage system must be replaced. Water seal, or passive, drainage, may be used instead of suction drainage once fluid drainage is minimal.

Routine repositioning of patients on bed rest facilitates fluid drainage. Sometimes, blood or transudative fluid pools in the pleural space as a result of the patient lying in a certain position for an extended period. If so, a large quantity of fluid (e.g., 400–500 mL) may drain rapidly into the chest drainage system when the patient is moved. When this amount of blood drains into the system, the patient is observed closely to ensure that the blood loss represents accumulated blood in the pleural space and not active bleeding. Active bleeding into the pleural space at a sustained rate of greater than 150 mL/h or more than 400 mL in 1 hour generally prompts operative exploration of the chest to identify and control the bleeding source.

A chest tube inserted for pneumothorax is generally connected to suction drainage until the chest radiograph demonstrates full lung expansion. Suction can usually be discontinued during periods of ambulation unless a large air leak is present. While suction is disconnected, water seal drainage allows continued egress of pleural air. When the patient returns to the room, suction is resumed.

Once the lung is fully expanded, apposition of the visceral and parietal pleurae facilitates cessation of the air leak whether or not suction is applied to the space. No controlled studies have documented that suction promotes air leak cessation, and it may in fact increase air leakage by increasing the alveolar-pleural pressure gradient (DeMeester & Lafontaine, 1990). In most instances of pneumothorax, the air leak has already sealed when the pleural space is drained or it stops within 12 to 24 hours; in 3% to 4% of patients, a fistula persists beyond this time (Deslauriers et al., 1989). After pulmonary resection procedures, air leakage is expected for several days.

Chest discomfort is common while a chest tube is in place. The degree of discomfort often increases when the lung reexpands and the visceral and parietal pleural surfaces are again in apposition. Although the patient may require more analgesia during this period, the pain indicates that the chest tube has been effective in achieving lung reexpansion. The patient should receive adequate analgesic medication to avoid chest wall splinting and hypoventilation.

During the occasional times when clamping a chest tube is indicated, tension pneumothorax can occur if an unsuspected air leak is present. Any time a clamp is in place, the nurse observes the patient for shortness of breath or chest pain that indicates pleural air accumulation (i.e., pneumothorax). If symptoms of pneumothorax occur, the clamp is removed to restore water seal or suction drainage and the physician is notified. If the patient's symptoms represent pneumothorax, bubbling will occur in the water seal chamber as soon as the clamp is released.

Chest roentgenograms are usually obtained daily during the period that chest tubes are in place. The roentgenogram allows definitive evaluation of the presence of air or fluid in the pleural space. A chest film is also obtained within several hours after converting from suction to water seal drainage to make

sure that the lung remains expanded. In most instances, chest tubes remain in place for less than a week. However, if a chest tube is in place for longer, the occlusive dressing is removed and replaced so that the insertion site can be inspected for evidence of infection. Dressing changes are then performed every 48 to 72 hours until the tube is removed.

CHEST TUBE REMOVAL

Chest tubes are removed when (1) fluid drainage is less than 100 to 150 mL/d and (2) there has been no evidence of an air leak after 24 to 48 hours of water seal drainage. Some thoracic surgeons prefer to clamp a tube for several hours before its removal. This simulates having no tube in place. It allows detection of a slow air leak that causes only occasional bubbling in the water seal chamber. Such a slow air leak may not be detected by intermittent assessment of the water seal chamber but could result in lung collapse after the tube is removed. A clamp is applied to the chest tube, and a chest roentgenogram is obtained to ensure that the lung remains expanded. If the chest roentgenogram demonstrates continued lung expansion, the tube is removed.

Removal of chest tubes in cardiothoracic surgical settings is sometimes performed by nurses who have been trained to perform the procedure. The optimal technique for chest tube removal in self-ventilating patients is a source of some controversy among thoracic surgeons. The underlying principle is prevention of air entry into the pleural space caused by involuntary patient inspiration in response to pain as the tube is withdrawn from the chest. Some surgeons believe there is less possibility of iatrogenic pneumothorax if the tube is withdrawn while the patient is performing a Valsalva maneuver after a deep inspiration; others advocate chest tube removal during a full exhalation.

With whichever technique is used, the nurse should be familiar with the principles involved and perform steps of the procedure in a consistent fashion. A clamp is applied to the chest tube to be removed. An occlusive dressing is prepared using petrolatum gauze and nonporous tape. The chest tube dressing and the suture holding the tube in place are removed. The patient is instructed to practice performing the chosen breathing technique. When the patient has demonstrated compliance with the breathing routine, he or she again breathes as instructed. The nurse holds the chest tube in one hand and with the other holds the prepared sterile dressing over the insertion site. The tube is removed quickly but smoothly while the chest tube entry site is occluded by manual compression of the dressing over the site. Adhesive tape is applied by a second nurse to form an occlusive dressing. A chest roentgenogram is obtained within several hours to ensure that tube removal has not caused pneumothorax.

If two pleural chest tubes with insertion sites in close proximity to one another are to be pulled, both tubes are clamped and pulled together. If a second chest tube connected by a "Y" connector to the same drainage system is to remain in the chest, it is clamped while the first tube is pulled. The remaining chest tube is then reattached to the drainage system with a straight connector and the clamp is removed.

In mechanically ventilated patients, chest tube removal is performed by two persons. One delivers and sustains an inspiration, using a self-inflating ventilation bag; a second person removes the tube during the sustained inspiration and applies the dressing. In thin, frail individuals and in those with impaired healing, a pursestring suture may be used to close the chest tube insertion incision at the time of tube removal. Suture closure of the insertion site ensures that recurrent pneumothorax does not result from air entry through the chest tube tract (Douglas, 1992).

The occlusive dressing remains in place for 48 hours to prevent pneumothorax due to air entering the pleural cavity through the chest tube tract in the subcutaneous tissue. After this time, the tract has usually closed and a dressing is no longer required. Occasionally, small amounts of residual fluid in the pleural space continue to drain through the chest tube insertion site for several days after the occlusive dressing has been removed. If so, the site is covered with a gauze dressing until drainage ceases. The patient is instructed to bathe normally and change the dressing daily or more frequently, depending on the amount of drainage.

SPECIAL SITUATIONS

MASSIVE AIR LEAK

A *massive air leak* is said to exist when air is entering the pleural space so rapidly that it causes continuous bubbling in the water seal chamber with suction drainage. Massive air leaks occur most commonly in patients receiving mechanical ventilation with high levels of positive end-expiratory pressure. When alveolar rupture occurs in these patients, positive-pressure ventilations and positive end-expiratory pressure facilitate rapid leakage of air through the visceral disruption into the pleural space.

Patients with massive air leaks are dependent on continuous suction drainage to control the rapid egress of air into the pleural space. If the rate of air leakage is greater than can be evacuated by the chest drainage system, the lung fails to reexpand. The patient may also develop *subcutaneous emphysema* or tracking of air into subcutaneous layers of the face, neck, shoulders, or chest (Fig. 42-5). Subcutaneous emphysema is easily detectable by palpation; the soft tissue feels spongy and crunchy to the touch. Occasionally, air tracks into the fascial layer of the neck, distorting the vocal cords and producing a change in the pitch of the patient's voice. If subcutaneous emphysema is excessive, it may also extend down the abdomen into the scrotum, where it is generally prevented from extending into the thighs by the attachments of the inguinal ligament (Pairolero & Payne, 1991).

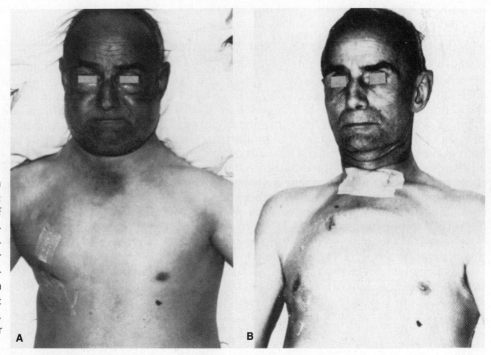

FIGURE 42-5. **(A)** Patient with subcutaneous emphysema; note swollen appearance of face and neck. **(B)** Same patient after subcutaneous emphysema resolved. (Eijgelaar A, 1991: Intrathoracic gas collections. In Webb WR, Besson A [eds]: Thoracic Surgery: Management of Chest Injuries, p. 35. St. Louis, Mosby–Year Book)

Continued lung collapse or development of subcutaneous emphysema indicates a need to better evacuate air from the pleural space. Additional water may be added to the suction chamber to increase the amount of suction, although this is limited by the size of the chamber. An *Emerson pump* (J. H. Emerson Co., Cambridge, MA), which can generate higher levels of negative suction, may be used alternatively. The insertion of an additional chest tube may also be required to evacuate air that is accumulating rapidly in the pleural space.

Critically ill patients who require mechanical ventilation and who have a massive air leak are often only marginally stable. Tension pneumothorax can occur despite a patent chest tube. Even momentary lung collapse due to discontinuation of suction or occlusion of the tube can result in hypotension or cardiac arrest. If the drainage system must be changed, it is advisable to have a physician in attendance. The equipment is prepared and a second physician or nurse assists so that the patient is disconnected from suction for only a matter of seconds. The tube is not clamped at any time during the drainage system change.

CHRONIC PLEURAL DRAINAGE

Infection of the pleural space occurs most often as a result of pyogenic pneumonia but can also develop as a complication of a thoracic operation, a subphrenic abscess, or chest trauma (Shields, 1994b). The accumulation of pus in the pleural space is termed *empyema thoracis*. Generally, the presence of purulent material causes an inflammatory response that fuses pleural margins around accumulated fluid, localizing the process into a contained pleural abscess (i.e., an empyema cavity) (Finkelmeier, 1986).

Empyema is often treated with chronic tube thoracostomy drainage until the cavity fills with granulation tissue, the remaining lung expands, the mediastinum shifts, and the cavity contracts and is obliterated (Alexander & Fetter, 1992). The closed chest drainage system can be converted to open drainage when loculation of the empyema cavity occurs, as evidenced by cessation of respiratory oscillations in the water seal chamber. Once this occurs, the tube is disconnected from the drainage system and a chest roentgenogram is obtained. If the patient remains without symptoms of pneumothorax and the chest film demonstrates continued lung expansion, the tube is left open to air.

When a chest tube is converted to open drainage in this manner, it is referred to as an *empyema tube*. The tube is generally severed so that only 2 to 3 inches extend outside the skin. After the tube has been cut, a large safety pin is inserted through the exposed portion of the tube and secured by tape to the chest wall so that the tube cannot migrate completely into the chest with respiratory pressure variations. The tube also remains sutured to the skin so that it does not slide out of the empyema cavity. Depending on the amount of drainage, an empyema tube is covered with a glove, ostomy pouch, or dressing.

If an empyema tube adequately drains the infected space, the patient remains afebrile and can usually be discharged from the hospital. If drainage from the tube is thick and purulent, it may be necessary for a family member or visiting nurse to irrigate the tube intermittently with saline solution so that it does not become occluded. The patient is instructed to reinsert the tube if it falls out to prevent closure of the skin opening. Over a period of weeks, the tube is gradually withdrawn from the cavity, an inch or so at a time. Tube repositioning prevents the tube from eroding the lung and permits cavity closure (Lawrence, 1989). A sinogram is sometimes obtained to document size of the remaining cavity.

PLEURAL SCLEROSIS

A common reason for placement of a chest tube is to evacuate a malignant pleural effusion. Several forms of advanced carcinoma are associated with recurring effusions, most commonly lung cancer, breast cancer, and lymphoma (Flye, 1989). As fluid accumulates in the pleural space, the patient experiences increasing shortness of breath. The fluid may be evacuated by a thoracentesis or chest tube thoracostomy, but it is likely to reaccumulate.

If chest tube thoracostomy drainage is performed, it is often accompanied by *pleural sclerosis*, a procedure designed to produce sterile pleuritis and obliteration of the pleural space (DeMeester & Lafontaine, 1990). The inflammatory reaction produced by pleural sclerosis causes visceral and parietal pleural surfaces to adhere to one another so that fluid cannot collect between them. If successful, the patient does not develop recurring effusion in the pleural space.

The procedure is performed when the effusion has been completely drained, as evidenced by less than 100 mL of drainage per day. Evacuating the fluid allows reexpansion of the lung so that parietal and visceral pleural surfaces are in apposition when the sclerosing agent is introduced (DeMeester & Lafontaine, 1990). A caustic agent such as doxycycline or bleomycin is injected by the physician through the tube into the pleural space. Chemical sclerosis is often painful. Parenteral narcotic analgesia is administered before introduction of the sclerosing agent and during the time that the sclerosing agent is within the pleural space. In addition, lidocaine is added to the sclerosing solution to provide topical anesthesia.

After insertion of the sclerosing agent, the tube is clamped for 6 to 8 hours. During the time that the tube is clamped and the solution is contained within the pleural space, the patient is instructed to turn from back to side to back every 2 hours. Repositioning allows the sclerosing agent to cover all the pleural surfaces. The chest tube clamp is then released, and the tube is left in place for several more days to pre-

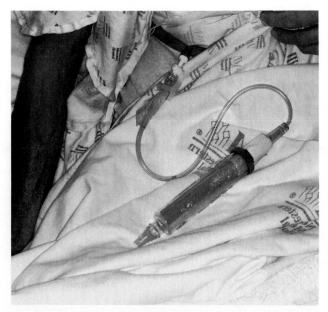

FIGURE 42-6. Chest drainage catheter in this patient with a persistent air leak has been connected to a Heimlich valve.

vent reaccumulation of fluid, maintain lung expansion, and allow the pleural surfaces to become adherent as a result of the induced chemical pleuritis. Pleural sclerosis is effective in preventing fluid reaccumulation in 80% to 85% of patients with malignant effusions (Ponn et al., 1991).

PNEUMOTHORAX ASSOCIATED WITH ACQUIRED IMMUNODEFICIENCY SYNDROME

Patients with acquired immunodeficiency syndrome often develop pneumothoraces in association with *Pneumocystis carinii* pneumonia (Fleisher et al., 1988). In these patients, healing processes are impaired and air leaks often persist, necessitating continued chest drainage for several weeks. If the air leak is small, a Heimlich valve may be substituted for the water seal chest drainage system. A *Heimlich valve* is a rigid extension tube designed to be connected to the chest tube. It contains a one-way flutter valve that allows air to escape from the chest tube to the atmosphere but prevents atmospheric air from entering the pleural space (Fig. 42-6). The chest tube and Heimlich valve are taped to the chest wall. The patient can be discharged from the hospital, ambulate freely, and wear clothing that obscures the chest tube from view.

REFERENCES

Alexander JC, Fetter JE, 1992: Postresectional empyema and bronchopleural fistula. In Wolfe WG (ed): Complications in Thoracic Surgery. St. Louis, Mosby—Year Book

Bojar RM, 1989: Postoperative care. In Bojar RM (ed): Manual of Perioperative Care in Cardiac and Thoracic Surgery. Boston, Blackwell Scientific Publications

Bolling SF, 1991: The management of complications of venous access monitoring and chest tubes. In Waldhausen JA, Orringer MB (eds): Complications in Cardiothoracic Surgery. St. Louis, Mosby—Year Book

Courad LL, Velly JF, N'Diaye M, 1990: Principles and techniques of chest drainage and suction. In Deslauriers J, Lacquet LK (eds): Thoracic Surgery: Surgical Management of Pleural Diseases. St. Louis, CV Mosby

DeMeester TR, Lafontaine E, 1990: The pleura. In Sabiston DC Jr, Spencer FC (eds): Surgery of the Chest, ed. 5. Philadelphia, WB Saunders

Deschamps C, Allen MS, Trastek VF, Pairolero PC, 1992: Postoperative management. Chest Surg Clin North Am 2: 713

Deslauriers J, Leblanc P, McClish A, 1989: Bullous and bleb diseases of the lung. In Shields TW (ed): General Thoracic Surgery, ed. 3. Philadelphia, Lea & Febiger

Douglas JM Jr, 1992: Complications related to patient positioning, thoracic incisions, and chest tube placement. In Wolfe WG (ed): Complications in Thoracic Surgery. St. Louis, Mosby—Year Book

Duhaylongsod FG, Wolfe WG, 1992: Complications of pulmonary resection. In Wolfe WG (ed): Complications in Thoracic Surgery. St. Louis, Mosby—Year Book

Elefteriades JA, Geha AS, 1985: Chest tubes. In House Officer Guide to ICU Care: The Cardiothoracic Surgical Patient. Rockville, MD, Aspen Publishers

Erickson RS, 1989a: Mastering the ins and outs of chest drainage—1. Nursing 89 19:37

Erickson RS, 1989b: Mastering the ins and outs of chest drainage–2. Nursing 89 19:47

Finkelmeier BA, 1986: Difficult problems in postoperative management. Crit Care Q 9:3

Fleisher AG, McElvaney G, Lawson L, et al., 1988: Surgical management of spontaneous pneumothorax in patients with acquired immunodeficiency syndrome. Ann Thorac Surg 45:21

Flye MW, 1989: Malignant pleural effusion. In Grillo HC, Austen WG, Wilkins EW, et al. (eds): Current Therapy in Cardiothoracic Surgery. Toronto, BC Decker

Fry WA, Paape K, 1994: Pneumothorax. In Shields TW (ed): General Thoracic Surgery, ed. 4. Baltimore, Williams and Wilkins

Glinz W, 1991: Intrathoracic fluid effusions. In Webb WR, Besson A (eds): Thoracic Surgery: Surgical Management of Chest Injuries. St. Louis, Mosby—Year Book

Hood RM, 1989: Post-injury and postoperative care of thoracic trauma. In Hood RM, Boyd AD, Culliford AT (eds): Thoracic Trauma. Philadelphia, WB Saunders

Joob AW, Hartz RS, 1994: General principles of postoperative care. In Shields TW (ed): General Thoracic Surgery, ed. 4. Baltimore, Williams & Wilkins

Keagy BA, Wilcox BR, 1989: Spontaneous pneumothorax. In Grillo HC, Austen WG, Wilkins EW, et al (eds): Current Therapy in Cardiothoracic Surgery. Toronto, BC Decker

Lawrence GH, 1989: Empyema and bronchopleural fistula. In Grillo HC, Austen WG, Wilkins EW, et al (eds): Current Therapy in Cardiothoracic Surgery. Toronto, BC Decker

Lim-Levy F, Babler SA, DeGroot-Kosolcharoen J, et al., 1986: Is milking and stripping chest tubes really necessary? Ann Thorac Surg 42:77

Miller KS, Sahn SA, 1987: Chest tubes: Indications, technique, management and complications. Chest 91:258

Munnell ER, 1991: Chest drainage in the traumatized patient. In Webb WR, Besson A (eds): Thoracic Surgery: Surgical Management of Chest Injuries. St. Louis, Mosby—Year Book

Pairolero PC, Payne WS, 1991: Postoperative care and complications in the thoracic surgery patient. In Baue AE, Geha AS, Hammond GL, et al. (eds): Glenn's Thoracic and Cardiovascular Surgery, ed 5. Norwalk, CT, Appleton & Lange

Ponn RB, Blancaflor J, D'Agostino RS, et al., 1991: Pleuroperitoneal shunting for intractable pleural effusions. Ann Thorac Surg 51:605

Ronan KP, Murray MJ, 1992: Perioperative assessment and mechanical ventilation. Chest Surg Clin North Am 2:745

Shields TW, 1994a: General features and complications of pulmonary resections. In Shields TW (ed): General Thoracic Surgery, ed. 4. Baltimore, Williams & Wilkins

Shields TW, 1994b: Parapneumonic empyema. In Shields TW (ed): General Thoracic Surgery, ed. 4. Baltimore, Williams & Wilkins

Symbas PN, 1989a: Pleural space sequelae from thoracic trauma. In Cardiothoracic Trauma. Philadelphia, WB Saunders

Symbas PN, 1989b: Chest drainage tubes. Surg Clin North Am 69:41

Waldhausen JA, Pierce WS, 1985: The physiology and management of chest injuries. In Johnson's Surgery of the Chest, ed. 5. Chicago, Year Book

43

CHAPTER

COMPLICATIONS OF THORACIC OPERATIONS

RESPIRATORY COMPLICATIONS
  Atelectasis
  Pneumonia
  Acute Respiratory Failure
CARDIOVASCULAR COMPLICATIONS
  Hemorrhage
  Cardiac Arrhythmias
  Myocardial Infarction
  Pulmonary Edema
INCISIONAL COMPLICATIONS
  Wound Infection
  Secondary Complications of Thoracotomy
    Incisions

COMPLICATIONS OF PULMONARY
    RESECTION
  Persistent Air Space
  Empyema
  Prolonged Air Leak and Bronchopleural
    Fistula
  Other Complications
COMPLICATIONS OF ESOPHAGEAL
    RESECTION
  Anastomotic Leak
  Chylothorax
  Postoperative Dysphagia

Significant complications after thoracic operations are relatively uncommon. The low incidence of morbidity and mortality may be attributed to a number of factors associated with contemporary perioperative management, including thorough preoperative evaluation of pulmonary, cardiac, and nutritional states; careful candidate selection for operative intervention; sophisticated perioperative hemodynamic monitoring; meticulous handling of tissue by the surgeon with preservation of adequate blood supply to areas of resection; and the availability of specialized nursing care in the postoperative period (Finkelmeier, 1986). Furthermore, the advent of limited pulmonary resections, thoracoscopic surgical techniques, and postoperative epidural analgesia have made thoracic surgical procedures possible in some patients who would formerly have been considered to have a prohibitive risk (Reilly et al., 1993).

Nevertheless, a variety of complications can occur, some of which have lethal or debilitating conse-

quences. The most important determinant of postoperative morbidity is the preoperative condition of the patient, particularly the patient's pulmonary and cardiac status. Thoracic operations are most often performed for resection of malignant neoplasms. Because smoking is a risk factor for both lung and esophageal cancer, many patients have a long smoking history and underlying chronic obstructive pulmonary disease. Associated major medical illnesses, such as coronary artery disease or diabetes, are also commonly present because lung and esophageal cancer typically occur in middle-aged or elderly individuals.

Patients with esophageal cancer usually have dysphagia and some degree of esophageal obstruction. Weight loss and debilitation may have occurred unless the tumor is detected early. In addition, since alcohol abuse is a risk factor for esophageal cancer, patients with tumors of the esophagus may have hepatic dysfunction or cardiomyopathy.

Betsy Finkelmeier: CARDIOTHORACIC SURGICAL NURSING.
© 1995 J.B. Lippincott Company.

RESPIRATORY COMPLICATIONS

Respiratory complications are one of the most common sources of morbidity in thoracic surgical patients. Postoperative deterioration in pulmonary function and gas exchange can be expected after any major surgical procedure as a result of (1) a reduction in vital capacity, tidal volume, and functional residual capacity, (2) a diminution of the normal sighing mechanism that helps to maintain lung volume and pulmonary compliance, (3) an alteration in the central respiratory drive secondary to narcotic administration, and (4) restricted ventilation due to immobility and pain (Todd, 1994). Specific factors associated with thoracic operations that predispose to postoperative respiratory impairment are displayed in Table 43-1. Pulmonary dysfunction can complicate any thoracic operation but is most likely after pulmonary resection operations (i.e., when a portion or all of a lung is removed).

ATELECTASIS

Atelectasis is the most common type of postoperative pulmonary dysfunction, with a reported incidence ranging from 10% to 70% (Piccione & Faber, 1991). Some degree of atelectasis is inevitable because of a decrease in functional residual capacity after thoracotomy (Joob & Hartz, 1994). The use of general anesthesia, division of chest wall musculature, immobility, and administration of narcotics for pain control all compromise the patient's ability to intermittently hyperexpand the lungs as would occur normally. In addition, many thoracic operations are performed using single lung ventilation, in which the ipsilateral lung is maintained in a deflated state during the operation to improve exposure.

Postoperative atelectasis usually occurs in a lobar or segmental pattern. The presence of collapsed portions of lung tissue decreases pulmonary compliance, increases the work of breathing, and produces areas of poor ventilation with resultant ventilation–perfusion mismatch (Bojar et al., 1989a). Clinical manifestations of atelectasis include fever, tachypnea, and diminished breath sounds on auscultation. Acute shortness of breath and a variable degree of cyanosis may occur with massive atelectasis (Shields, 1994).

Consistent performance of prescribed pulmonary hygiene interventions is essential to minimize postoperative atelectasis. In most cases, incentive spirometry, coughing, and deep breathing are sufficient to clear secretions and expand atelectatic airways. Atelectasis associated with respiratory insufficiency must be treated with more aggressive interventions, such as nasotracheal suctioning, endotracheal intubation, mechanical ventilation, or intermittent bronchoscopy for lavage and deep suctioning.

PNEUMONIA

Pneumonia remains a significant cause of morbidity after thoracic operations. It is most common in patients who require prolonged intubation or who are immunocompromised. Other causes of postoperative pneumonia include unrelieved atelectasis and aspiration of liquid gastric contents into the lungs (Pairolero & Payne, 1991). Esophageal resection for cancer and chest wall resection are thoracic operations associated with a higher incidence of pneumonia. Patients who undergo esophageal resection may have a poor preoperative nutritional status, chronic low-grade aspiration, poor gastric emptying, and operative disruption of normal esophageal sphincter mechanisms; major chest wall resections place the patient at greater risk by significantly compromising postoperative ventilatory function (Nelson & Moran, 1992).

Postoperative pneumonia is usually bacterial. Common causative organisms include *Hemophilus influenzae*, pneumococcus, and *Staphylococcus aureus* (Kaiser, 1990). Treatment consists of organism-specific antibiotic therapy, pulmonary hygiene interventions, and respiratory support as indicated by the patient's condition.

ACUTE RESPIRATORY FAILURE

Acute respiratory failure is defined as a clinical state in which oxygen delivery and alveolar gas exchange are inadequate to support tissue oxygenation. The most common cause of postoperative respiratory failure is retention of pulmonary secretions secondary to shallow breathing, ineffective cough, and splinting of the chest wall. Other less common etiologic factors include pneumonia and pulmonary edema. Acute respiratory failure is most common after major pulmonary resection operations in patients with underlying obstructive pulmonary disease. Despite preoperative clinical assessment and pulmonary function testing,

---

TABLE 43-1. FACTORS CONTRIBUTING TO RESPIRATORY IMPAIRMENT IN PATIENTS WHO UNDERGO THORACIC OPERATIONS

Underlying obstructive pulmonary disease
Single lung ventilation*
Physiologic consequences of thoracotomy incision
Excessive lung resection†
Acute injury to remaining lung†
Prolonged intubation
Inadequate pain control
Indwelling nasogastric tube‡
Excessive sedation
Fluid overload
Aspiration
Multiple transfusions of blood products

* Anesthetic technique used in many thoracic operations.
† Pulmonary resection operations.
‡ Esophageal resection operations.

it is not possible to predict with certainty a patient's ability to withstand removal of a portion or all of a lung.

Acute respiratory failure often develops insidiously over hours or days. Clinical signs of a deteriorating respiratory status include (1) tachypnea; (2) dyspnea and the use of accessory muscles of respiration; (3) decreasing arterial oxygen tension and decreasing, then increasing arterial carbon dioxide tension; (4) tachycardia; (5) pallor and diaphoresis; and (6) anxiety, disorientation, or obtundation (Hawthorne, 1992). Once the patient develops acute respiratory distress, endotracheal intubation and institution of mechanical ventilation are usually necessary. Frequent endotracheal suctioning is instituted to clear secretions and reexpand airways. Etiologic factors, such as pneumonia or pulmonary edema, are treated appropriately, and enteral alimentation is begun. Ventilatory support is continued until the patient demonstrates pulmonary function adequate for self-ventilation. If respiratory failure persists for more than 2 weeks, a tracheostomy is generally performed to avoid potential complications of prolonged endotracheal intubation.

The most severe form of respiratory failure is *adult respiratory distress syndrome* (ARDS). It is characterized by progressive hypoxemia and decreasing pulmonary compliance in the absence of fluid overload (Todd, 1992). ARDS usually follows an episode of sepsis or shock that produces changes in capillary membrane permeability and the release of bronchoconstricting mediators. The primary therapy for ARDS is mechanical ventilatory support. High FiO_2 and positive end-expiratory pressure levels are usually necessary to sustain adequate oxygenation. Contributing factors, such as pneumonia, atelectasis, pulmonary edema, or anemia, are identified and corrected with appropriate therapy. ARDS is associated with a 40% or greater mortality rate, and patients who do survive require prolonged intensive care (Todd, 1992).

CARDIOVASCULAR COMPLICATIONS

HEMORRHAGE

Hemorrhage is uncommon after thoracic operations if adequate hemostasis is achieved in the operating room before closing the chest. In patients who undergo pulmonary resection, significant bleeding sometimes arises from oozing small blood vessels in areas of denuded lung parenchyma, particularly when incomplete fissures have been divided by blunt dissection or when pleural adhesions have been manually separated (Elefteriades & Geha, 1985). Postoperative hemorrhage can also occur due to a coagulopathy caused by an underlying coagulation abnormality or liver failure (Pairolero & Payne, 1991). Rarely, disruption of a pulmonary artery or vein

anastomosis occurs, causing precipitous, massive hemorrhage.

The degree of postoperative blood loss is evaluated by frequent observation of chest tube output, as well as by serial hematocrit levels and radiographic evidence of hemothorax. If no chest tube is in place (e.g., after pneumonectomy), excessive bleeding is detected by roentgenographic demonstration of an abnormally large fluid collection in the operative hemithorax or by clinical signs of impending hypovolemic shock. Postoperative coagulopathy is treated with administration of platelets, fresh frozen plasma, or cryoprecipitate to restore adequate coagulation. In a patient with normal coagulation, continued blood loss of greater than 150 mL/h generally prompts operative reexploration to identify and control the source of bleeding. In the rare case of massive hemorrhage, the surgeon may need to reopen the chest incision in the intensive care unit and digitally compress the bleeding vessel to save the patient's life. The patient is then transported to the operating room for exploration and closure of the incision under sterile conditions.

Adequate evacuation of a hemothorax is important. Blood accumulating in the chest can compromise respiratory function. In addition, residual hemothorax provides an excellent medium for growth of bacteria and may lead to empyema and entrapment of the lung in a collapsed state.

CARDIAC ARRHYTHMIAS

Cardiac arrhythmias are common during the postoperative period. They occur most often in patients who are older than 50 years of age, who have preexisting cardiovascular disease, and who undergo pneumonectomy or esophageal surgery (Pairolero & Payne, 1991). The most frequently occurring arrhythmia is supraventricular tachycardia, in particular, atrial fibrillation. Supraventricular tachycardia is usually easily treated with standard pharmacologic agents. Digoxin is typically selected as the agent of choice. Other antiarrhythmic medications that may be used to treat postoperative supraventricular tachycardia include procainamide, verapamil, or diltiazem. Propranolol or other beta-blocking medications that may produce bronchospasm are less commonly used because of the prevalence of obstructive lung disease in patients who require thoracic surgery.

Sinus tachycardia is another common postoperative arrhythmia. It is usually provoked by a hypermetabolic state, such as occurs with fever, anxiety, pain, or anemia. Once the precipitating factor is corrected, the arrhythmia usually subsides. Ventricular arrhythmias are less common after thoracic operations. They generally indicate an acute problem requiring treatment, such as hypoxemia, hypokalemia, or myocardial ischemia. Lidocaine may be used to suppress ventricular ectopy while the causative factor is identified and treated.

MYOCARDIAL INFARCTION

Perioperative myocardial infarction occurs in approximately 3% of patients who undergo thoracotomy; it is most likely in patients older than 65 years of age and those with a history of coronary artery disease or preoperative evidence of myocardial ischemia or infarction (Bojar et al., 1989a). At greatest risk are patients who have sustained a preoperative myocardial infarction within 3 months of the thoracic operation (Shields, 1993). Ischemic events are most likely in the early postoperative period when major alterations occur in adrenergic activity, plasma catecholamine levels, body temperature, pulmonary function, fluid balance, and pain (Mathisen & Wain, 1992).

Perioperative myocardial infarction is suggested by characteristic chest discomfort or electrocardiographic abnormalities. A 12-lead electrocardiogram and serial creatine kinase isoenzyme measurements are obtained to confirm the diagnosis. Appropriate anti-ischemia medications and supportive therapy are instituted.

PULMONARY EDEMA

Pulmonary edema can occur as a result of excessive perioperative intravenous hydration or because of underlying heart disease. It represents an imbalance in hydrostatic and oncotic fluid pressures, along with altered capillary wall permeability. Fluid moves into the interstitial tissue of the lungs, collapsing or flooding alveoli. Blood flowing through capillaries adjacent to nonventilated alveoli passes without an exchange of oxygen, thus impairing blood gas exchange (Pairolero & Payne, 1991).

Pulmonary edema typically occurs soon after mechanical ventilation is discontinued or 24 to 48 hours after the operation, when fluid administered intraoperatively and that has entered interstitial tissue (i.e., the "third space") returns to the vascular system (Goldman & Braunwald, 1992). It is manifested by tachypnea, anxiety, restlessness, and acute respiratory insufficiency. Treatment includes administration of diuretic agents to remove excess fluid and supplemental oxygen to enhance oxygenation. Intubation and mechanical ventilation with positive end-expiratory pressure may be necessary depending on the degree of associated respiratory failure.

INCISIONAL COMPLICATIONS

WOUND INFECTION

Wound infection is uncommon after thoracotomy because of the excellent blood supply to the thoracic cage and the immunologic competence of the pleural space (Douglas, 1992). Infections that do occur usually result from contamination during operation or develop in patients with risk factors for infection, such as diabetes, chronic corticosteroid therapy, an immunocompromised state, or obesity (Trastek et al., 1992). The most frequent causative organism for infection of surgical wounds is *Staphylococcus aureus* (Kaiser, 1990).

Incisional infections are most often superficial. They are manifested by incisional drainage and erythema, swelling, and tenderness of surrounding subcutaneous tissue. Fever and an elevated white blood cell count are other typical findings. Fluid expressed from the incision is cultured to identify the causative organism. Treatment consists of intravenous antibiotic therapy and local wound care. The subcutaneous layer of the infected segment of the incision is opened to allow adequate drainage. Necrotic tissue is debrided as necessary, and the wound is cleansed and redressed several times daily.

Rarely, deep wound infection occurs and causes *dehiscence*, or separation, of the entire wound. In extreme cases, the muscle and ribs may separate, leading to collapse of the underlying lung and acute respiratory insufficiency. Emergent operative exploration is necessary to debride nonviable tissue, irrigate the pleural cavity, and reclose the ribs, chest wall, and usually the skin (McLaughlin, 1991).

SECONDARY COMPLICATIONS OF THORACOTOMY INCISIONS

Occasionally, complications develop that are secondarily related to a surgical incision. Complications specifically associated with lateral thoracotomy incisions include (1) traction injury to the brachial plexus from overextension of the shoulder, (2) neurovascular injury at the elbow from inadequate padding of the elbow, (3) a "winged scapula" (abnormal protrusion of the scapula) from division of the long thoracic nerve or from excessive posterior retraction, and (4) numbness in the medial aspect of the upper arm and axilla from intercostobrachial nerve injury (Warren, 1989).

COMPLICATIONS OF PULMONARY RESECTION

PERSISTENT AIR SPACE

A *persistent air space* is a potential complication of pulmonary resection operations. When a large portion but not all of a lung is removed, the volume of remaining lung may be inadequate to completely fill the hemithorax and an air space remains. Persistent air spaces are unusual because of several compensatory mechanisms that help obliterate a residual space after lobectomy or bilobectomy. The remaining lobe or lobes overexpand, the diaphragm on the operative side moves up, the ipsilateral intercostal spaces narrow, and the mediastinum shifts toward the operative side (Joob & Hartz, 1994).

Postoperative interventions that help avoid a persistent air space include deep breathing exercises and other pulmonary hygiene measures that promote expansion of atelectatic segments. In some cases, endotracheal suctioning and serial bronchoscopy may be necessary to fully expand collapsed portions of lung. Maintaining suction to the pleural space also promotes full lung expansion. Apposition of the visceral and parietal pleura over as great an area as possible facilitates adherence between the two surfaces (Townsend & Westaby, 1989).

Occasionally, an air space persists despite these compensatory mechanisms and preventive interventions. Factors that contribute to a residual air space include a large or persistent air leak; a resection that includes two lobes on the right or that leaves only the basal segments of the lower lobe; pulmonary fibrosis; disease in the remaining lung that limits expansion; incomplete decortication; postoperative atelectasis; and a fixed mediastinum due to radiation or prior inflammation (Piccione & Faber, 1991). A persistent air space causes no clinical sequelae in most patients and gradually disappears over a period of months (Shields, 1994). However, the presence of a residual space is worrisome because of the potential for development of an empyema.

EMPYEMA

An *empyema* (i.e., an infection of the pleural space) is a potential complication of any thoracic operation but is most likely after pneumonectomy or when a residual air space remains after a partial lung resection. A prolonged air leak or bronchopleural fistula may also contribute to development of postoperative empyema (Alexander & Fetter, 1992). Empyemas are more common after pulmonary resection performed for inflammatory disease than after operations for tumor resection (Shields, 1994). The most frequent causative organisms are *Staphylococcus aureus* and *Pseudomonas aeruginosa* (Pairolero et al, 1990; Alexander & Fetter, 1992).

Signs of pleural space infection include fever, purulent chest tube drainage, elevated white blood cell count, and roentgenographic evidence of an air–fluid level. If empyema is suspected, fluid from the pleural space is cultured to identify the causative pathogen. The primary therapy for empyema is effective drainage of the infected space by chest tube thoracostomy. Organism-specific antimicrobial therapy is also instituted. As the infective process in the pleural space evolves, the inflammatory response fuses pleural margins around accumulated fluid, localizing the process into a contained pleural abscess (i.e., an empyema cavity) (Finkelmeier, 1986). Chronic drainage of the cavity with one or more chest tubes may be necessary to achieve its obliteration.

Once areas of pleural fusing around the cavity develop sufficiently to keep the lung adherent to the chest wall, the chest tube or tubes may be disconnected from the water seal drainage system. A chest roentgenogram is obtained to ensure that the lung remains expanded with the cavity open to air. If so, the chest tube(s) is severed 1 to 2 inches from the skin surface and sutured in place. Depending on the amount of drainage, a dressing or ostomy pouch is applied over the tube(s).

Empyema tubes are generally in place for several weeks or months. The size of the cavity may be evaluated intermittently by sinogram (i.e., the injection of a small amount of contrast material into the cavity followed by radiographic examination). As cavity size diminishes, the tube(s) is gradually advanced to prevent its erosion into the lung and to allow closure of the cavity. A tube remains in the cavity until the intrapleural space is nearly eradicated to prevent leaving a closed cavity that is likely to become reinfected. In the case of a very large cavity or if a drainage tube cannot be adequately secured, a portion of rib may be resected to create a larger opening. A larger tube can then be placed through the bed of the resected rib. Alternatively, an *Eloesser's flap* (i.e., an epithelial-lined drainage tract) may be surgically created.

Depending on the specific circumstances, a surgical procedure is sometimes necessary to facilitate eradication of an empyema cavity. In patients with empyema after partial lung resection, the inflammatory fibrin reaction around the cavity can compress and entrap lung tissue, preventing the lung from expanding to obliterate the cavity (Alexander & Fetter, 1992). If so, *decortication* (i.e., removal of the visceral pleura) may be necessary to allow the underlying lung to reexpand fully.

If the remaining lung is inadequate to fill the space or if parenchymal fibrosis prevents lung reexpansion, a vascularized *muscle flap* may be translocated to the empyema cavity to obliterate the cavity. The chest wall muscles (e.g., pectoralis major or latissimus dorsi) are generally used to create a muscle flap. All have a single dominant blood supply, and their proximity to the pulmonary hilus makes it possible for these muscles to be rotated and transposed to most intrathoracic locations (Pairolero et al., 1992). Alternatively, a *thoracoplasty* may be performed to reduce the volume of an empyema cavity and facilitate healing. A thoracoplasty consists of removal of the skeletal support of a portion of the chest wall. Empyema after pneumonectomy may be treated with a *Claggett procedure;* after the cavity is adequately drained and cultures are negative, it is filled with an antibiotic solution and the drainage window is surgically closed.

PROLONGED AIR LEAK AND BRONCHOPLEURAL FISTULA

Air leakage is almost always present after operations in which a portion of a lung is removed. Air leaks generally originate in areas where incomplete fissures were divided or from denuded parenchyma that has been separated from areas where it adhered to the undersurface of the chest wall. Air leaks typically cease after several days but uncommonly persist for more than a week.

Most prolonged air leaks represent inadequate or failed closure of distal bronchioles or alveolar spaces and are termed *bronchoalveolar-pleural fistulae* (Rice & Kirby, 1992). They are generally associated with incomplete lung reexpansion and a residual pleural space. Prolonged air leakage is treated with continued chest tube drainage. Suction is usually maintained until the lung is fully expanded. Once this occurs, the chest tube may be converted to water seal drainage without suction until the air leak ceases.

Less commonly, a *bronchopleural fistula,* or persistent air leak from a proximal bronchus into the pleural space, occurs after pulmonary resection. Two pathophysiologic concepts help explain failure of a bronchial anastomosis to heal properly. First, blood supply to the bronchus is variable and may be compromised during the operative dissection; second, the tubular cartilaginous structure of the bronchus causes it to have a normal tendency to spring open (Allen et al., 1992). Bronchopleural fistulae are more likely after pneumonectomy than after lesser pulmonary resections; most common is a bronchopleural fistula after right pneumonectomy (Shields, 1994).

Factors that increase the risk for development of a bronchopleural fistula include tuberculosis or other pulmonary infection; nutritional depletion; intraoperative technical problems such as devascularization, contamination, improper closure, or inadequate length of the remaining bronchial stump; preoperative radiation; and trauma to the bronchial anastomosis from postoperative endotracheal suctioning (Kirsch et al., 1975). Careful intraoperative bronchial dissection, meticulous closure, and coverage of the bronchial stump with pericardium, pericardial fat, pleura, or intercostal muscle are surgical techniques that lessen the likelihood of bronchopleural fistula development (Bojar et al., 1989b).

An early bronchopleural fistula (within the first or second postoperative day) generally represents a technical problem with the surgical closure of the remaining bronchial segment; late bronchopleural fistula (8 to 10 days after operation) can occur due to (1) failed bronchial healing secondary to a lack of viable tissue coverage overlying the anastomotic site or (2) rupture of the anastomosis caused by infection of the pleural space (Shields, 1994). The incidence of bronchopleural fistula has decreased in recent years, but associated mortality remains high (Allen et al., 1992).

A bronchopleural fistula is manifested by a persistent, large air leak. If the rate of air leakage exceeds that which can be evacuated through the chest tubes, the patient develops *subcutaneous emphysema* as air tracks through subcutaneous tissue planes in the neck, shoulders, and chest. In severe cases, subcutaneous emphysema may extend into the arms, abdomen, and groins. The presence of subcutaneous em-

physema indicates a need to better evacuate pleural air, either by increasing the amount of suction to existing chest tubes or by placing an additional tube. No specific treatment is required for subcutaneous emphysema itself, which gradually dissipates over the course of several days.

Patients who have undergone pneumonectomy generally do not have a chest tube in place after surgery. Consequently, the development of a bronchopleural fistula causes a decrease in the postpneumonectomy space fluid level and progressive subcutaneous emphysema. The patient typically expectorates moderate or large amounts of gelatinous, serosanguineous material that has accumulated in the postpneumonectomy space during the days after the operation. The immediate consequence of a postpneumonectomy bronchopleural communication may be flooding of the remaining lung with fluid expectorated from the operative hemithorax. The patient is positioned with the operative side down, and emergent chest tube thoracostomy is performed. Intubation and mechanical ventilation may also be necessary. An associated empyema often develops since the postpneumonectomy space provides an excellent medium for growth of pathogenic organisms introduced into the space through the fistula.

Management of bronchopleural fistula is complex and depends on timing of fistula development, degree of infection in the pleural space, and presence of remaining pulmonary parenchyma (i.e., whether bronchopleural fistula occurs after pneumonectomy or lobectomy). Despite these variables, therapy is guided by three basic principles: (1) adequate pleural drainage, (2) closure of the fistula, and (3) obliteration of the residual pleural space (Allen et al., 1992).

Bronchopleural fistulae sometimes heal spontaneously, requiring only chest tube drainage of the pleural space. Surgical intervention may be necessary for a large or persistent fistula. The bronchial stump is closed and covered with transposed muscle, omentum, or pericardial fat. A concomitant surgical procedure, such as a chest wall muscle flap or thoracoplasty, may be necessary to obliterate an associated empyema cavity.

OTHER COMPLICATIONS

Patients who have undergone pneumonectomy may develop *postpneumonectomy pulmonary edema*. It is usually related to overhydration but can occur even with restricted perioperative fluid administration. Because one lung is absent, the entire cardiac output from the right side of the heart travels through the pulmonary vasculature of the remaining lung only. Pulmonary edema develops when fluid entering the peribronchial spaces exceeds the capacity of the lymphatic channels to drain the fluid. Pulmonary compliance decreases, increasing the work of respiration. Progressive dyspnea and hypoxemia develop as alveoli fill with fluid. If not detected and treated early, the condition is usually fatal. Treatment includes morphine, diuretics, and ventilatory support (Shields, 1994).

Cardiac herniation is mechanical displacement and entrapment of the heart through an iatrogenic defect in the pericardium. The pericardial defect is created during pulmonary resection procedures that necessitate opening the pericardial sac to ligate pulmonary hilar blood vessels. Cardiac herniation is a rare complication, most commonly associated with intrapericardial pneumonectomy (Piccione & Faber, 1991). It produces acute hemodynamic instability because mechanical compression of the great vessels decreases cardiac filling and cardiac output. If diagnosed, the patient is immediately positioned on the side opposite the pneumonectomy in an attempt to return the heart to the pericardial sac and relieve the cardiac malposition (Mathisen & Wain, 1992). Emergent surgical reexploration is then performed to reduce the herniation and repair the defect in the pericardium with a patch graft.

A rare complication of lobectomy is *lobar torsion,* or rotation of a remaining lobe on its bronchovascular pedicle. Lobar torsion may develop secondary to excessive intraoperative traction or may occur spontaneously. The diagnosis is suggested by radiographic findings and is confirmed during bronchoscopy by the appearance of the twisted lobar bronchus (Wagner & Nesbitt, 1992). Surgical exploration is performed to relieve the torsion and, if necessary, resect the affected lobe.

If lobar torsion is unrecognized, the lobar artery or vein may be injured, leading to *lobar infarction* and *gangrene.* Clinical manifestations of lobar gangrene include a persistent air leak, fever, and foul-smelling sputum (Bojar et al., 1989b). Surgical reexploration is performed to resect the necrotic lung tissue.

COMPLICATIONS OF ESOPHAGEAL RESECTION

ANASTOMOTIC LEAK

Operations in which part or all of the esophagus must be removed necessitate replacement of the resected esophageal segment with stomach or, less commonly, colon or small intestine. Depending on the visceral substitute chosen, the surgical procedure requires either one or three anastomoses to restore continuity to the gastrointestinal tract.

Esophagectomy with esophagogastrostomy is the most commonly performed esophageal resection operation. It includes repositioning of the stomach in the thorax to replace the resected esophagus. Because the stomach can be elongated to reach the upper chest without disrupting its distal continuity with the duodenum, only a single visceral anastomosis is necessary. This anastomosis, between the proximal stomach and the esophageal remnant, may be either in the mediastinum or neck. When a segment of colon is used for esophageal replacement (*esophagectomy with colon interposition*), it must be completely removed from its normal anatomic position to be translocated to the thorax. Consequently, three anastomoses are required to perform the procedure: (1) colon to proximal esophagus, (2) colon to stomach, and (3) reanastomosis of the two remaining bowel segments from which the colon was harvested.

The principal complication specifically related to esophageal resection is disruption of the esophageal anastomosis with leakage of nonsterile esophageal contents into the surrounding tissues. Esophageal anastomoses are particularly susceptible to disruption because, in contrast to other viscera, the esophageal wall has no serosal layer but consists only of mucosa and submucosa. In addition, arterial blood supply is variable and can be segmental; if blood flow to an esophageal anastomosis is compromised, ischemic necrosis can result (Wolfe & Sebastian, 1992). Other factors that increase the risk of anastomotic disruption include preoperative irradiation, residual tumor at the anastomotic site, poor nutritional status, and distal blockage (gastric outlet obstruction). Some authors report a higher incidence of anastomotic leaks when a cervical anastomosis is performed (Daniel et al., 1992; Huang, 1994). Others have noted a similar incidence for cervical and mediastinal anastomoses (Lam et al., 1992).

Because of the potential for postoperative anastomotic disruption, nasogastric suction is maintained and oral nourishment withheld for 5 to 7 days after esophageal resection. Nutrition is provided enterally by jejunostomy or by intravenous alimentation. To protect integrity of the anastomosis, the nasogastric tube is usually not manipulated and, if a proximal anastomosis is present, endotracheal suctioning is avoided. Before removing the nasogastric tube and instituting oral nourishment, a contrast esophagogram is performed to detect esophageal disruption and leakage. Also, a pleural chest tube is left in place until integrity of the anastomosis is demonstrated by the postoperative contrast study. After confirmation of esophageal integrity, a diet is resumed slowly, beginning with liquids and a mechanical soft diet before advancing to regular foods.

If anastomotic disruption does occur, nonsterile digestive fluids and bacteria leak into the periesophageal spaces, causing diffuse cellulitis and localized or extensive suppuration (Ellis, 1990). Morbidity and mortality from an anastomotic leak in the neck are less than with a thoracic anastomotic leak. Cervical anastomotic leaks may not produce associated symptoms. The localized infection can often be managed with local drainage, nasogastric suction, maintenance of an NPO status, and organism-specific antibiotics.

Infection in the thorax is more difficult to manage because of resultant mediastinitis. Sepsis, chest pain, and subcutaneous emphysema are typical manifestations. Surgical exploration of the chest is generally necessary to establish adequate drainage of the infection. Death occurs in as many as 50% of patients who develop disruption of an intrathoracic esophageal anastomosis (Shields, 1989).

CHYLOTHORAX

Chylothorax is the accumulation of fat-rich lymphatic fluid in the pleural space as a result of disruption of the thoracic duct or one of its branches. The thoracic duct is the largest lymphatic channel in the body (Wolfe & Sebastian, 1992) (Fig. 43-1). Because its primary function is the transport of digestive fat from the liver and intestinal tract to the venous system, lymphatic fluid contained in the thoracic duct is rich in fat and protein (Miller, 1994). Injury to the thoracic duct may occur during almost any thoracic operation, but proximity of the duct to the esophagus makes the complication more common after procedures that necessitate mobilization of the esophagus.

Chylothorax is manifested by drainage of large amounts of milky fluid through the chest tubes after resumption of oral nourishment in the postoperative

period. The primary consequence of the complication is nutritional depletion, particularly hypoproteinemia. Chylothorax is of most concern in patients with underlying nutritional depletion due to preoperative esophageal obstruction (Orringer, 1991).

Treatment consists of reducing chyle production by dietary restriction of long-chain fatty acids. Nourishment is provided in the form of a clear liquid or low-residue, elemental diet or intravenous hyperalimentation. Chest tube drainage is maintained until drainage is less than 100 mL/d. Chylothorax usually resolves with dietary fat restriction and chest tube drainage. If it persists, operative ligation of the disrupted lymphatic channel is performed.

POSTOPERATIVE DYSPHAGIA

Esophageal resection may be associated with *postoperative dysphagia*, resulting from the loss of normal peristaltic function of the esophagus. Neither stomach nor colon functions as effectively in the chest as does the native esophagus in transporting food. Consequently, patients may experience discomforting symptoms associated with eating, such as a sensation of early fullness, postprandial regurgitation, or a dumping syndrome, consisting of postprandial sweating, diarrhea, or both (Morton et al., 1991; Collard et al., 1992). Modifications in the amount and type of food ingested may be required to avoid dysphagia and other unpleasant symptoms. The patient is instructed to eat smaller meals, chew food thoroughly, and maintain an upright position during and after meals. These modifications also decrease the likelihood of postoperative aspiration.

Postoperative dysphagia sometimes results from the development of an *esophageal stricture* at the anastomotic site. Factors contributing to stricture formation include anastomotic leakage, tumor recurrence, tension on the suture line, and esophagitis (Bojar et al., 1989b). Strictures are treated with bougienage (i.e., mechanical dilatation) of the anastomosis. It may be necessary to perform dilatation several times or chronically to relieve symptoms.

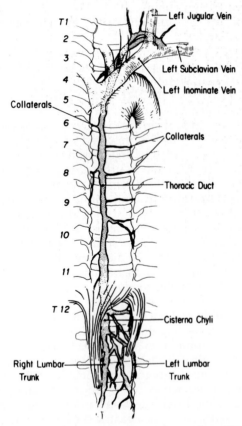

FIGURE 43-1. The most common course and position of the thoracic duct. (DeMeester TR, Lafontaine E, 1990: The pleura. In Sabiston DC Jr, Spencer FC [eds]: Surgery of the Chest, ed. 5, p. 455. Philadelphia, WB Saunders)

REFERENCES

Alexander JC, Fetter JE, 1992: Postresectional empyema and bronchopleural fistula. In Wolfe WG (ed): Complications in Thoracic Surgery. St. Louis, Mosby–Year Book

Allen MS, Deschamps C, Trastek VF, Pairolero PC, 1992: Bronchopleural fistula. Chest Surg Clin North Am 2:823

Bojar RM, Murphy RE, Payne DD, Diehl JT, 1989a: Postoperative care. In Manual of Perioperative Care in Cardiac and Thoracic Surgery. Boston, Blackwell Scientific Publications

Bojar RM, Murphy RE, Payne DD, Diehl JT, 1989b: Management of postoperative complications. In Manual of Perioperative Care in Cardiac and Thoracic Surgery. Boston, Blackwell Scientific Publications

Collard JM, Otte JB, Reynaert M, Kestens PJ, 1992: Quality of life three years or more after esophagectomy for cancer. J Thorac Cardiovasc Surg 104:391

Daniel TM, Fleisher KJ, Flanagan TL, et al., 1992: Transhiatal esophagectomy: A safe alternative for selected patients. Ann Thorac Surg 54:686

Douglas JM, 1992: Complications related to patient positioning, thoracic incisions, and chest tube placement. In Wolfe WG (ed): Complications in Thoracic Surgery. St. Louis, Mosby–Year Book

Elefteriades JA, Geha AS, 1985: Problems following noncardiac thoracic surgery. In House Officer Guide to ICU Care: The Cardiothoracic Surgical Patient. Gaithersburg, MD, Aspen Publishers

Ellis FH Jr, 1990: Disorders of the esophagus in the adult. In Sabiston DC Jr, Spencer FC (eds): Surgery of the Chest, ed. 5. Philadelphia, WB Saunders

Finkelmeier BA, 1986: Difficult problems in postoperative management. Crit Care Q 9:3

Goldman L, Braunwald E, 1992: General anesthesia and noncardiac surgery in patients with heart disease. In Braunwald E (ed): Heart Disease: A Textbook of Cardiovascular Medicine, ed. 4. Philadelphia, WB Saunders

Hawthorne MH, 1992: Recognition of thoracic surgical complications: A nursing perspective. In Wolfe WG (ed): Complications in Thoracic Surgery. St. Louis, Mosby–Year Book

Huang GJ, 1994: Replacement of the esophagus with the stomach. In Shields TW (ed): General Thoracic Surgery, ed. 4. Baltimore, Williams & Wilkins

Joob AW, Hartz RS, 1994: General principles of postoperative care. In Shields TW (ed): General Thoracic Surgery, ed. 4. Baltimore, Williams & Wilkins

Kaiser AB, 1990: Use of antibiotics in cardiac and thoracic surgery. In Sabiston DC Jr, Spencer FC (eds): Surgery of the Chest, ed. 5. Philadelphia, WB Saunders

Kirsch M, Rotman H, Behrendt D, et al., 1975: Complications of pulmonary resection. Ann Thorac Surg 20:215

Lam TC, Fok M, Cheng SW, Wong J, 1992: Anastomotic complications after esophagectomy for cancer. J Thorac Cardiovasc Surg 104:395

Mathisen DJ, Wain JC Jr, 1992: Cardiac complications following pulmonary resection. Chest Surg Clin North Am 2:793

McLaughlin JS, 1991: Positional and incisional complications of thoracic surgery. In Waldhausen JA, Orringer MB (eds): Complications in Cardiothoracic Surgery. St. Louis, Mosby–Year Book

Miller JI, 1994: Chylothorax. In Shields TW (ed): General Thoracic Surgery, ed. 4. Baltimore, Williams & Wilkins

Morton KA, Karwande SV, Davis RK, et al., 1991: Gastric emptying after gastric interposition for cancer of the esophagus or hypopharynx. Ann Thorac Surg 51:759

Nelson ME, Moran JF, 1992: Post-thoracotomy pneumonia. In Wolfe WG (ed): Complications in Thoracic Surgery. St. Louis, Mosby–Year Book

Orringer MB, 1991: Complications of esophageal resection and reconstruction. In Waldhausen JA, Orringer MB (eds): Complications in Cardiothoracic Surgery. St. Louis, Mosby–Year Book

Pairolero PC, Arnold PG, Trastek VF, et al., 1990: Postpneumonectomy empyema. J Thorac Cardiovasc Surg 99:958

Pairolero PC, Deschamps C, Allen MS, Trastek VF, 1992: Postoperative empyema. Chest Surg Clin North Am 2:813

Pairolero PC, Payne WS, 1991: Postoperative care and complications in thoracic surgery. In Baue AE, Geha AS, Hammond GL, et al. (eds): Glenn's Thoracic and Cardiovascular Surgery, ed. 5. Norwalk, CT, Appleton & Lange

Piccione W Jr, Faber LP, 1991: Management of complications related to pulmonary resection. In Waldhausen JA, Orringer MB (eds): Complications in Cardiothoracic Surgery. St. Louis, Mosby–Year Book

Reilly JJ, Mentzer SJ, Sugarbaker DJ, 1993: Preoperative assessment of patients undergoing pulmonary resection. Chest 103:342S

Rice TW, Kirby TJ, 1992: Prolonged air leak. Chest Surg Clin North Am 2:803

Shields TW, 1994: General features and complications of pulmonary resections. In Shields TW (ed): General Thoracic Surgery, ed. 4. Baltimore, Williams & Wilkins

Shields TW, 1989: Resection of the esophagus. In Shields TW (ed): General Thoracic Surgery, ed. 3. Philadelphia, Lea & Febiger

Shields TW, 1993: Surgical therapy for carcinoma of the lung. Clin Chest Med 14:121

Todd TR, 1992: The adult respiratory distress syndrome. Chest Surg Clin North Am 2:769

Todd TR, 1994: Ventilatory support of postoperative surgical patients. In Shields TW (ed): General Thoracic Surgery, ed. 4. Baltimore, Williams & Wilkins

Townsend ER, Westaby S, 1989: Space problems during and after lung resection. In Grillo HC, Austen WG, Wilkins EW, et al. (eds): Current Therapy in Cardiothoracic Surgery. Toronto, BC Decker

Trastek VF, Pairolero PC, Allen MS, Deschamps C, 1992: Unusual complications of pulmonary resection. Chest Surg Clin North Am 2:853

Wagner RB, Nesbitt JC, 1992: Pulmonary torsion and gangrene. Chest Surg Clin North Am 2:839

Warren WH, 1989: Lateral thoracotomy: Technique, indications, and complications. In Grillo HC, Austen WG, Wilkins EW, et al. (eds): Current Therapy in Cardiothoracic Surgery. Toronto, BC Decker

Wolfe WG, Sebastian MW, 1992: Complications following esophagectomy and esophagogastrectomy. In Wolfe WG (ed): Complications in Thoracic Surgery. St. Louis, Mosby–Year Book

44

POSTOPERATIVE CHEST ROENTGENOGRAM INTERPRETATION

THE PORTABLE CHEST ROENTGENOGRAM
  Technique and Patient Positioning
  Guidelines for Review
INTRATHORACIC CATHETERS, TUBES,
  AND DEVICES
TYPICAL POSTOPERATIVE ALTERATIONS
  Thoracic Operations
  Cardiac Operations

COMMON ABNORMALITIES
  Densities in the Pulmonary Parenchyma
  Fluid Collections
  Air Collections

The chest roentgenogram is an invaluable diagnostic tool in the daily care of cardiothoracic surgical patients. A preoperative chest roentgenogram is obtained shortly before every elective cardiac or thoracic operation to detect abnormalities that might alter the planned surgical therapy. This preoperative film also provides a baseline for comparison with postoperative films. During the postoperative period, chest roentgenograms are typically obtained (1) immediately after intrathoracic operations, (2) daily while the patient is critically ill, (3) after placement of intrathoracic catheters or tubes, (4) to detect pneumothorax after chest tube removal, (5) to provide radiologic evaluation of the patient's readiness for discharge from the hospital, and (6) if there is an unexplained deterioration in the patient's cardiopulmonary status.

Postoperative chest roentgenograms are often available for review by nurses who work in cardiothoracic surgical recovery or intensive care units. The nurse at the bedside may be the first to view a chest roentgenogram that demonstrates new clinical information. A basic knowledge of normal radiographic structures, position of intrathoracic catheters and tubes, and common postoperative abnormalities provides nurses in these settings with additional information that can enhance patient management. With appropriate physician consultation, the nurse can facilitate timely modifications in therapy based on radiographic findings. The ability to correlate radiographic findings with the patient's clinical status also increases the nurse's understanding of intrathoracic anatomy and pathophysiology. This chapter provides general information about portable roentgenograms and guidelines for recognizing normal postoperative alterations and common intrathoracic abnormalities of acute clinical significance.

THE PORTABLE CHEST ROENTGENOGRAM

TECHNIQUE AND PATIENT POSITIONING

Most chest roentgenograms available for viewing by nurses are obtained at the patient's bedside using portable equipment. An anteroposterior (AP) projection is used. That is, the x-ray tube is positioned in front of the patient's chest and the film cassette behind the patient's back. The x-ray beam passes through the patient from front to back. An AP projection is opposite that used for standard posteroanterior (PA) chest roentgenograms taken in a radiology department in which the x-ray beam passes through the patient from back to front.

A portable chest roentgenogram is of lesser quality than one obtained using equipment available in a radiology department. Also, AP and PA roentgenograms in the same patient are not comparable since an AP technique enlarges the shadow of the anteriorly positioned heart (Squire & Novelline, 1988a). Despite these limitations, a portable AP chest film provides a useful radiographic view of the thorax for clinical decision-making in patients too ill to be transported away from the nursing unit.

To provide the maximal amount of diagnostic information from a portable roentgenogram, consistent attention to technique and patient position is essential since it significantly influences the appearance of intrathoracic structures. Portable roentgenograms in hemodynamically stable patients are taken with the patient sitting fully upright in the bed. The diaphragms are lower when the patient is upright and the lungs are more fully expanded than when the patient is in a supine position and the diaphragms are pushed upward by abdominal viscera (Matthay & Sostman, 1990). Ideally, the patient's chest is perfectly perpendicular to the x-ray tube; if not, a lordotic projection is obtained in which the heart appears larger and indistinct and the height of the lung fields is decreased (Huseby, 1989). It may not be possible to position a patient whose condition is unstable in an upright position, so the roentgenogram is obtained with the patient supine.

Chest roentgenograms are generally taken at the end of a full inspiration to most clearly demonstrate intrathoracic structures, particularly the lungs. If the inspiratory effort is not good, the elevated diaphragms may cause a transverse appearance of the heart and give the pulmonary vasculature a falsely engorged appearance. Rotation of the patient can also distort the appearance of the heart and hilar areas and cause the lung fields to appear different in density.

GUIDELINES FOR REVIEW

A roentgenogram of the adult chest displays the heart, lungs, bony thorax, and soft tissues of the chest wall. The various structures are reviewed in a sequential fashion, examining each for abnormalities. The observed radiographic findings must be correlated with clinical information about the patient. For example, when comparing a roentgenogram obtained after extubation with a prior film obtained during mechanical ventilation, the lessened quantity of air in the lungs may make the roentgenogram look worse while the patient is actually physiologically better (Milne, 1980).

The bones, soft tissue, heart and great vessels, and lungs all produce different radiographic densities (Fig. 44-1). Bone, which is densest, creates the lightest, or most radiodense, shadow; lung, which is largely air, appears lucent, or black (Huseby, 1989). Examination of *thoracic bony structures* (ribs, sternum, vertebrae, clavicles, and scapulae) is not particularly relevant for cardiothoracic surgical nurses. Except in victims of chest trauma, it is unusual to detect an abnormality of acute clinical significance. The *soft tissues*, which create a radiodense shadow surrounding the bony thorax, are also generally normal. The most common soft tissue abnormality, subcutaneous emphysema, occurs infrequently and is described later in the chapter.

The *mediastinal shadow* is the radiodense area between the right and left lung fields. The *heart* and *great vessels* are the primary structures that create the mediastinal shadow. They are responsible for all of the profiles that bulge to the right and left of the spine (Squire & Novelline, 1988b). The right heart border, which extends slightly to the right of the thoracic spine, is formed predominantly by the right atrium. The left heart border comprises the aortic arch, pulmonary artery, left atrial appendage, and left ventricle. The majority of the cardiac mass lies in the left hemithorax.

The *trachea* can usually be seen in the mediastinal shadow as an air-filled structure located slightly to the right of the midline. The *main bronchi* are somewhat smaller in diameter than the trachea; the right mainstem bronchus continues downward from the trachea more vertically than the left in adults and divides into two main branches (Juhl, 1993). The shadows of other mediastinal structures, such as the esophagus, thymus, and lymph nodes, merge with one another and are superimposed upon the shadows of the spine, heart, and sternum (Squire & Novelline, 1988b).

Mediastinal width cannot be accurately assessed on AP roentgenograms because of mediastinal widening that occurs secondary to technique. On a PA roentgenogram, the simplest method of estimating mediastinal width is to determine the *cardiothoracic ratio* (i.e., the width of the cardiac silhouette at its widest diameter near the diaphragm as compared with the width of the chest) (Squire & Novelline, 1988c). The normal cardiac silhouette on a PA roentgenogram is less than or equal to one half of the width of the thoracic cavity.

Mediastinal shift (i.e., shifting of the trachea and other midline structures) is an important radiologic finding that can be caused by a variety of pathologic conditions. For example, an abnormality associated with volume loss, such as atelectasis, produces shifting of midline structures toward the affected side of the thorax. Conversely, space-occupying abnormali-

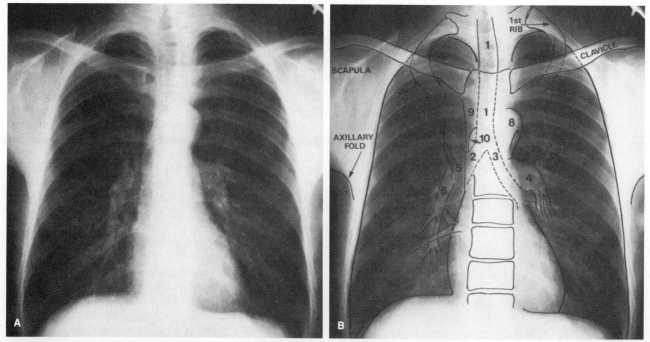

FIGURE 44-1. **(A)** Normal chest roentgenogram in posteroanterior projection. **(B)** Same radiograph with normal anatomic structures numbered or labeled: *1*, trachea; *2*, right main bronchus, *3*, left main bronchus; *4*, left pulmonary artery; *5*, right upper lobe pulmonary vein; *6*, right interlobar artery; *7*, right lower and middle lobe vein; *8*, aortic knob; and *9*, superior vena cava. (Fraser RG, Pare JAP, Pare PD, et al., 1988: The normal chest. In Diagnosis of Diseases of the Chest, ed. 3, p. 287. Philadelphia, WB Saunders)

ties (e.g., pneumothorax or pleural effusion) may shift the trachea and mediastinal shadow away from the affected side.

The *lung fields* occupy most of the right and left hemithorax. The lungs are examined primarily for areas of abnormally increased density or lucency. The normally expanded lungs appear predominately translucent, or black. Fine white linear shadows, known as *lung markings*, are visible throughout the lung fields and represent pulmonary blood vessels. These pulmonary vascular markings normally appear primarily in the bases with scant vascular markings in the upper lung fields (Sider, 1986). Lung markings should be visible extending to all edges of the thorax.

The heaviest and widest lung markings on either side of the heart shadow are created by the major pulmonary arteries and veins (Squire & Novelline, 1988d). These large pulmonary arteries and veins, and to a lesser extent nearby bronchi, form the complex shadow on either side of the heart known as the *pulmonary hilum* (Westra, 1990). The left hilum is higher in position than the right.

Interlobar fissures, created by the visceral pleura that lines each lobe, are usually not apparent on an AP roentgenogram unless fluid has collected within the fissure or a lobe is collapsed and therefore opacified (Freundlich & Bragg, 1992a). The *diaphragms* ap-

pear on the roentgenogram as smooth, dome-shaped structures that are in sharp contrast to the radiolucent lungs above (Juhl, 1993). The junction of the diaphragm and chest wall on either side of the thorax is known as the *costophrenic angle* or *sulcus* and should appear as a sharply defined angle.

INTRATHORACIC CATHETERS, TUBES, AND DEVICES

Postoperative cardiothoracic surgical patients typically have several intrathoracic catheters and tubes; each plays an important role in facilitating recovery from the operation. Radiopaque markings make these catheters and tubes visible on the chest roentgenogram and allow confirmation of proper positioning (Fig. 44-2). In addition, implanted prosthetic devices, such as cardiac valves or pacemakers, may also be identifiable on the postoperative roentgenogram.

An *endotracheal tube* is identified by a radiopaque line at the distal end of the tube, which should appear in the midtrachea 2 to 5 cm above the carina. The carina is most accurately located on the roentgenogram by following the inferior wall of the left mainstem bronchus medially until it joins the right mainstem bronchus (Goodman, 1983a). If the distal end of

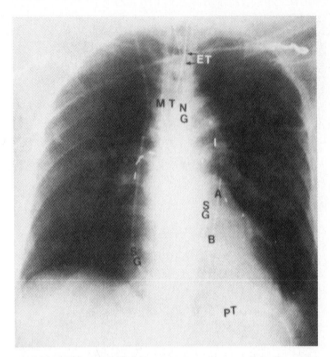

FIGURE 44-2. Portable chest roentgenogram taken after coronary artery bypass operation demonstrating position of endotracheal tube (*ET*), mediastinal chest tube (*MT*), nasogastric tube (*NG*), pulmonary artery catheter (*SG*), intra-aortic balloon catheter (*A-B*), and pericardial chest tube (*PT*). (Sider L, 1986: Interpretation of the postoperative chest radiograph. Crit Care Q 9:73)

an endotracheal tube is too high, accidental extubation is more likely. If the tube is positioned so that the end is distal to the carina, extending into the right mainstem bronchus, the left lung or right upper lobe is not ventilated and becomes atelectatic.

A *pulmonary artery catheter* can be traced on the roentgenogram through the superior vena cava, right atrium, and right ventricle. The tip of the catheter, positioned in a branch of the right or left main pulmonary artery, is apparent overlying the lung shadow on that side. If the tip is coiled in the right ventricle, pulmonary artery pressures cannot be measured and the patient may develop ventricular arrhythmias from mechanical irritation of the ventricle. If the tip is positioned too far peripherally in one of the pulmonary artery branches, it can totally occlude the vessel, leading to pulmonary ischemia or infarction. A *central venous catheter* is generally positioned so that the catheter tip is in the right atrium or superior vena cava. It should appear on the roentgenogram on the right side of the mediastinal shadow approximately halfway down the right heart border.

Temporary pacing leads, usually placed on the atrial and ventricular epicardium during cardiac operations, appear as thin coiled wires superimposed over the heart shadow. An *intra-aortic balloon catheter* appears on the roentgenogram as a radiodense line to the left of the spine (Sider, 1986). The tip of the balloon catheter, which is positioned just distal to the left subclavian artery, should appear below the aortic knob. A *nasogastric tube* is identified by the radiodense marking demonstrating the tip and side hole of the tube below the diaphragm and within or past the gastric lumen (Umali & Smith, 1991).

A *mediastinal chest tube* is identified by a radiodense line superimposed on the mediastinal shadow. A tube placed in the anterior mediastinum is visible parallel to the sternum; a posterior tube lies between the inferior heart border and diaphragm (Goodman, 1980). A *pleural chest tube* placed to evacuate pneumothorax is positioned so that its drainage holes lie between the apex of the lung and the anterior chest wall. A pleural tube placed to drain fluid is positioned inferiorly and posteriorly in the pleural space. All drainage holes should be positioned within the pleural cavity (Munnell, 1991). The last, or most proximal, side hole is identified on the chest roentgenogram by a short interruption in the radiodense line on the chest tube.

Implanted *cardiac valve prostheses* may or may not be visible on the chest roentgenogram, depending on the specific prosthesis. In most instances, the orientation of a radiodense valvular prosthesis reveals its position within the heart. The intracardiac position of cardiac valve prostheses can also be recognized by drawing an imaginary line from the right cardiophrenic border to the upper third of the left heart border (Sider, 1986). Prostheses implanted to replace atrioventricular (mitral or tricuspid) valves appear below this line, and those that replace semilunar (aortic) valves are visible above the line (Fig. 44-3).

A *permanent pacemaker* and *pacing leads* are easily visualized on a chest roentgenogram. A permanent pacemaker connected to transvenous leads is visible superimposed over the right or left upper lung field. A transvenous ventricular lead can be traced through the right side of the heart to its tip at the apex of the right ventricle, and an atrial lead appears superimposed on the right atrial shadow (Fig. 44-4). Permanent epicardial pacing leads are occasionally used; an epicardial lead attached to the right atrium appears at the edge of the right heart border, a right ventricular lead appears superimposed over the heart shadow, and a left ventricular lead appears at the edge of the left heart border. A pacemaker connected to epicardial leads is generally visible in the subcutaneous tissue of the upper abdomen. Infrequently, a pacemaker connected to epicardial leads is positioned in the subcutaneous tissue of the upper chest.

TYPICAL POSTOPERATIVE ALTERATIONS

THORACIC OPERATIONS

Patients who have undergone *thoracotomy* usually have two pleural chest tubes, one directed toward the apex of the lung and one toward the base (Fig. 44-5).

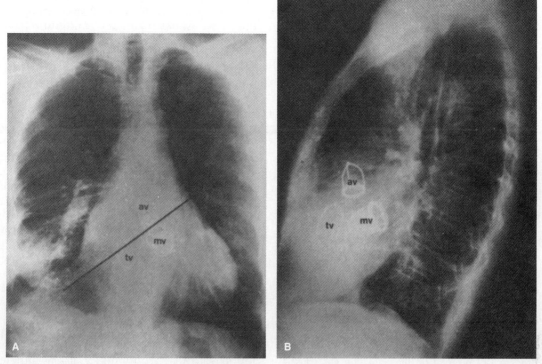

FIGURE 44-3. **(A)** Frontal roentgenogram showing location of implanted cardiac valve prostheses. An imaginary line can be drawn from the right cardiophrenic angle to the left upper heart border. The mitral valve (*mv*) and tricuspid valve (*tv*) prostheses are below this line; the aortic valve (*av*) prosthesis is above the line. **(B)** Appearance of the three valvular prostheses on a lateral roentgenogram. The mitral valve lies posterior to the tricuspid valve; the aortic valve is superior to both. (Sider L, 1986: Interpretation of the postoperative chest radiograph. Crit Care Q 9:76)

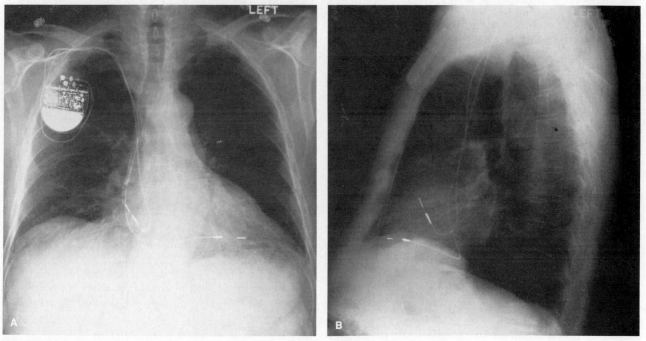

FIGURE 44-4. Posteroanterior **(A)** and lateral **(B)** chest roentgenograms illustrating the pulse generator and atrial and ventricular leads of a dual-chamber, transvenous permanent pacemaker. (Courtesy of Arthur Palmer, M.D.)

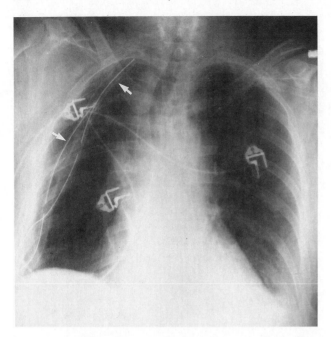

FIGURE 44-5. Portable chest roentgenogram obtained in early postoperative hours after right upper lobectomy. Two chest tubes have been positioned in the right pleural space (*arrows*). The loss of one lobe on the right side has caused tracheal deviation and narrowing of right-sided intercostal spaces. (Courtesy of Axel W. Joob, M.D.)

An endotracheal tube may also be present during the early postoperative hours. Areas where ribs have been surgically divided or resected are often apparent in the rib cage of the operative hemithorax. After *partial lung resection* (i.e., wedge resection, segmentectomy, or lobectomy) the chest roentgenogram ideally demonstrates full lung expansion on the operative side and minimal or no pleural fluid accumulation. Although small air leaks are typically present after pulmonary resection, there may be no radiographic evidence of pneumothorax because the chest drainage system usually prevents air accumulation in the pleural space. Often, a row of metallic staples, used to seal lung tissue that has been incised, is visible in the area of pulmonary resection.

After wedge resection or segmentectomy, an infiltrate representing hemorrhage, contusion, or atelectasis may be apparent in the involved lobe. After lobectomy, the remaining lobe or lobes overexpands to fill the space left by the resected lobe. The roentgenogram may demonstrate other compensatory changes as well that facilitate expansion of remaining lung to fill the operative hemithorax, including shifting of the mediastinum toward the operative side, narrowing of ipsilateral intercostal spaces, and elevation of the ipsilateral hemidiaphragm (Joob & Hartz, 1994) (Fig. 44-6). A small air space sometimes remains at the top of the operative hemithorax.

A chest roentgenogram in the early hours after *pneumonectomy* demonstrates a vacant hemithorax with little or no fluid, a fully expanded contralateral lung, and an approximately midline trachea (Goodman, 1983b). Often, no chest tube is in place or a clamped tube may be positioned in the empty pleural space. During the first several days after pneumonectomy, the roentgenogram provides an important means of assessing mediastinal position. Mediastinal shift toward either the operated or unoperated side may occur (Elefteriades & Geha, 1985). Gradual mediastinal shift toward the nonoperative side may indicate either atelectasis of the remaining lung or fluid accumulation in the operative hemithorax faster than air in the space can be resorbed (Goodman, 1980). Conversely, if air is resorbed more quickly than fluid is secreted into the empty space, the mediastinum may shift toward the operative side. Normally, the vacant hemithorax gradually fills with fluid over weeks or months until the pneumonectomy space is completely opacified by fluid or only a small air space at the top of the hemithorax remains (Fig. 44-7).

CARDIAC OPERATIONS

After *cardiac operations*, patients typically have an endotracheal tube, a pulmonary artery catheter, a cen-

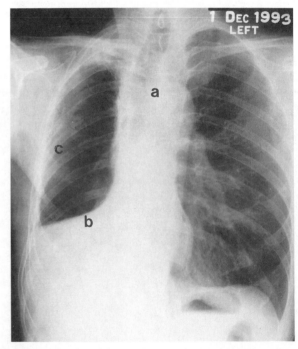

FIGURE 44-6. Posteroanterior roentgenogram after lobectomy of the right middle and lower lobes. Compensatory changes that facilitate expansion of the remaining upper lobe to fill the space include mediastinal shift (a) toward the operative hemithorax (note deviation of trachea to the right), elevation of right diaphragm (b), and narrowing of intercostal spaces on the right side (c). (Courtesy of Robert M. Vanecko, M.D.)

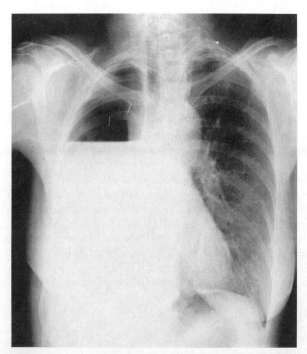

FIGURE 44-7. Posteroanterior roentgenogram obtained 1 week after right pneumonectomy demonstrates typical fluid accumulation in operative hemithorax. A subsequent roentgenogram several months later revealed further fluid accumulation with only a small residual air space at the top of the hemithorax. (Courtesy of Robert M. Vanecko, M.D.)

tral venous catheter, two mediastinal chest tubes, epicardial pacing wires, and a nasogastric tube. In patients with perioperative low cardiac output, an intraaortic balloon catheter may have been placed. A pleural chest tube may be present if one of the pleural spaces was opened. Rib fractures, particularly of the first or second rib, sometimes occur during median sternotomy and may be apparent on the postoperative roentgenogram (Chiles, 1992). Approximately 75% of patients have some degree of atelectasis in the left lower lobe of the lung; another 10% to 20% have bilateral atelectasis (Goodman, 1983b).

COMMON ABNORMALITIES

DENSITIES IN THE PULMONARY PARENCHYMA

Atelectasis

The most common cause of a parenchymal density in postoperative cardiothoracic surgical patients is *atelectasis*, that is, loss of lung volume due to collapse of the normally air-filled alveoli. Because the atelectatic area of lung no longer contains air, it appears as a white shadow within the lung field. The amount of atelectasis may be confined to several segments or may extend to an entire lobe or lung. A common form

of atelectasis in postoperative patients is *plate-like atelectasis* caused by collapse of small subsegmental areas of lung. Its name is derived from its characteristic appearance as a linear "plate-like" opacification in the lung field.

Sometimes, a lobar bronchus becomes obstructed with secretions causing opacification of an entire lobe (Fig. 44-8). Lobar atelectasis can often be detected by displacement of interlobar fissures in association with increased density of the collapsed lobe (Miller, 1994). *Air bronchograms,* or air-filled bronchi that stand out in contrast to an opacified segment of lung, may also be visible (Westra, 1990). A *silhouette sign* may assist in localizing a pulmonary opacity. It is present when a parenchymal abnormality obliterates the border of contiguous structures, such as the heart, aorta, or diaphragm (Juhl, 1993). For example, right middle lobe atelectasis obscures the right heart border whereas right lower lobe atelectasis obscures the right hemidiaphragm.

When a main bronchus is obstructed, the entire lung may become atelectatic and appear completely opaque (Chiles, 1992). The volume loss associated with large areas of atelectatic lung usually produces shifting of the trachea and mediastinum toward the affected side and elevation of the ipsilateral hemidiaphragm. The contralateral lung hyperinflates and appears excessively black (Sider, 1986).

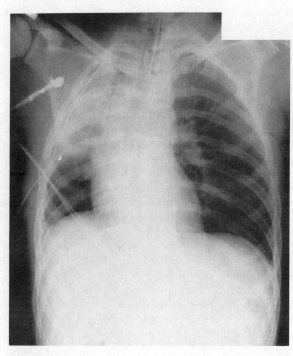

FIGURE 44-8. Right upper lobe atelectasis. Note opacification of right upper lung field and mediastinal shift (tracheal deviation) toward right hemithorax. Also apparent on the roentgenogram are a right pleural chest tube, an endotracheal tube, and a nasogastric tube. (Courtesy of Robert M. Vanecko, M.D.)

Consolidation

An abnormal parenchymal density may also represent *alveolar consolidation*, which is flooding of alveoli with fluid or material to the virtual exclusion of air (Freundlich & Bragg, 1992b). Alveolar consolidation may result from a variety of pathophysiologic entities, including pneumonia, pulmonary edema, aspiration, or intrapulmonary hemorrhage. *Pneumonia* is probably the most frequently observed cause of pulmonary consolidation in postoperative patients. Like atelectasis, pneumonia causes a focal opacity in the lung field. Depending on the stage of infection and organism involved, pneumonia can vary in appearance from a streaky, hazy area in the lung to a dense consolidation (Sider, 1986). Differentiation of pneumonia and atelectasis can be difficult, and sometimes both are present. Except in patients who require prolonged intubation and mechanical ventilation, most postoperative parenchymal densities represent atelectasis.

FLUID COLLECTIONS

Postoperative Hemorrhage

Hemorrhage in postoperative patients is always a concern and is one reason that patients undergoing cardiac or thoracic operations have portable chest roentgenograms on arrival in the postoperative intensive care or recovery unit. The degree of postoperative bleeding is best evaluated by quantification of blood loss in the chest drainage system. However, if the rate of bleeding is excessive or the tubes become occluded by clotted blood, blood accumulates in the chest. The roentgenogram may assist in establishing a diagnosis of postoperative hemorrhage by demonstrating mediastinal widening or hemothorax before clinical manifestations of hypovolemia develop. The chest roentgenogram is particularly important in detecting postoperative hemorrhage after pneumonectomy since a chest tube is usually not placed.

In patients undergoing cardiac operations, undrained blood collects in the mediastinal space, producing a widening of the mediastinal shadow on the chest film. Although mediastinal width on the preoperative PA and postoperative AP films are not comparable, comparison of two serial postoperative films may reveal an increasing mediastinal width. This finding, particularly if supported by clinical findings, is suggestive of mediastinal hemorrhage. A *hemothorax*, or blood in the pleural space, may also be present if one or both of the pleural spaces was opened during the operation.

In patients who have undergone pulmonary resection operations, blood that accumulates in the pleural space appears radiographically as a homogeneous opacity in a dependent position in the pleural cavity (Miller, 1994). Although a pleural fluid density appears the same whether it is blood (hemothorax), serous fluid (pleural effusion), pus (empyema), or chyle

(chylothorax), a new pleural fluid collection in the early postoperative hours can be assumed to be a hemothorax.

In most cases of acute hemothorax, the fluid moves freely in the pleural space with changes in the patient's position. Roentgenograms obtained for initial evaluation of a chest trauma patient or in the early postoperative period are usually taken in a supine position; blood in the pleural space layers out over the posterior surface of the lung field, producing a diffuse shadow that makes the affected lung appear denser than the lung on the opposite side (Fig. 44-9). If an upright roentgenogram is taken, the blood appears at the base of the lung, causing blunting of the normally sharply defined costophrenic angle. Excessive bleeding after pneumonectomy is manifested radiographically by a rapid increase in the fluid level in the operative hemithorax. The mediastinum and heart may be shifted toward the contralateral side.

Pleural Effusion

Patients who undergo coronary artery revascularization frequently develop serous *pleural effusions*, particularly on the left side, during the early postoperative period (Fig. 44-10). Large pleural effusions, especially if bilateral, may be overlooked on a supine film because they create diffuse opacifications of both hemithoraces (Moreno-Cabral et al., 1988). On an up-

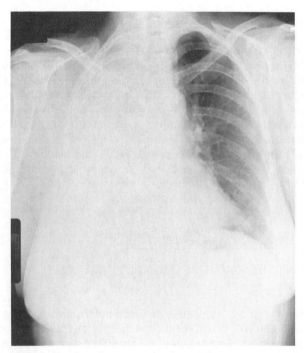

FIGURE 44-9. Supine chest roentgenogram demonstrating massive right hemothorax. With the patient in a supine position, the blood in the pleural space has layered out, opacifying the entire right lung field. (Courtesy of Robert M. Vanecko, M.D.)

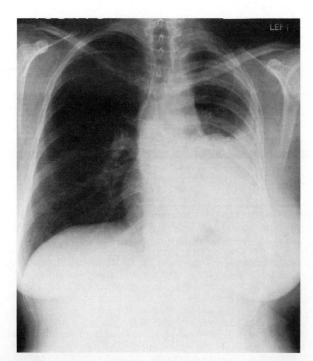

FIGURE 44-10. A moderate left-sided pleural effusion is apparent on this roentgenogram obtained with the patient in an upright position. (Courtesy of Robert M. Vanecko, M.D.)

right film, the fluid is easily apparent at the bases of the lungs. A *lateral decubitus* projection, taken with the patient lying on the right or left side, may also be helpful in diagnosing the presence and mobility of fluid in the pleural space (Freundlich & Bragg, 1992c). In the lateral decubitus view, the fluid forms a shadow parallel to the thoracic wall (Umali & Smith, 1991). Pleural fluid occasionally collects and is loculated in an interlobar fissure, causing the fissure to appear as a cigar-shaped opacity (Miller, 1994).

An unusual cause of postoperative pleural fluid accumulation after esophageal or pulmonary resection operations is operative injury of the thoracic duct with resultant *chylothorax*. Although not radiographically distinguishable from a transudative pleural effusion, chylothorax is easily diagnosed with thoracentesis or chest tube thoracostomy because of the characteristic milky appearance of the chylous fluid.

AIR COLLECTIONS

Pleural air accumulation (i.e., *pneumothorax*) produces a dark space devoid of the thin white lung markings that are normally present throughout the lung fields. The pleural air displaces the visceral pleura away from the parietal pleura lining the chest wall. The visceral pleura, which is not normally visualized, appears as a thin white line separating the lung and air-filled space (Chiles & Ravin, 1986) (Fig. 44-11).

A pneumothorax usually appears in nondependent areas of the pleural space unless the air is trapped or loculated beneath the lung. Consequently, in an upright chest roentgenogram, pneumothorax is typically seen at the apex of the lung. If the patient is in a supine position, air collects medially and anteriorly. A medial pneumothorax produces a lucent line next to the mediastinal shadow; an anterior air collection may not be visible without a cross-table lateral roentgenogram. If the pleural space contains fluid as well as air, the roentgenogram demonstrates an *air–fluid level* (i.e., a straight line separating the radiopaque fluid from the radiolucent air).

Pneumothorax is categorized according the estimated amount of the hemithorax that it occupies. A small cap of air above the apex of the lung is termed a 5% to 10% pneumothorax. A 100% pneumothorax is present if the entire lung is collapsed by pleural air; the lung appears as a small, opaque structure abutting the mediastinum, and the remaining hemithorax is radiolucent. A *tension pneumothorax* exists if mediastinal structures are shifted toward the opposite side. On the side of the tension pneumothorax, the lung appears compressed, the cardiac contour is flattened, and the hemidiaphragm may be inverted (Chiles, 1992).

Air occasionally accumulates in the subcutaneous tissues because a large air leak is present or because drainage of the pleural space is inadequate. *Subcutaneous emphysema* produces linear streaks of lucency outlining tissue planes or lucent bubbles within the soft tissues (Umali & Smith, 1991) (Fig. 44-12). Uncommonly, air may enter and collect within the mediastinum, producing a *pneumomediastinum*. Pneumo-

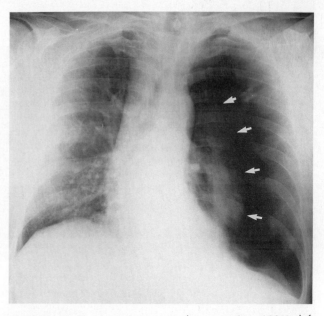

FIGURE 44-11. Roentgenogram demonstrating 100% left pneumothorax. Note edge of collapsed lung (*arrows*) and absence of lung markings beyond. (Courtesy of Robert M. Vanecko, M.D.)

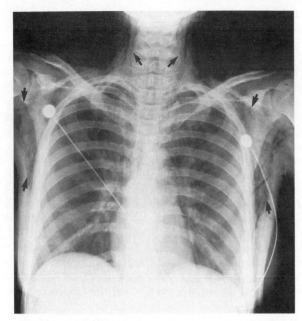

FIGURE 44-12. Chest roentgenogram in a patient with significant subcutaneous emphysema. Note translucent streaking in the subcutaneous tissue of the chest wall and neck (*arrows*). (Courtesy of Robert M. Vanecko, M.D.)

mediastinum produces a sharp, lucent line separate from and outlining the aorta, great vessels, heart, or paravertebral soft tissues (Sider, 1986).

REFERENCES

Chiles C, 1992: Radiologic recognition of complications of thoracic surgery. In Wolfe WG (ed): Complications in Thoracic Surgery. St. Louis, Mosby–Year Book

Chiles C, Ravin CE, 1986: Radiographic recognition of pneumothorax in the intensive care unit. Crit Care Med 14:677

Elefteriades JA, Geha AS, 1985: Problems following noncardiac thoracic surgery. In House Officer Guide to ICU Care: The Cardiothoracic Surgical Patient. Gaithersburg, MD, Aspen Publishers

Freundlich IM, Bragg DG, 1992a: Anatomy. In Radiologic Approach to Diseases of the Chest. Baltimore, Williams & Wilkins

Freundlich IM, Bragg DG, 1992b: Alveolar consolidation. In Radiologic Approach to Diseases of the Chest. Baltimore, Williams & Wilkins

Freundlich IM, Bragg DG, 1992c: Introduction. In Radiologic Approach to Diseases of the Chest. Baltimore, Williams & Wilkins

Goodman LR, 1980: Postoperative chest radiograph: II. Alterations after major intrathoracic surgery. AJR 134:803

Goodman LR, 1983a: Pulmonary support and monitoring apparatus. In Goodman LR, Putman CE (eds): Intensive Care Radiology: Imaging of the Critically Ill, ed. 2. Philadelphia, WB Saunders

Goodman LR, 1983b: The post-thoracotomy radiograph. In Goodman LR, Putman CE (eds): Intensive Care Radiology: Imaging of the Critically Ill, ed. 2. Philadelphia, WB Saunders

Huseby JS, 1989: Radiologic examination of the chest. In Underhill SL, Woods SL, Froelicher ES, Halpenny CJ (eds): Cardiac Nursing, ed. 2. Philadelphia, JB Lippincott

Joob AW, Hartz RS, 1994: General principles of postoperative care. In Shields TW (ed): General Thoracic Surgery, ed. 4. Baltimore, Williams & Wilkens

Juhl JH, 1993: Methods of examination, anatomy, and congenital malformations of the chest. In Juhl JH, Crummy AB (eds): Paul and Juhl's Essentials of Radiologic Imaging. Philadelphia, JB Lippincott

Matthay RA, Sostman HD, 1990: Chest imaging. In George RB, Light RW, Matthay MA, Matthay RA (eds): Chest Medicine, ed. 2. Baltimore, Williams & Wilkins

Miller WT, 1994: Roentgenographic evaluation of the lungs and chest. In Shields TW (ed): General Thoracic Surgery, ed. 4. Baltimore, Williams & Wilkens

Milne EN, 1980: Chest radiology in the surgical patient. Surg Clin North Am 60:1503

Moreno-Cabral CE, Mitchell RS, Miller DC, 1988: Perioperative care. In Manual of Postoperative Management of Adult Cardiac Surgery. Baltimore, Williams & Wilkins

Munnell ER, 1991: Chest drainage in the traumatized patient. In Webb WR, Besson A (eds): Thoracic Surgery: Surgical Management of Chest Injuries. St. Louis, Mosby–Year Book

Sider L, 1986: Interpretation of the postoperative chest radiograph. Crit Care Q 9:71

Squire LF, Novelline RA, 1988a: An invitation to think three-dimensionally. In Fundamentals of Radiology, ed. 4. Cambridge, MA, Harvard University Press

Squire LF, Novelline RA, 1988b: Study of the mediastinal structures. In Fundamentals of Radiology, ed. 4. Cambridge, MA, Harvard University Press

Squire LF, Novelline RA, 1988c: The heart. In Fundamentals of Radiology, ed. 4. Cambridge, MA, Harvard University Press

Squire LF, Novelline RA, 1988d: The lung itself. In Fundamentals of Radiology, ed. 4. Cambridge, MA, Harvard University Press

Umali CB, Smith EH, 1991: The chest radiographic examination. In Rippe JM, Irwin RS, Alpert JS, Fink MP (eds): Intensive Care Medicine, ed. 2. Boston, Little, Brown & Co

Westra D, 1990: Conventional chest radiography. In Sperber M (ed): Radiologic Diagnosis of Chest Disease. New York, Springer-Verlag

INDEX

Page numbers followed by *f* indicate figures; those followed by *t* indicate tabular material.